Introductory Textbook of Psychiatry

Third Edition

Introductory Textbook of Psychiatry

Third Edition

Nancy C. Andreasen, M.D., Ph.D.
Andrew H. Woods Professor of Psychiatry
Director, Mental Health Clinical Research Center
The University of Iowa College of Medicine
Iowa City, Iowa

Donald W. Black, M.D.
Professor of Psychiatry
The University of Iowa College of Medicine
Iowa City, Iowa

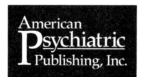

Washington, DC
London, England

Copyright © 2001 American Psychiatric Publishing, Inc.
ALL RIGHTS RESERVED
Manufactured in the United States of America on acid-free paper

04 03 02 01   4 3 2 1
Third Edition

American Psychiatric Publishing, Inc.
1400 K Street, N.W.
Washington, DC 20005
www.appi.org

Diagnostic criteria and other DSM-IV-TR material included in this book are reprinted with permission from the *Diagnostic and Statistical Manual of Mental Disorders,* Fourth Edition, Text Revision. Washington, DC, American Psychiatric Association, 2000. Copyright © 2000 American Psychiatric Association.

Library of Congress Cataloging-in-Publication Data
Andreasen, Nancy C.
   Introductory textbook of psychiatry / Nancy Andreasen, Donald W. Black.--3rd ed.
      p. ; cm.
   Includes bibliographical references and index.
   ISBN 0-88048-946-4 (hardcover : alk paper) -- ISBN 1-58562-036-X (pbk.: alk. paper)
      1. Psychiatry. I. Black, Donald W., 1956- II. Title.
   [DNLM: 1. Mental Disorders. WM 100 A557i 2001]
   RC454 .A427 2001
   616.89--dc21
                    00-067401

British Library Cataloguing in Publication Data
A CIP record is available from the British Library.

Contents

SECTION 1

Background

CHAPTER 1

The Global Burden of Mental Illness:

CHAPTER 2

CHAPTER 3

CHAPTER 4

CHAPTER 5

SECTION 2

Psychiatric Disorders

CHAPTER 6

CHAPTER 7

CHAPTER 8

CHAPTER 9

CHAPTER 10

CHAPTER 11

CHAPTER 12

CHAPTER 13

CHAPTER 14

SECTION 3

Special Topics

CHAPTER 25

SECTION 4

Treatments

CHAPTER 26

CHAPTER 27

Preface to the Third Edition

It has now been more than 13 years since we wrote the first edition of the *Introductory Textbook of Psychiatry*. Our major goal was to write a user-friendly textbook for persons just being introduced to the field of psychiatry. The main target audience traditionally has been third- or fourth-year medical students rotating through psychiatry, as well as psychiatric residents in their first and second years of training. Over the years, we have received positive feedback from others new to psychiatry, including social work and nursing students, physician assistant students, and even laypersons who simply wanted to learn more about their illnesses or those that ran in their families.

We thought then, and still do, that there was a need for an introductory textbook that presented psychiatry as a field exploding with knowledge, not one mired in the past. We thought it vital for students to be exposed to the broad range of psychiatric disorders and to gain a working knowledge of the fundamentals necessary for the practice of psychiatry, such as interviewing. We also thought students should understand the history of the field, neurobiological theories about the mental illnesses, and knowledge about the kinds of laboratory tests and evaluations helpful in assessing these disorders. Feedback from many people has indicated that the book largely succeeded in what we set out to do. Based on this feedback, we have made some further improvements. In the second edition, we added several new chapters, case vignettes, and illustrations and tables to help make some of the concepts more understandable.

In the current edition, we added even more case vignettes, useful illustrations, and tables and included exciting new findings about the specific psychiatric disorders. Chapter 22, which covers psychiatric aspects of human immunodeficiency virus, has perhaps changed the most because knowledge about this epidemic—which shows no signs of abating—has increased exponentially. Chapter 27, which covers somatic treatments, has been largely rewritten to reflect the burgeoning knowledge about new drug treatments, particularly antidepressants. For example, in the last few years, a great deal has been learned about the cytochrome P450 system, which can contribute to untoward drug interactions that clinicians must understand.

Of course, a large part of putting together the third edition involved careful rewriting and editing to ensure that the book remains readable, interesting, and understandable. Outdated information has been deleted, and new information has been integrated. References have been updated, as have the recommendations, or "clinical pearls." A unique aspect of the book, the Appendix, has been maintained to give students access to some of the common questionnaires originally developed for use. Increasingly, these quantitative methods are being integrated into routine clinical care as well because they are so helpful for understanding and assessing patients. For example, the Mini-Mental State Exam (MMSE), a brief questionnaire used internationally, allows clinicians to quickly assess the cognitive functioning of individuals. The MMSE has become such an important assessment tool that students learning about cognitive disorders need to be familiar with it. We have added the Beck Depression Inventory, commonly used to assess severity of depressive symptoms. Many clinicians who treat depression have patients fill out the self-report questionnaire at each visit to obtain an objective measure of the patient's condition.

Over the years, some students have told us that the book is too long or that it does not provide enough of a "cookbook." Some students seem to prefer pocket-sized tomes because they provide basic information without requiring much effort. We never sought to create such a book because we believe that even on a brief rotation, students should have access to more comprehensive information about psychiatry and psychiatric disorders. We understand that most medical students have brief rotations and cannot read the entire book, but we believe the book should be sufficiently broad to satisfy students who wish to gain a wide exposure to the field.

For these reasons, we offer recommendations about how students and psychiatry clerkship directors should use the book. Because clerkships differ substantially in content from school to school, it makes sense for clerkship directors to assign specific chapters or pages to read. The book can be broken down into learning modules to complement the needs of the particular program. Assignments can be expanded or shortened as appropriate, and the clerkship director always has the option of providing supplementary reading materials, course outlines, or papers from the peer-reviewed literature. We suggest the following model curriculum as a starting point:

- Chapter 2, "Diagnosis and Classification," pp. 21–44. These pages explain the purpose of diagnosis and classification in psychiatry.
- Chapter 3, "Interviewing and Assessment," pp. 45–90. These pages concern the major components of the psychiatric interview.
- Chapter 5, "The Neurobiology of Mental Illness," pp. 133–180. These pages cover important theories on brain function, neurotransmitters systems, and genetics thought to underlie most mental illnesses.
- Chapter 6, "Cognitive Disorders," pp. 183–210. These pages cover delirium and dementia.
- Chapter 7, "Schizophrenia," pp. 211–250. Schizophrenia is sufficiently important that students should read the entire chapter.
- Chapter 9, "Mood Disorders," pp. 269–314. Again, the mood disorders are so important that students should read the entire chapter.
- Chapter 10, "Anxiety Disorders," pp. 315–346. Students should be aware of the most important anxiety disorders.
- Chapter 14, "Alcohol-Related Disorders," pp. 403–422. Alcoholism is so important that students should read the entire chapter.
- Chapter 27, "Somatic Treatments," pp. 709–760. These pages cover the antipsychotics, antidepressants, mood stabilizers, and anxiolytics, all important for students to know.

Optional readings include

- Chapter 12, "Somatoform and Related Disorders," pp. 363–388. These pages cover somatization disorder.
- Chapter 18, "Eating Disorders," pp. 515–530. Students are encouraged to read the entire chapter.
- Chapter 21, "Suicide and Violent Behavior," pp. 553–568. Students should have a basic understanding of suicidal behavior.

With this edition, we aim to be responsive to feedback that we continue to receive. We view the book as a work in progress because there will always be ways to improve it. Furthermore, psychiatry is a dynamic and changing field, which is ultimately based on two of the most exciting fields in biomedicine—neuroscience and molecular genetics—and, therefore, this book must steadily change as well. Recommendations are always welcome. Occasional errors creep into books of this size, and we are always grateful when these are pointed out to us.

Preface to the Second Edition

Only four years have elapsed since the publication of the first edition of this textbook in 1991. Yet the worlds of medicine and psychiatry have changed with astonishing rapidity during that short interval, and the changes appear likely to accelerate.

Health care reform, viewed by many as health care destruction, is transforming the way that physicians treat their patients and organize their practices. Primary care is recovering recognition as the heart of medicine, and specialization is becoming less valued. If this reduces fragmentation of care, for patients a frustration at best and a bane at worst, medical care will be improved. On the other hand, managed care also appears to be making unwanted and sometimes undesirable intrusions into decision making. As physicians, we believe that the health and well-being of our patients should be our guiding compass, and economic incentives (including our own) should be secondary. We refuse to consider this position old-fashioned or naive.

Where does psychiatry stand in this rapidly changing environment? Although it is not a primary care discipline to the same extent as pediatrics or internal medicine, it will play a major role in a health care system that emphasizes the importance of primary care. Mental illnesses, after all, are very common. Only physicians in laboratory specialties such as pathology or radiology can avoid encountering the patients who have them. Family practitioners, internists, surgeons, pediatricians, and obstetrician/gynecologists are all certain to have to work with patients with depression or substance abuse almost daily. Other mental illnesses, such as schizophrenia, Alzheimer's disease, and anorexia nervosa, are also extremely common. The primary care physician must be able to diagnose mental illnesses on a regular basis and either treat them or refer patients to a psychiatrist as appropriate. In either situation a good grasp of psychiatry is mandatory. The treating psychiatrist, on the other hand, will also no doubt increasingly deliver more primary care to the patients in his or her practice. Just as the obstetrician/ gynecologist is the only physician that many women see regularly, thereby de facto becoming a primary care provider, a psychiatrist is also often the only physician that many patients see regularly. The distinction between psychiatry and primary care is likely to become increasingly blurred as psychiatrists assume more responsibility for the general health of the patients whom they see regularly.

The field of psychiatry has experienced many exciting new developments that permit it to be responsive to these challenges. Forty years ago, mental illnesses were untreatable and hopeless. The modern psychiatrist has a large arsenal of effective medications and other treatments, which now give most mental illnesses a better prognosis than cancer or cardiac disease. Further, the past few years have produced many new medications that are further enhancing our ability to care for patients. Just during the short interval since the first edition of this book, we have acquired risperidone for schizophrenia, paroxetine for obsessive-compulsive disorder, and venlafaxine for depression. Psychotherapeutic techniques also continue to be refined and better matched to the disorders for which they are most effective, as in the case of interpersonal psychotherapy for depression. In the area of diagnosis, the fourth edition of the *Diagnostic and Statistical Manual of Mental Disorders* (DSM-IV) was published in 1994, continuing the tradition of providing precise, objective, and optimally validated methods for defining and diagnosing mental illnesses.

The scientific basis of psychiatry also continues to grow and develop. Neuroimaging techniques now give us a direct window on the brain, permitting us to see with our own eyes the underlying physiology of mental activities such as remembering, feeling sadness, or making a decision. The psychiatrist using these techniques to map the brain is engaged in a voyage of discovery not unlike that of the early explorers who sought a trade route to India and instead discovered America. Textbooks of neuroscience are already being rewritten as truisms based on the older lessons of lesion studies or Brodmann cytoarchitectonics are found to be wrong. The chemical systems of the brain are also being remapped, and the mechanisms of drug action in the in vivo intact brain are being discovered. We can now visualize how the medications that we prescribe block various classes of receptors in the brain and exert their therapeutic effects. The 1990s have been declared the decade of the brain, and rightly so. Neuroscience and psychiatry are exploring the last uncharted territory in the human body. It is an incredibly exciting time to work in these fields.

Inevitably, all this growth in knowledge has required the appearance of a second edition of our textbook. Each chapter has been extensively updated to provide the most current information available about the various disorders and their treatments. Several new chapters have been added and additional topics are covered, including legal issues in psychiatry, sleep disorders, impulse control disorders, and violence. We have been gratified by the response to the first edition by our readers, who provided many helpful comments and criticisms that we have collected and responded to as best we can. Our medical students deserve special thanks, for they have proved to be a fertile testing ground—a focus group, if you will—to explore new ideas for further improving the book. Among the changes we have incorporated: more tables, additional case examples (and follow-up news on some of our first edition patients!), more complete coverage of mental disorders described in the DSM, and use of the latest criteria.

We have also been gratified that our book has enjoyed widespread acceptance and is used all over the United States, as well as in many foreign countries. Although some critics have suggested that the book is "biological," we refuse to be pigeonholed. If a descriptive term must be used, we prefer the terms *objective, empirical,* or *scientific.* Granted, we do not advocate slavish or unthinking adherence to outdated theory. Nor do we advocate uncritical acceptance of poorly grounded "facts." An objective, practical, and dynamic approach has shaped our approach to patient care: if well-grounded data exist to guide us, we shall use them. Where data do not exist, we shall use common sense, seeking new knowledge continuously and using it as it becomes available.

Psychiatry is sometimes considered fuzzy, imprecise, or not accountable. One of our objectives in this book has been to convey to students of all types that psychiatry is not only exciting, fun, and interesting, but also that it can be (and usually is) clearheaded, careful, and credible. After all, the reliability of diagnosing schizophrenia is higher than that of diagnosing rheumatoid arthritis, not to mention systemic lupus or multiple sclerosis. The cost-effectiveness of treating depression and mania is well established, and the treatment is far more gratifying to administer than treatments for stroke, back pain, or many forms of cancer. Of course, some trendy or silly ideas are sometimes put forth by psychiatrists, thereby calling into question the credibility of the field as a whole. But the majority provide the type of competent and well-founded diagnosis and treatment that we believe this book advocates. Psychiatry as a field and the illnesses that it treats are far from silly. These illnesses are common, important, potentially devastating, and often gratifyingly responsive to good care and management.

Our hope is that students reading this book will learn to share our excitement about the practice of psychiatry and our curiosity about its scientific foundations. We psychiatrists have a unique opportunity to spend time with our patients, to get to know them personally, and to work with an interdisciplinary team. Modern psychiatrists wear many hats. They must understand diagnosis, pathophysiology, and the latest drug therapies; at the same time, psychiatrists must possess empathy, be able to counsel and comfort distraught patients, and learn to help patients function in their day-to-day lives. A typical day's work may involve prescribing medication to a depressed patient, helping a teenager come to grips with the effect of having an alcoholic parent, and guiding a severely handicapped schizophrenic patient toward receiving needed social services. All this is not easy, but it can be enormously rewarding, particularly when students are able to follow their patients long enough to observe that for most the treatment actually works! Nothing is more satisfying than restoring a disabled person to independent functioning or a suffering person to freedom from mental pain.

We encourage students to read the introductory chapters first, to gain a working background of concepts and vocabulary and to learn interviewing techniques. Students should then feel free to skip around and read chapters or sections of chapters that apply to their particular patients—or sections that are simply interesting and fun to read. Enjoy!

Preface to the First Edition

Students sometimes begin working in psychiatry with a set of preconceptions about what it is, preconceptions shaped by the fact that information about psychiatry is omnipresent in popular culture. Taxi drivers, CEOs, teachers, and ministers often feel qualified to offer information and advice about how to handle "psychiatric problems," even though they may be unaware of distinctions as fundamental as the difference between psychiatry and psychology. These two disciplines are blurred together in the popular mind, and the term *psychiatry* evokes a potpourri of associations—Freud's couch, Jack Nicholson receiving electroconvulsive therapy in *One Flew Over the Cuckoo's Nest,* or Dr. Ruth discussing sexual adjustment on television. These images and associations tend to cloak psychiatry with an aura of vagueness, imprecision, muddleheadedness, and mindless coercion. It is unfortunate that such preconceptions are so pervasive, but fortunate that most of them are in fact in error, as students who use this book in conjunction with studying psychiatry in a clinical setting will soon discover.

What is psychiatry? It is the branch of medicine that focuses on the diagnosis and treatment of mental illnesses. Some of these illnesses are very serious, such as schizophrenia, Alzheimer's disease, or the various mood disorders. Others may be less serious, but still very significant, such as adjustment disorders or personality disorders. Psychiatry differs from psychology by virtue of its medical orientation. Its primary focus is illness or abnormality, as opposed to normal psychological functioning; the latter is the primary focus of psychology. Of course, abnormal psychology is a small branch within psychology, just as understanding normality is necessary for the psychiatrist to recognize and treat abnormal functioning. As a discipline within medicine, the primary purposes of psychiatry are to define and recognize illnesses, to identify methods for treating them, and ultimately to develop methods for discovering their causes and implementing preventive measures.

Psychiatry during the last decade of the twentieth century may be the most exciting discipline within medicine. Contemporary psychiatry is exciting for a variety of reasons. First, psychiatrists are specialists who work with the most interesting organ within the body, the brain. The brain is intrinsically fascinating because it controls nearly all aspects of functioning within the rest of the body, as well as the way people interact with and relate to one another. Psychiatry has received enormous support during recent years through the burgeoning of neuroscience, which has provided psychiatrists with the tools by which they can understand brain anatomy, chemistry, and physiology, thereby gradually developing a scientific base that will permit them to understand human emotion and behavior and to develop methods for treating abnormalities in these domains.

Yet, as psychiatry evolves into a relatively high-powered science, it remains a very clinical and human branch within medicine, and therefore a very rewarding field for students who have chosen medicine because they wish to have contact with patients. The clinician working in psychiatry must spend time with his or her patients and learn about them as human beings as well as individuals who have illnesses or problems. Learning the life stories of individual people is fun and interesting; as one colleague once said, "It amazed me when I realized that I would get paid for asking people things that everybody always wants to know about anyway!"

Finally, psychiatry has enormous breadth. As a scientific discipline, it ranges from the highly detailed facts of molecular biology to the abstract concepts of the mind. As a clinical discipline, it ranges from the absorbingly complex disturbances that characterize illnesses such as schizophrenia to the understandable fearfulness shown by young children when they must separate from their parents and attend school or be left with a baby-sitter. It can be very scientific and technical, as in the frontier-expanding research currently occurring in molecular genetics or neuroimaging; but it can also be very human and personal, as when a clinician listens to a patient's story and experiences the pleasure of being able to offer help by providing needed insights or even simple encouragement and support.

This book is intended as a tool to help you learn from your patients and from your teachers. We have tried to keep it simple, clear, and factual. References are provided for students who want to explore in more depth the topics covered in the various chapters. We have written this book primarily for medical students and residents during the first several years of their training, although we anticipate that it may also be useful to individuals seeking psychiatric training from the perspectives of other disciplines such as nursing or social work. We hope that, using this book as a tool, students of all ages and types will learn to enjoy working with psychiatric patients and with the art and science of contemporary psychiatry as much as we do.

SECTION 1

Background

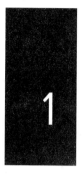

The Global Burden of Mental Illness

From Biblical Times to the Twenty-First Century

What curiosity, that delicate little plant, needs more than anything, besides stimulation, is freedom.

Albert Einstein

In 1990, two investigators at Harvard University, working in collaboration with the World Health Organization (WHO), published a pivotal book titled *The Global Burden of Disease.* This book captured the attention of leaders in the medical community because it provided the first objective summary of the costs of various types of illness to society throughout the world. The authors wanted to estimate the cost of illnesses in a manner that would not overrepresent wealthy developed nations, where the costs of health care are greater in part because more money is available to spend. They created a new measurement called disability-adjusted life-years (DALYs). DALYs are a combined measure of time lost as a result of premature mortality and time lived with the disability. A loss of one DALY is equivalent to the loss of 1 year of life for one person.

This interesting book has told us a great deal about both the economics and the demographics of diseases. Its data are broken down by age, by classes of disease, and by developed and developing countries. The book shows, for example, that infectious diseases are still creating a heavy disease burden in developing countries, whereas the burden in wealthier nations has shifted to diseases that affect older individuals, such as cardiovascular disease. These results are interesting but not surprising.

The head-turning fact in *The Global Burden of Disease* is the cost exacted by mental illnesses. Table 1–1 lists the 10 leading causes of disability in the world among persons who are between ages 15 and 44 years. To almost everyone's surprise, a mental illness—unipolar major depression—is the costliest illness in the world. Furthermore, a total of four mental illnesses are in the top 10: depression, alcohol use, manic-depressive (bipolar) illness, and schizophrenia. Because self-inflicted injuries (i.e., suicide) also are a consequence of mental illness, 5 of the 10 leading causes of disability are due to psychiatric problems.

The message is clear. At the beginning of the twenty-first century, physicians cannot afford to ignore mental illnesses. Every physician must become educated in diagnosis and treatment of these illnesses. We also must build a stronger cadre of clinical and basic scientists who will join in an effort to determine the mechanisms causing mental illness and to develop more effective treatments.

TABLE 1–1.   The 10 leading causes of disability in the world

Type of disability	Cost (in DALYs)	Cumulative % of cost
Unipolar major depression	42,972	10.3
Tuberculosis	19,673	14.9
Road traffic accidents	19,625	19.6
Alcohol use	14,848	23.2
Self-inflicted injuries	14,645	26.7
Manic-depressive (bipolar) illness	13,189	29.8
War	13,134	32.9
Violence	12,955	36.0
Schizophrenia	12,542	39.0
Iron deficiency anemia	12,511	42.0

Note.   DALYs=disability-adjusted life-years.

Why did the message of the global burden of mental illness come as such a shock? Why has the biomedical community failed to recognize the importance of psychiatric disorders until so recently?

Many of the answers to these questions are historical. People in contemporary society have confused ideas and attitudes about the nature of mental illness, largely because these disorders have been stigmatized and "swept under the rug." This has not always been the case. In some times and places, mental illnesses were described and treated as biomedical illnesses that affected one organ of the body—the brain. In other times, however, they were seen as diseases of the soul or spirit, a just punishment inflicted by a righteous god. As indicated in this textbook, mental illnesses now are understood as disorders of the mind that arise from disordered processes in the brain. They affect individuals, but they also affect how those individuals relate to others within the social networks that link everyone together. In the twenty-first century, mental illnesses are being intensively studied with the powerful new tools of neuroscience and molecular biology. Students of psychiatry are living in an exciting time, a time when the global burden of mental illness is widely recognized and when basic scientists and clinicians have joined together in the goal of eradicating the burden of the costliest disorders in contemporary society.

A review of the history of psychiatry is helpful in highlighting both progress and setbacks in the understanding and definition of mental illnesses.

Mental Illness in Biblical and Classical Times

Mental illnesses are among the first diseases to have been recognized as discrete illnesses. The concept of cancer or even congestive heart failure is relatively new compared with the concept of mental illness. Perhaps the oldest medical document in existence, the Eber Papyrus (probably composed in 1900 B.C.), contains references to specific syndromes such as depression. Biblical writings also contain descriptions of individuals with major mental illnesses; for example, in I Samuel, Saul is portrayed as falling into a serious depression, for which he is treated with soothing music.

By classical times, a full classification of mental illnesses had been developed. These included melancholia (depression), mania (a variety of psychotic states), delirium (mental confusion accompanied by fever), and hysteria (sudden unexplained episodes of somatic illness involving pain, sensory loss, paralysis, etc.). Although Greek and Roman physicians generally recognized these as major classes of mental illness, they could not agree on their specific causes. Hippocrates, for example, argued that mental illnesses, as well as all other cognitive and emotional functions, derived principally from the brain. Galen and his followers believed that mental illnesses were due to imbalances in quantities of body fluids. Melancholia, for example, was due to an excess of black bile, whereas other abnormalities arose from imbalances in the other three main fluids or humors of the body (blood, phlegm, and yellow bile). Still others argued for an "organ theory" of disease and believed that specific dysfunctions could be attributed to abnormalities in specific organs; delirium or mania, for example, were brain abnormalities, whereas hysteria was caused by a wandering uterus.

Although physicians in classical times had their major or minor differences about both the nosology and the pathophysiology of major mental illnesses, they rather consistently shared the belief that these illnesses were physical in nature. Although the Greeks developed highly sophisticated theories about the nature of the spirit, soul, or mind, they nevertheless believed that illnesses such as mania or melancholia were the result of aberrations in the body rather than in the soul or spirit. This led in turn to humane practices for the treatment of serious mental illnesses, involving rest and peaceful surroundings.

Medieval and Renaissance Attitudes

As Roman civilization declined and finally fell, enlightened attitudes about mental illness declined as well. The barbarian tribes that conquered Rome had no interest in maintaining learning or education, leading to massive destruction of the libraries that summarized classical knowledge about science and literature. Europe gradually struggled out of these "Dark Ages," largely through the influence of the Christian church, but the new prevailing worldview was not conducive to enlightenment about human illness in general or mental illness in particular. The emphasis was on saving souls, not bodies.

In this environment, mentally ill persons often were believed to be possessed by the Devil rather than to have some form of illness. Witches, warlocks, and demons in disguise were very real to the people of the Middle Ages. Various types of misfortune or suffering often were perceived as just punishments meted out through divine intervention as a consequence of sinful behavior. Thus, it was easy to believe that a person who fell into the deep despondency of depression, and who was experiencing a delusion of sin and guilt, was spiritually rather than physically ill. A person with the agitation and mental confusion that often accompany severe psychosis could easily be seen as possessed by diabolical forces. Such individuals often were "treated" through the church rather than through medicine, and many were tortured or burned at the stake. The church published texts, such as the *Malleus Maleficarum* (or the *Hammer of Witches*), to explain how such possessed individuals could be identified and killed, because they were considered dangerous to society. As late as the seventeenth century, the reigning monarch in England, James I, wrote a book on this topic, *Demonologie*. The last witch was hanged in England in 1684, but witch trials continued in the United States in Salem, Massachusetts, into the eighteenth century.

The Renaissance, the rebirth of interest in classical learning that began in Italy in the fifteenth century and spread throughout the rest of Europe during the next 100 years, brought a refreshing new light to this rather dim atmosphere. Artists rediscovered the study of anatomy, forbidden by the church, in order to better depict the human body. Authoritarian teachings were questioned. The new physics of Copernicus and Galileo displaced humans and the earth from the center of the universe. Doctors began to believe what their eyes and their inferences taught them, in contrast to arbitrary dogma that was obviously in error.

A few brave voices began to suggest that mental illnesses were diseases rather than forms of possession and bewitchment. In 1584, Reginald Scot published *The Discoverie of Witchcraft*, in which he argued that individuals accused of witchcraft were not in fact possessed by demons but were instead mentally ill and that their own descriptions of being possessed represented false products of their fevered imaginations and thus should be considered as delusions. Two years later, in 1586, a physician, Timothy Bright, published the first textbook about mental illness to appear in English, *The Treatise of Melancholie*. In this book, he described the classic symptoms of depression and their tendency to alternate with the periods of being "high" (in a way that anticipated later descriptions of bipolar disorder) and argued that the symptoms of mental illness were "naturall perturbations" that "altered either brayne or hart." Although these revolutionary ideas did not instantly gain wide acceptance, the foundations of modern psychiatry were being laid.

The Dawn of Scientific Psychiatry

Serious mental illnesses tended to be relatively chronic and incapacitating, especially in an era when no good treatments were available. If mentally ill persons were not burned at the stake, some other disposition had to be made. Hospitals or asylums were an alternative solution. To refer to the institutions created for the mentally ill during the seventeenth and eighteenth centuries as hospitals or asylums is, however, by and large a misnomer. In fact, patients were typically incarcerated, and many were not only locked in but also locked up in chains. Making matters worse, often distinctions were not clearly made between the mentally ill, the criminal, the mentally retarded, and the economically unfortunate. The desire to spare the rich from being forced to observe the suffering of the poor, the handicapped, or the seriously ill seems to be a persistent human failing, although hardly an appealing one.

The seeds of skepticism and doubt sown during the Renaissance flowered into rebellion and revolution during the era of the Enlightenment in the eighteenth century. All over the world, the weak, deprived, and powerless sought to take back their rights and to seize authority from the rich and powerful. The United States led the way with the first revolution of modern times, declaring all men to be created equal. The revolutionary movement in America sparked others in France, Italy, and elsewhere.

Philippe Pinel, a leader of the French Revolution, usually is considered the founding father of modern psychiatry. In 1793, he was named director of the Bicêtre, the hospital in Paris for insane men. Soon afterward, he instituted a grand, symbolic change by removing the chains that bound the patients to the walls at the Bicêtre and instituted a new type of treatment that he referred to as "moral treatment." (This meant treating patients in ways that were morally and ethically sensitive rather than attempting to teach them "morality.") He was later made director of the corresponding hospital for women, the Salpêtrière. In addition to attempting to treat patients with kindness and decency, Pinel tried to approach the study of the mentally ill scientifically. He describes his efforts in his *Treatise on Insanity* (1806):

> I, therefore, resolved to adopt that method of investigation which has invariably succeeded in all the departments of natural history, viz. To notice successively every fact, without any other object than that of collecting materials for future use; and to endeavor, as far as possible, to divest myself of the influence, both of my own prepossessions and the authority of others. (p. 2)

The *Treatise on Insanity* contains detailed case histories of individual patients so clearly described that they are instantly diagnosable as "classic cases" of what we now call schizophrenia or bipolar disorder 200 years later.

In addition to introducing psychotherapy, in the form of moral treatment, and stressing the importance of empirical observation, Pinel applied the scientific method to the study of psychiatry. He established epidemiological methods for recording numbers of cases, instituted follow-up studies so that the natural history of diseases could be observed, and used whatever scientific technology he had at hand to understand the pathophysiology of mental diseases. His approaches became the standard methods in most enlightened psychiatric facilities throughout Europe and the United States in the nineteenth century.

Thus, a new specialty within medicine was created, consisting of physicians who chose to specialize in the care of mentally ill patients. They became known as *psychiatrists,* which means literally "physicians who heal the mind." Psychiatry was one of the first disciplines within medicine to identify itself as a specialty. This was no doubt a consequence of both the large numbers of patients with mental illness and the special needs and challenges that they presented.

Psychiatry also got off to an early start in the United States. Perhaps because the creation of the United States was based on the ideals of the Enlightenment (most of the Founding Fathers such as Franklin, Washington, and Jefferson were adherents of the ideals of the Age of Reason), American attitudes toward mental illness were very progressive early in United States history. Benjamin Rush, a physician who specialized in the care of mentally ill persons, also signed the Declaration of Independence and founded the first psychiatric hospital in America more than 200 years ago (the Pennsylvania Hospital). The American Psychiatric Association was founded more than 150 years ago, in 1844, and its official journal, *The American Journal of Psychiatry,* is the oldest medical specialty journal in the United States and one of the oldest medical journals as well. The American Psychiatric Association was created through the collaboration of 13 people who were in charge of hospitals specifically dedicated to the care of the mentally ill; they agreed to meet regularly and to share their experiences in caring for patients with illnesses that caused them to lose their capacity to reason clearly. In this era, nearly every physician was a family practitioner. But even at that time, it was recognized that caring for mentally ill persons required special skills. The early writings of these 13 founders of the American Psychiatric Association contain an interesting combination of emphasis on empirical description, the study of neuroanatomy, and the value of compassion.

The First Era of Neuroscience

While psychiatry was establishing itself as a medical specialty, a new subdivision within science also was emerging. During the nineteenth century, clinical observations and technological developments converged to create an era when the brain was studied scientifically for the first time.

Some of the landmark achievements of the first era of neuroscience are summarized in Table 1–2. One major aspect was the mapping of specific cortical functions in the human brain. The initial observations focused on the specificity of language systems in the brain, beginning in 1837 with the observation of Marc Dax that left-sided injury tended to be associated with aphasia and right-sided injury with hemiparesis. A steady progression of discoveries ensued. More specific language functions were mapped, as Paul Broca observed that posterior frontal lesions led to impaired speech but intact comprehension, and Carl Wernicke observed that more posterior lesions in the parietal cortex (now recognized as language association regions) led to impaired comprehension with fluent but garbled and incomprehensible speech. Well-defined motor and sensory regions were subsequently recognized as well. The vast area of the frontal cortex, anterior to the central sulcus, was observed to mediate a variety of higher cognitive and emotional functions that distinctly differentiate human personality and behavior, such as social judgment, long-term planning, and the capacity to form close emotional attachments.

TABLE 1–2. Some major discoveries in the first era of neuroscience

Year	Discovery
1837	Dax: The lateralization of language
1861	Broca: The identification of "Broca's area"
1868	Harlow: The description of Phineas Gage and the role of the frontal cortex
1870	Fritsch and Hitzig: The lateralization of motor function
1876	Wernicke: The localization of language comprehension
1909	Brodmann: Mapping of cortical cytoarchitecture
1920s	Penfield: Mapping of cognitive and motor functions with microelectrodes
1921	Foix: The localization of Parkinson's disease in the substantia nigra
1937	Papez: The description of the limbic system

These various observations about human cerebral specialization were achieved through a combination of clinical observation and developments in the basic sciences. Most of the observations about language function were made through the study of stroke patients, and the role of the prefrontal cortex in governing human personality was first identified through the famous case of Phineas Gage, who sustained a major lesion to his frontal lobes in an accident. (This case is further discussed in Chapters 5 and 6.) The motor cortex was mapped through the developing science of neurophysiology.

Basic neuroscience also was making major strides, as the brain was being studied systematically for the first time: anatomically, microscopically, and functionally. A variety of staining techniques were developed that permitted scientists to examine the cellular structure of the brain and begin to explore the neural networks that connected various regions. Nissl, Golgi, and Weigert provided methods for visualizing neuronal cell bodies, axons, and dendrites. Subsequently, Brodmann used these staining techniques to systematically map structural differentiation within the brain and to relate it to specific types of cortical function. His detailed maps of differentiations in cell layers and structures permitted the identification of the more primitive paleocortex (such as is found in the limbic system) as distinct from the neocortex and also permitted the identification of different types of cell layers in cortical regions specialized for different functions, such as sensory perception or motor activity.

These advances did not escape the notice of forward-looking individuals in the new discipline of psychiatry. While still a student and trainee, young Sigmund Freud attempted to develop a new staining technique for nerve cells, which was never successful; later he wrote a treatise on aphasia in children and worked in pharmacology by examining the potential therapeutic effects of cocaine.

One of the greatest departments of psychiatry of all time was assembled in Munich at the turn of the century under the leadership of Emil Kraepelin who, like Philippe Pinel, was a major founding father of modern psychiatry. If Pinel was the founder of the psychosocial tradition in psychiatry, Kraepelin was the founder of the neuroscience tradition.

Emil Kraepelin and some of the members of his Department of Psychiatry in Munich are shown in Figure 1–1. (Brodmann, also a member of this department for a time, is not in this particular picture.) Kraepelin had made a commitment to study psychiatry from the time he was in his late teens. He began his career in Dorpat, a city in the Baltic region that was part of Russia at the time. (It is now Tartu in Estonia.) He then progressed to become a professor in Heidelberg and later in Munich. His vision of psychiatry was that it should combine careful clinical description with good basic neuroscience. His own interest was cognitive psychology, and he did some of the earliest work examining the effects of drugs on learning and memory. He also had the vision to recognize the importance of neuropathology and brain science, however, and he recruited some of the best scientific minds available to work with him to identify the mechanisms of major mental illnesses. At its peak,

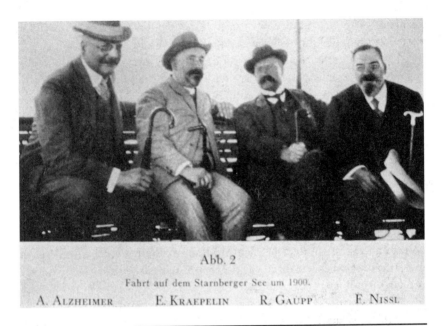

Abb. 2

Fahrt auf dem Starnberger See um 1900.

A. Alzheimer   E. Kraepelin   R. Gaupp   F. Nissl

FIGURE 1–1.   Emil Kraepelin, seated with other members of his Department of Psychiatry, near the Starnberger lake. From left to right: Alzheimer, Kraepelin, Gaupp, and Nissel (circa 1908).
Source.   Reprinted from Hippius H: *Kraepelin's Memoirs.* New York, Raven, 1989, p. 257. Used with permission.

his team included Kraepelin himself, Alzheimer, Brodmann, Nissl, and several less-well-known scientists. The productivity of this group is remarkable. Perhaps even more remarkable is the fact that most of these men were active clinicians who cared for patients during the day and worked in their laboratories at night. All were close friends, and all shared the goal of unraveling the mechanisms of the incapacitating brain diseases that eventually came to be known as schizophrenia, Alzheimer's disease, paranoia, and manic-depressive (bipolar) illness.

Kraepelin himself was a superb clinician and teacher who provided us with the classification of major mental illnesses that is still used. He combined information about age at onset with the natural history and longitudinal course of disorders to differentiate dementia praecox (now referred to as schizophrenia) from dementia in elderly persons (now referred to as Alzheimer's disease), paranoia (now referred to as delusional disorder), and manic-depressive illness (now referred to as bipolar disorder). He did this by observing that some individuals develop intellectual deterioration at a young age and fail to recover, whereas others develop this deterioration relatively late in life; he decided that the former had a discrete illness that he referred to as dementia praecox, whereas the latter had a very different illness because of their long period of intact functioning before the onset of dementia. He distinguished between dementia praecox and bipolar disorder because the former had a relatively chronic course leading to deterioration, whereas the latter was typically episodic with full remission between episodes of psychosis.

As Kraepelin and others within his department laid out this nosological structure, they applied the techniques of neuroscience to the study of postmortem brain specimens from patients they had known during life. Alzheimer observed that elderly demented patients had characteristic neuropathological lesions consisting of plaques and tangles; these became the neuropathological indicator of what is now known as Alzheimer's disease. Similar characteristic lesions were sought in patients with schizophrenia and bipolar disorder, but none were found, although occasional abnormalities were noted in both frontal and temporal regions. Kraepelin and his group were convinced that the major mental illnesses would ultimately be understood in terms of aberrations in neural functions. The goals that they set for themselves at the turn of the nineteenth century remain those that we have set for ourselves at the turn of the twentieth century.

In this era, achievements also were being made for the first time in the domain of somatic therapy. Working in Vienna, another contemporary of Freud and Kraepelin, Wagner von Jauregg, accidentally observed in 1887 that infection with malaria had a beneficial effect on patients with psychosis. This observation eventually led him to conduct a formal set of experiments 20 years later in which he infected with malaria a group of patients who had syphilis, a disorder largely under the care of psychiatrists because of its severe cognitive, behavioral, and emotional symptoms. The treatment was so effective that Wagner von Jauregg was later awarded a Nobel Prize for this discovery in 1927. Malarial treatment for syphilis remained a standard part of the therapeutic armamentarium until the discovery of penicillin. In the early twentieth century, other relatively crude and nonspecific treatments also were developed. These included the introduction of insulin shock therapy as a treatment for psychosis by Manfred Sakel in 1927 and the later development of electroshock therapy by Cerletti and Bini in 1938. Although most of the older forms of somatic therapy have now been supplanted by more specific methods of modulating brain chemistry through medications (see Chapter 27), electroconvulsive therapy is still widely used and highly effective in a small subgroup of psychiatric patients who primarily have severe mood disorders.

The Development of Psychoanalysis

Psychoanalysis was developed in the late nineteenth and early twentieth centuries. Because of the widespread popular appeal of psychoanalysis, its history is much better known than that of the neuroscientific traditions of psychiatry. It is important to realize, however, that psychoanalysis actually had its beginnings within the tradition of neuroscience. Sigmund Freud, the founder of the psychoanalytic method, spent his early career thinking about cerebral specialization, higher cortical functions, and their relation to the symptoms of mental illness. He embodied this thinking in a treatise, *A Project for a Scientific Psychology* (1895), in which he suggested that most specific symptoms of mental illness could be understood in terms of brain mechanisms.

Methods for investigating brain-behavior relationships remained relatively limited in the early twentieth century, however, consisting largely of neuroanatomy and neuropathology, with only a modest amount of neuropharmacology and neurophysiology. Thus, Freud himself turned to another fruitful avenue, the observation of clinical phenomena combined with speculations and hypotheses about their underlying psychic mechanisms. Unlike Kraepelin and his group, Freud was less interested in symptoms of psychosis and more interested in the symptoms referred to as *conversion* or *hysterical phenomena*. These symptoms consisted of peculiar unexplained pains and paralyses experienced by many individuals in the early twentieth century.

Freud's earliest thoughts on this subject, contained in *Studies in Hysteria* (co-authored with Josef Breuer), included the fundamental ideas that were the basis for what was later to become the extensive field of psychoanalysis. On the basis of his own experience in treating patients who had the sudden onset of paralyses or seizures with no obvious physical cause, he speculated that these symptoms could be the result of some type of trauma that occurred early in life and remained embedded in the psyche and caused irritation: "The memory of the trauma acts like a foreign body which long after its entry must continue to be regarded as an agent that is still at work" (p. 3). He observed that releasing these embedded memories, either through hypnosis or through free association, sometimes led to the remission of symptoms. This led to Freud and Breuer's famous pronouncement: "Hysterics suffer mainly from reminiscences" (p. 4).

These early ideas led to the extensive development of theories of psychological structure and function, such as the id, ego, and superego, as well as a variety of psychotherapeutic methods for manipulating psychological structures and functions and reducing symptoms. Psychoanalysis also extensively explored human sexuality, a courageous step at a time when most people were bound by rigid Victorian inhibitions about what they were allowed to say, think, and do. Because of its imagination and courage, the work of Freud and his disciples gained widespread respect. The methods that he developed for clinical management of milder psychiatric syndromes gained popularity and are still in use today, mostly in modified form.

The Second Era of Neuroscience

The term *neuroscience* did not in fact exist during the nineteenth or early twentieth century. Kraepelin, Alzheimer, Nissl, and Brodmann would have described themselves as "brain scientists." By the early to mid-twentieth century, however, a new array of techniques had been developed that permitted brain scientists to go far beyond the simple processes of examining neurons under the microscope or studying the gross structure of the brain. Developments in neuropharmacology, neurochemistry, molecular biology, and a variety of other related fields have been extraordinary. These developments led to the founding of a society of neuroscience in 1970 so that scientists working in the diverse areas related to the nervous system could meet and communicate with one another. By the mid-1990s, the Society for Neuroscience had gained more than 20,000 members, making it one of the largest scientific organizations in the United States. The vast array of techniques now available for studying the nervous system has rekindled the strong connections between psychiatry and neuroscience. Many psychiatrists believe that the dream (shared by Kraepelin and Freud) of understanding mental phenomena in terms of neural mechanisms now lies within our reach.

The growth of knowledge and expertise in neuroscience can be easily summarized by examining the history of Nobel Prize awards since their inception. Table 1–3 lists Nobel Prizes awarded in neuroscience and psychiatry. Early awards were given for microscopic techniques and for clinical achievements. Two awards, the prize to Wagner von Jauregg for malarial treatment of syphilis and to Moniz for the development of prefrontal leukotomy to treat schizophrenia, were purely clinical. Others were given more recently in basic areas that laid important foundations for clinical applications, such as Axelrod's studies of neurotransmission within the catecholamine system. The listing in Table 1–3 indicates that there has been a steady increase in prizes awarded in the area of neuroscience during the past several decades.

For any Nobel Prize given in any single year, there are of course dozens

TABLE 1–3.   Nobel Prizes awarded in neuroscience and psychiatry

Year	Investigators	Discovery
1906	Camillo Golgi and Santiago Ramón y Cajal	Work on structure of the nervous system
1927	Julius Wagner von Jauregg	Discovery of the therapeutic importance of malaria inoculation in dementia paralytica
1932	Edgar D. Adrian and Sir Charles Scott Sherrington	Discoveries regarding function of the neurons
1936	Sir Henry H. Dale and Otto Loewi	Discoveries relating to the chemical transmission of nerve impulses
1944	Joseph Erlanger and Herbert S. Gasser	Research on the differentiated function of single nerve fibers
1949	Antonio Egas Moniz	Discovery of therapeutic value of leukotomy in certain psychoses
1963	Sir John C. Eccles, Sir Alan Lloyd Hodgkin, and Andrew F. Huxley	Study of the transmission of nerve impulses along a nerve fiber (or relation between inhibition of nerve cells and repolarization of a cell's membrane)
1970	Julius Axelrod, Sir Bernard Katz, and Ulf von Euler	Discoveries concerning the chemistry of nerve transmission
1971	Earl Wilbur Sutherland Jr.	Study of hormones, the chemical substances that regulate virtually every body function
1977	Rosalyn S. Yalow	Radioimmunoassay
1977	Roger C.L. Guillemin and Andrew V. Schally	Production of peptide hormones in the brain
1979	Earl Hounsfield and Sir Allan M. Cormack	Development of computed tomography scanning
1981	Roger Sperry, David H. Hubel, and Tosten N. Wiesel	Studies on the function of the corpus callosum (split brain research, functions of left and right hemispheres); discoveries of the organization of the visual system
1986	Rita Levi-Montalcini and Stanley Cohen	Discovery of nerve growth factor
1994	Stanley Prusiner	Discovery of prions
2000	Arvid Carlsson, Paul Greengard, and Eric Kandel	Studies of neurotransmission and memory formation

of other equally deserving individuals who have made major contributions to science and clinical practice. For example, Nobel Prizes have not been awarded for positron-emission tomography, a far more powerful imaging technique than computed tomography, or for either antipsychotic drugs or antidepressants, which have been far more lasting and powerful ameliorators of human suffering than prefrontal leukotomy. Nevertheless, this list of Nobel laureates indicates that our knowledge base in neuroscience and in its clinical applications has been steadily advancing.

Within psychiatry as a specialized discipline, the major sources of impact from neuroscience have been neuropharmacology and neurochemistry. Coupled with the overall development in neuroscience, the discovery of relatively potent pharmacological treatments for major mental illnesses has also served to reawaken interest in clinical neurobiology. The discovery of chlorpromazine by Delay and Deniker in 1952 indicated that drugs could be developed that would have a powerful calming effect on psychotic and agitated patients. This discovery led rapidly to the development of a variety of antipsychotic drugs that are used for the treatment of psychosis. By the late 1950s, a second new specific class of medications had been developed, the antidepressants, the prototype of which is imipramine. Antianxiety drugs such as meprobamate also were developed. By the early 1960s, it had become clear to psychiatrists that an entire new discipline, psychopharmacology, was at their feet and that this discipline provided a powerful alternative to the techniques of psychotherapy that had been their major means of treating patients up to this point. Psychopharmacology (also referred to as neuropharmacology or neuropsychopharmacology) was clearly not only a tool for treatment but also a tool for studying brain chemistry and for developing new classifications of diseases based on patients' responses to specific drugs that manipulated specific classes of chemicals within the brain.

These developments have placed psychiatry squarely within the traditions of medicine and neuroscience at the beginning of the third millennium. To interest in neuropharmacology have been added neuroimaging and molecular biology. Modern students of psychiatry must simultaneously view their patients on multiple planes: as human beings who have particular symptoms (psychological), as individuals living within a social and cultural context (social), as products of the genetic endowments given to them by their parents and coded in their chromosomes (genetic-molecular), and as individuals whose ideas and emotions are both the product and the producers of a complex set of chemical events in their brains (neurochemical-neuroanatomical).

The Mind/Body Problem in Psychiatry

As this summary of the history of psychiatry indicates, people have not consistently agreed about the origins of mental illness or the appropriate areas of expertise for the clinicians who treat mental illness. Although the historical origins of psychiatry are clearly biological, in that the first individuals to identify and define mental illness in classical times believed that these illnesses were physical in origin, for many centuries people also have believed that mental illnesses were caused by a disease of the spirit or psyche. From the Middle Ages through the eighteenth or nineteenth century, the mentally ill were perceived as spiritually or morally diseased. Although the bulk of contemporary psychiatrists no longer hold this belief, literally centuries of misunderstanding must be forgotten or eliminated. Old ideas do not die easily, and consequently, mental illnesses tend to be stigmatized or misunderstood. The role of psychiatry is confused as well. Many laypersons still view psychiatrists as literally doctors of the mind or soul.

This misunderstanding also has been enhanced by the long-standing controversy about the relationship between the mind and the body. Many religions teach that there is a soul or spirit that exists independently of the body and that survives it after death. People who think concretely and metaphorically tend to see the soul or spirit as a tiny ghost sitting somewhere in the body (usually in the brain in modern thinking) and moving or guiding its actions. The existence of the spirit or soul is fundamentally a philosophical or religious issue, not a scientific or medical one. There is simply no way to prove or disprove the existence of the soul and its continuing existence after death. That is a matter of faith.

It is clear that, on at least one level, what is commonly referred to as the *mind* is simply the summation of various electrical and chemical events occurring in the brain. Thinking, believing, remembering, feeling, tasting, and all the other cognitive, sensory, and behavioral functions that human beings experience are fundamentally determined at the molecular level, within a context of neural networks. These events do not exist independently of external environmental influences but rather are influenced by and reactive to them. Head injuries damage neurons and cause new networks to be developed. Perceptions and experiences are encoded and remembered, and this learning and memory affect later cognitive events. Thus, mental phenomena, often referred to as *mind*, can and must be understood in terms of the brain.

The study of psychiatry, the branch of medicine devoted to the study of mental illnesses, is, therefore, a discipline dedicated to the investigation of abnormalities in brain function. The clinical appearance of these abnormalities may be florid and obvious, as in the case of psychosis. The abnormalities may be subtle and mild, as in the case of personality disorders. Ultimately, the drive of modern psychiatry is to develop a comprehensive understanding of normal brain function at levels that range from mind to molecule and to determine how aberrations in these normal functions (produced either endogenously through genetic coding or exogenously through environmental influences) lead to the development of symptoms of mental illnesses.

Bibliography

Ackerknecht EH: Short History of Psychiatry. New York, Hafner, 1968

Alexander FG, Selesnick ST: The History of Psychiatry: An Evaluation of Psychiatric Thought and Practice From Prehistoric Times to the Present. New York, Harper & Row, 1966

Andreasen NC: The Broken Brain: The Biological Revolution in Psychiatry. New York, Harper & Row, 1984

Andreasen NC (ed): Am J Psychiatry 151 (Sesquicentennial Edition suppl, June), 1994

Breuer J, Freud S: Studies in Hysteria (1883–1895). Translated by Brill AA. New York, Nervous and Mental Disease Publishing, 1936

Gilman SL: Seeing the Insane. New York, Wiley, 1982

Kraepelin E: Lectures on Clinical Psychiatry. London, Bailliere, Tindall & Cox, 1904

Murray CJL, Lopez AD: The Global Burden of Disease. Boston, MA, Harvard University Press, 1996

Pichot P: A Century of Psychiatry. Paris, Editions Roger Dacosta, 1983

Pinel P: A Treatise on Insanity. London, Messrs Cadell & Davies, Strand, 1806

Rush B: Two Essays on the Mind. Philadelphia, PA, Charles Cist, 1786

Zilboorg G: A History of Medical Psychology. New York, WW Norton, 1941

Self-Assessment Questions

1. Describe Greek attitudes toward mental illness. What were the four humors?
2. Describe attitudes toward mentally ill persons during the Middle Ages. How long ago was the last witch known to be tormented or burned at the stake?
3. Describe the ideas and accomplishments of Philippe Pinel.
4. Who was Emil Kraepelin? Name two eminent neuroscientists who were members of his department.

5. Wagner von Jauregg and Moniz received Nobel Prizes for clinical achievements. What were they? Describe two more recent achievements that received Nobel Prizes and that provide a link between neuroscience and psychiatry.

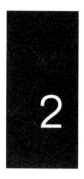

2 Diagnosis and Classification

Knowledge keeps no better than fish.

Alfred North Whitehead

Beginning students of psychiatry are often puzzled about what is expected of them when they are asked to make a diagnosis. This is because two major traditions for observing and understanding patients have historically coexisted within psychiatry: the biomedical model and the psychodynamic model. The biomedical model is closely allied with general medicine and stresses diagnosing discrete illnesses or disorders. The psychodynamic model, conversely, stresses the importance of understanding the patient's symptoms and behavior in terms of underlying psychological processes (referred to as psychodynamics). A psychiatrist applying the biological or medical model attempts to determine whether the patient has one of the group of commonly recognized disorders, such as schizophrenia or bipolar disorder, and then plans the care of the patient accordingly, often by prescribing medications. A psychiatrist applying the psychodynamic model attempts to understand why the patient presents with a particular complaint, often in terms of relationships with parents or early life experiences, and then seeks to help the patient change his or her maladaptive behavior or reduce his or her psychological pain by helping him or her understand and readjust these dynamics. This is often done with psychotherapy.

Although these two traditions were once relatively polarized, they have become increasingly unified in the modern practice of psychiatry, which usually stresses the importance of an integrated *biopsychosocial model*. This model emphasizes the importance of evaluating all aspects of a patient's symptoms and experiences: examining both biological and psychological processes as they occur within a particular social and personal context. The heart of this examination begins, however, with attempting to recognize the particular pattern of symptoms and experiences that leads to the diagnosis of a specific psychiatric disorder based on a nomenclature and classification system that has been developed with considerable care and rigor during the past two decades. This system, known as the *Diagnostic and Statistical Manual of Mental Disorders*, Fourth Edition (DSM-IV), provides the basis for diagnosis and classification in psychiatry. In 2000, a text revision of DSM-IV was published, DSM-IV-TR, that updated the text but did not change the essential criteria for diagnosis.

The Fundamental Purpose of Diagnosis and Classification

The fundamental purpose of diagnosis and classification is to isolate a group of discrete disease entities, each of which is characterized by a distinct pathophysiology and/or etiology. Ideally, all diseases in medicine would be defined in terms of etiology. For most illnesses, however, we do not know or understand the specific etiology. By and large, a full understanding of etiology is limited to the infectious diseases, in which the etiology is exposure to some infectious agent to a degree sufficient that the body's immune mechanisms are overwhelmed. (And even in this instance, our knowledge of immune mechanisms is incomplete.) We also understand the etiology of a variety of hereditary metabolic diseases, such as phenylketonuria (PKU). We have been able to define these diseases in terms of a specific metabolic defect (e.g., failure to metabolize phenylalanine) and have traced that metabolic defect down to a specific genetic locus that produces an abnormal protein. The case of PKU, however, illustrates how complex the search for causes can actually be. We now know that there are two forms of PKU; both are characterized by failure to metabolize phenylalanine, but they involve two different enzymes within the metabolic pathway. Thus, even for a simple disease with a recognized metabolic defect, increasing knowledge can also increase complexity. Now this simple disease must be understood as two different diseases with two different specific causes at the molecular level.

For most diseases, however, our understanding is at the level of pathophysiology rather than etiology. Diseases are defined in terms of the mechanisms that produce particular symptoms, such as infarction in the myocardium, inflammation in the joints, or abnormal regulation of insulin production.

In the areas of pathophysiology and etiology, psychiatry has more uncharted territory than the rest of medicine. Most of the disorders or diseases diagnosed in psychiatry are *syndromes:* collections of symptoms that tend to occur together and that appear to have a characteristic course and outcome. Much of the current investigative research in psychiatry is directed toward the goal of identifying the pathophysiology and etiology of major mental illnesses, but this goal has been achieved for only a few disorders (Alzheimer's disease, multi-infarct dementia, Huntington's disease, and substance-induced syndromes such as amphetamine-related psychosis or Wernicke-Korsakoff syndrome).

Purposes of Diagnosis in Psychiatry

Even though they do not contain information about specific mechanisms or causes for an identified group of symptoms, diagnoses in psychiatry serve a variety of important purposes. Thus, making a careful diagnosis is as fundamental in psychiatry as it is in the remainder of medicine.

Diagnosis helps to simplify our thinking and reduce the complexity of clinical phenomena in psychiatry. Psychiatry is a diverse field, and symptoms of mental illness encompass a broad range of emotional, cognitive, and behavioral abnormalities. The use of diagnoses introduces order and structure to this complexity. Disorders are divided into broad classes based on common features (e.g., psychosis, substance abuse, dementia, anxiety). The overall structure of the current psychiatric classification system used in this text is summarized in Table 2–1. Within each of the major classes, specific syndromes are then further delineated (e.g., dividing substance-related disorders in terms of the type of substance involved, dividing the dementias into Alzheimer's disease and vascular dementia). The existence of broad groups of diagnostic categories, subdivided into specific disorders, creates a structure within the apparent chaos of clinical phenomena and makes mental illnesses easier to learn about and understand. Although diagnoses are not necessarily defined in terms of etiology or pathophysiology, they are typically defined in terms of syndromal clinical features. Thus, this creation of order out of chaos does not misrepresent reality in the process of facilitating understanding.

TABLE 2–1.   DSM-IV-TR classification

Disorders usually first diagnosed in infancy, childhood, or adolescence
Mental retardation
  Mild
  Moderate
  Severe
  Profound
  Severity unspecified
Learning disorders
  Reading disorder
  Mathematics disorder
  Disorder of written expression
  Learning disorder not otherwise
    specified
Motor skills disorder
  Developmental coordination disorder
Communication disorders
  Expressive language disorder
  Mixed receptive-expressive
    language disorder
  Phonological disorder
  Stuttering
  Communication disorder not
    otherwise specified
Pervasive developmental disorders
  Autistic disorder
  Rett's disorder
  Childhood disintegrative disorder
  Asperger's disorder
  Pervasive developmental disorder
    not otherwise specified
Attention-deficit and disruptive
  behavior disorders
  Attention-deficit/hyperactivity
    disorder
  Attention-deficit/hyperactivity
    disorder not otherwise specified
  Conduct disorder
  Oppositional defiant disorder

Disruptive behavior disorder not
    otherwise specified
Feeding and eating disorders of infancy
  or early childhood
  Pica
  Rumination disorder
  Feeding disorder of infancy or early
    childhood
Tic disorders
  Tourette's disorder
  Chronic motor or vocal tic disorder
  Transient tic disorder
  Tic disorder not otherwise specified
Elimination disorders
  Encopresis
  Enuresis
Other disorders of infancy, childhood,
  or adolescence
  Separation anxiety disorder
  Selective mutism
  Reactive attachment disorder of
    infancy or early childhood
  Stereotypic movement disorder
  Disorders of infancy, childhood, or
    adolescence not otherwise
    specified

**Delirium, dementia, and amnestic and
other cognitive disorders**
Delirium
  Delirium due to a general medical
    condition
  Substance-induced delirium
  Delirium due to multiple etiologies
  Delirium not otherwise specified
Dementia
  Dementia of the Alzheimer's type
  Vascular dementia
  Dementia due to HIV disease

TABLE 2–1. DSM-IV-TR classification (*continued*)

Delirium, dementia, and amnestic and other cognitive disorders (*continued*)

    Dementia due to head trauma

    Dementia due to Parkinson's disease

    Dementia due to Huntington's disease

    Dementia due to Pick's disease

    Dementia due to Creutzfeldt-Jakob disease

    Dementia due to other general medical conditions

    Substance-induced persisting dementia

    Dementia due to multiple etiologies

    Dementia not otherwise specified

  Amnestic disorders

    Amnestic disorder due to a general medical condition

    Substance-induced persisting amnestic disorder

    Amnestic disorder not otherwise specified

  Other cognitive disorders

Mental disorders due to a general medical condition

  Catatonic disorder due to a general medical condition

  Personality change due to a general medical condition

  Mental disorder not otherwise specified due to a general medical condition

Substance-related disorders

  Substance abuse

  Substance intoxication

  Substance withdrawal

  Alcohol-related disorders

  Amphetamine (or amphetamine-like)–related disorders

  Caffeine-related disorders

  Cannabis-related disorders

  Cocaine-related disorders

  Hallucinogen-related disorders

  Inhalant-related disorders

  Nicotine-related disorders

  Opioid-related disorders

  Phencyclidine (or phencyclidine-like)–related disorders

  Sedative-, hypnotic-, or anxiolytic-related disorders

  Polysubstance-related disorder

  Other (or unknown) substance-related disorders

Schizophrenia and other psychotic disorders

  Schizophrenia

    Paranoid type

    Disorganized type

    Catatonic type

    Undifferentiated type

    Residual type

  Schizophreniform disorder

  Schizoaffective disorder

  Delusional disorder

  Brief psychotic disorder

  Shared psychotic disorder (folie à deux)

  Psychotic disorder due to a medical condition

  Substance-induced psychotic disorder

  Psychotic disorder not otherwise specified

TABLE 2–1.   DSM-IV-TR classification *(continued)*

Mood disorders
  Mood episodes
    Major depressive episode
    Manic episode
    Mixed episode
    Hypomanic episode
  Depressive disorders
    Major depressive disorder
    Dysthymic disorder
    Depressive disorder not otherwise
      specified
  Bipolar disorders
    Bipolar I disorder
    Bipolar II disorder
    Cyclothymic disorder
    Bipolar disorder not otherwise
      specified
  Other mood disorders
    Mood disorders due to a general
      medical condition
    Substance-induced mood disorder
    Mood disorder not otherwise
      specified

Anxiety disorders
  Panic attack
  Agoraphobia
  Panic disorder without agoraphobia
  Panic disorder with agoraphobia
  Agoraphobia without history of panic
    disorder
  Specific phobia
  Social phobia
  Obsessive-compulsive disorder
  Posttraumatic stress disorder
  Acute stress disorder
  Generalized anxiety disorder

  Anxiety disorder due to a general
    medical condition
  Substance-induced anxiety disorder
  Anxiety disorder not otherwise
    specified

Somatoform disorders
  Somatization disorder
  Undifferentiated somatoform disorder
  Conversion disorder
  Pain disorder
  Hypochondriasis
  Body dysmorphic disorder
  Somatoform disorder not otherwise
    specified

Factitious disorders

Dissociative disorders
  Dissociative amnesia
  Dissociative fugue
  Dissociative identity disorder
  Depersonalization disorder
  Dissociative disorder not otherwise
    specified

Sexual and gender identity disorders
  Sexual dysfunctions
    Sexual desire disorders
    Sexual arousal disorders
    Orgasmic disorders
    Sexual pain disorders
    Sexual dysfunction due to a general
      medical condition
    Substance-induced sexual
      dysfunction
    Sexual dysfunction not otherwise
      specified

TABLE 2–1. DSM-IV-TR classification *(continued)*

Sexual and gender identity disorders *(continued)*

  Paraphilias
    Exhibitionism
    Fetishism
    Frotteurism
    Pedophilia
    Sexual masochism
    Sexual sadism
    Transvestic fetishism
    Voyeurism
    Paraphilia not otherwise specified
  Gender identity disorders
    Gender identity disorder
    Gender identity disorder not otherwise specified
  Sexual disorder not otherwise specified

Eating disorders
  Anorexia nervosa
  Bulimia nervosa
  Eating disorder not otherwise specified

Sleep disorders
  Primary sleep disorders
    Dyssomnias
    Parasomnias
  Sleep disorders related to another mental disorder
  Sleep disorder due to a general medical condition
  Substance-induced sleep disorder

Impulse-control disorders not elsewhere classified
  Intermittent explosive disorder
  Kleptomania
  Pyromania
  Pathological gambling
  Trichotillomania
  Impulse-control disorder not otherwise specified

Adjustment disorders

Personality disorders
  Paranoid personality disorder
  Schizoid personality disorder
  Schizotypal personality disorder
  Antisocial personality disorder
  Borderline personality disorder
  Histrionic personality disorder
  Narcissistic personality disorder
  Avoidant personality disorder
  Dependent personality disorder
  Obsessive-compulsive personality disorder
  Personality disorder not otherwise specified

Other conditions that may be a focus of clinical attention

Psychiatric diagnoses facilitate communication between clinicians. When physicians give a patient's symptoms a specific diagnosis, such as bipolar disorder, they are making a specific statement about the clinical picture with which that particular patient presents. A diagnosis concisely summarizes information for all other clinicians who subsequently examine the patient's records or to whom the patient is referred. A diagnosis of bipolar disorder, for example, indicates that

- The patient has had at least one episode of mania.
- During that episode of mania, the patient experienced a characteristic group of symptoms such as elated mood, increased energy, racing thoughts, rapid speech, grandiosity, and poor judgment.
- The patient probably has had episodes of depression as well, characterized by sadness, insomnia, decreased appetite, feelings of worthlessness, and other typical depressive symptoms.

The use of diagnostic categories gives clinicians a kind of "shorthand" through which they can summarize large quantities of information relatively easily.

Diagnoses help to predict the outcome of the disorder. Many psychiatric diagnoses are associated with a characteristic course and outcome. For example, bipolar disorder is usually episodic, with periods of relatively severe abnormalities in mood interspersed with periods of near normality or complete normality. Most patients with bipolar disorder have a relatively good outcome. Some other types of disorders, such as schizophrenia or personality disorders, typically have a more chronic course. Diagnoses are a useful way of summarizing the clinician's expectations about the patient's course of illness in the future.

Diagnoses are often used to decide on an appropriate treatment. As psychiatry has advanced clinically and scientifically, relatively specific treatments for particular disorders or groups of symptoms have been developed. For example, antipsychotic drugs are typically used to treat psychoses. Thus, they are used for disorders such as schizophrenia, in which psychosis is typically prominent, as well as forms of mood disorder in which psychotic symptoms occur. A diagnosis of mania suggests the use of medications such as lithium carbonate or valproate. Some relatively targeted medications are now available, such as the serotonin reuptake inhibitors for obsessive-compulsive disorder.

Diagnoses are used to assist in the search for pathophysiology and etiology. Clinical researchers use diagnoses to reduce heterogeneity in their samples and to separate groups of patients who may share a common mechanism or cause that produces their symptoms. Patients who share a relatively specific set of symptoms, such as severe schizophrenia characterized by negative symptoms, are often hypothesized to have a disorder that is mechanistically or etiologically distinct. Knowledge about specific groupings of clinical symptoms can be related to knowledge about brain specialization and function in order to formulate hypotheses about the neurochemical or anatomical substrates of a particular disorder. Ideally, the use of diagnoses defined on the basis of the clinical picture will lead ultimately to diagnoses that serve the fundamental purpose of identifying causes.

Other Purposes of Diagnosis

Beyond these clinical uses, diagnostic systems also have other purposes. Although physicians prefer to conceptualize their relationships with patients in terms of care and treatment, diagnoses are used by other health care providers, attorneys, epidemiologists, and insurance companies. Each time a clinician makes a diagnosis and records it, he or she must do so with an awareness of the other nonclinical uses to which it may be put.

Diagnoses are used to monitor treatment and to make decisions about reimbursement. As care has become increasingly managed, predetermined guidelines (diagnosis-related groups) have been set that define the length of a hospitalization or treatment course for a specific diagnosis. In some regions, physicians or their assistants must spend hours speaking on the telephone or writing letters if their patient's course of treatment appears to exceed the preset guidelines. This situation will probably not change the physician's diagnosis, but it has certainly changed the autonomy that physicians once enjoyed.

Diagnoses are used by attorneys in malpractice suits and in other litigation. Although psychiatrists are the least sued among medical specialists, lawsuits are a concern for all specialists in our litigious society. Some diagnoses, such as major depression, carry with them a clear set of risks, such as suicide. Clinicians must be aware of those risks and clearly document that they have provided appropriate care. As the DSM has made the diagnostic system of psychiatry more open and available, both lawyers and patients have learned much more about psychiatric nosology. A physician called into court must expect to defend a recorded diagnosis with appropriate documentation that the various criteria have been assessed and are met.

Diagnoses are used by health care epidemiologists to determine the incidence and prevalence of various diseases throughout the world. Diagnoses recorded in hospital or clinic charts are translated into a standard system established by the World Health Organization (WHO), the International Classification of Diseases (ICD). This system is used to track regional differences in disease patterns, as well as changes over time.

Diagnoses are used to make decisions about insurance coverage. A carelessly made diagnosis, be it of hypertension or major depression, may make it difficult for a patient to obtain life insurance or future health care insurance. Diagnoses also are sometimes used to make decisions about employment, admission to college, and other important opportunities. Because mental illnesses may be subject to discrimination and misunderstanding, these diagnoses involve a particular risk. The clinician obviously must walk a fine line—perhaps impossibly fine.

Development of the Diagnostic and Statistical Manual of Mental Disorders

The process of diagnosis in psychiatry is partially simplified by the fact that the national professional organization to which most psychiatrists in the United States belong, the American Psychiatric Association, has formulated a manual that summarizes all of the diagnoses used in psychiatry, specifies the symptoms that must be present to make a given diagnosis, and organizes these diagnoses together into a classification system. This manual is titled the *Diagnostic and Statistical Manual of Mental Disorders* (DSM). Over the years, it has undergone four major revisions (DSM-I, DSM-II, DSM-III, and DSM-IV). Currently, diagnoses in psychiatry are based on DSM-IV, which was revised during the 1990s and published in 1994. As mentioned previously, a text revision of DSM-IV, DSM-IV-TR, was published in 2000.

Psychiatry is the only specialty in medicine that has so consistently and comprehensively formalized the diagnostic processes for the disorders within its domain. This precision and structure are particularly important in psychiatry because psychiatry lacks recognized etiologies for most disorders as well as specific laboratory diagnostic tests. Consequently, diagnosis relies largely on the patient's presenting symptoms and history. Without such structure, the diagnostic process could become confused and fuzzy.

The impetus to organize a DSM began during World War II. For the first time, psychiatrists from all over the United States were brought together in clinical settings that required them to communicate clearly with one another. It became apparent that diagnostic practices varied widely throughout the United States, no doubt reflecting a diversity of training. After World War II, the Veterans Administration attempted to design a relatively comprehensive diagnostic system for its own use. Shortly thereafter, the American Psychiatric Association convened a task force to develop a diagnostic manual for use in all of American psychiatry. The product was DSM-I, which was published in 1952. The second edition, DSM-II, was published in 1968.

Compared with DSM-III and DSM-IV, the more recent manuals, DSM-I and DSM-II were relatively simple. The definitions of disorders and the overall classification system were designed by a small group of clinicians who convened, discussed their clinical experiences, and decided together on appropriate categories and defining features. Definitions tended to be brief, descriptive, and relatively vague. For example, the definition of manic-depressive illness in DSM-II was as follows:

Manic-Depressive Illnesses (Manic-Depressive Psychoses)
   These disorders are marked by severe mood swings and a tendency to remission and recurrence. Patients may be given this diagnosis in the absence of a previous history of affective psychosis if there is no obvious precipitating event. This disorder is divided into three major subtypes: manic type, depressed type, and circular type. (p. 8)

These handbooks were relatively small. DSM-I contained 132 pages, and DSM-II contained 119 pages.

DSM-III, by contrast, represented a major change—and, most clinicians would concur, a major improvement. Because of their vagueness and imprecision, the definitions in DSM-I and DSM-II did not adequately fulfill many of the purposes summarized earlier in this chapter. In particular, the descriptions were not specific enough to facilitate communication among clinicians and to delineate one disorder from another. Although the purpose of DSM-I and DSM-II was to ensure that a psychiatrist in Peoria, Illinois, meant the same thing by a diagnosis of schizophrenia as did a psychiatrist on Park Avenue in New York City or in Laguna Beach, California, this was clearly not the case.

Several research investigations had examined diagnostic agreement among clinicians. They made it clear that different clinicians using DSM-I or DSM-II guidelines would give different diagnoses to the same patient. Naturally, this lack of consensus and agreement about how to diagnose symptoms called the credibility of psychiatry into question. These research studies of poor agreement, completed during the 1960s, coincided with the development of relatively specific new medications such as antipsychotics and antidepressants. When relatively specific treatments for particular disorders became available, it was clearly important to define the disorders well so that appropriate treatment would be prescribed.

When the Task Force on DSM-III was appointed in 1972, its members decided to set a new agenda for the development of the DSMs. Many members of this task force were eminent researchers with expertise in disciplines such as pharmacology and genetics. Thus, they were especially aware of the importance of diagnostic precision. At their first meetings, they decided to formulate a set of rules by which they would abide:

1. They would attempt to formulate specific diagnostic criteria that would be as objective as possible to define each of the disorders included in the manual.
2. They would make their decisions about defining criteria and overall organizational structure on the basis of existing research data whenever possible.
3. They would not resort to anecdotal approaches or simple clinical opinion if at all possible.
4. They would include a glossary to define terms used in the text.
5. In addition to the criteria, they would provide clinicians with information that would assist them in understanding specific disorders better, such as population frequency, gender ratio, and longitudinal course.
6. They would provide a set of references that would support their decisions.

Apart from the last rule, which was not feasible because of the large quantity of references that would have been needed, these rules were followed relatively closely.

When DSM-III finally appeared in 1980, it was widely recognized as a major innovation. Although some clinicians complained that it was boring or dull, most appreciated its objectivity. For the first time, the methods by which a psychiatric diagnosis could be made were relatively clear. The process has been somewhat facetiously referred to as the "Chinese-menu approach" to diagnosis. Most of the time, the criteria require that a specified subset from a listed group of symptoms be present in order to make a diagnosis (e.g., select "two from column one and three from column two," as on some Chinese restaurant menus). For example, in contrast to the rather vague definition of manic-depressive illness above, the DSM-III definition of major depressive disorder was as follows:

Diagnostic Criteria for Major Depression

A. One or more major depressive episodes
B. Has never had a manic episode

Diagnostic Criteria for Major Depressive Episode

A. Dysphoric mood or loss of interest or pleasure in all or almost all usual activities and pastimes. The dysphoric mood is characterized by symptoms such as the following: depressed, sad, blue, hopeless, low, down in the dumps, irritable. The mood disturbance must be prominent and relatively persistent, but not necessarily the most dominant symptom, and does not include momentary shifts from one dysphoric mood to another dysphoric mood, e.g., anxiety to depression to anger, such as are seen in states of acute psychotic turmoil. (For children under 6, dysphoric mood may have to be inferred from a persistently sad facial expression.)

B. At least four of the following symptoms have been present nearly every day for a period of at least 2 weeks (in children under 6, at least three of the first four).

   1. poor appetite or significant weight loss (when not dieting) or increased appetite or significant weight gain (in children under 6, consider failure to make expected weight gains)
   2. insomnia or hypersomnia
   3. psychomotor agitation or retardation (but not merely subjective feelings of restlessness or being slowed down) (in children under 6, hypoactivity)
   4. loss of interest or pleasure in usual activities, or decrease in sexual drive not limited to a period when delusional or hallucinating (in children under 6, signs of apathy)
   5. loss of energy; fatigue
   6. feelings of worthlessness, self-reproach, or excessive or inappropriate guilt (either may be delusional)
   7. complaints or evidence of diminished ability to think or concentrate, such as slowed thinking, or indecisiveness not associated with marked loosening of associations or incoherence
   8. recurrent thoughts of death, suicidal ideation, wishes to be dead, or suicide attempt

C. Neither of the following dominates the clinical picture when an affective syndrome is absent (i.e., symptoms in criteria A and B above):

   1. preoccupation with a mood-incongruent delusion or hallucination (see definition below)
   2. bizarre behavior

D. Not superimposed on schizophrenia, schizophreniform disorder, or a paranoid disorder

E. Not due to any organic mental disorder or uncomplicated bereavement (pp. 213–214, 218)

DSM-III was the first effort by a medical specialty to provide a comprehensive and detailed diagnostic manual in which all disorders were defined by highly specific criteria. DSM-III was a hefty tome—494 pages long—and changed the practice of psychiatry in many ways. In general, it introduced substantial improvements in psychiatric diagnosis, which have been carried forward in DSM-IV, published in 1994, and the recent DSM-IV text revision.

The DSM system, as represented by all versions since DSM-III, has been an effective treatment for some of the previous muddleheadedness of psychiatric diagnosis. But this treatment has not been without some untoward side effects as well.

Advantages and Disadvantages of the DSM System

The DSM system has many advantages, which can be summarized as follows:

The DSM system has substantially improved the reliability of diagnosis. Reliability, a biometric concept, refers to the ability of two observers to agree on what they see. It is measured by a variety of statistical methods, such as percent agreement, correlation coefficients, and the kappa statistic, which corrects for chance agreement. The reliability of DSM-III was assessed in field trials and found to be relatively good. Even more extensive field trials and reliability studies were done for DSM-IV. These have been extensively summarized in the DSM Sourcebooks (1994–1998). The kappa statistics for most diagnoses are approximately 0.8 or greater, which is considered very good. By contrast, percent agreements (which are not corrected for chance agreement) for major disorders such as depression or schizophrenia had been estimated as low as 20%–30% in several studies completed before DSM-III was available.

The DSM system has clarified the diagnostic process and facilitated history taking. Because DSM-IV-TR specifies exactly which symptoms must be present to make a diagnosis, as well as the characteristic course of disorders whenever this is appropriate, it is highly objective. During the 1970s, many psychiatrists received predominantly psychodynamic training, which deemphasized a medical approach to diagnosis. This approach stressed the importance of recognizing underlying psychological processes rather than objective signs and symptoms. Although clinically useful, this approach is more subjective, is difficult to teach to beginners, and requires substantial training. The DSM system provided a simpler approach that brought signs and symptoms back to the forefront of evaluation. Its criteria systematically specify which signs must be observed and which symptoms must be inquired about. This structured approach also makes it an excellent teaching tool for medical students and residents.

The DSM system has clarified and facilitated the process of differential diagnosis. Because it is so explicit, DSM-IV-TR helps clinicians decide which symptoms must be present to rule in or to rule out a particular diagnosis. For example, it specifies that a diagnosis of schizophrenia cannot be made if a full mood syndrome is present. Likewise, a diagnosis cannot be made if some type of drug of abuse, such as amphetamine, has led to the presence of psychotic symptoms. Not only are differential diagnostic issues embedded in the criteria, but the text of each DSM also contains a relatively detailed discussion of the differential diagnosis for each disorder.

Every paradise has its serpent and poisoned apple. Every treatment has its unwanted side effects. Thus, the DSM system also has certain problems and disadvantages.

The increased precision sometimes gives clinicians and researchers a false sense of certainty about what they are doing. The DSM criteria are simple provisional agreements, arrived at by a group of experts, on what characteristic features must be present to make a diagnosis. Although the criteria are based on data whenever possible, the available data are often inadequate for building the criteria totally on a scientific database. Thus, the selection of signs and symptoms is often relatively arbitrary. The diagnoses themselves are certainly arbitrary. They will remain arbitrary as long as we are ignorant about pathophysiology and etiology. Medical students and residents often crave certainty (as do many physicians long out of training), and so they want very much to believe that a given DSM diagnosis refers to some "real thing." Thus, the DSM system sometimes leads clinicians to lapse into petty and pointless debates about whether a patient "really" is depressed if he or she does or does not meet the DSM criteria. The criteria should be seen for what they are: useful tools that introduce structure but are arbitrary in essence. They should be applied with a healthy sense of skepticism.

The DSM system may sacrifice validity for reliability. *Reliability* refers to the capacity of individuals to agree on what they see, whereas *validity* refers to the capacity to make useful predictions. In particular, the validity of a medical diagnostic system refers to its ability to predict prognosis and outcome, response to treatment, and ultimately etiology. Put simply, reliability refers to whether something can be measured precisely, whereas validity refers to whether it is worth measuring at all. Psychodynamically oriented clinicians have objected that the DSM system has sacrificed some of psychiatry's most clinically important concepts because psychodynamic explanations and descriptions are generally excluded from DSM. Biologically oriented psychiatrists have objected to the lack of validity in DSM as well. In this instance, they point to the arbitrary nature of the definitions, which are not rooted in information about biological causes.

The DSM system may encourage clinicians to treat diagnosis as no more than a checklist and forget about the patient as a person. When psychiatry was primarily psychodynamically oriented, psychiatrists viewed establishing rapport with the patient as a major goal, and they spent a great deal of time becoming familiar with the personal life history of each patient. DSM-IV-TR can be used to streamline clinical interviews because it encourages the use of a checklist of symptoms in making a diagnosis. There is nothing wrong with the checklist approach, but the initial diagnostic interview should include many more aspects of the patient's life as well. The psychodynamic approach was correct in emphasizing the importance of rapport and knowing the patient as a unique person. The opportunity to establish a close doctor-patient relationship, based on asking about many facets of a person's life, makes psychiatry a particularly interesting and enjoyable specialty in medicine—at least for those physicians who are genuinely interested in having a caring and human relationship with their patients.

Overview of DSM Nosology

As Table 2–1 indicates, the various psychiatric diagnoses are divided among a substantial number of main categories or headings. A more detailed description of the various diagnoses under these headings appears in Sections 2 and 3 of this book.

   Disorders usually first diagnosed in infancy, childhood, or adolescence include a large variety of conditions that typically begin before adulthood. They include developmental disorders such as mental retardation and a variety of specific learning, motor skills, and communication disabilities. They also include pervasive developmental disorders such as autism and other related conditions. The attention-deficit and disruptive behavior disorders include some of the most common conditions seen in children, such as attention-deficit/hyperactivity disorder and conduct disorders. The category also includes disorders involving motor activity that occur in children (e.g.,

Tourette's disorder and other tic syndromes) and disorders of basic biological processes such as eating and elimination. Some disorders that are often observed in children and adolescents, such as depression or schizophrenia, are not classified here because the preponderance of individuals with these diagnoses are adults, and the clinical syndromes are essentially the same in both children and adults.

Delirium, dementia, and amnestic and other cognitive disorders include the various dementias such as Alzheimer's disease, vascular dementia, Huntington's disease, and Creutzfeldt-Jakob disease. This category also includes delirium, which is subspecified according to its cause (e.g., secondary to a general medical condition or to some type of drug). The common theme in this particular category is that a cause or pathophysiological mechanism usually is clearly recognized. It may be a pathogen such as human immunodeficiency virus (HIV), a drug such as alcohol, or a general medical illness such as myxedema. The disorders in this category also are characterized by abnormalities in higher cortical functions such as memory or abstract thinking.

Substance-related disorders include the various conditions that occur as a consequence of substance use. These syndromes are subdivided into abuse, intoxication, and withdrawal, on the basis of the pattern of use, the acuity of recent dose, and the presence of physiological dependence. The specific type of drug being used or abused also is identified.

Schizophrenia and other psychotic disorders include a group of conditions characterized by the presence of abnormalities in perception (hallucinations) and in inferential thinking (delusions) and other symptoms that reflect difficulties in distinguishing between what is real and what is unreal and that are referred to as *psychotic*. Schizophrenia is a severe psychotic disorder that is among the most common psychiatric disorders. A variety of other psychotic conditions are also classified in this category, such as substance-induced psychosis.

Mood disorders are also among the most common conditions seen in psychiatry. They are divided into two broad groups. The bipolar conditions are characterized by at least one episode of mania (and typically episodes of depression as well), whereas the depressive disorders involve only depression (and therefore are sometimes referred to as unipolar disorders).

Anxiety disorders also include a variety of very common conditions, such as panic disorder, agoraphobia, social phobia, obsessive-compulsive disorder, posttraumatic stress disorder, and generalized anxiety disorder.

Somatoform disorders represent a category in which the patient has a variety of physical complaints for which no specific etiology can be found.

They include conversion disorder (e.g., unexplained paralyses, seizures), hypochondriasis, and somatization disorder (a disorder characterized by multiple somatic complaints and sometimes referred to as Briquet's syndrome).

Factitious disorders are feigned disorders in which the patient produces the symptoms intentionally; either physical or psychological symptoms may be feigned.

Dissociative disorders are a group of conditions that are relatively uncommon, although they have been diagnosed with increasing frequency during recent years. They include dissociative identity disorder (formerly called multiple personality disorder), dissociative fugue, dissociative amnesia, and depersonalization disorder. The essential feature of these disorders is a disturbance in identity, memory, or consciousness that cannot be explained on a physical basis.

Sexual and gender identity disorders include conditions often referred to as sexual deviations (paraphilias), such as exhibitionism, pedophilia, sexual masochism, and sexual sadism. They also include specific sexual dysfunctions, such as difficulty in achieving erection or orgasm, premature ejaculation, and dyspareunia. Gender identity disorder, formerly referred to as transsexualism, is also included.

Eating disorders include anorexia nervosa and bulimia nervosa. Patients with anorexia nervosa have a pathological desire to be excessively thin and develop a syndrome characterized by weight loss and emaciation. Those with bulimia nervosa maintain normal weight but use vomiting as a way to control the effects of binge-eating behavior.

Sleep disorders are divided into dyssomnias and parasomnias. The dyssomnias are disorders of initiating or maintaining sleep, such as insomnia and hypersomnia. The parasomnias include more "psychological" conditions, such as nightmares, sleep terrors, and sleepwalking. These conditions are particularly common in children but are grouped with the sleep disorders to maintain consistency.

Impulse-control disorders include a variety of conditions involving poor impulse control, such as kleptomania, pathological gambling, and pyromania.

Adjustment disorders include a group of disorders involving a painful or maladaptive reaction to some specific stress, such as divorce, marital discord, or loss of a job. The adjustment disorders are further subdivided according to the patient's symptoms, such as anxiety, depression, or physical complaints.

Personality disorders refer to conditions in which the personality traits become maladaptive. The personality disorders are divided into three clusters. Cluster A consists of personality disorders that are symptomatically (and perhaps etiologically) related to psychotic disorders, such as paranoid, schizoid, and schizotypal personality disorders. Cluster B includes personality disorders sometimes referred to as "acting out." People with these personality disorders are often somewhat difficult to deal with because they are erratic, unpredictable, overemotional, and self-centered. They include antisocial, borderline, histrionic, and narcissistic personality disorders. Cluster C consists of personality disorders characterized by fearfulness and anxiety. They include avoidant, dependent, and obsessive-compulsive personality disorders.

The Multiaxial System

The DSM classification system is multiaxial. The term *multiaxial* refers to a system that characterizes patients in multiple ways so that the clinician is encouraged to evaluate all aspects of the patient's health and social background. The five axes used to code patient characteristics are summarized in Table 2–2.

TABLE 2–2. Multiaxial system of DSM-IV and DSM-IV-TR

Axis I	Clinical disorders
	Other conditions that may be a focus of clinical attention
Axis II	Personality disorders
	Mental retardation
Axis III	General medical conditions
Axis IV	Psychosocial and environmental problems
Axis V	Global assessment of functioning

Axis I is used to indicate the major syndromes, such as schizophrenia, bipolar disorder, and panic disorder. If several diagnoses are present, all can be noted.

Axis II is used to code disorders that arise relatively early in life and persist; specifically, mental retardation and personality disorders are coded on this axis. This is seen as a way of calling the clinician's attention to these conditions, which are often ignored (particularly the personality disorders). Patients may of course have both Axis I and Axis II diagnoses (e.g., major depressive disorder and borderline personality disorder).

Axis III is used to code the various medical conditions the patient has (e.g., hypertension, diabetes, thyroid disease) that may be relevant to his or her care. Axis III is an important component of diagnosis because it calls the clinician's attention to medical conditions that might interact with the patient's various psychiatric disorders. It also alerts the clinician that the patient might be taking medications to treat these conditions that could interact with any psychoactive drugs prescribed.

Axis IV codes the various psychosocial and environmental problems that may interact with the patient's psychiatric and general medical illnesses. Whenever possible, the clinician notes the specific stressor and codes its level of severity. Axis IV serves to alert the clinician to any personal factors that might be relevant to the patient's diagnosis (e.g., the exacerbation of depression produced by living with an alcoholic spouse) or that raise problems in care and management (e.g., homelessness). The coding for the severity of psychosocial and environmental problems, along with some typical examples that serve as anchor points, is summarized in Table 2–3.

TABLE 2–3. DSM-IV-TR severity of psychosocial stressors scale

		Examples of stressors	
Code	Term	Acute events	Enduring circumstances
1	None	No acute events that may be relevant to the disorder	No enduring circumstances that may be relevant to the disorder
2	Mild	Broke up with boyfriend or girlfriend; started or graduated from school	Family arguments; job dissatisfaction; residence in high-crime neighborhood
3	Moderate	Marriage; marital separation; loss of job; retirement; miscarriage	Marital discord; serious financial problems; trouble with boss; being a single parent
4	Severe	Divorce; birth of first child	Unemployment; poverty
5	Extreme	Death of spouse; serious physical illness diagnosed; victim of rape	Serious chronic illness in self or child; ongoing physical or sexual abuse
6	Catastrophic	Death of child; suicide of spouse; devastating natural disaster	Captivity as hostage; concentration camp experience
0	Inadequate information, or no change in condition		

TABLE 2–4. DSM-IV Global Assessment of Functioning (GAF) Scale

Consider psychological, social, and occupational functioning on a hypothetical continuum of mental health–illness. Do not include impairment in functioning due to physical (or environmental) limitations.

Code (Note: Use intermediate codes when appropriate, e.g., 45, 68, 72.)

100 Superior functioning in a wide range of activities, life's problems never seem to get out of hand,
| is sought out by others because of his or her many positive qualities. No symptoms.
91

90 Absent or minimal symptoms (e.g., mild anxiety before an exam), good functioning in all areas,
| interested and involved in a wide range of activities, socially effective, generally satisfied with
81 life, no more than everyday problems or concerns (e.g., an occasional argument with family members).

80 If symptoms are present, they are transient and expectable reactions to psychosocial stressors
| (e.g., difficulty concentrating after family argument); no more than slight impairment in social,
71 occupational, or school functioning (e.g., temporarily falling behind in schoolwork).

70 Some mild symptoms (e.g., depressed mood and mild insomnia) OR some difficulty in social,
| occupational, or school functioning (e.g., occasional truancy, or theft within the household),
61 but generally functioning pretty well, has some meaningful interpersonal relationships.

60 Moderate symptoms (e.g., flat affect and circumstantial speech, occasional panic attacks) OR
| moderate difficulty in social, occupational, or school functioning (e.g., few friends, conflicts
51 with peers or co-workers).

50 Serious symptoms (e.g., suicidal ideation, severe obsessional rituals, frequent shoplifting) OR
| any serious impairment in social, occupational, or school functioning (e.g., no friends, unable
41 to keep a job).

40 Some impairment in reality testing or communication (e.g., speech is at times illogical, obscure,
| or irrelevant) OR major impairment in several areas, such as work or school, family relations,
31 judgment, thinking, or mood (e.g., depressed man avoids friends, neglects family, and is unable to work; child frequently beats up younger children, is defiant at home, and is failing at school)

30 Behavior is considerably influenced by delusions or hallucinations OR serious impairment in
| communication or judgment (e.g., sometimes incoherent, acts grossly inappropriately, suicidal
21 preoccupation) OR inability to function in almost all areas (e.g., stays in bed all day; no job, home, or friends)

20 Some danger of hurting self or others (e.g., suicide attempts without clear expectation of death;
| frequently violent; manic excitement) OR occasionally fails to maintain minimal personal
11 hygiene (e.g., smears feces) OR gross impairment in communication (e.g., largely incoherent or mute).

10 Persistent danger of severely hurting self or others (e.g., recurrent violence) OR persistent
| inability to maintain minimal personal hygiene OR serious suicidal act with clear expectation
1 of death.

0 Inadequate information.

The rating of overall psychological functioning on a scale of 0–100 was operationalized by Luborsky in the Health-Sickness Rating Scale (Luborsky L: "Clinicians' Judgments of Mental Health." *Archives of General Psychiatry* 7:407–417, 1962). Spitzer and colleagues developed a revision of the Health-Sickness Rating Scale called the Global Assessment Scale (GAS) (Endicott J, Spitzer RL, Fleiss JL, Cohen J: "The Global Assessment Scale: A Procedure for Measuring Overall Severity of Psychiatric Disturbance." *Archives of General Psychiatry* 33:766–771, 1976). A modified version of the GAS was included in DSM-III-R as the Global Assessment of Functioning (GAF) Scale.

Axis V provides a global assessment of the overall level of functioning and psychological health of the patient. It includes various indices of social, psychological, and occupational functioning. These are coded on the Global Assessment of Functioning (GAF) Scale, which ranges from 1 to 90, with 90 representing absent or minimal symptoms. The GAF Scale is summarized in Table 2–4. (The use of this scale provides the clinician with some indication of the patient's overall prognosis, because high-functioning individuals typically have a better outcome.)

How to Become Familiar With the DSM System

The DSM system is obviously large and complex. Beginning clinicians should not attempt to master everything at once. Rather, they should focus on the major and common conditions that are frequently seen either in psychiatric practice or in primary care settings. They should become very familiar with the diagnostic criteria for a few common conditions, such as schizophrenia, major depression, dementia, anxiety disorders, and personality disorders. A few sets of symptom criteria (e.g., major depression) should be committed to memory, simply because they are used so often in so many different clinical settings. The system is too vast to commit all of it to memory, however, and so the clinician should not feel concerned about the need to refer back to the criteria frequently when evaluating patients' symptoms and making diagnoses.

Bibliography

American Psychiatric Association: Diagnostic and Statistical Manual: Mental Disorders. Washington, DC, American Psychiatric Association, 1952

American Psychiatric Association: Diagnostic and Statistical Manual of Mental Disorders, 2nd Edition. Washington, DC, American Psychiatric Association, 1968

American Psychiatric Association: Diagnostic and Statistical Manual of Mental Disorders, 3rd Edition. Washington, DC, American Psychiatric Association, 1980

American Psychiatric Association: Diagnostic and Statistical Manual of Mental Disorders, 4th Edition. Washington, DC, American Psychiatric Association, 1994

American Psychiatric Association: Diagnostic and Statistical Manual of Mental Disorders, 4th Edition, Text Revision. Washington, DC, American Psychiatric Association, 2000

Feighner JP, Robins E, Guze SB, et al: Diagnostic criteria for use in psychiatric research. Arch Gen Psychiatry 26:57–63, 1972

Feinstein AR: ICD, POR, and DRGs: unsolved scientific problems in the nosology of clinical medicine. Arch Intern Med 148:2269–2274, 1988

Kendler KS: Toward a scientific psychiatric nosology: strengths and limitations. Arch Gen Psychiatry 47:969–973, 1990

King LS: Medical Thinking: A Historical Preface. Princeton, NJ, Princeton University Press, 1982

Pincus HA, Frances A, Davis WW, et al: DSM-IV and new diagnostic categories: holding the line on proliferation. Am J Psychiatry 149:112–117, 1992

Robins E, Guze SB: Establishment of diagnostic validity in psychiatric diagnosis: its application to schizophrenia. Am J Psychiatry 126:983–987, 1970

Spitzer RL, Endicott J, Robins E: Research diagnostic criteria: rationale and reliability. Arch Gen Psychiatry 35:773–782, 1978

Spitzer RL, Williams JBW, Skodol AE: DSM-III: the major achievements and an overview. Am J Psychiatry 137:151–164, 1980

Widiger TA, Frances AJ, Pincus HA, et al: DSM-IV Sourcebook, Vols 1–4. Washington, DC, American Psychiatric Association, 1994

Wilson M: DSM-III and the transformation of American psychiatry—a history. Am J Psychiatry 150:399–410, 1993

Wing JK, Cooper JE, Sartorius N: The Measurement and Classification of Psychiatric Symptoms. Cambridge, MA, Cambridge University Press, 1974

World Health Organization: International Statistical Classification of Diseases and Related Health Problems, 10th Revision. Geneva, Switzerland, World Health Organization, 1992

Self-Assessment Questions

1. What is the overall purpose of diagnosis and classification in medicine generally? Give several examples of diseases for which this purpose has been achieved. Describe the extent to which it has been achieved in psychiatry.
2. Describe some of the specific purposes of psychiatric diagnosis.
3. Describe some of the changes introduced by DSM-III.
4. Define the concepts of reliability and validity.
5. Describe the advantages of the DSM approach. What are some of its disadvantages?
6. What is meant by the term *multiaxial?* List the five axes that are included in DSM-IV-TR.

3 Interviewing and Assessment

Festina lente.
Make haste slowly.

A Latin proverb

Because so much of psychiatric diagnosis depends at present on clinical history, the ability to interview and to take an accurate history is one of the most fundamental skills in psychiatry. Demands placed on the interviewer will vary, depending on the type of illness the patient has and its severity. Patients with milder syndromes, such as anxiety disorders or personality disorders, are usually more capable of describing their symptoms and history clearly and articulately. The severely ill depressed, manic, or psychotic patient presents a real challenge. These patients may speak in a disorganized manner, be very distractible, be uninterested or uncooperative, or even be mute. Clinicians may have to depend on informants, such as family members or friends, in addition to the patient.

Interviewing Techniques

Although the demands of the interview may vary depending on the patient and his or her illness, some techniques are common to most interviewing situations.

Establish rapport as early in the interview as possible. It is often best to begin by asking the patient about himself or herself—what kind of work he or she does, where he or she goes to school, what he or she is studying, how old he or she is, whether he or she is married or single, and what kinds of things he or she does for fun. Questions about these topics should not be asked in a manner that seems to "grill" the patient, but rather in a way that indicates that the interviewer is genuinely interested in getting to know the patient. The overall tone of the opening of the interview should, therefore, convey warmth and friendliness. After rapport has been established, the interviewer should then inquire about what kind of problem the patient has been having, what brought him or her to the clinic, or why he or she came into the hospital.

Determine the patient's chief complaint. Sometimes this complaint will be helpful and explicit (e.g., "I've been feeling very depressed," or "I've been having a pain in my head that other doctors can't explain"). At other times, the chief complaint may be relatively vague and require several follow-up questions (e.g., "I don't know why I'm here—my family brought me," or "I've been having trouble at work"). When the replies are not particularly explicit, the interviewer will need to follow up his or her initial questions with others that will help determine the nature of the patient's problem (e.g., "What kinds of things have been bothering your family?" "What kind of trouble at work?"). The initial portion of the interview, devoted to eliciting the chief complaint, should take as long as is necessary to determine the patient's primary problem. When the patient is a clear, logical informant, he or she should tell his or her story as freely as possible without interruption. When he or she is a relatively poor informant, the interviewer will need to be active and directive.

Use the chief complaint to develop a provisional differential diagnosis. As in the rest of medicine, once the patient's primary problem has been determined, the interviewer begins to construct in his or her mind a range of explanations as to the specific diagnosis that might lead to that particular problem. For example, if the patient indicates that he or she has been hearing voices, the differential diagnosis includes a variety of disorders that produce this type of psychotic symptom, such as schizophrenia, schizophreniform disorder, psychotic mania, substance abuse involving hallucinogens, and alcoholic hallucinosis. Being able to develop a differential diagnosis, of course, requires some knowledge of the various types of psychiatric disorders and their characteristic symptoms. As in the rest of medicine, skill in making a differential diagnosis increases with knowledge and experience. Overall, however, it may be comforting to realize that the fundamental process of interviewing and diagnosing is the same in psychiatry as it is in internal medicine or neurology.

Rule the various diagnostic possibilities out or in by using more focused and detailed questions. The existence of DSM-IV-TR is particularly helpful in this regard. If the patient's chief complaint has suggested three or four different possible diagnoses, the interviewer can determine which is most relevant by referring to the diagnostic criteria for those disorders. Thus, the interviewer determines what additional symptoms are present besides those already enumerated when the chief complaint was elicited. The interviewer inquires about the course and onset of the symptoms and about the existence of physical or psychological precipitants such as drugs, alcohol, or personal losses.

Follow up vague or obscure replies with enough persistence to accurately determine the answer to the question. Some patients, particularly psychotic patients, have great difficulty answering questions clearly and concisely. They may say "yes" or "no" to every question asked. When a pattern of this sort is observed, the patient should be repeatedly asked to describe his or her experiences as explicitly as possible. For example, if the patient says that he or she hears voices, he or she should be asked to describe them in more detail—whether they are male or female, what they say, and how often they occur. The greater the level of detail the patient is able to provide, the more confident the clinician can feel that the symptom is truly present. Because making a diagnosis of schizophrenia or other major psychiatric disorder has important prognostic implications, the clinician should not hastily accept an answer that suggests vaguely that the patient may have a particular symptom of a disorder.

Let the patient talk freely enough to observe how tightly his or her thoughts are connected. Most patients should be allowed to talk for at least 3 or 4 minutes without interruption in the course of any psychiatric interview. The very laconic patient, of course, will not be able to do this, but most can. The coherence of the pattern in which the patient's thoughts are presented may provide major clues to the type of problem that he or she is experiencing. For example, patients with mania, schizophrenia, and depression may have any one of a variety of types of "formal thought disorder" (see section "Definitions of Common Signs and Symptoms and Methods for Eliciting Them" later in this chapter). Coherence of thought also may be helpful in making a differential diagnosis between dementia and depression.

Use a mixture of open and closed questions. Interviewers can learn a great deal about patients by mixing up their types of questions, just as a good pitcher mixes up his pitches. Open-ended questions permit the patient to ramble and become disorganized, whereas closed questions determine whether the patient can come up with the specifics when pressed. These are important indicators as to whether the patient is conceptually disorganized or confused, whether he or she is being evasive, or whether he or she is answering randomly or falsely. The content of the questions should be mixed as well. For example, at some point in the interview, the interviewer will probably want to drop his or her objective style of interviewing and focus on some personal topic that is affect-laden, such as sexual or interpersonal relationships. These questions will give the interviewer important clues about the patient's capacity to show emotional responsiveness. Evaluating the patient's mood and affect is a fundamental aspect of the psychiatric evaluation, just as is evaluating the coherence of his or her thinking and communication.

Do not be afraid to ask about topics that you or the patient might find difficult or embarrassing. Beginning interviewers sometimes find it difficult to ask about topics such as sexual relationships, sexual experiences, or even use of alcohol or drugs. Yet all this information is part of a complete psychiatric interview and must be included. Nearly all patients expect doctors to ask these questions and are not offended. Likewise, beginning interviewers are sometimes embarrassed to ask about symptoms of psychosis, such as hearing voices. To the interviewer, these symptoms seem so "crazy" that the patient might be insulted by being asked about them. Again, however, information of this type is basic and cannot be avoided. If John Hinckley Jr.'s psychiatrist had been more aggressive in inquiring about delusions, a diagnosis of schizophrenia might have been made before the assassination attempt on President Reagan occurred, and a great deal of misery could thereby have been avoided. If the patient seems "obviously" not psychotic, questions about psychotic symptoms still should be asked—and in an unapologetic manner. If the patient seems amused or annoyed, then the interviewer can explain that he or she must cover all kinds of questions to provide a comprehensive evaluation of each patient.

Do not forget to ask about suicidal thoughts. This is another topic that may seem to fall into the "embarrassing" category. Nevertheless, suicide is a common outcome of many psychiatric illnesses, and it is incumbent on the interviewer to ask about it. The subject can be broached quite tactfully by a question such as "Have you ever felt life isn't worth living?" The topic of suicide can then be approached gradually, leading to questions such as "Have you ever thought about taking your life?" Further tips on interviewing the suicidal patient are provided in Chapter 21.

Give the patient a chance to ask questions at the end. From the patient's point of view, there is nothing more frustrating than being interviewed for an hour and then ushered out of the office or examining room with his or her own questions unanswered. The questions that patients ask often tell a great deal about what is on their mind (or not on their mind). Thus, these questions may be quite helpful in the differential diagnostic process. Even if not helpful, they are significant to the patient and therefore intrinsically important.

Conclude the initial interview by conveying a sense of confidence and, if possible, of hope. Thank the patient for providing so much information. Compliment him or her, in whatever way it can be done sincerely, on having told his or her story well. Indicate that you now have a much better understanding of his or her problems, and conclude by stating that you will do what you can to help him or her. If you already have a relatively good idea that his or her problem is one that is amenable to treatment, explain that to the patient. At the end of the initial interview, if you are uncertain about diagnosis or treatment, indicate that you have learned a great deal but that you need to think about the problem some more and perhaps gather more information before arriving at a recommendation.

Components of a Psychiatric Interview and Assessment

An initial psychiatric evaluation serves several purposes. One is to formulate an impression as to the patient's diagnosis or differential diagnosis and to begin to generate a treatment plan. The second purpose is to produce a written document for the patient's record that contains information organized in a standard, readable, and easily interpretable way. The initial interview is often therapeutic as well, in that it permits the clinician to establish a relationship with the patient and to reassure him or her that help will be provided.

The outline of that written record is summarized in Table 3–1. As the table indicates, a standard psychiatric evaluation is very similar to the eval-

TABLE 3–1.   Outline of the psychiatric evaluation

Identification of patient and informants

Chief complaint

History of present illness

Past history

Family history

Social history

General medical history

Mental status examination

General physical examination

Neurological examination

Diagnostic impression

Treatment and management plan

uations used in the rest of medicine, with some minor modifications. The content of the present illness and past history is focused primarily on psychiatric symptoms, and the family history includes more information about psychiatric illnesses in the family. Family history and social history also include more sociodemographic and personal information than is recorded in the standard medical history. The mental status examination is typically included only in psychiatric and neurological evaluations.

Identification of Patient and Informants

Identify the patient by stating his or her age, handedness, race, gender, marital status, and occupational status. Indicate whether the patient was the sole informant or whether additional history was obtained from family members or previous psychiatric records. Indicate whether the patient was self-referred, was brought in at the request of family members, or was referred by a physician; if the latter two, specify which family members or physician. In addition, indicate how reliable the informant appears to be.

Chief Complaint

Begin by stating the patient's chief complaint in his or her own words. An additional sentence or two of amplifying information also may be provided, particularly if the patient's chief complaint is relatively vague.

History of Present Illness

Provide a concise history of the illness or problem that brought the patient in for treatment. Begin by describing the onset of the symptoms. If this is the patient's first episode, first psychiatric evaluation, or first hospital admission, that should be stated early in the history of the present illness. Indicate how long ago the first symptoms began, the nature of their onset (e.g., acute, insidious), and whether the onset was precipitated by any particular life events or problems. If the latter, these events or problems should be described in some detail. Likewise, medical conditions that may have served as precipitants should be described. If drug or alcohol abuse was a potential precipitant, that also should be noted.

The evolution of the patient's various symptoms should be described. A systematic summary of all symptoms present, in a form useful for making a differential diagnosis of the present illness, should be provided. This listing of symptoms should reflect the criteria included in DSM-IV-TR and should specify both which symptoms are present and which symptoms are absent. The description of symptoms should not be limited to those included in the DSM-IV-TR diagnostic criteria, however, because these typically do not provide a full description of the range of symptoms that patients have (i.e., they are minimal, not comprehensively descriptive). The description of the present illness also should indicate the degree of incapacity that the patient is experiencing as a consequence of his or her symptoms, as well as the influence of the symptoms on his or her personal and family life. Any treatments the patient has received for the present illness should be noted, including dosages, duration of treatment, and effectiveness of the specific medications because these will often dictate the next step.

Past History

The past history has two main components: history of psychiatric illness and personal history.

History of psychiatric illness provides a summary of past illnesses, problems, and their treatment. In patients with complex histories and chronic psychiatric illnesses, this portion of the history will be quite extensive. It should begin by noting the number of past hospitalizations or episodes and the age at which the patient was first seen for psychiatric evaluation. Thereafter, past episodes should be described in chronological order, with some information about duration of episodes, types of symptoms present, severity of symptoms, and treatments received (and response to treatment). If a characteristic pattern is present (e.g., episodes of mania are always followed by episodes of depression, or past depressive episodes have consistently responded to a particular medication), this pattern should be noted because it provides useful prognostic information. If the patient's memory for past symptoms is relatively poor, this should also be noted. If the bulk of the past history is obtained from old records rather than from the patient himself or herself, this should be recorded. Confirmation by family members of types and patterns of symptoms and number of episodes also should be noted.

Personal history provides a concise narrative description of the patient's life history. It includes information about where the patient was born, where he or she grew up, and the nature of his or her early life adjustment. Any problems during childhood, such as temper tantrums, school phobia, or delinquency, should be noted. The patient's relationships with his or her parents and siblings should be described. Psychosexual development, such as age at first sexual experience, also should be described. Information about familial religious or cultural attitudes that is relevant to the patient's condition should be noted. Educational history should be summarized, including information about how many years of school the patient completed, how well he or she performed, and what his or her academic interests were. Some description should be provided of his or her interest and participation in extracurricular activities and his or her interpersonal relationships during adolescence and early adulthood. Work history and military history also should be summarized. Certain areas may need more emphasis and detail, depending on the chief complaint and diagnostic formulation.

Family History

The age and occupation of both parents and all siblings should be noted, as should the age and education or occupation of all children (if applicable). If any of these first-degree relatives has a history of any mental illness, the specific illness should be mentioned, along with information about treatment, hospitalization, and long-term course and outcome. It may be necessary to describe specific disorders because many patients will not recognize alcoholism or criminality, for example, as emotional problems: "Do any blood relatives have a history of alcoholism, criminality, drug abuse, severe depression, or suicide attempts or suicide? Have any ever had psychiatric hospitalization or institutionalization? Have any ever taken 'nerve pills' or seen psychiatrists, psychologists, or counselors?" The interviewer should obtain as much information as possible about mental illness in second-degree relatives as well. Any relevant information about the family's social, cultural, or educational background also may be included in this section of the interview. It is often helpful to draw pedigrees in complicated cases.

Social History

The social history section contains a summary of the patient's current social situation. It summarizes marital status, occupation, and income. The location of his or her residence should be described, as well as the specific family members who live with the patient. This section of the history should provide information about the various social supports currently available to the patient. Habits (e.g., smoking, use of alcohol) should be recorded as well.

General Medical History

The patient's current and past state of health should be summarized. Any existing illness for which the patient is currently receiving treatment should be noted, as well as the types of treatments, medications, and their doses. Allergies, past surgeries, traumatic injuries, or other serious medical illnesses should be summarized. Head injuries, headaches, seizures, and other problems involving the central nervous system are particularly relevant.

Mental Status Examination

The mental status examination is the psychiatric equivalent of the physical examination in medicine. It includes a comprehensive evaluation of the patient's appearance, thinking and speech patterns, and so forth. It is described in more detail below.

The components of the mental status examination are summarized in Table 3–2. Some portions of the mental status examination are determined simply by observing the patient (e.g., appearance, affect). Others are determined by asking the patient relatively specific questions (e.g., mood, abnormalities in perception). Still others are assessed by asking the patient a specified set of questions (e.g., memory, general information). The interviewer should develop his or her own repertoire of techniques to assess functions such as memory, general information, and calculation. He or she should consistently use this same repertoire for all patients so that he or she develops a good sense of the range of normal and abnormal responses in individuals of various ages, educational levels, and psychopathological states.

Appearance and Attitude

Describe the patient's general appearance, including grooming, hygiene, and facial expression. Note whether the patient looks his or her stated age, younger, or older. Note type and appropriateness of dress. Describe whether the patient's attitude is cooperative, guarded, angry, or suspicious.

TABLE 3–2.   Outline of the mental status examination

Appearance and attitude

Motor activity

Thought and speech

Mood and affect

Perception

Orientation

Memory

General information

Calculations

Capacity to read and write

Visuospatial ability

Attention

Abstraction

Judgment and insight

Motor Activity

Note the patient's level of motor activity. Does he or she sit quietly, or is he or she physically agitated? Note any abnormal movements, tics, or manner-isms. If relevant, evaluate for and note any indications of catatonia, such as waxy flexibility (see below). Determine whether any indications of tardive dyskinesia or any other abnormal movements are present.

Thought and Speech

Psychiatrists often speak about "thought disorder" or "formal thought dis-order." This concept refers to the patient's pattern of speech, from which ab-normal patterns of thought are inferred. It is, of course, not possible to evaluate thought directly. Note the rate of the patient's speech—whether it is normal, slowed, or pressured. Indicate whether his or her speech indicates a pattern of thought that is logical and goal oriented or whether any of a va-riety of abnormalities in form of thought is present (e.g., derailment, inco-herence, poverty of content of speech). Summarize the content of the thought, noting in particular any delusional thinking that is currently ob-served. Any delusions should be described in detail. (If this has already been done in the history of the present illness, that can be noted with a simple statement such as "Delusions were present as described above.")

Mood and Affect

The term *mood* refers to an emotional attitude that is relatively sustained; it is typically determined through the patient's own self-report, although some inferences can be made from the patient's facial expression. Note whether the patient's mood is neutral, euphoric, depressed, anxious, or irritable.

Affect is inferred from emotional responses that are usually triggered by some stimulus. Affect refers to the way that a patient conveys his or her emotional state, as perceived by others. The examiner watches the response of the patient's face to a joke or a smile, determines whether the patient shows appropriate or inappropriate emotional reactions, and notes the degree of reactivity of emotion. Affect is typically described as full, flat, blunted, or inappropriate. Flat or blunted affect is inferred when the patient shows very little emotional response and seems emotionally dulled, whereas inappropriate affect refers to emotional responses that are not appropriate to the content of the discussion, such as silly laughter for no apparent reason.

Perception

Note any abnormalities in perception. The most common perceptual abnormalities are hallucinations: abnormal sensory perceptions in the absence of an actual stimulus. Hallucinations may be auditory, visual, tactile, or olfactory. Sometimes hypnagogic or hypnopompic hallucinations occur when the patient is falling asleep or waking from sleep; these are not considered true hallucinations.

Orientation

Describe the patient's level of orientation. Normally, this includes orientation to time, place, and person. Orientation is assessed by asking the patient to describe the day, date, year, time, place where he or she is currently residing, and his or her name and identity.

Memory

Memory is divided into very short term, short term, and long term. All three types should be described. Very-short-term memory involves the immediate registration of information, which is usually assessed by having the patient repeat back immediately a series of digits or three pieces of information (e.g., the color green, the name Mr. Williams, and the address 1915 High Street). The examiner determines whether the patient can recall these items immediately after he or she is told them. If the patient has difficulty, he or she should be given the items repeatedly until he or she is able to register them.

If he or she is unable to register them after three or four trials, this should be noted. The patient should then be warned that he or she will be asked to recall these items in 3–5 minutes. His or her ability to remember them after that time interval is an indication of his or her short-term memory. Long-term memory is assessed by asking the patient to recall events that occurred in the past several days, as well as events that occurred in the more remote past, such as months or years ago.

General Information

General information is assessed by asking the patient a specific set of questions covering topics such as the names of the last five presidents, current events, or information about history or geography. The patient's fund of general information should be noted in relation to his or her level of educational achievement. This is particularly important in assessing the possibility of dementia.

Calculations

The standard test of calculations is serial 7s. This test involves having the patient subtract 7 from 100, then 7 from that product, and so on for at least five subtractions. Some chronic patients become relatively well trained on this exercise, so it is a good idea to have other tools in one's repertoire. One that is quite useful involves asking the patient to make calculations necessary in daily living (e.g., "If I went to the store and bought six oranges, priced at three for a dollar, and gave the clerk a $10 bill, how much change would I get back?"). Calculations can be modified for the patient's educational level. Poorly educated patients may need to calculate serial 3s. Likewise, real-life calculations can be simplified or made more complicated.

Capacity to Read and Write

The patient should be given a simple text and asked to read it aloud. He or she also should be asked to write down a specific sentence, either of the examiner's choice or of his or her own choice. The patient's ability to read and write should be assessed relative to his or her level of education.

Visuospatial Ability

The patient should be asked to copy a figure. This figure can be quite simple, such as a square inside a circle. An alternative task is to ask the patient to draw a clock face and set the hands at some specified time, such as 20 minutes to 3 o'clock.

Attention

Attention is assessed in part by several of the above tasks, such as calculations or clock setting. Additional tests of attention can be used, such as asking the patient to spell a word backward (e.g., world). The patient also can be asked to name five things that start with a specific letter, such as *d*. The latter is also a good test of cognitive and verbal fluency.

Abstraction

The patient's capacity to think abstractly can be assessed in a variety of ways. One favorite method is asking the patient to interpret proverbs, such as "A rolling stone gathers no moss" or "Don't cry over spilt milk." Alternatively, the patient can be asked to identify commonalities between two items (e.g., "How are an apple and an orange alike?", "How are a fly and a tree alike?").

Judgment and Insight

Assess the patient's overall judgment and insight by noting how realistically he or she has assessed his or her illness and his or her various life problems. Insight can be ascertained relatively directly. Does the patient understand that he or she is ill? Does the patient express a need for treatment? Judgment may not be as easily assessed, but the patient's recent choices and decisions will help in its determination. Sometimes simple questions may be helpful. The following are frequently used: "If you found a stamped, addressed envelope, what would you do?" and "If you were in a movie theater and smelled smoke, what would you do?"

General Physical Examination

The general physical examination should follow the standard format used in the rest of medicine, covering organ systems of the body from head to foot. Examinations of patients of the opposite sex (e.g., male physician examining a female patient) should be chaperoned.

Neurological Examination

Likewise, a standard neurological examination should be done. A detailed neurological evaluation is particularly important in psychiatric patients to rule out focal signs that might explain the patient's symptoms.

Diagnostic Impression

The clinician should note his or her diagnostic impression based on all five DSM-IV-TR axes whenever possible. When appropriate, more than one diagnosis should be made. When the diagnosis is uncertain, the qualifier *provisional* should be added. Not infrequently, it is difficult to make a definitive diagnosis at the time of the index evaluation. When this situation occurs, differential diagnostic possibilities should be listed.

Treatment and Management Plan

The treatment and management section will vary, depending on the level of diagnostic certainty. If the diagnosis is quite uncertain, the first step in treatment and management will involve additional assessments to determine the diagnosis with more certainty. Thus, the treatment and management plan may include a list of laboratory tests appropriate to assist in the differential diagnosis listed above. Alternatively, when the diagnosis is straightforward, a specific treatment plan can be outlined, including a proposed medication regimen, plans for vocational rehabilitation, a program for social skills training, marital counseling, or other ancillary treatments appropriate to the patient's specific problems.

Definitions of Common Signs and Symptoms and Methods for Eliciting Them

A vast panoply of signs and symptoms can characterize major mental illnesses. The following are some of the more common signs and symptoms that are seen in relatively severe psychiatric disorders. They include symptoms seen in psychotic states, mood syndromes, and anxiety states. Where appropriate, some suggested questions are provided that can be used to probe for these symptoms. Those in parentheses are follow-up questions.

Symptoms That Frequently Occur in Psychotic Illnesses

The term *psychosis* has several different meanings, which may be especially confusing to beginning students. In the broadest sense, the term refers to the group of symptoms that characterize the most severe mental illnesses, such as schizophrenia or mania, and that involve an impairment in the ability to make judgments about the boundaries between what is real and unreal (sometimes called "an impairment in reality testing"). At a more operational level, psychosis refers to a specific group of symptoms that are common in these severe disorders. In the narrowest sense, psychosis is synonymous with having delusions and hallucinations. A somewhat broader operational definition also includes bizarre behavior, disorganized speech ("positive formal thought disorder"), and inappropriate affect.

Another way to classify some of the major symptoms of severe mental illnesses is to divide them into two broad groups: positive and negative. *Positive symptoms* represent an exaggeration or distortion of functions that are normally present (e.g., perception, inferential thinking). They include delusions, hallucinations, disorganized speech, bizarre or disorganized behavior, and inappropriate affect. The first two are evaluated by questioning and the final three by observation. Sometimes this group of positive symptoms is further subdivided into two dimensions. The *psychotic dimension* includes delusions and hallucinations, whereas the *disorganized dimension* includes disorganized speech and behavior and inappropriate affect. *Negative symptoms* are characterized by a diminution or loss of functions that are normally present, such as fluency of speech or emotional expression. Negative symptoms are common in psychosis but also may occur in nonpsychotic illnesses such as depression. They include alogia, affective blunting, avolition-apathy, anhedonia-asociality, and attentional impairment. The first two of these are evaluated primarily by observation and the last three by interviewing.

Some of the negative symptoms may be difficult to distinguish from the effects of antipsychotic medications used to treat psychotic illnesses. These medications often produce parkinsonian side effects and akinesia, which look quite similar to some of the common negative symptoms such as affective blunting or avolition. Sometimes negative symptoms are also difficult to distinguish from depressive symptoms, particularly anhedonia. It has been suggested that clinicians should attempt to determine whether negative symptoms are *secondary* (i.e., due to antipsychotics or depression) or *primary* (i.e., intrinsic to the illness). As is discussed in the chapter on schizophrenia (Chapter 7), negative symptoms are thought to reflect some type of fundamental neural abnormality occurring in schizophrenia; disentangling primary from secondary negative symptoms could be important in the search for this abnormality. At a practical clinical level, however, this distinction may be difficult to make reliably.

Delusions

Delusions represent an abnormality in content of thought. They are false beliefs that cannot be explained on the basis of the subject's cultural background. Although delusions are sometimes defined as *fixed false beliefs,* in their mildest form delusions may persist for only weeks to months, and the subject may question his or her beliefs or doubt them. The subject's behavior may or may not be influenced by his or her delusions. The assessment of the severity of individual delusions and of the global severity of delusional thinking should take into account their persistence, their complexity, the extent to which the subject acts on them, the extent to which the subject doubts them, and the extent to which the beliefs deviate from those that nonpsychotic people might have.

Persecutory delusions.   People with persecutory delusions believe that they are being conspired against or persecuted in some way. Common manifestations include the belief that one is being followed, that one's mail is being opened, that one's room or office is bugged, that the telephone is tapped, or that police, government officials, neighbors, or fellow workers are harassing the subject. Persecutory delusions are sometimes relatively isolated or fragmented, but sometimes the person has a complex system of delusions involving both a wide range of forms of persecution and a belief that there is a well-designed conspiracy behind them: for example, that the patient's house is bugged and that he or she is being followed because the government wrongly considers him or her a secret agent of a foreign government. This delusion may be so complex that it explains almost everything that happens to him or her.

- *Have you had trouble getting along with people?*
- *Have you felt that people are against you?*
- *Has anyone been trying to harm you in any way?*
- *(Do you think people have been plotting against you?)*

Delusions of jealousy.   The patient believes that his or her mate is having an affair with someone. Miscellaneous bits of information are construed as "evidence." The person usually goes to great effort to prove the existence of the affair, searching for hair in the bedclothes, the odor of shaving lotion or smoke on clothing, or receipts or checks indicating that a gift has been bought for the lover. Elaborate plans are often made to trap the two together.

- *Have you worried that your (husband, wife, boyfriend, girlfriend) might be unfaithful to you?*
- *(What evidence do you have?)*

Delusions of sin or guilt.   The patient believes that he or she has committed some terrible sin or done something unforgivable. Sometimes the patient is excessively or inappropriately preoccupied with things he or she did wrong as a child, such as masturbating. Sometimes the patient feels responsible for causing some disastrous event, such as a fire or an accident, with which he or she in fact has no connection. Sometimes these delusions have a religious flavor, involving the belief that the sin is unpardonable and that the subject will suffer eternal punishment from God. Sometimes the patient simply believes that he or she deserves punishment by society. The patient may spend a good deal of time confessing these sins to whoever will listen.

- *Have you felt that you have done some terrible thing?*
- *Is there anything that's bothering your conscience?*
- *(What is it?)*
- *(Do you feel you deserve to be punished for it?)*

Grandiose delusions. The patient believes that he or she has special powers or abilities. He or she may think that he or she is actually some famous person, such as a rock star, Napoleon, or Christ. He or she may believe he or she is writing some definitive book, composing a great piece of music, or developing some wonderful new invention. The patient is often suspicious that someone is trying to steal his or her ideas, and he or she may become quite irritated if his or her abilities are doubted.

- *Do you have any special powers, talents, or abilities?*
- *Do you feel you are going to achieve great things?*

Religious delusions. The patient is preoccupied with false beliefs of a religious nature. Sometimes these exist within the context of a conventional religious system, such as beliefs about the Second Coming, the Anti-Christ, or possession by the Devil. At other times, they may involve an entirely new religious system or a pastiche of beliefs from a variety of religions, particularly Eastern religions, such as ideas about reincarnation or Nirvana. Religious delusions may be combined with grandiose delusions (if the subject considers himself or herself a religious leader), delusions of guilt, or delusions of being controlled. Religious delusions must be outside the range of beliefs considered normal for the patient's cultural and religious background.

- *Are you a religious person?*
- *(What was your religious training as a child?)*
- *Have you had any unusual religious experiences?*
- *Have you become closer to God?*

Somatic delusions. The patient believes that somehow his or her body is diseased, abnormal, or changed. For example, he or she may believe that his or her stomach or brain is rotting, that his or her hands have become en-

larged, or that his or her facial features are unusual or misshapen (dysmorphophobia). Sometimes somatic delusions are accompanied by tactile or
other hallucinations, and when this occurs, both should be considered to be
present. (For example, a patient believes that he has ball bearings rolling
about in his head, placed there by a dentist who filled his teeth, and can actually hear them clanking against one another.)

- *Is there anything wrong with the way your body is working?*
- *Have you noticed any change in your appearance?*

Ideas and delusions of reference.   The patient believes that insignificant
remarks, statements, or events refer to him or her or have some special
meaning for him or her. For example, the patient walks into a room, sees
people laughing, and suspects that they were just talking about him or her
and laughing at him or her. Sometimes items read in the newspaper, heard
on the radio, or seen on television are considered to be special messages to
the subject. In the case of ideas of reference, the patient is suspicious but recognizes that his or her idea may be erroneous. When the patient actually believes that the statements or events refer to him or her, then this is
considered a delusion of reference.

- *Have you walked into a room and thought that people were talking
  about you or laughing at you?*
- *Have you seen things in magazines or on TV that seem to refer to you
  or contain a special message for you?*
- *Have you received special messages in any other ways?*

Delusions of being controlled.   The patient has a subjective experience
that his or her feelings or actions are controlled by some outside force. The
central requirement for this type of delusion is an actual strong subjective
experience of being controlled. It does not include simple beliefs or ideas,
such as that the subject is acting as an agent of God or that friends or parents
are trying to coerce him or her into something. Rather, the patient must describe, for example, that his or her body has been occupied by some alien
force that is making it move in peculiar ways or that messages are being sent
to his or her brain by radio waves and causing him or her to experience particular feelings that he or she recognizes are not his or her own.

- *Have you felt that you were being controlled by some outside force?*
- *Do you feel that any person or force is controlling you?*
- *(Do you feel like a puppet on a string?)*

Delusions of mind reading.   The patient believes that people can read his or her mind or know his or her thoughts. This is different from thought broadcasting (see below) in that it is a belief without a percept. That is, the patient subjectively experiences and recognizes that others know his or her thoughts, but he or she does not think that they can be heard out loud.

- *Have you had the feeling that people could read your mind or know what you are thinking?*

Thought broadcasting/audible thoughts.   The patient believes that his or her thoughts are broadcast so that he or she or others can hear them. Sometimes the patient experiences his or her thoughts as a voice outside his or her head; this is an auditory hallucination as well as a delusion. Sometimes the subject feels that his or her thoughts are being broadcast, although he or she cannot hear them himself or herself. Sometimes he or she believes that his or her thoughts are picked up by a microphone and broadcast on the radio or television.

- *Have you heard your own thoughts out loud, as if they were a voice outside your head?*
- *Have you felt that your thoughts were broadcast so that other people could hear them?*

Thought insertion.   The patient believes that thoughts that are not his or her own have been inserted into his or her mind. For example, the patient may believe that a neighbor is practicing voodoo and planting alien sexual thoughts into his or her mind. This symptom should not be confused with experiencing unpleasant thoughts that the patient recognizes as his or her own, such as delusions of persecution or guilt.

- *Have you felt that thoughts were being put into your head by some outside force or person?*

Thought withdrawal.   The patient believes that thoughts have been taken away from his or her mind. He or she is able to describe a subjective experience of beginning a thought and then suddenly having it removed by some outside force. This symptom does not include the mere subjective recognition of alogia.

- *Have you felt that your thoughts were taken away by some outside force or person?*

Hallucinations

Hallucinations represent an abnormality in perception. They are false perceptions occurring in the absence of an identifiable external stimulus. They may be experienced in any of the sensory modalities, including hearing, touch, taste, smell, and vision. True hallucinations should be distinguished from illusions (which involve a misperception of an external stimulus), hypnagogic and hypnopompic experiences (which occur when a patient is falling asleep and waking up, respectively), or normal thought processes that are exceptionally vivid. If the hallucinations have a religious quality, then they should be judged within the context of what is normal for the patient's social and cultural background. The patient always should be asked to describe the hallucination in detail. The term *pseudohallucinations* refers to hallucinations that the patient reports but that have no identifiable percept (e.g., the patient "sees things that aren't there" but is unable to describe any actual specific perceptions). Pseudohallucinations are more fully discussed in Chapter 13.

Auditory hallucinations.   The patient has reported voices, noises, or sounds. The most common auditory hallucinations involve hearing voices speaking to the patient or calling his or her name. The voices may be male or female, familiar or unfamiliar, and critical or complimentary. Typically, patients with schizophrenia experience the voices as unpleasant and negative. Hallucinations involving sounds other than voices, such as noises or music, should be considered less characteristic and less severe.

- *Have you heard voices or other sounds when no one is around or when you couldn't account for them?*
- *(What did they say?)*

Voices commenting.   These hallucinations involve hearing a voice that makes a running commentary on the patient's behavior or thought as it occurs.

- *Have you heard voices commenting on what you are thinking or doing?*
- *(What do they say?)*

Voices conversing.   These hallucinations involve hearing two or more voices talking with each other, usually discussing something about the patient.

- *Have you heard two or more voices talking with each other?*
- *(What do they say?)*

Somatic or tactile hallucinations.   These hallucinations involve experiencing peculiar physical sensations in the body. They include burning sensations, tingling, and perceptions that the body has changed in shape or size.

- *Have you had burning sensations or other strange feelings in your body?*
- *(What were they?)*

Olfactory hallucinations.   The patient experiences unusual smells that are typically quite unpleasant. Sometimes the patient may believe that he or she himself or herself smells. This belief should be considered a hallucination if the patient can actually smell the odor himself or herself but should be considered a delusion if he or she believes that only others can smell the odor.

- *Have you experienced any unusual smells or smells that others don't notice?*
- *(What were they?)*

Visual hallucinations.   The patient sees shapes or people that are not actually present. Sometimes these are shapes or colors, but most typically they are figures of people or humanlike objects. They also may be characters of a religious nature, such as the Devil or Christ. As always, visual hallucinations involving religious themes should be judged within the context of the patient's cultural background.

- *Have you had visions or seen things that other people cannot?*
- *(What did you see?)*

Bizarre or Disorganized Behavior

The patient's behavior is unusual, bizarre, or fantastic. The information for this symptom will sometimes come from the patient, sometimes come from other sources, and sometimes come from direct observation. Bizarre behavior due to the immediate effects of intoxication with alcohol or drugs should not be considered a symptom of psychosis. Social and cultural norms must be considered in making the determination of bizarre behavior, and detailed examples should be elicited and noted.

Clothing and appearance. The patient dresses in an unusual manner or does other strange things to alter his or her appearance. For example, he or she may shave off all his or her hair or paint parts of his or her body different colors. His or her clothing may be quite unusual; for example, he or she may choose to wear some outfit that appears generally inappropriate and unacceptable, such as a baseball cap backward with rubber galoshes and long underwear covered by denim overalls. The patient may dress in a fantastic costume representing some historical personage or a person from outer space. He or she may wear clothing completely inappropriate to the climatic conditions, such as heavy wools in summer.

- *Has anyone made comments about the way you look?*
- *(What did they say?)*

Social and sexual behavior. The patient may do things that are considered inappropriate according to usual social norms. For example, he or she may masturbate in public, urinate or defecate in inappropriate receptacles, walk along the street muttering to himself or herself, or begin talking to people whom he or she has never before met about his or her personal life (as when riding on a subway or standing in some public place). He or she may drop to his or her knees praying and shouting or suddenly sit in an unusual position when in the midst of a crowd. He or she may make inappropriate sexual overtures or remarks to strangers.

- *Have you done anything that others might think is unusual or that has called attention to yourself?*
- *(What did you do?)*
- *Has anyone complained or commented about your behavior?*
- *(Why did they complain or comment?)*

Aggressive and agitated behavior. The patient may behave in an aggressive, agitated manner, often quite unpredictably. He or she may start arguments inappropriately with friends or members of his or her family, or he or she may accost strangers on the street and begin haranguing them angrily. He or she may write letters of a threatening or angry nature to government officials or others with whom he or she has some quarrel. Occasionally, patients may perform violent acts such as injuring or tormenting animals or attempting to injure or kill human beings.

- *Have you been unusually angry or irritable with anyone?*
- *(How did you express your anger?)*
- *(Have you done anything to try to harm animals or people?)*

Ritualistic or stereotyped behavior.   The patient may develop a set of repetitive actions or rituals that he or she must perform over and over. Sometimes he or she will attribute some symbolic significance to these actions and believe that they are either influencing others or preventing himself or herself from being influenced. For example, he or she may eat jelly beans every night for dessert, assuming that different consequences will occur, depending on the color of the jelly beans. He or she may have to eat foods in a particular order, wear particular clothes, or get dressed in a certain order. He or she may have to write messages to himself or herself or to others over and over, sometimes in an unusual or occult language.

- *Are there any things that you do over and over?*
- *Are there any things that you have to do in a certain way or in a particular order?*
- *(Why do you do it?)*
- *(Does it have any special meaning or significance?)*

Disorganized Speech (Positive Formal Thought Disorder)

Disorganized speech, which is also referred to as positive formal thought disorder, is fluent speech that tends to communicate poorly for a variety of reasons. The patient tends to skip from topic to topic without warning; to be distracted by events in the nearby environment; to join words together because they are semantically or phonologically alike, even though they make no sense; or to ignore the question asked and answer another. This type of speech may be rapid, and it frequently seems quite disjointed. It has sometimes been referred to as *loose associations*. Unlike alogia (negative formal thought disorder; see subsection "Alogia" later in this chapter), a wealth of detail is provided, and the flow of speech tends to have an energetic rather than an apathetic quality to it.

To evaluate thought disorder, the patient should be permitted to talk without interruption for as long as 5 minutes. The interviewer should observe closely the extent to which the patient's sequencing of ideas is well connected. The interviewer also should pay close attention to how well the patient can reply to various types of questions, ranging from simple ("When were you born?") to more complicated ("Why did you come to the hospital?"). If the ideas seem vague or incomprehensible, the interviewer should prompt the patient to clarify or elaborate.

Derailment (loose associations).   The patient has a pattern of spontaneous speech in which the ideas slip off the track onto another that is clearly but obliquely related or onto one completely unrelated. Things may be said in juxtaposition that lack a meaningful relationship, or the patient may shift idiosyncratically from one frame of reference to another. At times, there may be a vague connection between the ideas, and at other times, none will be apparent. This pattern of speech is often characterized as sounding "disjointed." Perhaps the most common manifestation of this disorder is a slow, steady slippage, with no single derailment being particularly severe, so that the speaker gets farther and farther off the track with each derailment without showing any awareness that his or her reply no longer has any connection with the question that was asked. This abnormality is often characterized by lack of cohesion between clauses and sentences and by unclear pronoun references.

> *Interviewer: Did you enjoy college?*
> *Subject: Um-hm. Oh hey well I, I oh, I really enjoyed some communities. I tried it, and the, and the next day when I'd be going out, you know, um, I took control like uh, I put, um, bleach on my hair in, in California. My roommate was from Chicago and she was going to the junior college. And we lived in the Y.W.C.A., so she wanted to put it, um, peroxide on my hair, and she did, and I got up and I looked at the mirror and tears came to my eyes. Now do you understand it—I was fully aware of what was going on but why couldn't I, I…why the tears? I can't understand that, can you?*

Tangentiality.   The patient replies to a question in an oblique, tangential, or even irrelevant manner. The reply may be related to the question in some distant way, or the reply may be unrelated and seem totally irrelevant.

> *Interviewer: What city are you from?*
> *Subject: Well, that's a hard question to answer because my parents…I was born in Iowa, but I know that I'm white instead of black, so apparently I came from the North somewhere and I don't know where, you know, I really don't know whether I'm Irish or Scandinavian, or I don't, I don't believe I'm Polish, but I think I'm, I think I might be German or Welsh.*

Incoherence (word salad, schizophasia).   The patient has a pattern of speech that is essentially incomprehensible at times. Incoherence is often accompanied by derailment. It differs from derailment in that in incoherence the abnormality occurs within the level of the sentence or clause, which contains words or phrases that are joined incoherently. The abnormality in derailment involves unclear or confusing connections between larger units, such as sentences or clauses. This type of language disorder is relatively rare. When it occurs, it tends to be severe or extreme, and mild forms are quite uncommon. It may sound quite similar to Wernicke's aphasia or jargon aphasia, and in these cases the disorder should only be called incoherence definitively when history and laboratory data exclude the possibility of a past stroke and clinical testing for aphasia has negative results.

> *Interviewer:* What do you think about current political issues like the energy crisis?
>
> *Subject:* They're destroying too many cattle and oil just to make soap. If we need soap when you can jump into a pool of water, and then when you go to buy your gasoline, my folks always thought they should, get pop but the best thing to get, is motor oil, and, money. May, may as, well go there and, trade in some, pop caps and, uh, tires, and tractors to grup, car garages, so they can pull cars away from wrecks, is what I believed in.

Illogicality. The patient has a pattern of speech in which conclusions are reached that do not follow logically. Illogicality may take the form of non sequiturs (meaning "it does not follow"), in which the patient makes a logical inference between two clauses that is unwarranted or illogical. It may take the form of faulty inductive inferences. It may also take the form of reaching conclusions based on faulty premises without any actual delusional thinking.

> *Subject:* Parents are the people that raise you. Anything that raises you can be a parent. Parents can be anything—material, vegetable, or mineral—that has taught you something. Parents would be the world of things that are alive, that are there. Rocks—a person can look at a rock and learn something from it, so that would be a parent.

Circumstantiality. The patient has a pattern of speech that is very indirect and delayed in reaching its goal ideas. In the process of explaining something, the speaker brings in many tedious details and sometimes makes parenthetical remarks. Circumstantial replies or statements may last for many minutes if the speaker is not interrupted and urged to get to the point. Interviewers will often recognize circumstantiality on the basis of needing to interrupt the speaker to complete the process of history taking within an allotted time. When not called circumstantial, these people are often referred to as long-winded.

Although it may coexist with instances of poverty of content of speech or loss of goal, circumstantiality differs from poverty of content of speech in containing excessive amplifying or illustrative detail and from loss of goal in that the goal is eventually reached if the person is allowed to talk long enough. It differs from derailment in that the details presented are closely related to some particular goal or idea and that the particular goal or idea must, by definition, eventually be reached (unless the patient is interrupted by an impatient interviewer).

Pressure of speech.   The patient has an increase in the amount of spontaneous speech as compared with what is considered ordinary or socially customary. The patient talks rapidly and is difficult to interrupt. Some sentences may be left uncompleted because of eagerness to get on to a new idea. Simple questions that could be answered in only a few words or sentences are answered at great length so that the answer takes minutes rather than seconds and indeed may not stop at all if the speaker is not interrupted. Even when interrupted, the speaker often continues to talk. Speech tends to be loud and emphatic. Sometimes speakers with severe pressure will talk without any social stimulation and talk even though no one is listening. When patients are receiving antipsychotics or lithium, their speech is often slowed down by medication, and then it can be judged only on the basis of amount, volume, and social appropriateness. If a quantitative measure is applied to the rate of speech, then a rate greater than 150 words per minute is usually considered rapid or pressured. This disorder may be accompanied by derailment, tangentiality, or incoherence, but it is distinct from them.

Distractible speech.   During the course of a discussion or an interview, the patient stops talking in the middle of a sentence or idea and changes the subject in response to a nearby stimulus, such as an object on a desk, the interviewer's clothing or appearance, and so forth.

> Subject: *Then I left San Francisco and moved to…where did you get that tie? It looks like it's left over from the '50s. I like the warm weather in San Diego. Is that a conch shell on your desk? Have you ever gone scuba diving?*

Clanging.   The patient has a pattern of speech in which sounds rather than meaningful relations appear to govern word choice, so that the intelligibility of the speech is impaired and redundant words are introduced in addition to rhyming relationships. This pattern of speech also may include punning associations, so that a word similar in sound brings in a new thought.

> Subject: *I'm not trying to make a noise. I'm trying to make sense. If you can make sense out of nonsense, well, have fun. I'm trying to make sense out of sense. I'm not making sense [cents] anymore. I have to make dollars.*

Catatonic Motor Behavior

Catatonic motor symptoms are not common and should only be considered present when they are obvious and have been directly observed by the clinician or some other professional.

Stupor. The patient has a marked decrease in reactivity to the environment and reduction of spontaneous movements and activity. The patient may appear to be aware of the nature of his or her surroundings.

Rigidity. The patient shows signs of motor rigidity, such as resistance to passive movement.

Waxy flexibility. The patient maintains postures into which he or she is placed for at least 15 seconds.

Excitement. The patient has apparently purposeless and stereotyped excited motor activity not influenced by external stimuli.

Posturing and mannerisms. The patient voluntarily assumes an inappropriate or a bizarre posture. Manneristic gestures or tics also may be observed. These involve movements or gestures that appear artificial or contrived, are not appropriate to the situation, or are stereotyped and repetitive. (Patients with tardive dyskinesia may have manneristic gestures or tics, but these should not be considered manifestations of catatonia.)

Inappropriate Affect

The patient's affect expressed is inappropriate or incongruous, not simply flat or blunted. Most typically, this manifestation of affective disturbance takes the form of smiling or assuming a silly facial expression while talking about a serious or sad subject. For example, the patient may laugh inappropriately when talking about thoughts of harming another person. (Occasionally, patients may smile or laugh when talking about a serious subject that they find uncomfortable or embarrassing. Although their smiling may seem inappropriate, it is due to anxiety and therefore should not be rated as inappropriate affect.)

Alogia

Alogia is a general term coined to refer to the impoverished thinking and cognition that often occur in patients with schizophrenia (from the Greek *a*, "no"; *logos*, "mind, thought"). Subjects with alogia have thinking processes that seem empty, turgid, or slow. Because thinking cannot be observed directly, it is inferred from the patient's speech. The two major manifestations of alogia are nonfluent empty speech (poverty of speech) and fluent empty speech (poverty of content of speech). Blocking and increased latency of response also may reflect alogia.

Poverty of speech. The patient has a restricted *amount* of spontaneous speech, so that replies to questions tend to be brief, concrete, and unelaborated. Unprompted additional information is rarely provided. Replies may be monosyllabic, and some questions may be left unanswered altogether. When confronted with this speech pattern, the interviewer may find himself or herself frequently prompting the patient to encourage elaboration of replies. To elicit this finding, the examiner must allow the patient adequate time to answer and to elaborate his or her answer.

> *Interviewer: Can you tell me something about what brought you to the hospital?*
> *Subject: A car.*
> *Interviewer: I was wondering about what kinds of problems you've been having. Can you tell me something about them?*
> *Subject: I dunno.*

Poverty of content of speech. Although the patient's replies are long enough so that speech is adequate in amount, it conveys little information. Language tends to be vague, often overabstract or overconcrete, repetitive, and stereotyped. The interviewer may recognize this finding by observing that the patient has spoken at some length but has not given adequate information to answer the question. Alternatively, the patient may provide enough information but require many words to do so, so that a lengthy reply can be summarized in a sentence or two. This abnormality differs from circumstantiality in that the circumstantial patient tends to provide a wealth of detail.

> *Interviewer: Why is it, do you think, that people believe in God?*
> *Subject: Well, first of all because he, uh, he are the person that is their personal savior. He walks with me and talks with me. And uh, the understanding that I have, um, a lot of people, they don't readily, uh, know their own personal self. Because, uh, they ain't, they all, just don't know their personal self. They don't, know that he uh—seemed like to me, a lot of 'em don't understand that he walks and talks with 'em.*

Blocking. The patient's train of speech is interrupted before a thought or an idea has been completed. After a period of silence, which may last from a few seconds to minutes, the person indicates that he or she cannot recall what he or she has been saying or meant to say. Blocking should be judged to be present only if a person voluntarily describes losing his or her thought or if, on questioning by the interviewer, the person indicates that that was his or her reason for pausing.

> *Subject:* So I didn't want to go back to school so I…(1-minute silence while the patient stares blankly).
> *Interviewer:* What about going back to school? What happened?
> *Subject:* I dunno. I forgot what I was going to say.

Increased latency of response.   The patient takes a longer time to reply to questions than is usually considered normal. He or she may seem distant, and sometimes the examiner may wonder whether he or she has heard the question. Prompting usually indicates that the patient is aware of the question but has been having difficulty formulating his or her thoughts to make an appropriate reply.

> *Interviewer:* When were you last in the hospital?
> *Subject:* (30-second pause) A year ago.
> *Interviewer:* Which hospital was it?
> *Subject:* (30-second pause) This one.

Perseveration.   The patient persistently repeats words, ideas, or phrases so that once a patient begins to use a particular word, he or she continually returns to it in the process of speaking. Perseveration differs from "stock words" in that the repeated words are used in ways inappropriate to their usual meaning. Some words or phrases are commonly used as pause-fillers, such as "you know" or "like." These should not be considered perseverations.

> *Interviewer:* Tell me what you are like—what kind of person you are.
> *Subject:* I'm from Marshalltown, Iowa. That's 60 miles northwest, northeast of Des Moines, Iowa. And I'm married at the present time. I'm 36 years old; my wife is 35. She lives in Garwin, Iowa. That's 15 miles southeast of Marshalltown, Iowa. I'm getting a divorce at the present time. And I am at present in a mental institution in Iowa City, Iowa, which is 100 miles southeast of Marshalltown, Iowa.

Affective Flattening or Blunting

Affective flattening or blunting manifests itself as a characteristic impoverishment of emotional expression, reactivity, and feeling. Affective flattening can be evaluated by observation of the patient's behavior and responsiveness during a routine interview. The evaluation of affective expression may be influenced by the patient's use of prescription drugs because the parkinsonian side effects of antipsychotics may lead to masklike facies and diminished associated movements. Other aspects of affect, such as responsivity or appropriateness, will not be affected, however.

Unchanging facial expression.   The patient's face does not change expression, or changes less than normally expected, as the emotional content of the discourse changes. His or her face appears wooden, mechanical, and frozen. Because antipsychotics may partially mimic this effect, the interviewer should be careful to note whether the patient is taking medication.

Decreased spontaneous movements.   The patient sits quietly throughout the interview and shows few or no spontaneous movements. He or she does not shift position, move his or her legs, or move his or her hands or does so less than normally expected.

Paucity of expressive gestures.   The patient does not use his or her body as an aid in expressing his or her ideas through means such as hand gestures, sitting forward in his or her chair when intent on a subject, or leaning back when relaxed. Paucity of expressive gestures may occur in addition to decreased spontaneous movements.

Poor eye contact.   The patient avoids looking at others or using his or her eyes as an aid in expression. He or she appears to be staring into space even when he or she is talking. The interviewer should consider the quality as well as the quantity of eye contact.

Affective nonresponsivity.   The patient fails to smile or laugh when prompted. This function may be tested by smiling or joking in a way that would usually elicit a smile from a psychiatrically normal individual.

Lack of vocal inflections.   While speaking, the patient fails to show normal vocal emphasis patterns. Speech has a monotonic quality, and important words are not emphasized through changes in pitch or volume. The patient also may fail to change volume with changes of content, so that he or she does not drop his or her voice when discussing private topics or raise it as he or she discusses things that are exciting or for which louder speech might be appropriate.

Avolition-Apathy

Avolition-apathy manifests itself as a characteristic lack of energy and drive. Patients become inert and are unable to mobilize themselves to initiate or persist in completing many different kinds of tasks. Unlike the diminished energy or interest of depression, the avolitional symptom complex in schizophrenia usually is not accompanied by saddened or depressed affect. The avolitional symptom complex often leads to severe social and economic impairment.

Grooming and hygiene. The patient pays less attention to grooming and hygiene than is normal. Clothing may appear sloppy, outdated, or soiled. He or she may bathe infrequently and not care for his or her hair, nails, or teeth—leading to manifestations such as greasy or uncombed hair, dirty hands, body odor, or unclean teeth and bad breath. Overall, the appearance is dilapidated and disheveled. In extreme cases, the patient may even have poor toilet habits.

Impersistence at work or school. The patient has difficulty in seeking or maintaining employment (or doing schoolwork) as appropriate for his or her age and gender. If a student, he or she does not do homework and may even fail to attend class. Grades will tend to reflect this. If a college student, he or she may have registered for courses but dropped several or all of them. If of working age, the patient may have found it difficult to work at a job because of an inability to persist in completing tasks and apparent irresponsibility. He or she may go to work irregularly, wander away early, fail to complete expected assignments, or complete them in a disorganized manner. He or she may simply sit around the house and not seek any employment or seek it only in an infrequent or desultory manner. If a homemaker or a retired person, the patient may fail to complete chores, such as shopping or cleaning, or complete them in an apparently careless and half-hearted way. If in a hospital or an institution, he or she does not attend or persist in vocational or rehabilitative programs effectively.

- *Have you been able to (work, go to school) during the past month?*
- *Have you been attending vocational rehabilitation or occupational therapy sessions (in the hospital)?*
- *What have you been able to do?*
- *(Do you have trouble finishing what you start?)*
- *(What kinds of problems have you had?)*

Physical anergia. The patient tends to be physically inert; he or she may sit in a chair for hours at a time and not initiate any spontaneous activity. If encouraged to become involved in an activity, he or she may participate only briefly and then wander away or disengage himself or herself and return to sitting alone. He or she may spend large amounts of time in some relatively mindless and physically inactive task such as watching television or playing solitaire. His or her family may report that he or she spends most of his or her time at home "doing nothing except sitting around." Either at home or in an inpatient setting, he or she may spend much of his or her time sitting in his or her room.

- *How have you been spending your time?*
- *Do you have any trouble getting yourself going?*

Anhedonia-Asociality

Anhedonia-asociality encompasses the patient's difficulties in experiencing interest or pleasure. It may express itself as a loss of interest in pleasurable activities, an inability to experience pleasure when participating in activities normally considered pleasurable, or a lack of involvement in social relationships of various kinds.

Recreational interests and activities.   The patient may have few or no interests, activities, or hobbies. Although this symptom may begin insidiously or slowly, there will usually be some obvious decline from an earlier level of interest and activity. Patients with relatively milder loss of interest will engage in some activities that are passive or nondemanding, such as watching television, or will show only occasional or sporadic interests. Patients with the most extreme loss will appear to have a complete and intractable inability to become involved in or enjoy activities. The evaluation in this area should take both the quality and the quantity of recreational interests into account.

- *What do you do for enjoyment?*
- *(How often do you do those things?)*
- *Have you been attending recreational therapy?*
- *(What have you been doing?)*
- *(Do you enjoy it?)*

Sexual interest and activity.   The patient may show a decrement in sexual interest and activity or enjoyment as would be judged healthy for the patient's age and marital status. Individuals who are married may manifest disinterest in sex or may engage in intercourse only at the partner's request. In extreme cases, the patient may not engage in sex at all. Single patients may go for long periods without sexual involvement and make no effort to satisfy this drive. Whether married or single, patients may report that they subjectively feel only minimal sex drive or that they take little enjoyment in sexual intercourse or in masturbatory activity even when they engage in it.

- *What has your sex drive been like?*
- *Have you been able to enjoy sex lately?*
- *(What is your usual sexual outlet?)*
- *(When was the last time?)*

Ability to feel intimacy and closeness. The patient may be unable to form intimate and close relationships of a type appropriate for his or her age, gender, and family status. In the case of a younger person, this area should be evaluated in terms of relationships with the opposite sex and with parents and siblings. In the case of an older person who is married, the relationship with the spouse and with children should be evaluated, whereas older unmarried individuals should be judged in terms of relationships with the opposite sex and any family members who live nearby. Patients may show few or no feelings of affection to available family members, or they may have arranged their lives so that they are completely isolated from any intimate relationships, living alone and making no effort to initiate contacts with family or members of the opposite sex. If the patient is gay or lesbian, then relationships with members of the same sex may be evaluated as indications of an ability to feel intimacy and closeness.

- *Do you feel close to your family (husband, wife, children)?*
- *Is there anyone outside your family who you feel especially close to?*
- *(How often do you see [them, him, her]?)*

Relationships with friends and peers. Patients also may be relatively restricted in their relationships with friends and peers of either gender. They may have few or no friends, make little or no effort to develop such relationships, and choose to spend all or most of their time alone.

- *Do you have many friends?*
- *(Are you very close to them?)*
- *(How often do you see them?)*
- *(What do you do together?)*
- *Have you gotten to know any patients in the hospital?*

Attention

Attention is often poor in patients with severe mental illnesses. The patient may have trouble focusing his or her attention, or he or she may be able to focus only sporadically and erratically. He or she may ignore attempts to converse with him or her, wander away while in the middle of an activity or a task, or appear to be inattentive when engaged in formal testing or interviewing. He or she may or may not be aware of his or her difficulty in focusing his or her attention.

Social inattentiveness.   While involved in social situations or activities, the patient appears inattentive. He or she looks away during conversations, does not pick up the topic during a discussion, or appears uninvolved or disengaged. He or she may abruptly terminate a discussion or a task without any apparent reason. He or she may seem "spacey" or "out of it." He or she may seem to have poor concentration when playing games, reading, or watching television.

Inattentiveness during mental status testing.   The patient may perform poorly on simple tests of intellectual functioning despite adequate education and intellectual ability. This should be assessed by having the patient spell *world* (or some equivalent five-letter word) backward and by serial 7s (at least a tenth-grade education) or serial 3s (at least a sixth-grade education) for a series of five subtractions.

Manic Symptoms

Euphoric mood.   The patient has had one or more distinct periods of euphoric, irritable, or expansive mood, not due to alcohol or drug intoxication.

- *Have you been feeling extremely good or high—clearly different from your normal self?*
- *(Do your friends or family think this is more than just feeling good?)*
- *Have you felt irritable and easily annoyed?*
- *(How long has this mood lasted?)*

Increase in activity.   The patient shows an increase in involvement or activity level associated with work, family, friends, sex drive, new projects, interests, or activities (e.g., telephone calls, letter writing).

- *Are you more active or involved in things compared with the way you usually are?*
- *(How about at work, at home, with your friends, or with your family?)*
- *(What about your involvement in hobbies or other interests?)*
- *Have you been unable to sit still, or have you had to be moving or pacing up and down?*

Racing thoughts/flight of ideas. The patient has the subjective experience that his or her thinking is markedly accelerated. For example, "My thoughts are ahead of my speech."

- *Have your thoughts been racing through your mind?*
- *Do you have more ideas than usual?*

Inflated self-esteem. The patient has increased self-esteem and appraisal of his or her worth, contacts, influence, power, or knowledge (may be delusional) as compared with his or her usual level. Persecutory delusions should not be considered evidence of grandiosity unless the patient feels persecution is due to some special attributes (e.g., power, knowledge, or contacts).

- *Do you feel more self-confident than usual?*
- *Do you feel that you are a particularly important person or that you have special talents or abilities?*

Decreased need for sleep. The patient needs less sleep than usual to feel rested. (This rating should be based on the average of several days rather than a single severe night.)

- *Do you need less sleep than usual to feel rested?*
- *(How much sleep do you ordinarily need?)*
- *(How much sleep do you need now?)*

Distractibility. The patient's attention is too easily drawn to unimportant or irrelevant external stimuli. For example, the patient gets up and inspects some item in the room while talking or listening, shifts his or her topic of speech, and so forth.

- *Are you easily distracted by things around you?*

Poor judgment. The patient shows excessive involvement in activities that have a high potential for painful consequences that are not recognized (e.g., buying sprees, sexual indiscretions, foolish business investments, reckless giving).

- *Have you done anything that caused trouble for you or your family or friends?*

- *Looking back now, have you done anything that showed poor judgment?*
- *Have you done anything foolish with money?*
- *Have you done anything sexually that was unusual for you?*

Depressive Symptoms

Dysphoric mood.   The patient feels sad, despondent, discouraged, or unhappy; significant anxiety or tense irritability also should be rated as a dysphoric mood. The evaluation should be made irrespective of length of mood.

- *Have you been having periods of feeling depressed, sad, or hopeless? When you didn't care about anything or couldn't enjoy anything?*
- *Have you felt tense, anxious, or irritable?*
- *(How long did this last?)*

Change in appetite or weight.   The patient has had significant weight loss. This should not include dieting, unless the dieting is associated with some depressive belief that approaches delusional proportions.

- *Have you had any changes in your appetite—either increase or decrease?*
- *Have you lost or gained much more weight than is usual for you?*

Insomnia or hypersomnia.   Insomnia may include waking up after only a few hours of sleep, as well as difficulty in getting to sleep. Patterns of insomnia include *initial* (trouble going to sleep), *middle* (waking in the middle of the night but eventually falling asleep again), and *terminal* (waking early—e.g., 2:00 A.M. to 5:00 A.M.—and remaining awake).

- *Have you had trouble sleeping?*
- *(What was it like?)*
- *(Do you have trouble falling asleep?)*
- *(Do you wake up too early in the morning?)*
- *Have you been sleeping more than usual?*
- *How much sleep do you get in a typical 24-hour period?*

Psychomotor agitation.   The patient is unable to sit still, with a need to keep moving. (Do not include mere subjective feelings of restlessness.) Objective evidence (e.g., hand wringing, fidgeting, pacing) should be present.

- *Have you felt restless or agitated?*
- *Do you have trouble sitting still?*

Psychomotor retardation. The patient feels slowed down and experiences great difficulty moving. (Do not include mere subjective feelings of being slowed down.) Objective evidence (e.g., slowed speech) should be present.

- *Have you been feeling slowed down?*

Loss of interest or pleasure. The patient has loss of interest or pleasure in usual activities or a decrease in sexual drive. This may be similar to the anhedonia seen in psychosis. In the depressive syndrome, loss of interest or pleasure is invariably accompanied by intense, painful affect, whereas in psychosis, the affect is often blunted.

- *Have you noticed a change in your interest in things you normally enjoy?*
- *(What have you been less interested in?)*

Loss of energy. The patient has a loss of energy, becomes easily fatigued, or feels tired. These energy comparisons should be based on the person's usual activity level whenever possible.

- *Have you had a tendency to feel more tired than usual?*
- *(Have you been feeling as if all your energy is drained?)*

Feelings of worthlessness. In addition to feelings of worthlessness, the patient may report feelings of self-reproach or excessive or inappropriate guilt. (Either may be delusional.)

- *Have you been feeling down on yourself?*
- *Have you been feeling guilty about anything?*
- *(Could you tell me about some of the things for which you feel guilty?)*

Diminished ability to think or concentrate. The patient complains of diminished ability to think or concentrate, such as slowed thinking or indecisiveness; not associated with marked derailment or incoherence.

- *Have you had trouble thinking?*
- *What about your concentration?*
- *Have you had trouble making decisions?*

Recurrent thoughts of death/suicide.   The patient has thoughts about death and suicide, plus possible wishes to be dead and/or suicide attempts.

- *Have you been thinking about death or about taking your own life?*
- *(How often have these thoughts occurred?)*
- *(What were you thinking of doing?)*

Distinct quality to mood.   The patient's depressed mood is experienced as distinctly different from the kind of feelings experienced after the death of a loved one. If the patient has not lost a loved one, ask him or her to compare the feelings with those after some significant personal loss appropriate to his or her age and experience.

- *The feelings of (sadness) you are having now—are they the same as the feelings you would have had when someone close to you died, or are they different?*
- *(How are they similar or different?)*

Nonreactivity of mood.   The patient does not feel much better, even temporarily, when something good happens.

- *Do your feelings of depression go away or get better when you do something you enjoy, such as talking with friends, visiting your family, or (mention some favorite recreation)?*

Diurnal variation.   The patient's mood shifts during the course of the day. Some patients feel terrible in the morning but feel steadily better as the day goes on and even near normal in the evening. Others feel good in the morning and worse as the day progresses.

- *Is there any time of the day that is especially bad for you?*
- *(Do you feel worse in the morning? In the evening?)*
- *(Or is it about the same all the time?)*

Anxiety Symptoms

Panic attacks.   The patient has discrete episodes of intense fear or discomfort in which a variety of symptoms occur, such as shortness of breath, dizziness, palpitations, or shaking.

- *Have you ever experienced a sudden attack of panic or fear, in which you felt extremely uncomfortable?*

- *(How long did it last?)*
- *(Did you notice any other symptoms occurring at the same time?)*
- *(Did you feel as if you were going to die or go crazy?)*

Agoraphobia. The patient has a fear of going outside (literally "a fear of the marketplace"). In many patients, however, the fear is more generalized and involves being afraid of being in a place or situation from which escape might be difficult.

- *Have you ever been afraid of going outside, so that you tended to just stay home all the time?*
- *Have you been afraid of getting caught or trapped somewhere, so that you would be unable to escape?*

Social phobia. The patient has a fear of being in some social situation where he or she will be seen by others and may do something that he or she might find to be humiliating or embarrassing. Some common social phobias include fear of public speaking, fear of eating in front of others, or fear of using public bathrooms.

- *Do you have any special fears, such as a fear of public speaking?*
- *Of eating in front of others?*

Specific phobia. The patient is afraid of some specific circumscribed stimulus. Specific phobias often involve animals, such as snakes or insects; they also involve seeing blood, being at high places, or being afraid to fly on airplanes.

- *Do you have any other specific fears?*
- *Are you afraid of snakes?*
- *The sight of blood?*
- *Air travel?*

Obsessions. The patient experiences persistent ideas, thoughts, or impulses that are unwanted and experienced as unpleasant. The patient tends to ruminate and worry about them. The patient may try to ignore or suppress them but typically finds this difficult. Some common obsessions include repetitive thoughts of performing some violent act or becoming contaminated by touching other people or public objects.

- *Are you ever bothered by persistent ideas that you can't get out of your head, such as being dirty or contaminated?*
- *(Can you give me some specific examples?)*

Compulsions.   The patient has to perform specific acts over and over in a way that he or she recognizes to be senseless or inappropriate. Usually, the compulsions are performed to ease some worry or obsession or to prevent some feared event from occurring. For example, a patient may have the worry that he or she has left the door unlocked and have to return over and over to check it. Obsessions about contamination may lead to repetitive hand washing. Obsessions about thoughts of violence may lead to ritualistic behavior designed to prevent injury to the person about whom violence has been imagined.

- *Do you have any acts that you have to perform over and over, such as washing your hands or checking the stove?*
- *(Can you give me some examples?)*

Interviews and Rating Scales for Research

To standardize research assessments, a variety of interviews and rating scales have been developed. Typically, these interviews and rating scales have been rigorously evaluated to document that they have excellent reliability, making them relatively precise instruments for measurement and assessment.

Structured Interviews

Nine major structured interviews are currently available for psychiatric research. They are listed in Table 3–3. Each of these has various strengths and weaknesses. All use a structured or systematic approach to eliciting information about the patient's current and past history.

The *Present State Examination (PSE)*, developed by John Wing in England in the 1960s, is the oldest of the structured psychiatric interviews. Its time frame is limited to symptoms present during the past month, making it unsatisfactory for lifetime diagnoses. It cannot be used to make DSM-IV-TR diagnoses without substantial adaptations and additions. Consequently, it is used infrequently in American research.

The *Schedule for Affective Disorders and Schizophrenia (SADS)* became available in the 1970s and was the first well-developed American structured interview. It includes two sections, one evaluating the current condition and a second evaluating symptoms occurring during the patient's lifetime. Thus,

TABLE 3–3.   Structured interviews

Present State Examination (PSE)

Schedule for Affective Disorders and Schizophrenia (SADS)

Diagnostic Interview Schedule (DIS)

Structured Clinical Interview for Diagnosis (SCID)

Comprehensive Assessment of Symptoms and History (CASH)

Composite International Diagnostic Interview (CIDI)

Mini-International Neuropsychiatric Interview (MINI)

Structured Interview for the Diagnosis of DSM-IV Personality Disorders (SIDP-IV)

Personality Disorders Examination (PDE)

it gives broad coverage of symptoms and history. It was developed before DSM-III, however, and cannot be used to make DSM-IV-TR diagnoses. It has its own set of diagnostic criteria, the Research Diagnostic Criteria.

The *Diagnostic Interview Schedule (DIS)* was designed largely to do epidemiological field studies of large populations. Unlike the PSE and the SADS, it does not require interviewers with experience in working with psychiatric patients. Although it is well suited for large-scale epidemiological studies, its coverage is relatively sparse for working with actual patients who have relatively severe psychiatric syndromes.

The *Structured Clinical Interview for Diagnosis (SCID)* was the first interview designed specifically to apply DSM criteria to psychiatrically ill patients. Its focus is largely on making diagnoses, and it therefore primarily includes information listed in the DSM diagnostic criteria. It is concise and user friendly but incomplete in its coverage. Several versions of the SCID are available, which focus on different aspects of psychopathology (e.g., psychoses, anxiety disorders, personality disorders). The specific version chosen will depend on the interests of the investigator.

The *Comprehensive Assessment of Symptoms and History (CASH)* was developed in the 1980s. Because diagnostic criteria have been changing rapidly during the past few years, the CASH was designed to provide a broad coverage of symptoms so that investigators would have a comprehensive database that could be adapted to different diagnostic systems. It includes a current and a past section. It also includes structured sections to assess sociodemographic history, handedness, memory impairment, negative symptoms, and a variety of other aspects of clinical descriptions that are not included in the structured interviews listed above.

The *Composite International Diagnostic Interview (CIDI)*, based on the DIS, was developed for use in cross-sectional epidemiological research by the World Health Organization. The questions are modular in design, so researchers can choose diagnostic categories of interest to them. It is designed to be used by lay interviewers.

The *Mini-International Neuropsychiatric Interview (MINI)* was developed in the 1990s. It was designed to meet the need for a short (15 minutes to administer) but accurate structured psychiatric interview for multicenter clinical trials and epidemiological studies. The MINI is based on the DSM-IV criteria. Because it is brief and relatively easy to administer, it may be useful in nonresearch clinical settings.

The *Structured Interview for the Diagnosis of DSM-IV Personality Disorders (SIDP-IV)* was developed as a complement to the other structured interviews designed to make Axis I diagnoses. It provides a structured interview that permits clinicians and investigators to make assessments for diagnosis of personality syndromes according to DSM-IV criteria.

The *Personality Disorders Examination (PDE)* also was developed by the World Health Organization; it is designed for cross-sectional research on personality disorders. Unlike the CIDI and the DIS, it is intended for use by experienced clinicians.

Rating Scales

Rating scales typically are designed to provide a rapid and concise assessment of a specific aspect of psychopathology. Most rating scales have been developed for use in clinical drug trials or other situations in which investigators want to assess a change in the patient's status by taking repeated measurements over time (usually at weekly intervals). Table 3–4 lists some of the rating scales that are commonly used in psychiatric research of this type. Copies of each of these scales appear in the Appendix.

The *Brief Psychiatric Rating Scale (BPRS)* is the oldest rating scale. It was developed in the 1960s and used factor analysis to sift through a broad array of symptoms seen in psychiatric patients and generate a relatively small number of factors. These include things such as conceptual disorganization, hostility, and social withdrawal. The BPRS is still widely used, although most of the items rated are relatively abstract compared with the specific symptoms currently used to assess psychopathology.

The *Scale for the Assessment of Negative Symptoms (SANS)* and the *Scale for the Assessment of Positive Symptoms (SAPS)* were designed to provide more complete coverage of the symptoms of psychosis than is provided by

TABLE 3–4. Rating scales

Brief Psychiatric Rating Scale (BPRS)

Scale for the Assessment of Negative Symptoms (SANS)

Scale for the Assessment of Positive Symptoms (SAPS)

Hamilton Rating Scale for Depression (HRSD)

Beck Depression Inventory (BDI)

Hamilton Anxiety Scale

Yale-Brown Obsessive Compulsive Scale (Y-BOCS)

Abnormal Involuntary Movement Scale (AIMS)

Simpson-Angus Scale

Mini-Mental State Exam (MMSE)

Global Assessment Scale (GAS)

the BPRS. The SANS is the only scale currently in wide use that assesses negative symptoms. These scales rate the phenomena that clinicians are accustomed to assessing, such as delusions, hallucinations, and positive formal thought disorder.

The *Beck Depression Inventory (BDI)* focuses on cognitive symptoms of depression, unlike the HRSD. It is probably the most widely used depression inventory.

The *Hamilton Rating Scale for Depression (HRSD)* is also one of the oldest rating scales. It was specifically designed to provide a quantitative measurement of symptoms of depression that would be sensitive to change. Like the BPRS, it was developed shortly after the discovery of psychoactive drugs and was a standard instrument used to assess the efficacy of new antidepressants as they were developed.

The *Hamilton Anxiety Scale* performs a similar function to the HRSD for assessing anxiety. It is also widely used in clinical drug trials and as an overall assessment instrument.

The *Abnormal Involuntary Movement Scale (AIMS)* was developed to determine whether patients had developed abnormal movements characteristic of tardive dyskinesia. It is currently widely used in antipsychotic trials.

The *Simpson-Angus Scale* is also widely used and is similar to the AIMS, but it focuses more specifically on the side effects of antipsychotics, such as parkinsonian symptoms or akathisia.

The *Mini-Mental State Exam (MMSE)* is a brief questionnaire designed to assess cognitive status. It provides quantitative measurements of orientation, memory, calculations, and other aspects of the systematic mental status examination. It is a quantitative scale with a perfect score of 30 points. It is now widely used as a simple, rapid method for assessing abnormalities in mental status.

The *Global Assessment Scale (GAS)* is a 100-point scale (0=extremely poor, 100=superior) that is included in a variety of structured interviews, such as the SADS or the CASH. It is very similar to the Global Assessment of Functioning (GAF) Scale (described in Chapter 2), which was derived from the GAS. This scale provides a brief, simple way of assessing the patient's level of functioning and severity of psychopathology. Because the GAS is quite sensitive to change, it is frequently used as an overall index of the patient's improvement over time.

The *Yale-Brown Obsessive Compulsive Scale (Y-BOCS)* is commonly used to assess obsessive-compulsive symptoms. Its sensitivity to change makes it particularly useful for clinical treatment studies. It has been modified to evaluate other syndromes, including dysmorphobia, compulsive buying, and pathological gambling.

Bibliography

American Psychiatric Association: Diagnostic and Statistical Manual of Mental Disorders, 3rd Edition. Washington, DC, American Psychiatric Association, 1980

American Psychiatric Association: Diagnostic and Statistical Manual of Mental Disorders, 4th Edition. Washington, DC, American Psychiatric Association, 1994

Andreasen NC: Thought, language, and communication disorders, I: clinical assessment, definition of terms, and evaluation of their reliability. Arch Gen Psychiatry 36:1315–1321, 1979

Andreasen NC: Negative symptoms in schizophrenia: definition and reliability. Arch Gen Psychiatry 39:784–788, 1982

Andreasen NC: The Scale for the Assessment of Negative Symptoms (SANS). Iowa City, The University of Iowa, 1983

Andreasen NC: The Scale for the Assessment of Positive Symptoms (SAPS). Iowa City, The University of Iowa, 1984

Andreasen NC: Comprehensive Assessment of Symptoms and History (CASH). Iowa City, The University of Iowa, 1985

Andreasen NC, Flaum M, Arndt S: The Comprehensive Assessment of Symptoms and History (CASH): an instrument for assessing psychopathology and diagnosis. Arch Gen Psychiatry 49:615–623, 1992

Arndt S, Alliger RJ, Andreasen NC: The distinction of positive and negative symptoms: the failure of a two-dimensional model. Br J Psychiatry 158:317–322, 1991

Beck AT, Ward CH, Mendelson M, et al: An inventory of measuring depression. Arch Gen Psychiatry 4:53–63, 1961

Department of Health, Education, and Welfare: Abnormal Involuntary Movement Scale. Washington, DC, Alcohol, Drug Abuse and Mental Health Administration, 1974

Endicott J, Spitzer RL: A diagnostic interview: the Schedule for Affective Disorders and Schizophrenia (SADS). Arch Gen Psychiatry 35:837–844, 1978

Endicott J, Spitzer RL, Fleiss JL, et al: The Global Assessment Scale: a procedure for measuring overall severity of psychiatric disturbance. Arch Gen Psychiatry 33:766–771, 1976

Folstein MF, Folstein SE, McHugh P: Mini-Mental State: a practical method for grading the cognitive state of patients for the clinician. J Psychiatr Res 12:189–198, 1975

Goodman WK, Price LH, Rasmussen SA, et al: The Yale-Brown Obsessive-Compulsive Scale I: development, use, and reliability. Arch Gen Psychiatry 46:1006–1011, 1989

Hamilton M: The assessment of anxiety states by rating. Br J Psychiatry 32:50–55, 1959

Hamilton M: A rating scale for depression. J Neurol Neurosurg Psychiatry 23:56–62, 1960

Overall J, Gorham D: Brief Psychiatric Rating Scale. Psychol Rep 10:799–812, 1962

Robins LN, Helzer JE, Croughan J, et al: National Institute of Mental Health Diagnostic Interview Schedule: its history, characteristics, and validity. Arch Gen Psychiatry 38:381–389, 1981

Robins LN, Wing J, Wittchen HV, et al: The Composite International Diagnostic Interview—an epidemiological instrument for use in conjunction with different diagnostic systems and in different cultures. Arch Gen Psychiatry 45:1069–1077, 1988

Sheehan DV, Lecrubier Y, Sheehan KH, et al: The MINI-International Neuropsychiatric Interview (MINI): the development and validation of a structured diagnostic psychiatric interview for DSM-IV and ICD-10. J Clin Psychiatry 59 (suppl 20):22–33, 1998

Simpson GM, Angus JWS: A rating scale for extrapyramidal side effects. Acta Psychiatr Scand Suppl 212:11–19, 1970

Spitzer RL, Williams JBW, Gibbon M: The Structured Clinical Interview for DSM-III (SCID), I: history, rationale, and description. Arch Gen Psychiatry 49:624–629, 1992

Stangl D, Pfohl B, Zimmerman M, et al: A structured interview for DSM-III personality disorders: a preliminary report. Arch Gen Psychiatry 42:591–596, 1985

Wing JK: A standard form of psychiatric Present State Examinations (PSE) and a method for standardizing the classification of symptoms, in Psychiatric Epidemiology. Edited by Hare EH, Wing JK. London, Oxford University Press, 1970, pp 93–108

Self-Assessment Questions

1. Describe the way in which the patient's chief complaint can be used to take a history and to develop a differential diagnosis.
2. Describe several techniques that are important for concluding the initial interview with a patient.
3. Enumerate the components of a standard psychiatric history, giving each of the main headings of the overall outline.
4. Summarize the major components of the mental status examination.
5. Enumerate the five positive symptoms of psychosis. Give examples of some typical kinds of delusions and hallucinations.
6. List the five common negative symptoms.
7. Enumerate and define some of the symptoms observed in depression.
8. Enumerate and define some of the symptoms observed in mania.
9. Enumerate and define some of the symptoms observed in anxiety disorders.

4 Laboratory Tests

There is no observer outside the experiment.

Heisenberg

Although psychiatry places a greater emphasis on careful history taking and assessment than do most other medical specialties, laboratory tests are also growing in importance. Because so much has been discovered about the neural substrates of mental illnesses during the past several decades, psychiatrists have begun to identify tests of brain structure and function that may provide useful information to help guide diagnosis and treatment. Few current laboratory tests have a sensitivity and specificity equivalent to that of a glucose tolerance test for diabetes or a serum thyroxin test for myxedema or thyrotoxicosis. Tests of this type are available for only a few disorders (e.g., Alzheimer's disease), and even in these few instances their diagnostic validity is still not firmly established. Nevertheless, some type of laboratory workup will be appropriate for many psychiatric patients to establish baseline levels of function, to rule out confounding medical conditions, or to evaluate the presence of toxins that may cause symptoms of mental illness.

In the current era of cost-consciousness, laboratory tests should not be ordered unnecessarily, but they also should not be avoided if needed. Psychiatric patients require the same type of careful and high-quality workup as do patients who are evaluated for cardiac, pulmonary, or renal symptoms. Although psychiatric patients' symptoms may appear to be "in their minds," they may actually be mediated by processes affecting their brains or arising from other bodily organs. The rationale for obtaining laboratory tests will depend on the clinical presentation and should be tailored to the needs of the individual patient and the setting in which he or she is seen.

Some laboratory tests usually should be ordered for patients admitted to a psychiatric unit, although the laboratory workup may be quite simple. The need for laboratory evaluations among outpatients will vary, depending on the age of the patient, the type of symptoms with which he or she presents, and the type of treatment plan. Young, healthy individuals who have received a medical evaluation within the past few years and who have relatively mild psychiatric symptoms probably will need nothing. However, even among outpatients, some laboratory assessments may be necessary in patients who are elderly or who present with severe or complex problems, particularly when the differential diagnosis suggests some medical cause for the presenting symptoms.

Most laboratory procedures conducted for psychiatric patients are done for one of five purposes:

1. To complete a general medical workup of the sort done routinely for any hospital admission
2. To rule out some nonpsychiatric cause of the presenting symptoms
3. To conduct a specific workup appropriate for a specific treatment that has been planned (e.g., a workup before conducting electroconvulsive therapy [ECT])
4. To obtain information that will assist in making a differential diagnosis among several different mental illnesses
5. To assist in determining pathophysiology, estimating prognosis, and formulating a treatment plan

Each of these purposes, and the relevant laboratory procedures, is discussed in more detail below.

General Medical Workup

Standards as to what is considered an appropriate general medical workup may vary in different hospital settings. In general, however, most patients admitted to a hospital receive a set of screening laboratory evaluations. Typically, these consist of a complete blood count, urinalysis, serum electrolytes, liver enzymes (i.e., aspartate aminotransferase, alanine aminotransferase), serum creatinine, blood urea nitrogen (BUN), and sometimes a chest film or electrocardiogram (ECG). The relevance of the latter two depend in part on the patient's age, smoking history, and overall physical condition. Given that many patients with mental illnesses have a history of heavy smoking, an evaluation of pulmonary and cardiac status may be appropriate. Female patients need a Papanicolaou test, and women older than 45 should be evaluated with mammography at periodic intervals. The inpatient psychiatrist should assume responsibility for ensuring that appropriate laboratory screens are obtained, taking into account whether the patient has had any of these evaluations recently.

A psychiatrist who is seeing outpatients at regular intervals also should assume responsibility for ensuring that his or her patients receive annual general medical workups, including appropriate histories, physical examinations, and laboratory tests. In some cases, the psychiatrist assumes the role of a primary care physician because he or she is the physician whom the patient sees most frequently. The psychiatrist usually will assume primary responsibility for conducting a physical and neurological examination in an inpatient setting and will obtain referrals to a specialist if questions arise. In an outpatient setting the responsibility will vary depending on the working environment and regional mores. The psychiatrist working in a general medical clinic or health maintenance organization (HMO) will share the responsibility, whereas psychiatrists in solo practice or a specialty group usually will conduct a physical and neurological examination, order appropriate tests, and interpret them. (Some psychiatrists who practice only psychotherapy may, however, prefer to refer their patients to an internist or family practitioner because of concerns that the physical contact may interfere with the process of psychotherapy.) Overall, the rule that fragmenting care across multiple specialists gives patients poor service holds as much for patients with mental illnesses as it does for patients with other types of illness. Consequently, the psychiatrist should maintain good general medical skills and be prepared to handle simple and routine medical problems.

Laboratory Tests to Rule Out Nonpsychiatric Causes of Symptoms

Many diagnoses in psychiatry are diagnoses of exclusion. That is, they are typically made after it has been determined that the patient's symptoms are not due to some other specific medical or neurological disorder. Historically, psychiatrists would say that they were ruling out "organic" causes of the symptoms. In fact, disorders were divided into those that were "organic" (i.e., physically based) and those that were "functional" (i.e., mentally based). This phraseology has clearly become outdated, however, because diseases such as schizophrenia and bipolar disorder almost certainly have a specific organic cause, rooted in aberrations in brain chemistry or circuitry. Consequently, this outmoded distinction has been abandoned in DSM-IV and its recent text revision, DSM-IV-TR.

Table 4–1 lists a variety of conditions commonly considered in the differential diagnosis of serious mental illnesses such as the dementias, schizophrenia, bipolar disorder, and the various anxiety disorders. In general, when DSM-IV-TR states that "the disturbance is not due to a general medical condition," one of the group of disorders in Table 4–1 is to be ruled out. These various disorders are discussed in more detail under the differential diagnosis of the various conditions presented in Section II of this volume ("Psychiatric Disorders"). If one of these conditions is being seriously considered, the psychiatrist often will order a screening test. If the results are suggestive of a neurological or general medical diagnosis, then the clinician usually will consult with another medical specialist to select additional laboratory tests and interpret them.

TABLE 4–1.   Conditions commonly considered in the differential diagnosis of major mental illnesses

Multi-infarct dementia

Subdural hematoma

Normal-pressure hydrocephalus

Tumors

Human immunodeficiency virus (HIV)–related dementia

Temporal lobe epilepsy

Endocrine/metabolic disorders

Exposure to toxins

Vitamin deficiency syndromes (e.g., pernicious anemia)

Other central nervous system infections (e.g., syphilis)

Substance-induced symptoms

Neuropsychiatric effects of medical treatment (e.g., potassium deficiency from diuretics, fatigue from propranolol, digitalis toxicity, phenytoin toxicity)

Patients with multi-infarct dementia, subdural hematoma, normal pressure hydrocephalus, tumors, and human immunodeficiency virus (HIV)–related dementia all may present with confusion, memory impairment, personality change, poor attention and drive, tearfulness and depression, or suspiciousness and even frank psychosis. The most common psychiatric illnesses that must be differentiated from these conditions include Alzheimer's disease, schizophrenia and related psychotic conditions (e.g., schizophreniform disorder, delusional disorder), and the various mood disorders.

Neuroimaging provides the most efficient method for ruling out most of these conditions. A simple computed tomography (CT) scan may be sufficient. Magnetic resonance imaging (MRI) is more effective because it permits the identification of small focal lesions, which may represent old infarcts and which typically appear as areas of increased signal intensity. The white matter lesions of multiple sclerosis also are readily seen with MRI, and patients with HIV-related dementia may show similar small focal lesions. Because of its excellent resolution and three-dimensional capacity, MRI is particularly useful for identifying tumors. Tumors typically appear bright on MRI when T2-weighted sequences (specific scanning sequences that are especially sensitive for detecting abnormal tissue but poorer for seeing structure) are used.

As is described in more detail below, Alzheimer's disease represents a special case in neuroimaging evaluations. With functional imaging techniques such as single photon emission computed tomography (SPECT) and positron-emission tomography (PET), 70%–80% of the patients with Alzheimer's disease show a characteristic decrease in metabolic function or cerebral blood flow in posterior temporoparietal regions. Alzheimer's disease appears at present to be the only major mental illness that shows this characteristic pattern of hypometabolic function; thus, functional imaging techniques such as SPECT or PET may be particularly useful in differentiating Alzheimer's disease from other disorders that present with confusion and intellectual deterioration. Other laboratory tests, such as the electroencephalogram (EEG) and neuropsychological assessment, also may be useful in evaluating this particular group of "rule outs."

Temporal lobe epilepsy (TLE) typically presents with dissociative-like episodes or personality changes such as hyperreligiosity, hypergraphia (writing prolifically), hyposexuality, temper outbursts, and occasionally mood or psychotic-like symptoms. Thus, its differential diagnosis includes the various dissociative disorders, obsessive-compulsive personality disorder, antisocial personality disorder, conduct disorders, and the mood and psychotic disorders. Because TLE is caused by an electrical and functional disturbance in the brain, it is best evaluated by the laboratory tests that use the methods of neurophysiology or functional neuroimaging. The EEG is the test of choice because it is noninvasive, inexpensive, and relatively easy to administer. Nevertheless, the focal lesion in TLE may be deeply embedded inside the brain in the anterior poles of the temporal lobes or even the medial aspects of the temporal lobes. Because the EEG uses surface electrodes, it may not pick up seizure foci in these deep brain regions. Consequently, the assessment of TLE may require additional techniques, even when an EEG is used. Sleep deprivation may bring out focal abnormalities not noticed with a routine EEG, and nasopharyngeal leads are particularly appropriate if a diagnosis of TLE is being considered. PET scanning may also pick up focal regions of hypometabolic function, but this neuroimaging technique is not widely available and is much more costly.

Patients with endocrine disorders, exposure to toxins, vitamin deficiency syndromes (e.g., pernicious anemia), and other central nervous system (CNS) infections apart from the acquired immunodeficiency syndrome (AIDS) (e.g., syphilis) may present with fatigue, weakness, decreased drive, memory impairment, intellectual confusion, and personality change. Again, the most common psychiatric differential diagnoses are the various dementias, psychotic conditions, mood disorders, and a few anxiety or personality disorders. Hyperthyroidism is a common mimic of anxiety conditions, whereas myxedema is a common mimic of mood disorders. The other "rule outs" are considerably less common. These conditions are evaluated by a variety of specific assessment techniques, including serum triiodothyronine (T_3) and thyroxine (T_4), a complete blood count, serum assays for toxins, or a Venereal Disease Research Laboratory (VDRL) test for syphilis.

Finally, the clinician must attempt to determine whether a patient's presenting symptoms are the result of use of various street drugs or various medications prescribed by physicians, which are often all too readily available. Street drugs such as amphetamines, cocaine, and phencyclidine are special culprits in producing psychotic-like syndromes that resemble schizophrenia. Marijuana abuse leads to lethargy and withdrawal that may mimic depression, the negative symptoms of schizophrenia, or personality syndromes such as schizoid or schizotypal personality disorder. These drugs also may produce periods of feeling high that may mimic mood disorders. Use of street drugs, which is often denied by patients on interview, can be assessed through routine urine drug screens. Because of the substantial prevalence of substance abuse in contemporary American society, a urine drug screen should be nearly a routine diagnostic test for patients admitted as inpatients to psychiatric facilities.

Iatrogenic psychiatric disorders also are not uncommon. Patients who have received large quantities of prescribed drugs also may present with a variety of symptoms that mimic psychiatric disorders. Patients taking diuretics for hypertension may have a potassium deficiency that produces fatigue and that mimics depression. Propranolol may have similar effects. Digitalis toxicity and phenytoin (Dilantin) toxicity can produce fatigue and intellectual confusion that may mimic depression, psychosis, or dementia. Particularly in elderly patients, the clinician should maintain a high index of suspicion that symptoms that present as possible psychiatric disorders are in fact caused by prescribed medications. Anxiolytics and hypnotics, which are frequently prescribed by nonpsychiatric physicians, also can produce a variety of symptoms that mimic classic psychiatric disorders, such as confusion, lethargy, or withdrawal. Frequently, the diagnosis of a psychiatric condition due to prescribed drugs can be made simply from the history. Sometimes, however, laboratory tests are needed, for example, to establish low serum potassium levels or to obtain quantitative blood levels for prescribed medications such as digitalis.

Workups Pertaining to Specific Types of Psychiatric Treatments

Laboratory tests are used not only to assist in diagnosis and differential diagnosis but also to obtain information before instituting a particular treatment. Some treatments, such as ECT, have a modest risk associated with them. Therefore, it is desirable to obtain laboratory assessments to determine and document the patient's physical condition before the treatment, to rule out conditions that might be adversely affected by the treatment, and to establish baseline values for the patient before instituting treatment.

Electroconvulsive Therapy

As is discussed in more detail in the chapter on somatic therapies (Chapter 27), ECT is a relatively safe and highly effective treatment for some psychiatric disorders, such as severe depression. The actual physical convulsion involved is typically attenuated through the use of succinylcholine. Routine chemistries, including a complete blood count, serum electrolytes, and urinalysis, are obtained to rule out physical disorders that may contraindicate ECT. Spine films are no longer routinely obtained but may be indicated in elderly or arthritic patients before instituting ECT. Noticing signs of osteoporosis on spine films does not necessarily rule out the use of ECT when it is clinically appropriate, but it may suggest that a somewhat higher dose of succinylcholine is needed. An ECG usually is obtained to determine baseline cardiac status, because arrhythmias can occur during or after a treatment. Thus, when an elderly depressed patient has questionable signs of dementia, it is best to obtain a full dementia workup before ECT, including an EEG, because ECT itself may produce some EEG changes or memory impairment. Neuropsychological tests obtained after ECT also may be uninterpretable for several months.

Lithium Treatment

Lithium carbonate, which is used for the treatment of bipolar disorder, occasionally has adverse effects on both the thyroid gland and the kidney. Thus, it is desirable to obtain a urinalysis, serum electrolytes, BUN, serum creatinine, and serum T_3 and T_4 before instituting lithium treatment. Because lithium produces ECG changes, which are nonspecific and do not reflect cardiotoxicity, many clinicians often consider it worthwhile to obtain an ECG before prescribing lithium. This decision will be heavily dependent on the age and general health of the patient.

Whether the patient is taking a therapeutic level of lithium is also determined through a simple laboratory test to measure lithium blood levels. These are usually obtained twice weekly during the first few weeks of lithium treatment. Thereafter, they are typically obtained at regular intervals, such as every 6 months or every year, on an outpatient basis as long as the patient is taking lithium. Serum electrolytes, BUN, serum creatinine, and serum T_3 and T_4 levels also are typically rechecked at similar intervals. An elevated serum creatinine level should be followed up with a 24-hour creatinine clearance test.

Antipsychotic Treatment

Prescription of antipsychotic medications usually does not require any special workup. The major issue that arises in the use of antipsychotic treatments is determining the reasons for poor response, because approximately 25%–30% of the patients who receive antipsychotics are at least partially treatment refractory. When poor response occurs, the clinician will wonder whether the patient is taking the medication at all, whether the patient is experiencing toxic effects, or whether the dose is too low.

Several tests are available to help with these questions. First, blood levels can be obtained for two antipsychotics: haloperidol and clozapine. Assays can be obtained for other antipsychotics, but they have little meaning because these other antipsychotics produce many active metabolites and therefore make blood levels essentially uninterpretable. Furthermore, clear guidelines have not been established for the relation between blood levels and clinical response. Measurement of blood levels can be used, however, to determine whether the patient is taking any antipsychotic medication at all.

A second laboratory test that eventually may be useful for antipsychotics and other medications is genetic subtyping for the cytochrome P450 allele. The gene for this enzyme has been characterized, and its mutations have been identified. Depending on whether a person carries the wild-type allele or the mutated allele, drug metabolism rates will vary. People with two wild-type alleles will metabolize rapidly, those with one mutation will have slower metabolism, and those with two mutations will metabolize poorly. Although the test to detect this polymorphism is still too cumbersome and costly for routine use, determining whether a person is a slow or rapid metabolizer may become a clinically useful test in the future.

As described later in this chapter, both SPECT and PET can be used to visualize and measure the density of dopamine type 2 (D_2) receptors in the brain and their relative degree of blockade in response to treatment with antipsychotic drugs. These methods are not yet an established clinical laboratory test, but they have been extremely useful in determining the correct dose-response relations for antipsychotics. They may become useful in the future for tracking changes in the integrity of the dopamine system or other neurochemical systems in the human brain that are modulated by psychoactive drugs.

One antipsychotic medication, clozapine, routinely requires special laboratory tests. The first of the new atypical antipsychotics, clozapine is highly effective and has minimal extrapyramidal side effects. However, it has one significant adverse effect. A very small percentage of patients taking this drug develop blood dyscrasias. Because these emerge relatively quickly and can be fatal, clozapine requires regular monitoring of white blood cells with a complete blood count. Although this requirement may preclude the use of clozapine in some patients because of both cost and inconvenience, many patients are willing to tolerate these disadvantages because of clozapine's efficacy and minimal side effects.

The major adverse effects of antipsychotics are on the extrapyramidal system. These effects are more severe for the older conventional antipsychotics (see Chapter 27 for additional information). The development of tardive dyskinesia is the single most important serious long-term side effect. Its emergence can be monitored through regular physical examinations, during which the Abnormal Involuntary Movements Scale (AIMS; described in Chapter 3) is used to track the development of abnormal movements.

Antidepressant Treatment

Treatment with antidepressants also does not usually require any specific laboratory workup before instituting treatment. The decision about the use of laboratory tests in patients who will receive tricyclics or serotonin reuptake inhibitors (SRIs) will depend on the age and physical condition of the patient. Typically, no tests are obtained for healthy young adults. Because tricyclics may produce ECG changes, however, an ECG should be obtained before prescribing thse agents when there is any question that this test may be needed later on, as in older patients who have a possible cardiac abnormality. Because of the effects of tricyclics on the cardiovascular system, these medications have largely been supplanted by the newer antidepressants.

As with antipsychotic treatments, reasons for poor response or nonresponse can be an issue. Assays are available to monitor blood levels for some antidepressants, but no imaging techniques are as yet available. Therefore, in the case of poor response, the clinician usually must rely on individual judgment to make dose adjustments (see Chapter 27, "Somatic Treatments," for a more complete discussion of management of dosages of psychoactive medications).

Laboratory Procedures Used to Assist in Psychiatric Differential Diagnosis and Treatment Planning

In addition to the above highly specific indications for laboratory tests, a variety of tests may be obtained in psychiatric patients to assist in differential diagnosis or in understanding the nature and severity or the pathophysiology of the illness. Information about the pathophysiology can be helpful in counseling the patient and family about prognosis and in treatment planning. Some tests that are especially useful in this regard include the various neuroimaging procedures and various types of psychological tests. These may assist in determining the overall integrity of brain function, the presence of structural abnormalities, or the presence of generalized intellectual deficits or specific learning disabilities. Although very few of these tests give highly specific diagnostic information, they can sometimes assist in making a diagnosis and can be quite useful in treatment planning. As discussed earlier in this chapter, normal EEG results may rule out a condition such as TLE, and a SPECT scan will sharpen the differential diagnosis between depression and dementia. Nonspecific neural abnormalities are sometimes observed in patients with schizophrenia or bipolar disorder; when present, these suggest that the patient may be more sensitive to medication side effects and may be more refractory to treatment. Some of the laboratory tests that are especially useful for psychiatric differential diagnosis and treatment planning are described in detail below.

Overview of Laboratory Tests Frequently Used in Psychiatry

Neurophysiological Techniques

Electroencephalogram

The EEG is one of the oldest laboratory tests available to psychiatrists. Hans Berger, a psychiatrist who pioneered the development of the EEG, was the first person to record the electrical activity of the brain. Until the advent of structural imaging techniques, such as CT and MRI, EEG was the major method for evaluating abnormal brain activity produced by abnormalities such as tumors, head injuries, and seizures. CT and MRI now offer relatively benign methods for studying the brain in vivo to rule out the presence of diseased regions of tissue, but the EEG remains the simplest, most noninvasive method for evaluating seizures and metabolic dysfunctions.

The EEG measures electrical activity with a montage of electrodes scattered over the surface of the brain. An example of a typical montage appears in Figure 4–1. Electrical activity is recorded from leads connected to these surface electrodes; a typical modern EEG uses 16 leads. The electrical activity is then recorded on a polygraph, much like an ECG, and the pattern of activity is evaluated. Although computerized methods have been developed for reading EEGs, the best computer continues to be the human brain connected to the human eye.

EEG characteristics are described in terms of the frequency of the waveforms observed (measured in cycles per second [cps]). The normal human brain typically shows activity in either the beta (>12 cps) or the alpha (8–12 cps) range during the waking state. As individuals become drowsy, theta (4–8 cps) and delta (<4 cps) activity are observed. In the waking state, both theta and delta activity are considered abnormal in the healthy human brain. (Diffuse theta activity is sometimes seen in elderly individuals while awake, however.) Delta activity is clearly abnormal and represents sick or dying tissue.

Abnormalities observed on the EEG include spike and wave patterns, focal slowing, and diffuse slowing. Spike and wave patterns are typically seen in brains susceptible to seizures. The location of the spike may indicate

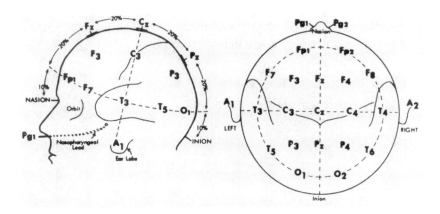

FIGURE 4–1. A typical electroencephalogram montage. Leads are arrayed in order to cover the entire brain, ranging from frontal to occipital.

the primary focus from which the seizure derives. The spikes of a brain predisposed to produce epileptic attacks are less often seen during the waking state. Consequently, EEGs are best obtained while the patient is asleep; sedation is often prescribed to induce sleep during the EEG so that abnormal seizure foci can be observed.

Encephalographers believe that a seizure disorder cannot be ruled out through a simple waking EEG. In addition, nasopharyngeal leads may be needed to identify a deep seizure focus. The tendency to manifest spike activities is suppressed by anticonvulsant medications, such as phenytoin. Thus, a patient with epilepsy may have normal EEG findings when he or she is appropriately medicated, particularly if only a waking EEG is obtained. Normal EEG results do not rule out the existence of a seizure disorder because the identification of spike and wave activity requires catching the brain during the elusive moments when spikes are occurring. Nevertheless, serial normal EEG findings obtained in sleeping, unmedicated individuals do make the diagnosis of a seizure disorder unlikely.

EEGs are very sensitive to metabolic dysfunctions and to the effects of various drugs. In the case of metabolic dysfunctions, the EEG may be the simplest method for determining that the patient's cognitive symptoms are due to some type of metabolic disorder. A variety of psychoactive drugs affect the EEG: lithium, for example, produces an increase in theta activity, whereas benzodiazepines produce rapid activity (i.e., beta activity). Sometimes the EEG provides a clinician with the first clue that a patient has been taking unprescribed medications or even medications prescribed by another physician. In a few rare instances, the EEG can serve as a useful test for ruling out psychiatric disorders that represent conversion phenomena or malingering. For example, the presence of photic driving (produced by visual stimulation with flashes of bright lights) on an EEG will rule out hysterical (i.e., conversion) blindness.

Sleep EEG (polysomnography) is a special type of electroencephalography involving the collection of electrical brain activity data during all-night sleep. During a normal full night's sleep, individuals go through a sleep cycle characterized by drowsiness (indicated by theta activity on the EEG) leading into alternating periods of rapid eye movement (REM) sleep and deep dreamless sleep (delta sleep). The healthy individual passes through approximately five such cycles during the course of a night's sleep. Polysomnography can be used to monitor a variety of sleep disorders that are often characterized by abnormal sleep patterns, such as those associated with depression. A short REM latency and reduced delta sleep are frequently observed in patients with depression. This abnormality occurs so frequently in depression that some investigators consider it a biological marker, but polysomnography is too time-consuming and expensive to be widely used to screen for this abnormality. Additional information about polysomnography and sleep disorders is found in Chapter 24 ("Sleep Disorders").

Evoked Potentials

Evoked potentials of various kinds also provide ancillary information. Evoked potentials are changes in brain electrical activity that are usually seen in specific regions in response to a stimulus, such as a particular kind of sound, instructions to monitor for a target displayed on a video screen, or some other type of cognitive or perceptual task. In contrast to a simple EEG, which is a general indicator of overall brain electrical activity, evoked potentials (also called *event-related potentials*) reflect the behavior of the brain while it is performing higher cognitive tasks. The most commonly used is the P300, a large positive wave usually seen 300 msec after the stimulus that was used to evoke it. The P300 is thought to reflect some aspect of the ability to focus attention. It appears to be decreased in schizophrenia, and abnormalities also have been reported in other disorders that involve cognitive dysfunctions.

These neurophysiological techniques are relatively crude compared with neuroimaging techniques such as CT, SPECT, and PET. Nevertheless, they may have clinical utility for several reasons. First, they do not involve any radiation exposure and are noninvasive. Therefore, they may be particularly valuable for studying brain activity in special populations, such as children. Second, they represent the only functional imaging technique (i.e., a technique that permits visualization of the brain performing particular functions or tasks) that has very fine temporal resolution. They can record events that occur in milliseconds, whereas the time window for SPECT and PET studies is seconds to hours. Third, they are simple to perform and, thus, inexpensive and accessible. Therefore, they may be used as a first-line assessment technique in some situations.

Structural Neuroimaging Techniques

Computed Tomography

CT scanning has been available since the early 1970s and was the first in vivo brain imaging technique to become widely used. Before CT, brain structure could be visualized only through the use of crude and invasive techniques such as pneumoencephalography.

The development of CT became possible only after the invention of efficient, high-speed computers. CT provides the prototype for most of the other neuroimaging techniques currently in use. In CT, an X-ray beam is passed through serial slices of the brain, and the degree of attenuation is measured when it emerges on the other side. The brain slice is divided into a series of tiny cubes (voxels or volume elements), and a number reflecting the degree of attenuation can be assigned to each of the voxels. These numerical codes are then assigned a shade of gray, reflecting the degree of X-ray attenuation, which gives a visual picture of brain structure. Cerebrospinal fluid, which attenuates least, appears darkest, whereas white matter, which attenuates most, appears lightest.

CT abnormalities may be seen in many mental disorders, including dementia, schizophrenia, alcoholism, anorexia nervosa, and perhaps some mood disorders. The types of abnormalities observed are nonspecific, in terms of both pathophysiology and diagnosis. The most typical findings are ventricular enlargement or cortical atrophy. A CT scan showing these types of abnormalities is seen in Figure 4–2. In general, these findings, when present, do not confirm a specific diagnosis because the same types of abnormalities may be present in many different disorders. Furthermore, in interpreting CT scans, the age of the individual must be taken into consideration. Neuronal loss and the development of ventricular enlargement and cortical atrophy appear to occur in healthy individuals as a part of the aging process. Thus, in interpreting CT scans in elderly individuals, it can often be difficult to decide whether the atrophy and ventricular enlargement seen on CT are within normal limits for an individual's age or whether they represent a pathological process. These same concerns about evaluating the effects of aging pertain to the interpretation of MRI scans as well.

Schizophrenia is the psychiatric illness that has been most extensively studied with CT scanning. More than 50 controlled CT studies have been conducted. As the summary of studies in Figure 4–3 indicates, most of these studies have shown that schizophrenic patients as a group tend to have an increase in ventricular size when compared with nonschizophrenic control subjects. Among the positive studies, the prevalence of extreme degrees of abnormality varied from study to study, ranging from as low as 5% to as high as 40%.

It is quite clear that ventricular enlargement is not seen in all schizophrenic patients. When present, ventricular enlargement appears to be correlated with a variety of other characteristics. Thus, a CT scan may provide the clinician with some information about long-term clinical course and prognosis. Schizophrenic patients with ventricular enlargement tend to have a lower level of educational achievement, often a more insidious onset, and indications of cognitive impairment when assessed neuropsychologically. They also may respond less well to antipsychotic medication, and some even appear to be worsened by it. Thus, their treatment should be managed somewhat more cautiously than that of patients whose CT scans indicate normal brain structure.

It has recently been observed that ventricular enlargement in schizophrenia probably does not represent a progressive neuronal loss, as occurs in Alzheimer's disease. Although very few studies have examined a single cohort of patients with serial scans over a 5- to 10-year period, ventricular size has been observed in a large group of schizophrenic patients with a broad range of ages. The results suggested that, unlike the changes associated with degenerative dementia, the brain changes in schizophrenia are not progressive over time, and in fact ventricular enlargement and prominent sulci are present early in the illness (i.e., at the time of first evaluation for symptoms). Furthermore, these brain abnormalities tend to be more prominent and severe in male patients. Because males are known to be much more vulnerable to birth injuries and developmental defects (e.g., males have a higher rate of learning disability, hyperactivity, and being spontaneously aborted), it seems likely that the finding of ventricular enlargement in young male schizophrenic patients presenting with their first episode reflects some type of cerebral injury that occurred relatively early in life and created a cerebral substrate that was more vulnerable to the development of schizophrenia in later years.

Studies of mood disorders have been more equivocal. Unlike schizo-

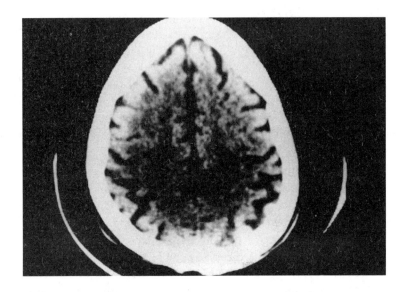

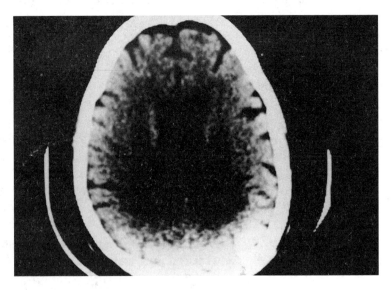

FIGURE 4–2. Computed tomography scan from an individual with schizophrenia. The slice on the **bottom** passes through the body of the ventricles and shows ventricular enlargement. Sulcal prominence is noted as well. The slice on the **top** is obtained from a higher level in the same individual brain and also shows prominent cortical sulci.

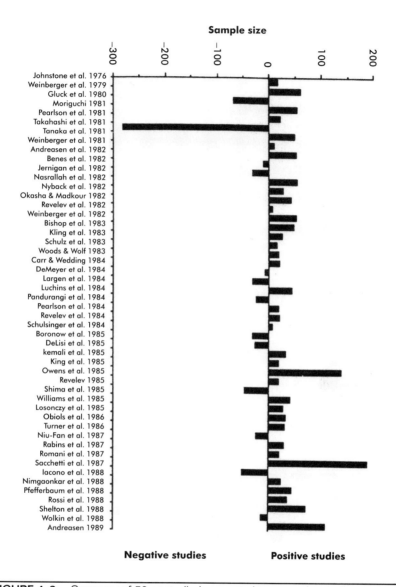

FIGURE 4–3. Summary of 50 controlled computed tomography studies evaluating the presence of ventricular enlargement in schizophrenia. Most of the studies reported ventricular enlargement.

Source. Reprinted from Andreasen NC, Swayze VW II, Flaum M, et al: "Ventricular Enlargement in Schizophrenia Evaluated With Computed Tomographic Scanning—Effects of Gender, Age, and Stage of Illness." *Archives of General Psychiatry* 47:1008–1015, 1990. Copyright 1990, American Medical Association. Used with permission.

phrenia, in which the preponderance of studies have indicated that the disorder is characterized by structural abnormalities, only about half of the studies of mood disorders have found abnormalities to be present. In general, sample sizes have been too small to evaluate age and gender effects. The existing data appear to suggest that a gender effect also exists in the presence of ventricular enlargement in patients with bipolar disorder, with males being more vulnerable. The ventricular enlargement seen in depressed patients may not exceed that which is normal for the aging process, making it appear that ventricular enlargement is not statistically increased in depressed patients when age is controlled for. This does not mean, of course, that ordering a CT scan is inappropriate in an elderly depressed patient because the differential diagnosis of dementia and depression is often a difficult one in this age group; a finding of substantial cortical atrophy and ventricular enlargement would definitely tip the balance in the direction of diagnosing dementia.

Magnetic Resonance Imaging

MRI has a substantial number of advantages over CT. The images produced through MRI are developed by placing the patient's brain or body in a magnetic field, which causes the hydrogen protons to be aligned and concentrates the force of the magnetic moment produced so that it is large enough to be measurable. Thereafter, the protons can be raised to a higher energy level through stimulation with a radiofrequency signal targeted to their own Larmor frequency; the relaxation, or decay, to the original energy state can then be measured as a signal that is produced from tissue voxels, much as in the case of CT.

Only a few risks are involved in the use of MRI scanning. Because of the presence of the magnetic field, patients whose bodies contain metal objects, such as aneurysm clips or metal plates in their skulls, cannot be imaged. Patients with pacemakers also must be excluded. Because patients must be placed inside a tubelike metal cavity to be scanned, there is some risk of experiencing claustrophobia. This can usually be minimized or eliminated with adequate patient preparation. A relatively new option is an open form of MRI that does not require the tube-like metal cavity; this may be advantageous for some patients.

In addition to being relatively risk-free, MRI has several other advantages. Unlike CT, whose images are limited to the transverse or transaxial plane, MRI permits reconstruction and visualization of images from the brain in all planes. Because of the brain's complex three-dimensional structure, multiple perspectives are very useful. Coronal cuts, in particular, are especially valuable for visualizing small subcortical structures of great interest to psychiatry, such as the caudate, putamen, amygdala, and hippocampus. Resolution is superb with MRI, producing "slices" of brain that look as if they were obtained in a pathology laboratory at postmortem. With CT scanning, it is difficult to see the posterior fossa because of the great density of bone in that region, but bony artifacts are not a problem with MRI, and posterior fossa structures are well visualized.

Both difficulties and advantages arise because many different imaging options are available. The technician can substantially change the type of pictures produced by altering imaging parameters such as repetition time or echo time. The actual image signal is a mixture of four components: the flow velocity, the proton density, and the relaxation of the protons in different three-dimensional planes (T1 and T2 relaxation times). Depending on the scanning sequence used, images can be weighted by enhancing the proton density component, the T1 component, or the T2 component. A scanning sequence may be selected to produce impressive anatomical resolution (e.g., a proton density image or a T1-weighted image), or a sequence may be selected that shows very poor anatomical resolution but displays clear, specific areas of tissue abnormality (e.g., T2-weighted images with a long echo time and repetition time).

Clinicians need to be aware of what they may be looking for when they decide to order an MRI scan. If they are looking for a tumor, multiple sclerosis plaques, or areas of microinfarction, they may prefer a T2-weighted image. If they are seeking a clear picture of the size and shape of the ventricles or the amygdala-hippocampus, they will prefer a T1-weighted image. The question to be answered should, therefore, be clearly stated on the order form used to request an MRI scan, so that the radiologist and technicians can use the appropriate sequence.

Advances in MRI technology now also permit clinicians to acquire MRI data three-dimensionally and to obtain very thin slices. This has created an opportunity to develop software that allows visualization of the surface anatomy of the brain through methods known as surface/volume rendering. Because the slices contain voxels that are "cubic" (i.e., about 1 mm in all three dimensions), the brain also can be resliced or resampled after acquisition. Clinicians with access to such software can now identify major landmarks on the brain surface, such as the central sulcus or sylvian fissure; cleave through planes to visualize regions such as the planum temporale or Heschl's gyrus; and resample their images so that they can simultaneously visualize the brain in three orthogonal planes. Figure 4–4 shows the ability to visualize brain surface anatomy and three orthogonal planes simultaneously by using image analysis software developed for this purpose in our Image Processing Laboratory at the University of Iowa in Iowa City. This software, BRAINS (Brain Research: Analysis of Images, Networks, and Systems), also permits automated measurements of subregions, measurement of surface features, and alignment of structural and functional images. Software of this type has essentially turned MRI into a tool that permits clinicians to do an anatomical postmortem in the antemortem state. Table 4–2 lists some of the basic problems inherent in the analysis and measurement of MRI images that are solved through the use of software such as BRAINS. Figure 4–5 illustrates its application to cleave along the sylvian fissure and to visualize the planum temporale in vivo.

TABLE 4–2.   Basic problems in image analysis

Defining boundaries of structures

Measuring volumes

Measuring physiological parameters (e.g., blood flow, receptor density)

Three-dimensional visualization

Integrating data from multiple modalities (e.g., magnetic resonance imaging, positron-emission tomography)

Because MRI is still a relatively new technique, generalizations about its clinical usefulness are in a continual state of evolution as new information is acquired. As might be expected, the presence of ventricular enlargement in schizophrenia also has been repeatedly confirmed with MRI. Various other specific anomalies also have been reported, such as partial agenesis of the callosum and decreased temporal lobe size. A summary of the types of abnormalities that have been observed in schizophrenia appears in Table 4–3. Figure 4–6 shows an image of a patient with schizophrenia who has agenesis of the corpus callosum. This is one of many different types of midline abnormalities or developmental anomalies that have an increased incidence in schizophrenia. Others include cavum septi pellucidi, ectopic gray matter, and changes in gray matter structures such as the thalamus or hippocampus. Many of these anomalies that have been seen with MRI are supported through independent observation of postmortem tissue and analyses of cell counts or cellular alignment.

Some patients with bipolar disorder have been reported to have an increased number of small regions of high signal intensity (referred to colloquially as *unidentified bright objects*). The clinical significance of unidentified bright objects is uncertain, both in bipolar disorder and in other syndromes

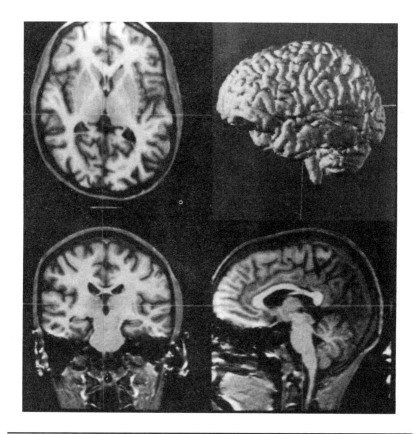

FIGURE 4–4.   A view of the brain surface, with resampling in three orthogonal planes, as produced by the software program BRAINS (Brain Research: Analysis of Images, Networks, and Systems). The capacity to simultaneously visualize anatomy in three planes and on the brain surface is extremely useful for understanding the interrelations between structures and their circuitry.

in which they are seen, such as the dementias; however, they almost certainly represent tiny areas of tissue loss, which result from microinfarctions in at least some cases.

Starvation, as occurs in anorexia nervosa and alcoholism, also often can result in characteristic abnormalities on MRI scan. Patients with anorexia who have fallen substantially below their normal weight typically have cortical atrophy, which reverses with adequate nutrition. An example of this process is shown in Figure 4–7. Younger alcoholic patients who are malnourished and dehydrated also may have reversible abnormal MRI findings. However, long-term severe alcohol abuse is likely to produce irreversible ab-

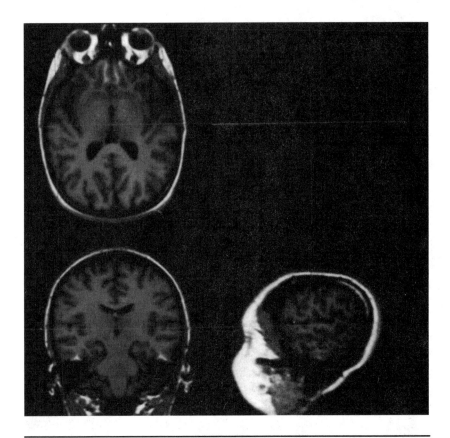

FIGURE 4–5.   A view of the planum temporale, produced by using the resampling feature of the software program BRAINS (Brain Research: Analysis of Images, Networks, and Systems). A plane has been drawn parallel to the sylvian fissure and the overlying parietal regions lifted off, much as would be done with a post-mortem dissection.

normalities. Maternal consumption of large quantities of alcohol during pregnancy may produce the fetal alcohol syndrome, which is characterized by craniofacial anomalies, decreased cerebral size, and sulcal/gyral anomalies such as pachygyria. A brain from a person with fetal alcohol syndrome is shown in Figure 4–8, along with a surface rendered from the brain of a person of similar age and gender who was not exposed in utero to alcohol for comparison. A variety of developmental anomalies also may be seen in individuals with autism.

The indications for ordering a structural imaging technique such as CT or MRI are summarized in Table 4–4. In general, clinicians will want to order

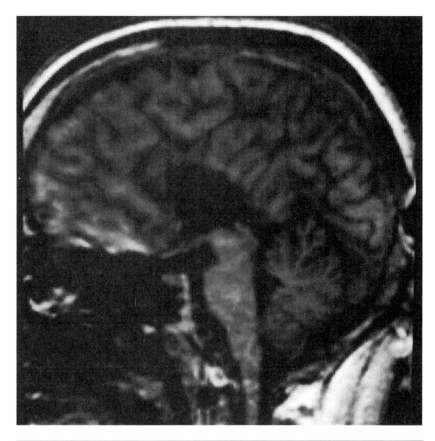

FIGURE 4–6. A midsagittal view of the brain from an individual with schizophrenia who has nearly complete agenesis of the corpus callosum.

one of these procedures when they need to rule out a physical cause for the patient's symptoms, such as a tumor or multiple sclerosis. Because of the rather substantial literature supporting the presence of structural abnormalities in schizophrenia, as well as their prognostic significance, it is probably appropriate to obtain a CT or an MRI scan in a young individual presenting with his or her first episode of psychosis. These techniques also may be used to monitor progressive loss of tissue in the dementias, as well as to observe the reversibility of structural changes in conditions such as anorexia nervosa or alcoholism.

As MRI has become increasingly available, physicians are faced with a decision as to whether to order a CT or an MRI first. Until recently, the choice was almost invariably CT, largely because of its wide availability and

TABLE 4–3.   Abnormalities commonly seen in schizophrenia

Ventricular enlargement

Prominent cortical sulci

Decreased cerebral size

Decreased frontal size

Decreased temporal size

Decreased hippocampal size

Decreased size of superior temporal gyrus

Decreased thalamic size

Increased caudate/putamen size

Midline developmental abnormalities

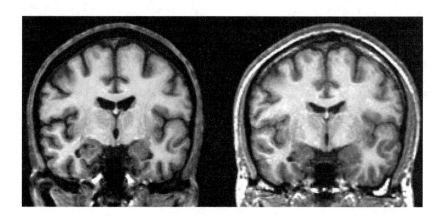

FIGURE 4–7.   A view of the brain surface and its internal contents shown in three orthogonal planes in an individual with anorexia nervosa. The image on the left shows the brain during starvation, and the image on the right shows the individual's brain after her weight had returned to normal. Note the reversal of brain shrinkage that occurs with weight normalization.

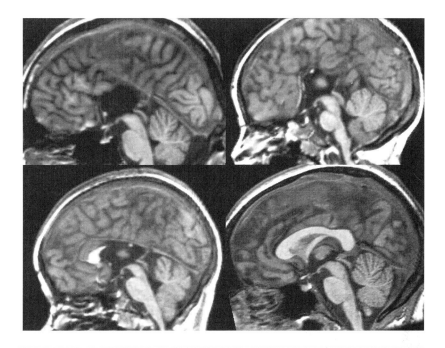

FIGURE 4–8. A view of the brain surface and its internal contents in an individual with fetal alcohol syndrome (**top**) and in a person of comparable age and gender who did not experience in utero exposure to alcohol (**bottom**). Note the marked decrease in cerebral size in the person with fetal alcohol syndrome.

inexpensiveness. Because MRI is a much superior imaging technique, however, it is has begun to supplant CT, particularly for the evaluation of psychiatric populations, in whom a detailed view of brain surface and subcortical regions may be very useful.

Functional Neuroimaging Techniques

The ability to visualize and measure the functional activity of the human brain has been one of the most exciting developments in psychiatry and neuroscience during the past decade. Although used relatively infrequently as clinical laboratory tests, these techniques have provided psychiatry with tools for understanding many facets of dysfunctional brain biology in mental illnesses. Because mental illnesses are in essence aberrations in mental phenomena (e.g., the occurrence of hallucinations, or the experience of a perception without a stimulus), they have provided psychiatry with an opportunity to identify the neural substrates of abnormal mental phenomena.

Through the extensive application of these functional imaging techniques during the past decade, we have learned a great deal about dysfunctions in neural circuitry that occur in mental illnesses. With the study of healthy volunteers, these techniques have also taught us a great deal about how the brain produces normal mental processes such as language, emotion, and consciousness.

TABLE 4–4.   Indications for ordering a computed tomography or magnetic resonance imaging scan

Confusion and/or dementia of unknown cause

First episode of a psychotic disorder of unknown etiology

First episode of a major mood disorder after age 50 years

Marked personality change after age 50 years

History of recent head trauma

Anorexia nervosa with marked weight loss

Alcoholism or other substance abuse disorder with signs or symptoms of cognitive deterioration

---

Functional neuroimaging includes three modalities: functional magnetic resonance (fMR), PET, and SPECT. All of these techniques are used to observe and measure regional metabolic and neurochemical functions and dysfunctions in the brain. fMR is used primarily to measure regional cerebral blood flow, although magnetic resonance techniques also can be used to examine chemical spectra in the brain regions (magnetic resonance spectroscopy [MRS]). SPECT is used to measure both regional cerebral blood flow and densities of neuroreceptors. PET was originally used to measure glucose utilization, as an indicator of brain metabolic activity. It is now used primarily to measure regional cerebral blood flow and density of neuroreceptors.

Functional Magnetic Resonance and Magnetic Resonance Spectroscopy

The recent expansion of magnetic resonance into the functional imaging domain has been a major breakthrough. Whereas conventional structural magnetic resonance depends on exploiting the paramagnetic properties of the hydrogen proton, fMR is based on the chemistry of hemoglobin, which is also paramagnetic. Essentially, fMR visualizes and measures the process of the conversion of hemoglobin to deoxyhemoglobin, an indicator of brain blood flow and, secondarily, brain metabolism. Because the human body has much less deoxyhemoglobin than hydrogen, the signal from deoxyhemoglobin is relatively weak. The ability to collect usable information from fMR depends, therefore, on increasing the signal-to-noise ratio by collecting the signal repetitively. Operationally, this means that a specific task is repeated multiple times. The ability to conduct fMR imaging depends not only on the recognition that deoxyhemoglobin can produce a magnetic resonance signal but also on the availability of high-speed computers that can process large amounts of numerical data.

Since the first magnetic resonance study of human mental activity was reported in *Science* in 1991, the technique has steadily improved. Early studies explored familiar territory. For example, visual and motor pathways in the brain are well understood. Therefore, the method was validated by demonstrating that the visual cortex will "light up" when a person looks at a flashing checkerboard. Likewise, the motor cortex is activated by tasks such as finger tapping, and one can see metabolic activity shift from the right hemisphere when the left finger is tapped to the left hemisphere when the right finger is tapped.

fMR is now the most widely used tool for the study of normal cognition and brain abnormalities in mental illnesses. fMR recently has been applied to study more complex mental functions such as memory, attention, emotion, and language perception and production. It has also been used to contrast brain metabolic activity in healthy volunteers with that in patients who have mental illnesses. Because fMR, like structural MRI, is relatively risk free, it has been particularly helpful for the study of children. fMR has now been used to examine brain abnormalities in childhood disorders such as hyperactivity and dyslexia. Brain dysfunctions in schizophrenia, mood disorders, and anxiety disorders also have been examined.

MRS is another extension of magnetic resonance technology to the functional domain. This application is similar to the use of MRS in physical chemistry. When MRS is applied to human functional neuroimaging, chemical spectra in the human brain can be visualized and measured. Any compound that contains a paramagnetic ion can be studied: phosphorus-31, carbon-13, fluorine-19, sodium-23, lithium-7, and hydrogen. Because MRS is somewhat more difficult to execute than fMR, the application of MRS to the study of mental illness is still in its infancy. However, MRS is a powerful tool for in vivo evaluation of brain chemistry. At present, it has been used for two purposes. First, MRS has been used to examine the composition of brain tissue in patients with mental illnesses to determine whether some type of pathological process is occurring. For example, several studies have reported abnormalities in the balance between phosphomonoesters (indicators of cell growth) and phosphodiesters (breakdown products reflecting neuronal decline or damage) in illnesses such as schizophrenia. Second, MRS has been used to study the brain uptake and metabolism of medications. For example, many psychoactive drugs contain carbon, fluorine, or lithium. As MRS continues to evolve, it may be used as an in vivo assay of drug uptake in the brain and provide a method for measuring dose-response characteristics.

Positron-Emission Tomography

PET scanning requires the use of radioactive isotopes, which must be synthesized on site. The tracers used are positrons (i.e., positively charged electrons), which are generated in a cyclotron and have short half-lives (2 minutes for oxygen-15, 30 minutes for carbon-11, approximately 2 hours for fluorine-18). Because of the technical requirements of an on-site cyclotron and a radiochemistry laboratory that can attach the positron-emitting isotopes to an informative molecule (e.g., glucose, a drug), PET is a relatively costly technique. Its clinical applications are limited, but it has been a workhorse tool in psychiatric research since the 1980s.

Its first application was the study of glucose utilization in the brain with fluorodeoxyglucose (FDG). Abnormal patterns of glucose utilization have been observed in a variety of disorders, such as seizures, tumors, stroke, Alzheimer's disease, schizophrenia, bipolar disorder, alcoholism and other forms of substance abuse, and obsessive-compulsive disorder. In addition, FDG was used in pioneering studies of cognitive activation, although this role has largely been ceded now to either fMR or PET studies of blood flow with a newer tracer, oxygen-15–labeled H_2O. FDG has important clinical applications in the presurgical evaluation of intractable seizures because it provides more specific focal localization than EEG. Studies of Alzheimer's disease have shown characteristic decreases in blood flow in posterior temporoparietal regions, which can sometimes be helpful in a differential diagnosis between Alzheimer's disease and depression.

Most PET studies of psychiatric and neurological patients during the past decade have used oxygen-15–labeled H_2O. It provides a measure of cerebral blood flow, which is closely linked to metabolic activity, so this tracer is now used to study the brain during the "resting" state and, more important, during a variety of mental tasks. Because oxygen-15 has a half-life of approximately 2 minutes, it can be used to take relatively short "snapshots" of mental activity over 20- to 40-second intervals, permitting repeated back-to-back studies. In these studies, the tasks are varied in small details, so that various kinds of mental activity can be divided into component parts. For example, the general construct of memory can be examined through multiple back-to-back studies within a single individual, with the tasks differing in their use of visual versus auditory memory or recall versus recognition. This technology has been widely used to map cognitive processes in healthy individuals and to determine the extent to which cognitive processing is disturbed in patients who have mental illnesses.

Studying the brain in persons with mental illness has led to many interesting findings. The most consistent theme in these studies is that one cannot localize a specific mental illness or a specific cognitive process to a single place. Instead, the brain works by using distributed circuits in which multiple and variable nodes are used depending on the nature of the task and the type of illness. For example, several investigators have examined patients with schizophrenia who were actively hallucinating. They found relatively expected flow abnormalities in the auditory temporal cortex but also observed abnormal flow in other interconnected regions, including the anterior cingulate and the thalamus. Although early studies of patients with schizophrenia that used FDG indicated decreased glucose utilization in prefrontal cortex, many more recent studies that used oxygen-15–labeled H_2O have indicated other abnormalities as well, with relatively consistent changes in thalamus, anterior cingulate, and cerebellum. Oxygen-15–labeled H_2O also has been used to study emotional processing in patients with mood disorders or anxiety disorders. These studies also have implicated a variety of regional circuit abnormalities, particularly in interconnected limbic areas such as the amygdala, hippocampus, anterior cingulate, and inferior frontal lobes.

One of the most important applications of PET has been the study of neurochemical systems in the brain. Most of these studies have labeled neuroreceptors with ligands that are well characterized pharmacologically and known to produce relatively specific blockade of receptor sites, such as the D_2 receptor or the serotonin type 2 (5-HT_2) receptor. For example, carbon-11 raclopride is a widely used ligand that permits quantitative measurement of D_2 receptor density. Early applications of this method involved mapping the distribution of neurochemical systems in the human brain and attempts to find abnormalities in receptor density in specific mental illnesses such as schizophrenia. More recently, however, the method has been applied to the study of dose-response relationships with very interesting results. These studies have indicated that a conventional antipsychotic drug, such as haloperidol, produces nearly complete blockade of D_2 receptors (considered to be the primary target of antipsychotic treatment for many years) in relatively small doses (approximately 6 mg). Other newer atypical antipsychotics, such as risperidone, also produce nearly complete blockade of D_2 receptors in low doses (approximately 4 mg) and also block 5-HT$_2$ receptors.

These research studies have had a major clinical effect because they have indicated that smaller doses of medications can produce a therapeutic effect. Clinicians have now reduced doses of antipsychotics from relatively high levels (e.g., 20 mg or more of haloperidol only a few years ago) to much lower doses, based on the evidence from these PET studies. In addition, these studies have been helpful in predicting doses at which extrapyramidal side effects are likely to occur. It has been established that a blockade of greater than 70%–80% is highly likely to produce significant extrapyramidal side effects.

Single Photon Emission Computed Tomography

The basic principles of both SPECT and PET are the same. They involve imaging the localization of radioactive isotopes in areas of high functional activity in the brain. In the case of SPECT, the isotopes are single photon emitters. These isotopes, such as technetium-99 and iodine-123, are stable and have relatively long half-lives. This characteristic makes them convenient for long-term storage and relatively handy to use. However, these molecules are not normally present in the human body, and they are relatively difficult to attach to informative compounds to make them suitable as imaging agents. When they are attached, there is some risk that the biological activity of the compound will be changed because of the introduction of the foreign isotope.

Whereas PET is costly and complex, SPECT offers convenience and ease of use as its major strengths. SPECT studies usually require the use of a triple-headed rotating gamma camera of the sort available in most nuclear medicine departments. Because the blood flow agents such as hexamethyl-propyleneamine oxime (HMPAO) are commercially available as well, SPECT is an imaging technique that can be used for evaluating psychiatric patients as needed.

SPECT has several clinical applications. It is well suited for documenting the occurrence of stroke because it provides a direct measure of cerebral blood flow. In addition, SPECT is often diagnostically useful for the differential diagnosis of depression and dementia in elderly patients. Patients with Alzheimer's disease have a relatively characteristic decrease in cerebral blood flow in posterior temporoparietal regions, whereas patients with depression have normal flow, a generalized decrease, or decreases in anterior regions. In any case, the flow patterns observed in Alzheimer's disease are relatively characteristic, reflecting the initial localization of plaques and tangles in temporal regions before the disease progresses and produces more widespread brain involvement. Patients with HIV-related dementia begin to develop patchy areas of decreased perfusion when the symptoms of dementia begin.

SPECT also has been adapted to the imaging of neuroreceptors. Although this application is currently used primarily for research, it offers the long-term possibility of providing a clinical test to track receptor blockade, adjust medication doses, and monitor for indicators of the development of tardive dyskinesia. Iodine-123 β–CIT is the tracer that has been developed to measure dopamine function. This tracer has been used to study the activity of the dopamine system in various disorders, including schizophrenia and substance abuse. In addition, a benzodiazepine tracer, iodine-123 iomazenil, also is available and has been used to study this neurochemical system in disorders such as substance abuse.

Neuroendocrine Techniques

Some mental illnesses, such as depression or anxiety disorders, have a variety of symptoms that suggest some type of neuroendocrinological abnormality. Just as frontal lobe tumor or TLE is important in the differential diagnosis of schizophrenia (thereby suggesting the importance of frontal and temporal abnormalities in that illness), so too adrenal and thyroid diseases provide important differential diagnoses for depression and anxiety disorders. Depression, in particular, has many symptoms suggestive of chronobiological dysregulation: insomnia, anorexia, and disrupted diurnal variation.

This recognition has been supported by nearly four decades of research in neuropsychoendocrinology. This research necessarily confronted many difficult methodological problems because of the well-recognized effects of stress on the endocrine system and the resultant difficulty in separating cause from effect. Nevertheless, a picture has emerged suggesting that some patients with major mental illnesses show clear neuroendocrine abnormalities.

One laboratory test that developed out of this research was the dexamethasone suppression test (DST) to assist in the diagnosis of depression. Typically, 1 mg of dexamethasone is given at 11:00 P.M., and blood samples are drawn the next day at 8:00 A.M., 4:00 P.M., and 11:00 P.M. If the patient "breaks through" the dexamethasone suppression, showing a serum cortisol level greater than 5 μg/dL, the test is considered positive. Approximately 40% of depressed patients have a positive ("abnormal") DST result; unfortunately, positive DST results are seen in many conditions, such as anorexia nervosa and other disorders characterized by weight loss. Although psychiatrists for a time hoped that they might have a relatively sensitive and specific laboratory test for severe depression, this is clearly not the case.

IQ Testing

IQ testing is a relatively simple "laboratory test" that has been used in psychiatry for many years. Generally, IQ testing is done with one of two standard tests: the Wechsler Adult Intelligence Scale—Revised (WAIS-R) or the Wechsler Intelligence Scale for Children—Revised (WISC-R). Both of these tests are revisions, developed in 1981 and 1974, respectively, based on earlier tests developed by David Wechsler in the 1950s.

These tests consist of 11 subscales, summarized in Table 4–5. Six of these tests measure verbal abilities, and five are considered performance tests. These tests are well normed, and the scoring has been devised so that the average individual will achieve a score of 100.

TABLE 4–5.   Subscales of the Wechsler Adult Intelligence Scale—Revised

Verbal tests	Performance tests
Information	Picture completion
Digit span	Picture arrangement
Vocabulary	Block design
Arithmetic	Object assembly
Comprehension	Digit symbol
Similarities	

Although the WAIS-R and WISC-R are frequently referred to as intelligence tests, and are used to generate Verbal, Performance, and Full-Scale IQs, their most powerful application is to observe the patterning of intellectual abilities that is reflected on the 11 subscales. Most psychiatrically normal individuals tend to have similar scores on all the subtests. Individuals who have various psychopathological conditions can show deviations from this pattern. For example, with normal aging, scores on the verbal items tend to remain relatively high, whereas scores on the performance items tend to decline; these are sometimes referred to as "hold" and "don't hold" tests because of their characteristic changes with aging. When an elderly individual shows very poor performance on both the verbal and the performance tests to a degree inconsistent with his or her past education, this pattern of findings is consistent with the diagnosis of dementia. Because motivation, attention, and effort are important parts of IQ testing, however, poor performance may be relatively nonspecific. A depressed individual also may perform poorly on the verbal tests because of disinterest and apathy, although typically these tests are affected less by depression than are the performance tests.

IQ testing also can be quite helpful in evaluating children and adolescents. The test may provide some index to specific intellectual deficits that may be interfering with the child's capacity to perform well in school. Again, erratic patterns are particularly helpful in assessment. For example, a child with specific learning disabilities may be performing very poorly in school, yet have normal or even high intelligence, indicating that he or she has the basic intellectual capacity to perform at a normal or high level if the specific learning disabilities can be minimized (e.g., reading disability, mathematics disability). Children with conduct disorders typically have higher scores on the performance tests than on the verbal tests.

Personality Testing

The most widely used personality test is the Minnesota Multiphasic Personality Inventory (MMPI), developed in the 1940s. The MMPI generates scores on nine scales: hypochondriasis, depression, hysteria, psychopathic deviance, masculinity/femininity, paranoia, psychasthenia (or anxiety), schizophrenia, and mania.

The MMPI was developed empirically, with the original intent of creating a measure of psychopathology. A list of symptom items was generated and then given to individuals with diagnoses of the various conditions that the scales measure. Psychiatrically normal individuals also were assessed. When groups of patients with a specific condition such as paranoia assented to specific items to a degree that differentiated them significantly from psychiatrically normal individuals, those items were considered to be markers for that diagnosis. For example, patients with diagnoses of schizophrenia often scored "yes" on the item "I sometimes think about things too terrible to mention."

The MMPI was originally developed to aid in diagnosis, but its widest use at present is more descriptive than diagnostic. As in the case of the WAIS-R, clinicians can learn much more by looking at profiles and patterns than they can by looking at a single peak. Thus, for example, a patient who is depressed may indeed score high on the depression scale, but a high score on the psychasthenia scale may suggest that the patient's depressive symptoms are largely neurotic and likely to be chronic. High scores on scales 1 and 3 (hypochondriasis and hysteria) coupled with a low score on scale 2 (depression) are consistent with acting-out personality disorders that are likely to be difficult to treat. Patients who score high on the hysteria, psychopathic deviance, and mania scales also are likely to have difficult personality problems (e.g., antisocial personality disorder, borderline personality disorder).

Although the MMPI is the most widely used personality inventory, several other tests have been developed. The Cattell-16 PF was developed as a more "pure" personality test because it did not attempt to base its profiles on individuals with diagnosed psychopathology. Rather, various psychiatrically normal individuals were evaluated with a preselected set of items; subsequently, the items were subjected to factor analysis, yielding a profile consisting of 16 personality factors. The Eysenck Personality Inventory, a more modest instrument, also was developed through factor analysis. It measures the dimensions of introversion, extraversion, and neuroticism. Although the Cattell-16 PF and the Eysenck Personality Inventory are sometimes used in personality research, the MMPI remains the most widely used instrument in clinical settings.

Neuropsychological Testing

Neuropsychological testing was developed as a method for assessing cognitive deficits believed to be neurally based. Originally, as was the case for the MMPI and the WAIS-R, assessment batteries were developed in the hope that they would assist in making a specific diagnosis. The premier example is the Halstead-Reitan Neuropsychological Test Battery, originally developed to assist in the differential diagnosis of dementia and specific neurological conditions. Again, it has become increasingly clear that no single test can bear the burden of making specific diagnoses that clinicians themselves find difficult to make. Thus, the area of neuropsychology also has turned recently toward the goal of examining profiles and patterns and attempting to identify specific kinds of abnormality.

Increasingly, neuropsychology attempts to assess a variety of specific cognitive functions, such as memory, attention, and fluency of thinking. A clinician assessing patients neuropsychologically will tailor the assessment to the types of problems that the specific patient is having to try to identify whether a specific area of deficit is present.

For example, a group of tests is available to assess aphasia. These evaluate the patient's capacity to comprehend verbal and written information, to follow commands, to process syntactically versus semantically, and to speak fluently. When a comprehensive assessment for aphasia is completed, the clinician can define the patient's specific areas of deficit. For example, he or she will be able to indicate that the patient has impaired fluency of expression and poor syntactic expression but intact syntactic comprehension, a pattern consistent with a posterior frontal lesion.

In addition, various specific neuropsychological tests are often used to assess other specific aspects of mental functions. Some of the most common, categorized according to the function they are thought to assess most prominently, are described below.

Attention

Attention may be impaired in dementia, psychotic disorders, or a variety of other mental illnesses, including mood disorders.

Continuous Performance Test (CPT). The CPT is perhaps the most widely used test of attention currently available. The CPT was originally developed to detect deficits in sustained alertness in patients with brain damage. Several different versions of this task are available, but most involve attentional tasks in which patients observe series of letters or numbers that are presented very briefly one at a time, with a relatively short interval in between, and the subject is asked to press a button each time a predesignated target stimulus appears in a random series.

Trail Making Test Part A and B. The trail making tests are widely used components of the Halstead-Reitan Neuropsychological Test Battery used to assess attention and sequencing. The individual is asked to connect items in a series (e.g., A to 1, B to 2) from among items randomly selected on a page.

Executive Functions

Executive functions are considered to be "higher cortical functions" and involve decision making, planning, and changing strategies for abstraction or conceptualizing. These functions are particularly likely to be impaired in dementia but also may be involved in schizophrenia. Although abnormalities may be noted in the mood disorders, they are likely to be reversible.

Wisconsin Card Sorting Test. This test is widely regarded as an important test for assessing problem-solving abilities and the capacity to alter response set. The test involves sorting cards according to color, shape, or number. Intermittently, the individual is corrected while using a sorting strategy and at that point must recognize that he or she needs to shift response set.

Stroop Test. The Stroop Test assesses capacity to shift response set, as well as attention and mental control.

Porteus Mazes Test. Porteus Mazes is a standard maze test, in which the ability of the subject to plan is challenged by the task of figuring out a path between the entrance and the exit of a maze.

Tower of London. The Tower of London is a planning task that requires the subject to develop a strategy for moving balls lined up on sticks from an initial position to a final goal position.

Fluency

Many patients with schizophrenia or depression have an impaired ability to generate spontaneous ideas or activities. Important clinical correlates are symptoms such as alogia and avolition. Several tests are used to assess fluency, which is also often considered a "frontal" function.

Controlled Oral Word Association Test. The Controlled Oral Word Association Test assesses the subject's verbal fluency by providing probes, such as asking the subject to name as many words as possible that start with the letter *D*. This test has been widely used as part of the Multilingual Aphasia Examination.

Category Fluency Test. The Category Fluency Test assesses the subject's fluency by asking him or her to name as many words as possible that belong to a specific semantic category (e.g., animals, fruits, vegetables). One minute is allowed for each category.

Verbal Memory

Because verbal memory is an important temporolimbic function, it may be important to assess its dimensions in patients with a variety of mental illnesses, especially dementia.

Logical memory (Wechsler Memory Scale). The Wechsler Memory Scale involves having the subject listen to a coherent story and then recall as many details of the story as possible. Both immediate and delayed recall are assessed.

Rey Auditory Verbal Learning Test. This test involves determining the subject's capacity to learn a list of words by rote. Both immediate memory and delayed recall are assessed. A learning curve also is established.

Paired Associate Learning. This somewhat more complicated memory task asks the subject to learn a list of words that are associated with a cue set of words (e.g., metal-iron, baby-cries).

Visual Reconstructive Memory

The following tests of visual reconstructive memory are frequently considered to assess right hemisphere function.

Rey-Osterreith Complex Figure. The Rey-Osterreith Complex Figure involves showing a complex figure to the subject, having him or her copy it, and having him or her draw it again from memory immediately and after a delay. Although this task is somewhat difficult to administer, it can be given in a reliable and standardized way by giving the subject colored pencils in a set sequence.

Benton Visual Retention Test. The widely used Benton Visual Retention Test examines the ability to copy and recall a variety of figures and shapes. (See Figure 4–9 for an illustration of one of the figures that the subject is asked to remember and draw.)

Working Memory

Working memory is defined as the capacity to hold information in a short-term buffer and to use it to perform a mental task. The classic example of working memory is learning a telephone number just long enough to dial it. After this process has been completed, the information is erased from the memory buffer. Working memory is impaired in a variety of mental illnesses, particularly schizophrenia.

Digit Span Test. The ability to recall a string of digits is a relatively simple clinical test of working memory, although it does not require the actual performance of "work." In a clinical setting, the clinician can use digit span to test for working memory by giving a patient increasingly long lists of digits that can be recalled either forward or backward.

N-back test. In an N-back test, the person is exposed to sequential pieces of information, with a set amount of time elapsing between each presentation. He or she is then asked to recall the information given just before the most recent presentation (a one-back test), the information two times before the most recent presentation (a two-back test), and so on. The N-back test has been used extensively in neuroimaging studies. A simple clinical N-back

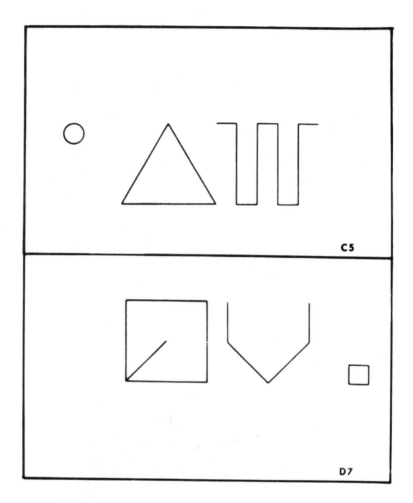

FIGURE 4–9. Examples of figures that patients are asked to copy and recall on the Benton Visual Retention Test.

test also can be used at the bedside by presenting the patient with a predetermined set of materials, such as lists of words or digits.

Motor Function

It may be important to assess motor function in patients with mental illnesses, both because motor slowness may be a correlate of some diagnoses such as depression and because of the motor side effects of antipsychotic medications.

Finger Oscillation Test. The Finger Oscillation Test measures tapping speed with the left and right hands. It gives a measure of overall motor speed as well as an assessment of lateral asymmetries in motor performance.

Purdue Pegboard Test. The Purdue Pegboard Test was developed to assess manual dexterity. Fine motor performance is assessed with the right hand, the left hand, and then both hands simultaneously. It provides a useful measure of lateralization.

Clinical Utility of Neuropsychological Tests

When a group of neuropsychological tests such as those described above is administered to an individual, the clinician obtains some sense of the person's overall patterns of abilities and deficits. Patients who have psychosis or depression often have a generalized impairment on all tests, although patients with schizophrenia may have specific regional deficits (e.g., frontal deficits) depending on their symptoms. Tests of verbal versus visual memory can be used to compare left and right hemisphere function and to isolate patterns of abnormality within a single hemisphere. Tests of memory are particularly useful in evaluating dementia and depression. Although depressed patients may score somewhat poorly on all tests because of a lack of interest and motivation, they typically do not have highly selective memory deficits. Following up a patient's performance on these tests over time also may assist in diagnosis because an improvement in performance accompanied by a clinical improvement in symptoms is supportive of the diagnosis of a reversible mental disorder, such as depression (as opposed to a dementia, in which a progressive course would be expected).

Bibliography

American Psychiatric Association: Diagnostic and Statistical Manual of Mental Disorders, 4th Edition. Washington, DC, American Psychiatric Association, 1994

American Psychiatric Association: Diagnostic and Statistical Manual of Mental Disorders, 4th Edition Text Revision. Washington, DC, American Psychiatric Association, 2000

Andreasen NC: Brain imaging: applications in psychiatry. Science 239:1381–1388, 1988

Andreasen NC: Brain Imaging, in American Psychiatric Press Review of Psychiatry, Vol 12. Edited by Oldham JM, Riba MB, Tasman A. Washington, DC, American Psychiatric Press, 1993, pp 309–511

Belliveau JW, Kennedy DN, McKinstry RC, et al: Functional mapping of the human visual cortex by magnetic resonance imaging. Science 254:716–719, 1991

Elster AD (ed): Magnetic Resonance Imaging: A Reference Guide and Atlas. Philadelphia, PA, JB Lippincott, 1986

Frackowiak RSJ, Friston KJ, Frith CD, et al: Human Brain Function. San Diego, CA, Academic Press, 1997

Gold PW, Goodwin FK, Chrousos GP: Clinical and biochemical manifestations of depression: relation to the neurobiology of stress, part 1. N Engl J Med 319:348–353, 1988

Gold PW, Goodwin FK, Chrousos GP: Clinical and biochemical manifestations of depression: relation to the neurobiology of stress, part 2. N Engl J Med 319:413–420, 1988

Kapur S, Zipursky R, Jones C, et al: Relationship between dopamine D_2 occupancy, clinical response, and side effects: a double-blind PET study of first episode schizophrenia. Am J Psychiatry 157:514–520, 2000

Kooi KA: Fundamentals of Electroencephalography. New York, Harper & Row, 1971

Krishnan KRR, Doraiswamy PM (eds): Brain Imaging in Clinical Psychiatry. New York, Marcel Dekker, 1997

Latchaw RE, Ugurbil K, Hu X: Functional MR imaging of perceptual and cognitive functions. Neuroimaging Clin N Am 5:193–205, 1995

Lezak MD: Neuropsychological Assessment, 3rd Edition. New York, Oxford University Press, 1990

Mazziotta JC, Toga AW, Frackowiak RSJ: Brain Mapping: The Disorders. San Diego, CA, Academic Press, 2000

Ogawa S, Lee T-M, Kay AR, et al: Brain magnetic resonance imaging with contrast dependent on blood oxygenation. Proc Natl Acad Sci U S A 87:9868–9872, 1990

Petersen SE, Fox PT, Posner MI, et al: Positron emission tomographic studies of the processing of single words. J Cogn Neurosci 1:153–170, 1989

Raz N, Gunning FM, Head D, et al: Selective aging of the human cerebral cortex observed in vivo: differential vulnerability of the prefrontal gray matter. Cereb Cortex 7:268–282, 1997

Reynolds CF, Kupfer DJ: Sleep research in affective illness: state of the art circa 1987. Sleep 10:199–215, 1987

Ribeiro SCM, Tandon R, Gruenhaus L, et al: The DST as a predictor of outcome in depression: a meta-analysis. Am J Psychiatry 150:1618–1629, 1993

Salibi N, Brown MA: Clinical MR Spectroscopy. New York, Wiley-Liss, 1998

Sedvall G, Farde L, Persson A, et al: Imaging of neurotransmitter receptors in the living human brain. Arch Gen Psychiatry 43:995–1005, 1986

Smith RC, Lange RC: Understanding Magnetic Resonance Imaging. Boca Raton, FL, CRC Press, 1997

Yudoksky SC, Hales RE (eds): The American Psychiatric Press Textbook of Neuropsychiatry, 3rd Edition. Washington, DC, American Psychiatric Press, 1997

Self-Assessment Questions

1. What are some of the conditions that must be considered in the differential diagnosis of serious mental illnesses? Describe ways in which
laboratory tests can be used in ruling out these disorders.
2. Describe the workup usually required prior to ECT.
3. Describe some special techniques that may be necessary to enhance the
power of EEG, particularly to detect seizure foci deep within the brain.
What is polysomnography?
4. Describe some applications of structural imaging techniques such as
CT scanning or MRI to the study of mental illnesses such as schizophrenia. Why must the clinician carefully specify the question that he
or she is asking before ordering an MRI scan?
5. What is *functional neuroimaging?* Describe some applications of functional neuroimaging to the evaluation of psychiatric patients.
6. What is the most widely used test to assess personality? What are its
major clinical applications?
7. What is *neuropsychological testing?* Name four different neuropsychological tests, and describe the cognitive functions that they are designed
to assess.

5 The Neurobiology of Mental Illness

Men ought to know that from the brain, and from the
brain only, arise our pleasures, joys, laughter, and jests,
as well as our sorrows, pains, griefs, and fears. Through
it, in particular, we think, see, hear...

Hippocrates

Understanding the machinery of our brains and minds occurs on many levels. While talking with patients and attempting to understand how their symptoms arise from the brain and mind, the student of psychiatry must think on many levels simultaneously. This challenge to achieve distributed parallel processing in real time while formulating a treatment plan that will relieve distressing symptoms is one of the things that makes psychiatry so interesting. Figure 5–1 summarizes this concept.

Psychiatry as a discipline begins with abnormal thoughts, feelings, experiences, and behavior. Understanding these abnormalities requires that we understand the mechanisms of normal behavior. Normal behavior must be conceptualized as the consequence of functional brain systems that mediate language, perception, memory, attention, emotion, and other mental systems. These functional mind/brain systems are more or less "hardwired" in the normal adult brain, although they are plastic and dynamic in the young developing brain.

The *functional* systems are the product of a set of *neural* systems or networks that communicate with one another electrically and chemically. Although the circuits within these neural networks also may be more or less

133

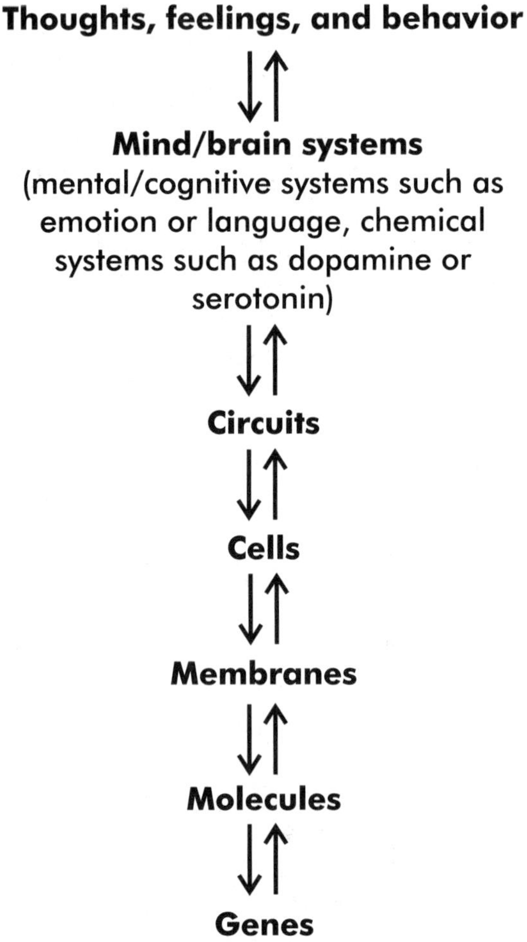

Thoughts, feelings, and behavior
↓↑

Mind/brain systems
(mental/cognitive systems such as
emotion or language, chemical
systems such as dopamine or
serotonin)
↓↑

Circuits
↓↑

Cells
↓↑

Membranes
↓↑

Molecules
↓↑

Genes

FIGURE 5–1.   A multilevel approach to understanding mental illnesses.

hardwired in the mature adult brain, in that long tracts and connections are established, the neurochemical circuits of the brain appear to be highly adaptable and subject to multiple modulatory influences and feedback loops. These neural circuits are in turn composed of cells that communicate with one another through chemical messengers such as dopamine, which in turn communicate through second-messenger systems. Instructions for synthesizing and metabolizing the molecular messengers of the mind are coded in the neuron's DNA within its nucleus, as are instructions for synthesizing the complex proteins that form the receptors embedded in cell membranes that serve as transducers for the molecular messengers. During the past several years, many of these receptors have been cloned, opening up the possibility that we can improve the medications that modulate brain chemistry.

Thus, psychiatry stretches from mind to molecule and from clinical neurobiology to molecular neurobiology as it attempts to understand how aberrations in thinking, behavior, and emotions are rooted in underlying biological mechanisms. Abnormalities in DNA can be studied directly through the developing techniques of molecular biology and molecular genetics, whereas the genetic transmission of illnesses within families must be determined through clinical assessment of affected and unaffected individuals. This process brings us back full circle from the molecule to the mind and from the laboratory to the clinic.

The upcoming decade will be an interesting and exciting time for students of psychiatry of all ages. Although we do not as yet have a complete map of the human brain that summarizes its various circuits, functions, and chemical anatomy, the maturation of neuroimaging technology during the past 10 years has substantially advanced our knowledge. In vivo imaging of brain structure and function has yielded substantial amounts of information that have led to a steady revision of earlier concepts and models that were based solely on lesion methods and postmortem data. Directly visualizing how the brain performs mental work during a functional magnetic resonance or positron-emission tomography (PET) imaging procedure is clearly more accurate than trying to infer indirectly how the brain/mind works by observing what it cannot do when parts are missing.

The process of "mapping the brain" is complemented by the process of "mapping the human genome." Both of these processes will be ongoing during the first decade of the twenty-first century. As information describing the brain at the level of systems (collected through in vivo neuroimaging) joins information from the level of molecules (collected through programs such as the Human Genome Project), enormous advances are certain to occur in our understanding of the mechanisms producing mental illness. This will lead both to improved treatments and to preventive measures. In this chapter, we provide a selective overview of a few topics from neurobiology that are relevant to understanding the effect these advances will have on the practice of psychiatry during the next few years.

Anatomical and Functional Brain Systems

The human brain can be divided into various systems that mediate many different cognitive, emotional, and perceptual functions, such as the motor system, the visual system, the auditory system, and the somatosensory cortical system. The systems that are of special interest to psychiatry are those that are particularly disturbed in mental illnesses. These systems represent some of the last frontiers in the study of the human brain. Four important anatomical systems are the prefrontal system, the limbic system, the basal ganglia system, and cerebellar feedback loops. Important functional systems include memory, language, attention, and executive functions.

Any method for dividing the brain into parts or systems is somewhat arbitrary. Anatomical systems are interconnected with one another and work interactively. Functional systems are also highly interdependent with one another and with the prefrontal, limbic, and basal ganglia systems as well. Furthermore, the division of the brain into anatomical and functional systems and neurochemical systems is also arbitrary. These oversimplifications are introduced purely for conceptual convenience, providing a strategy for reducing the overwhelming complexity of the central nervous system (CNS) to a level that permits discussion and analysis. Ultimately, however, a full understanding of the brain can be gained only by an ongoing process of analysis (or breakdown and simplification) and synthesis (or rebuilding and unifying).

The Prefrontal System and Executive Functions

The prefrontal system, or prefrontal cortex, is one of the largest cortical subregions in the human brain. Brodmann estimated that it constitutes 29% of the cortex in humans compared with 17% in chimpanzees, 7% in dogs, and 3.5% in cats. The relative development of the prefrontal cortex in various animal species is shown in Figure 5–2.

Because of the extraordinary development of the prefrontal cortex in humans, its function has been a focus of both speculation and investigation for many years. The lesion method provided an early landmark in the understanding of the prefrontal cortex through the case of Phineas Gage, a quarry worker who was accidentally injured by an explosion that drove an iron bar through his left frontal lobe. Gage survived the bizarre accident, but he sustained major personality changes, which were originally described by Harlow. Before the accident, Gage was conscientious, serious, and hardworking, but after the accident, he became immature, childlike, socially inappropriate, and irresponsible. This early initial report has been supplemented by a substantial literature based on studies of patients with frontal lobe tumors, traumatic injuries to the frontal lobes, and surgical treatments for epilepsy, psychosis, and obsessive-compulsive disorder. This work clearly indicates

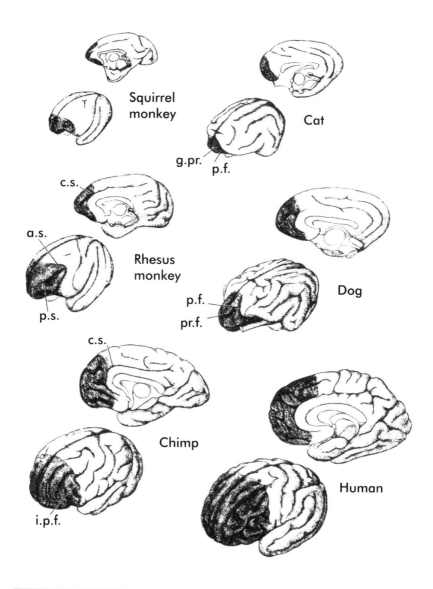

FIGURE 5–2. Phylogenetic development of the prefrontal cortex.
a.s.=arcuate sulcus; c.s.=cingulate sulcus; g.pr.=gyrus proreus; i.p.f.=inferior pre-central fissure; p.f.=presylvian fissure; pr.f.=proreal fissure; p.s.=principal sulcus.
Source. Reprinted from Fuster JM (ed): *The Prefrontal Cortex: Anatomy, Physiology, and Neuropsychology of the Frontal Lobes,* 2nd Edition. New York, Raven Press, 1989. Used with permission.

that substantial damage to the prefrontal cortex typically produces a syndrome quite similar to that of Gage. Although gross intelligence is not necessarily impaired by frontal lobe lesions (and actually may be improved in patients with severe psychosis), individuals with substantial frontal lobe injury lose other capacities such as volition, the ability to plan, and social judgment.

These clinical studies of humans have been supplemented during recent years by substantial neurophysiological studies of nonhuman primates that used techniques of neurophysiology, neuroanatomy, and neurochemistry. Primate studies have reinforced the conclusions from the earlier clinical work, indicating that the prefrontal cortex subserves a variety of major functions that permit us to integrate information from various sources, to plan and make decisions, and to generate new thoughts and ideas.

The prefrontal cortex is a massive association cortex receiving connections from all over the brain. An oversimplified schematic "wiring diagram" of its multiple connections is shown in Figure 5–3. Although the prefrontal cortex has been defined in many ways, perhaps the most widely accepted definition is based on its thalamic connections. According to this definition, the *prefrontal cortex* is the anterior (or rostral) brain region that receives projections from the medial dorsal nucleus of the thalamus. This definition identifies more or less homologous brain regions across a variety of species. In primates, the morphological boundaries are the arcuate sulcus, the inferior precentral sulcus, and the anterior cingulate gyrus. The cortical region thus defined typically has six layers, with pyramidal cells in layers three and five and granular cortex in layer four. In the more inferior portions of the prefrontal cortex, however, layer four becomes transitional.

The interconnections of the prefrontal cortex provide some clues about its functions. The medial dorsal thalamic projections have two components: magnocellular and parvicellular. The magnocellular component projects principally to the orbital and medial portions of the prefrontal cortex, whereas the parvicellular component projects to the dorsolateral portion of the prefrontal cortex. These different projections appear to be related to differences in function in these two parts of the prefrontal cortex. Two quite different types of frontal syndromes have been observed. Lesions to the orbital region of the prefrontal cortex tend to produce euphoria, hyperkinesis, and inappropriate social behavior, whereas lesions to the dorsolateral portion produce apathy, hypokinesis, and impaired cognitive performance.

The prefrontal cortex has reciprocal connections with most other parts of the neocortex, including somatic, auditory, and visual regions, suggesting that the prefrontal cortex is responsible for integrating information from a

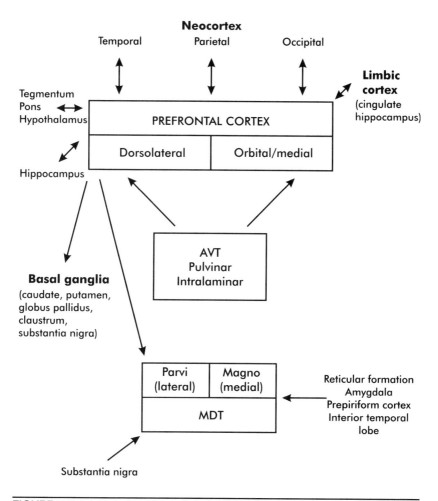

FIGURE 5–3. Interconnections of the prefrontal cortex.
AVT=anterior ventral thalamus; MDT=medial dorsal thalamus.
Source. Copyright 1986 Nancy C. Andreasen.

variety of sensory modalities. It also has direct reciprocal connections with the hippocampus and amygdala, indicating that it may play some role in integrating learning and memory, and with three other thalamic nuclei (anterior ventral, intralaminar, and pulvinar) and the tegmentum, pons, substantia nigra, and septal area. Although these connections are reciprocal, the prefrontal cortex is the only cortical region that sends direct projections to the hypothalamus and septal regions, suggesting a major role for the prefrontal cortex in the regulation of limbic functions. In addition, the orbitomedial portion of the prefrontal cortex sends direct, and unreciprocated, projections to the basal ganglia (caudate, putamen, globus pallidus, claustrum, and substantia nigra). These projections appear to be excitatory (i.e., glutamatergic); because of the possible importance of the dopamine-rich basal ganglia in mediating the symptoms of psychosis, and in developing side effects to long-term neuroleptic treatment such as tardive dyskinesia, this particular set of efferent fibers may suggest the mechanism by which the prefrontal cortex could interact with the basal ganglia and the thalamus to produce psychotic symptoms.

The above survey of anatomical connections suggests some of the functions of the prefrontal cortex. It is clearly a huge association region in the brain that integrates input from much of the neocortex, limbic regions, hypothalamic and brain-stem regions, and (via the thalamus) most of the rest of the brain. Its high degree of development in humans suggests that it may mediate a variety of specifically human functions often referred to as *executive functions,* such as high-order abstract thought, creative problem solving, and the temporal sequencing of behavior.

Lesion and trauma studies, supplemented by experimental studies in nonhuman primates, have substantially added to this view of the functions of the prefrontal cortex. It is now clear that the prefrontal cortex mediates numerous functions, including attention and perception, motility, temporal integration, and affect and emotion. Lesions to the prefrontal cortex can produce lowering of awareness, sensory neglect, distractibility, disorders of visual search and gaze control, difficulty in concentrating, hyperkinesis or hypokinesis (depending on the site of the lesion), difficulty in planning and completing sequential acts, difficulty in organizing speech, defective memory, defective control of interference, defective planning, and abnormalities in affect (apathy or euphoria).

Depending on the site of the lesion, some features may predominate, suggesting some specialization in the organization of the prefrontal cortex. Orbitomedial lesions produce the "euphoric syndrome," characterized by sporadically hypomanic affect, hyperactivity, distractibility, emotional shallowness, childish humor, antisocial behavior, and disinhibition of sexual drive and other basic instinctual drives. Dorsolateral lesions tend to produce an "apathetic syndrome," characterized by impoverished affect, hypokinesis, inattentiveness, decreased drive and initiative, impoverished speech, "pseudodepression," and impaired capacity to generate abstract concepts. Within both of these syndromes, however, lies a common core: impairment in the capacity to pursue goal-directed behavior based on the integration of environmental and internal cues. Most investigators believe that this function is the basic one pursued in the prefrontal cortex.

In vivo neuroimaging studies complement these lesion studies and have added to information about the functions of the prefrontal cortex. We now recognize that this large expanse in the human brain serves many different functions and is best conceptualized as composed of multiple nodules. In particular, many investigators have documented that the prefrontal cortex plays a major role in memory, which lesion studies previously suggested was primarily a function of limbic structures such as the hippocampus. Several PET studies have now shown that the prefrontal cortex (particularly the dorsolateral prefrontal cortex) is used for working memory and that different regions are used for encoding, retrieval, and novelty recognition. The inferior frontal cortex, including both orbital areas and the straight gyrus, is engaged during tasks that produce emotional arousal or permit the attribution of emotional significance to particular stimuli. Furthermore, functional imaging studies of patient populations indicate that different regions of the prefrontal cortex are abnormal in various mental illnesses. For example, patients with schizophrenia show decreased function in the dorsolateral prefrontal cortex during memory tasks and in inferior frontal regions during tasks that involve personal memories or the attribution of emotional significance. Patients with obsessive-compulsive disorder, which is characterized by excessive planning and overabstractness of thought, have increased flow in the inferior frontal cortex.

The Limbic System: The Anatomical Basis of Emotion

The word *limbic* comes from the Latin *limbus* (border). This term was first used by Broca to refer to the circular ring of tissue that appears to "hem" the prefrontal, parietal, and occipital neocortex when the brain is viewed from a midsagittal perspective. (He also called it the "great lobe of the hem.") Because the olfactory nerve is connected to both the superior (septal region) and the inferior (uncus, amygdala) portions of this reverse-C-shaped group of structures in the center of the brain, it was also known for a time as the *rhinencephalon* (nose brain). Cytoarchitectonic maps also showed that the cellular structure in these regions was paleocortex rather than neocortex.

The function of this "primitive" central brain region was assumed to be related to olfaction until the 1930s, when James Papez proposed another alternative. He introduced the idea of the *Papez circuit,* which is illustrated in Figure 5–4. He suggested that the major input to this circuit was not the olfactory portion of the brain but rather a group of association cortices that collected information from a variety of neocortical regions and then relayed this information to the Papez circuit in the limbic system. Papez suggested that the major function of this brain region was to experience and regulate emotion. Within the circuit, messages would flow from higher cortical regions to the cingulate gyrus, hippocampus, amygdala, mamillary bodies, and anterior thalamus. Papez suggested that emotions were concentrated in deeper structures such as the hippocampus, whereas awareness of them occurred in the cingulate gyrus.

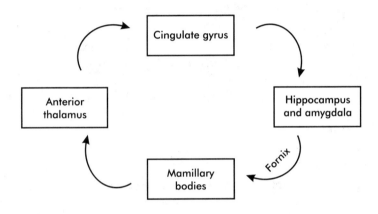

FIGURE 5–4.   The limbic system as conceptualized by Papez. In the "Papez limbic circuit," the cingulate gyrus, hippocampus, amygdala, mamillary bodies, and anterior thalamus interact to create a reverberating circuit in medial portions of the brain that process and produce emotions.
Source.   Andreasen 2001. Copyright 1984 Nancy C. Andreasen.

In his classic paper (in which he deduced the function of the limbic system in the absence of any actual data), Papez proposed that there are, in fact, three different "streams" within the limbic system. The stream of thought occurs when an emotion-provoking stimulus is perceived by the thalamus, and awareness of it is produced through the cingulate gyrus and lateral cortex. The stream of feeling occurs as a consequence of the association of the perception with past experiences in the mamillary bodies and hippocampus, mediated through the thalamus. The stream of movement occurs through a circuit connecting the thalamus to the corpus striatum and motor cortex, permitting a motor response to the emotional stimulus.

The work of Papez was subsequently supplemented by that of Paul Mac-Lean, Walle Nauta, and many others. There is still no consensus as to what constitutes a clear definition of the limbic system or of its components. As in other brain systems, boundaries can be defined on the basis of cytoarchitectonics, interconnections, or inputs. Nauta proposed, as a unifying concept, that the various structures in the limbic system share circuitry that connects them to the hypothalamus. He pointed out that the interconnections between the hypothalamus (via the mamillary bodies), the amygdala, the hippocampus, and the cingulate gyrus are reciprocal. The hypothalamus collects visceral sensory signals from the spinal cord and brain stem; input also comes to this circuit through two major neocortical association regions, the prefrontal cortex and the inferior temporal association cortex.

The limbic system is clearly of great importance for understanding human emotion and psychological experiences. Its various interconnections suggest that it integrates visceral sensations such as hunger and sexual drives with perceptions from the external environment by using input from multiple modalities (e.g., visual, sensory, and auditory cues). In addition, the limbic system appears to reference this information against previous experience, stored as memories, so that we can make judgments about the emotional significance or meaning of our perceptions and experiences.

Recent studies by Joseph LeDoux and Michael Davis have added substantially to our understanding of the role of the limbic system and its relation to a variety of psychiatric syndromes. In particular, the amygdala contributes importantly to survival mechanisms by permitting us to rapidly recognize dangerous stimuli. This circuit is used when we must react quickly to danger, such as when we see a bear approaching our campsite or a person waving a gun in a shopping mall. Such experiences are processed on a "fast track" that engages subcortical regions (thalamus and amygdala) and permits a rapid but crude response. In addition, a "slower track," which includes higher cortical regions such as the prefrontal cortex, is used to process emotional stimuli, and it may be applied secondarily to make a more refined reaction (e.g., recognizing that the gun is only a water pistol and therefore not dangerous). The hippocampus also plays a role in limbic responses, in that it appears to assess contextual cues that also permit the attribution of emotional significance.

These initial animal and lesion studies have been complemented by in vivo imaging studies of cerebral blood flow responses to frightening stimuli. These functional imaging studies have provided additional support to limbic models of emotion by indicating that the thalamus and amygdala are indeed activated when healthy volunteers are exposed to unpleasant or frightening stimuli. Furthermore, both PET and magnetic resonance imaging (MRI) studies have been done in patients who have mental illnesses that may occur as a consequence of exposure to aversive stimuli, such as posttraumatic stress disorder (PTSD). These studies indicated that patients with PTSD may in fact have structural changes in the brain involving decreased hippocampal size, probably as a consequence of chronic overstimulation with cortisol. It now appears that exposure to aversive stimuli lays down powerful memory traces that are difficult to extinguish and that are stored in limbic circuitry, thereby forming the basis for later emotional responses that may be either adaptive or pathological, depending on the nature of the initial exposure and later individual experiences.

The symptoms and subjective experiences of patients with temporal lobe epilepsy (TLE) also may provide some clues to the functions of this region. Such patients experience a variety of phenomena, including olfactory or gustatory hallucinations, déjà vu, derealization, and depersonalization. They also perform repetitive motoric acts that may be highly complex and that appear to rely on procedural memory. Patients with TLE have an increased rate of psychosis, and TLE is often considered to be a crude neurological model for the psychotic syndromes.

The Basal Ganglia System

At first impression, it might seem that the basal ganglia system has no relevance to psychiatry. The usual concept of the basal ganglia is that they primarily regulate and mediate motor activity. For a variety of reasons, however, it appears likely that the basal ganglia also may play a major role in the expression and regulation of emotion and cognition.

The major structures of the basal ganglia include the caudate, putamen, and globus pallidus. A triplanar view of the caudate and other basal ganglia structures, as seen on MRI scan, is shown in Figure 5–5. The substantia nigra, located in the midbrain, is not visualized. The caudate is a C-shaped mass of gray matter tissue that has its head at the lateral anterior borders of the frontal horns of the ventricles. It arches back posteriorly in a circular fashion and then curls forward again, ending in the amygdala bilaterally. Separated from it, and lateral to it, is the lentiform nucleus, so called because it is shaped like a lens. The medial portion of the lentiform nucleus, which is darker and more densely full of gray matter, is the putamen, and the globus pallidus is lateral to it. The caudate is separated from the lentiform nucleus by the anterior limb of the internal capsule, but the MRI scan shows clearly that bands of gray matter interconnect these two nuclei; posteriorly the lentiform nucleus is separated from the thalamus by the posterior limb of the internal capsule. Because these structures contain an intermixture of gray and white matter, they have a striped appearance in postmortem brains and on MRI scan, causing them to be referred to as the *corpus striatum* (striped body).

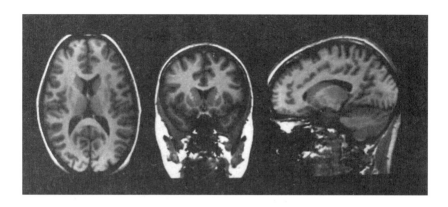

FIGURE 5–5. The basal ganglia as seen with magnetic resonance imaging. The triplanar resampling and visualization, achieved through locally developed software for image analysis (BRAINS, or Brain Research: Analysis of Images, Networks, and Systems), permits viewing of structures with a complex shape such as the caudate from three different angles, thus enhancing our capacity to understand brain anatomy three-dimensionally.
Source. Copyright 1993 Nancy C. Andreasen.

This brain region may be important to the understanding of mental illness for several reasons. First, several major syndromes involving abnormalities in these regions manifest psychiatric symptoms. Patients with Huntington's chorea, characterized by severe atrophy in the caudate nucleus, typically present with mental symptoms that are similar to those seen in patients with psychosis. Patients with Huntington's disease often develop delusional thinking, depression, and/or inappropriate impulsive behavior. They also develop severe dementia, occurring in the context of a previously normal personality. Parkinson's disease is another syndrome affecting the basal ganglia; it is caused by neuronal loss in the substantia nigra, the midbrain region of the basal ganglia that sends projections to the caudate, with dopamine as its primary neurotransmitter. MRI resolution is now sufficiently good that we can directly visualize the substantia nigra; a biplanar view appears in Figure 5–6. Unfortunately, this ability is not of great utility in monitoring the development of Parkinson's disease in predisposed individuals because symptoms do not begin to appear until most of the pigmented neurons have been lost. In Parkinson's disease, loss of pigmented neurons, and the associated loss of dopaminergic activity, produces a variety of symptoms similar to the negative symptoms of schizophrenia, including affective blunting and loss of volition. A mild dementia also may occur.

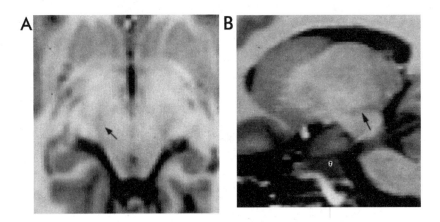

FIGURE 5–6. The substantia nigra as seen in (**A**) transaxial and (**B**) sagittal planes. The dark-pigmented neurons show up as a subtle dark shading (see **Arrows**).
Source. Copyright 1993 Nancy C. Andreasen.

A second reason that the basal ganglia may be of some relevance to the development of symptoms of major mental illnesses derives from their chemical anatomy. One set of cell bodies within the cerebral dopamine system resides in this system, within the pigmented neurons of the substantia nigra. The caudate and putamen contain a very high concentration of dopamine receptors, particularly dopamine type 2 (D_2) receptors. The efficacy of antipsychotic medications has been shown to be highly correlated with their ability to block D_2 receptors (see section "Neurochemical Systems" later in this chapter). Because D_2 receptors have a very high density in these regions, the caudate and putamen may be important sites for antipsychotic drug action and may play a role in generating psychotic symptoms such as delusions and hallucinations.

The Cerebellum and "Mental Coordination"

The cerebellum may seem totally irrelevant to a textbook of psychiatry. However, advances in our understanding of the function of the cerebellum during the past decade suggest that it too may play a key role in the circuitry of mental illness. A phylogenetic clue to the importance of the cerebellum derives from evolutionary biology. The human cerebellum, like the prefrontal cortex, is one-third larger than it is in chimpanzees. It also contains more neurons than the entire cerebral cortex. Both lesion and functional imaging studies suggest that the cerebellum is not simply a structure used to coordinate motor activity, as has been taught in medicine for many years, but also is used to coordinate mental functions such as attention, emotion, memory, and language.

Lesion studies indicate that loss of cerebellar tissue consistently produces a deficit in the ability to estimate time intervals or to imitate motor rhythms. Complementing these lesion studies, PET studies of healthy volunteers indicate that the cerebellum is activated in a broad range of mental tasks, including emotional attribution, language perception and production, focusing attention, and many kinds of memory functions. These observations suggest that the cerebellum probably performs the very basic function of keeping track of information within the context of time. It works as a *metron* that permits us to recognize where our bodies are moving in space and to make fine-grained adaptations (its motor function) and also to recognize where our thoughts are going in our minds and to correct and adjust our speech, attentional focus, or emotional responses (its mental function). As is described in more detail in Chapter 7, patients with schizophrenia have consistently been shown to have abnormalities in blood flow in the cerebellum and other components of circuits connected with it.

The Memory System

The memory system is a major functional brain system that may be impaired in some patients who have major mental illnesses. Deficits in learning and memory are the hallmark of the dementias. Although patients with psychoses do not typically have severe memory deficits, some investigators have speculated that the neural mechanisms of psychotic phenomena such as delusions and hallucinations might be based, at least in part, on either abnormal excitability or abnormal "wiring" in the neural circuitry involved in encoding, retrieval, and interpretation of memories. Within psychoanalytic theory, it has long been believed that the various neuroses, such as anxiety disorders and hysteria (i.e., somatization disorder), might represent the painful stimulus of repressed memories that have not been psychologically integrated. The process of psychotherapy certainly involves the process of learning, which is based on memory; patients who successfully complete a course of psychotherapy have learned new ways of thinking about themselves, understanding their past experiences, and relating to other people. Thus, the psychosocial treatment of mental illnesses probably also involves the memory system in the brain.

It is a truism that we still have a great deal to learn about learning and memory. Nevertheless, we have also learned a great deal during recent decades. For many years, cognitive psychologists have dedicated themselves to identifying the site or sites where memories are encoded, sometimes referred to as the "search for the engram." For example, Karl Lashley of Harvard University spent much of his career placing lesions in various parts of the brain in experimental animals, showing that no specific lesion could produce memory deficits, thereby suggesting that the brain was equipotential in its capacity for learning and memory. This situation changed radically, however, as the result of a single informative and very famous case, that of H.M. He was treated surgically for intractable epilepsy by removal of the anterior temporal poles bilaterally. Afterward, he was observed to have totally lost the capacity to remember any new information he was given, although his memory for information learned before the surgery was completely intact. This famous case focused attention on the gray matter structures located in the anterior poles of the temporal lobes, the amygdala and hippocampus, and on the possible importance of bilateral as opposed to unilateral lesions.

We now know, on the basis of the case of H.M. and a large quantity of other human and animal evidence, that unilateral lesions do not typically produce memory deficits but that bilateral lesions in certain specific locations can completely destroy learning and memory. We now suspect that some aspects of learning and memory are mediated in two brain regions, the hippocampus and the amygdala. A triplanar view of the hippocampus, as visualized with MRI, appears in Figure 5–7; as indicated in that figure, the hippocampus is a large elongated structure that reaches from the anterior temporal pole far back into more posterior brain regions.

Because the memory system appears to depend on the presence of multiple "backup files," identifying the circuitry involved has not been simple. For example, it was thought for several years that the hippocampus was a primary site for encoding memory and that the amygdala served very little function, based on evidence that bilateral removal of the amygdala alone did not impair learning and memory. Later, however, Mishkin observed that similar bilateral lesions to the hippocampus also did not impair the performance of macaques on visual recognition memory tasks. Thus, most recently, it has been concluded that both of these brain regions work together to store memories. Loss of both produces massive memory defects, whereas loss of one or the other produces relatively restricted abnormalities or even none.

However, the functions of these two nuclei are not simply duplicative. Current evidence suggests that the amygdala may work primarily to integrate memories learned from different modalities. For example, monkeys who have

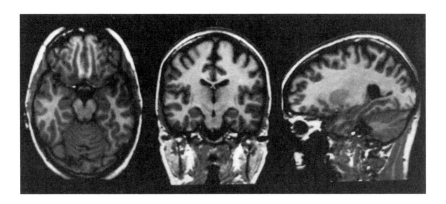

FIGURE 5–7.   A triplanar view of the hippocampus. Note its long posterior section as seen in the less familiar sagittal view (**right**).
Source.   Copyright 1993 Nancy C. Andreasen.

lesions in the amygdala cannot visually recognize objects that they have examined only by touch, whereas animals with lesions in the hippocampus can do so. The amygdala also plays an important role in social behavior, at least in nonhuman primates, because animals with lesions in the amygdala have difficulty recognizing social hierarchies, expressing aggression, experiencing fear, or demonstrating normal maternal behavior. The amygdala also plays an important role in facial recognition and facial perception.

These lesion studies were recently supplemented by PET scan studies of memory. With this in vivo method, the hippocampus and amygdala have been surprisingly difficult to activate in memory paradigms. The primary method for studying higher cortical functions with PET involves the use of oxygen-15–labeled H_2O, a tracer with a short half-life (2 minutes) that provides a measure of cerebral blood flow and that can be used in multiple back-to-back studies (usually eight) in a single individual. Thus, the person can be given multiple kinds of tasks that engage memory (e.g., verbal, visual, short-term, long-term), and the brain regions involved can be identified by measuring brain blood flow while the brain is being scanned as the individual performs the memory task. Each specific task usually is observed by using image subtraction (i.e., a baseline or control task is subtracted from the experimental task), and results from groups of individuals are usually averaged to produce a generalizable result and to improve the signal-to-noise ratio. This method permits the direct observation of brain physiology during the performance of specific mental work; therefore, it is particularly powerful. Brain regions that consistently increase blood flow during memory tasks include prefrontal and other association cortices and the cerebellum. These results complement the inferences concerning the mechanisms of memory that have been drawn from lesion studies. They suggest that learning and memory may be distributed and cortical, in addition to involving the hippocampus and amygdala.

Just as the brain regions that encode memories do not appear to be homogeneous or equipotential, so too memory itself is probably a diverse set of functions that are mediated in different ways. Typically, memory is now thought of as a multistage process. The first stage involves encoding, or placing a memory in a temporary storage buffer for a brief period. Working memory is a related, but different, concept. Working memory is the form that we use when we learn a telephone number long enough to dial it or a driver's license number long enough to write it down. Working memory is usually quickly discarded, however, whereas memories that are encoded are retained for longer periods so that they can pass on to the next phase, consolidation. Consolidated memories involve information that we have learned and retained for longer than a few minutes. Students reading this textbook at this moment are encoding, but they are also preparing to consolidate information so that they can retain it and use it at some later time (e.g., during an examination).

Normal human experience, as well as research in neuroscience, indicates that many techniques can be used to facilitate learning or consolidation of memory. These techniques include things such as repetition, rehearsal, and mnemonic devices. This type of memory is probably mediated by a different set of mechanisms that leads to long-term storage of information. Once such information is stored, some of it may be slowly lost.

The mechanisms mediating encoding versus consolidation are not clear, although an increasing consensus is developing that the mechanisms are different. Current research suggests that short-term memory (i.e., working memory, the process of encoding) probably involves activating short synaptic circuits through neurochemical transmission; this type of neural activity is both rapidly implemented and rapidly reversed. On the other hand, consolidation of memory probably involves a more permanent process, most likely through the development of a sequence of molecules that stores information. Eric Kandel, who was recently awarded the Nobel Prize, has conducted substantial work in this area with the gill withdrawal reflex in the *Aplysia* as a model. Kandel suggested that consolidation and storage of memory may depend on the synthesis of proteins and RNA in neurons that are synaptically connected during the time that short-term learning has been occurring; this type of process would represent a molecular consolidation of memory that could be permanently stored.

Eventually, the stored memories must be retrieved, another stage in the memory process. The process of retrieval can involve either recall or recognition, with the former being more difficult than the latter. *Retrieval* is the familiar process that we all go through when we search our minds to find the right word or the correct answer to a question. When we find what we are looking for, we have achieved successful retrieval. Recognizing the word or information as correct is called *ecphoria*. Sometimes, however, we attempt to retrieve and cannot find the correct memory. Ecphoria is the process that permits us to make this distinction.

The Language System

As far as we know, the capacity to communicate in a highly developed and complex language is limited to humans. Although porpoises, dolphins, and a few other creatures are believed to communicate specific messages to one another, humans alone appear to have a syntactically complex language that exists in both oral and written forms. The ability to record our history and to communicate scientifically and culturally has permitted us to repeatedly build complex civilizations and social systems, and perhaps to destroy them as well.

The capacity to communicate in oral and written language is facilitated by dedicated brain regions that probably occur only in humans. These language systems are localized in the neocortex. A simplified schematic diagram of the human brain circuitry traditionally considered to mediate language functions appears in Figure 5–8. Based on lesion studies, this system appears to be located almost totally in the left hemisphere in most individuals, although about one-third of left-handed persons use either their right hemisphere or both hemispheres to perform language functions.

Although the history of our understanding of the language system goes back to the nineteenth century, and specifically to the work of Broca and Wernicke (each of whom has a neocortical region that bears his name), much of our early understanding of the specialized detail of the language system derives from the work of Norman Geschwind and his colleagues in Boston, Massachusetts. Geschwind was one of the earliest neuroscientists to reawaken interest in hemispheric specialization and asymmetry, observing that the functional specialization in the brain is reflected at least partially in its anatomical structure. He observed that the planum temporale (the flat plane of the temporal lobe that is seen from the top when the cortex above is removed through dissection) is larger on the left side, reflecting the specialized development of the left hemisphere for language. (See Chapter 4,

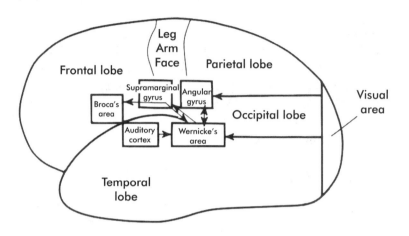

FIGURE 5–8. Interconnections of the language system.
Source. Andreasen 2001. Copyright 1984 Nancy C. Andreasen.

Figure 4–5 for a direct in vivo visualization of the planum temporale with the use of MRI.)

The left hemisphere contains three major language regions, as well as some subsidiary ones. Broca's area is the region dedicated to the production of speech. It contains information about the syntactical structure of language, provides the little words such as prepositions that tie the fabric of language together, and is the generator for fluent speech. Lesions to Broca's area, which occur in persons who have a stroke (often with an accompanying right hemiparesis), lead to halting, stammering, ungrammatical speech. Wernicke's area is often referred to as the auditory association cortex. It encodes the information that permits us to understand or interpret information presented to us in auditory form. The perception of sound waves, which encode speech, occurs through transducers in the ear that convert the information to neural signals. The signals are received in the auditory cortex, but the meaning of the specific signals cannot be understood (i.e., perceived as constituting words with specific meanings—as opposed, for example, to the wordless music of a symphony) without being compared with "templates" in Wernicke's area. An analogous process occurs when we understand written language. In this case, the information is collected through our eyes, relayed via the optic tracts to the primary visual cortex in the occipital lobe, and then forwarded to the angular gyrus, a visual association cortex that contains the information or templates that permit us to recognize language presented in visual form.

Various stroke syndromes have been described that represent specific damage to these specialized brain regions. For example, *Wernicke's aphasia* occurs as a result of damage to Wernicke's area and leaves individuals without the ability to understand what is said; this is a direct consequence of their loss of the auditory association cortex, which attributes meaning to the sound waves that they hear. In addition, individuals with Wernicke's aphasia lose the ability to speak coherently because they have lost the meaning of language; individuals with Wernicke's aphasia produce fluent, disorganized speech that is sometimes referred to as *word salad* or *jargon aphasia*. Wernicke's aphasia is sharply distinguished from *Broca's aphasia;* in the latter case, individuals can comprehend what is said to them but have a marked deficit in their ability to express themselves, a situation that typically leads to great frustration. Damage to the angular gyrus leads to loss of the ability to read and write, the two forms of language that are visually mediated, with no loss of auditory comprehension or spontaneous speech.

As in the case of memory, our understanding of the language system based on the study of stroke patients has been supplemented by PET studies. Again, the results suggest that the intact, functioning brain appears to perform language functions in a more complex manner than was suggested by lesion studies. Specifically, the strong left hemisphere dominance for language is being called into question. PET studies indicate that auditory language perception appears to occur bihemispherically and that blood flow also may increase in both hemispheres during language generation.

Patients with major mental illnesses have disruptions in their capacity to communicate with language. Some of these incapacities are similar to those observed in patients with the aphasias produced by stroke, but none is identical. Some patients with schizophrenia have very impoverished speech that is reminiscent of Broca's aphasia but lacks its halting, agrammatical quality. Likewise, some patients with schizophrenic or manic psychosis produce very disorganized, abundant speech similar to that produced by patients with Wernicke's aphasia, but (unlike patients with Wernicke's aphasia) they appear to have intact comprehension. Auditory hallucinations (hearing voices) are abnormal auditory perceptions of language; that is, the individual perceives auditory speech when none is present.

The Attention System

Attention is the cognitive process through which the brain identifies stimuli within the context of time and space and selects what is relevant for both input and output. We are bombarded continually with sensory information in multiple modalities, as well as with the information within our internal cognitive repertoire. A person driving a car on a busy highway is receiving information about other cars, the road, and the surrounding terrain from his or her visual system; auditory input from the car motor or the rush of other vehicles as they pass; and tactile input from hands on the steering wheel and the foot on the gas pedal and the physical sensations experienced by the rest of the body as the car grips the road or bounces and sways. The person also may be talking on a cellular phone, listening to music, or thinking about a recent conversation. Attention is the cognitive process that permits the person to suppress irrelevant stimuli (e.g., to ignore most of the landscape), to notice important stimuli (e.g., that the car in front is braking and slowing down suddenly), and to shift from one stimulus to another (e.g., from thoughts about the recent conversation to the traffic). If we lacked this capacity, we would be overwhelmed and bombarded with stimuli. Attention is sometimes compared to a spotlight, which the brain uses to highlight what is important to the survival, needs, or interests of the organism.

Attention may be the most "central" of the various cognitive systems; therefore, it is more difficult to study in isolation than the other systems described above. It is sometimes classified into different types:

- *Sustained attention* involves focusing for a prolonged period (as when studying for an examination).
- *Directed attention* involves consciously selecting a particular feature or stimulus from the large array available (as when a professor instructs students to notice a particular lesion that they may not have recognized on an X ray).
- *Selective attention* involves focusing attention on a stimulus that may have importance for personal or practical reasons (as when a person at a dinner party hears his or her name spoken in a nearby conversation).
- *Divided attention* involves focusing attention on several things at the same time, or in rapidly shifting sequence (as when the person at the dinner party tries to listen to two conversations at once).
- *Focused attention* involves directing attention to some particular stimulus or task (as when solving a mathematics problem or developing the outline for a paper to be written).

Attention appears to be mediated through multiple brain systems. Input to the brain is probably first provided by the *reticular activating system*, which arises in the brain stem. Midline circuitry passes this information through the thalamus, which appears to play a major role in gating or filtering. Many other brain regions also appear to play a major role in attention, including the cingulate gyrus, the hypothalamus, the hippocampus and amygdala, the prefrontal cortex, and the temporal, parietal, and occipital cortices. As Figure 5–3 shows, these regions are all interconnected.

Lesion studies have emphasized the phenomenon of *sensory neglect* or *hemineglect*, which was first described by Hughlings-Jackson. He observed a patient who ignored sensory input as a result of a lesion in the right parietal lobe. More recent studies have examined this abnormality in a variety of patients. Although the classic case involves an inability to focus spatial attention as a consequence of right parietal injury, neglect also may occur after injury to the left hemisphere.

Neuroimaging studies using PET have shown that the cingulate gyrus shows increases in cerebral blood flow during tasks that place heavy demands on the attention system, such as those that involve competition and interference between stimuli. They also have shown that blood flow can be shifted from one hemisphere to another as a consequence of directed attention; increased blood flow is seen in the right superior temporal gyrus as a consequence of instructions to listen to sounds in the left ear, and the increase shifts to the left superior temporal gyrus in response to instructions to attend to the right ear. Increasing the difficulty of the task through competing stimuli produces an increase in frontal flow as well.

Neurochemical Systems

In addition to the anatomical and functional systems described above, the brain consists of a group of neurochemical systems. These systems provide the "fuel" that permits the anatomical and functional systems to run (or run poorly, when an abnormality occurs). The neurochemical systems are not isomorphic with the anatomical and functional systems. Rather, they are interwoven and interdependent. Any anatomical subsystem within the brain usually runs on multiple classes of neurotransmitters. Clearly, this complexity of anatomical and neurochemical organization permits much greater fine tuning of the entire system.

Neuron, Synapse, Receptor, and Second Messenger

Neurons may have various structural configurations depending on the function they perform. They all consist of a cell body containing the nucleus and at least one axon of variable length that transfers from the cell body the propagation of electrical excitation that ultimately leads to the release of neurotransmitters that are located in terminals at the synapses. The cell body is surrounded by dendrites that enlarge the capacity of the cell body to receive information through synaptic input from other neurons. Likewise, axons may branch as they terminate and then produce multiple synaptic contacts.

Although the initial propagation of messages is electrical, communication at the synapse is chemical. It is mediated through a variety of substances recognized to be chemical messengers between neurons, or *neurotransmitters*. Neuroscientists have agreed for several decades on a set of criteria that defines "classic" neurotransmitters (Table 5–1). For a substance to be accepted as a neurotransmitter, investigators must establish that it is contained within the neuron, synthesized by the neuron, and released at the synapse and that it causes a reproducible physiological response. The classic neurotransmitters that meet these criteria are principally catecholamines and amino acids, such as dopamine, serotonin, acetylcholine, γ-aminobutyric acid (GABA), and glutamate.

TABLE 5–1.   Criteria for a "classic" neurotransmitter

1. It is synthesized in the neuron.

2. It is present in the presynaptic terminal and is released in an amount sufficient to exert a particular effect on a receptor neuron.

3. When applied exogenously (as drug) in reasonable concentrations, it mimics exactly the action of the endogenously released neurotransmitter.

4. A specific mechanism exists for removing it from its site of action, the synaptic cleft.

In addition to these classic neurotransmitters, chemical communication between regions also occurs through other neurotransmitters that have not yet been proved to meet all of the above criteria. It has now been recognized for nearly three decades that peptides are also synthesized in the CNS. Although the earliest peptides to be recognized were those that were clearly hormonal (e.g., adrenocorticotropic hormone [ACTH]), the discovery of endogenous opioid peptide neurotransmitters (endorphins) substantially expanded interest in peptide transmitters within the CNS. Because they are proteins (i.e., have their synthesis directed by nuclear DNA), the peptide neurotransmitters must be synthesized in the neuronal cell body rather than in the synapse. They are carried down to the synapse through storage vesicles, where they can then be released. Although some peptide neurotransmitters function in much the same way as the classic neurotransmitters, others serve as cotransmitters.

Although the belief in a single neuron–single neurotransmitter used to be universal, it is now recognized that many neurons contain at least two neurotransmitters. Often a classic neurotransmitter and a neuropeptide are coupled. For example, cholecystokinin (CCK) serves as a cotransmitter with the dopamine neurons that project to the cortex and limbic system (but not those that project to the basal ganglia). The peptide cotransmitters are generally thought to be modulatory or regulatory.

A schematic representation of a synapse appears in Figure 5–9, and an electron micrograph of an actual synapse is shown in Figure 5–10. The classic neurotransmitters are synthesized at the neuronal synapse from precursor molecules (e.g., tyrosine). The neurotransmitter molecules must be sequestered in vesicles to prevent breakdown by enzymes contained within the neuronal cytosol (e.g., by monoamine oxidase). Adequate quantities of neurotransmitter are maintained at the synapse through a variety of regulatory factors. Short-term monitoring to determine whether adequate quantities of the neurotransmitter are contained in vesicular storage is done through end-product inhibition. For example, tyrosine hydroxylase is the rate-limiting enzyme for the synthesis of dopamine and norepinephrine. If an adequate supply of norepinephrine is available at the terminal, it inhibits the activity of tyrosine hydroxylase, preventing further synthesis.

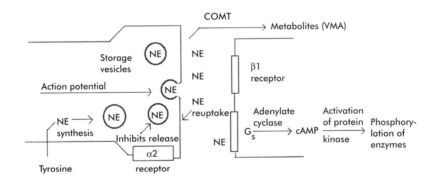

FIGURE 5–9. Schematic view of a synapse. This schematic drawing shows a simplified view of the cascade of events occurring during synaptic transmission, beginning with neurotransmitter release, stimulated through an action potential, and leading to the occupation of a receptor and the subsequent activation of second-messenger systems.

cAMP=cyclic adenosine monophosphate; COMT=catechol-*O*-methyltransferase; NE=norepinephrine; VMA = vanillylmandelic acid.

Source. Copyright 1993 Nancy C. Andreasen.

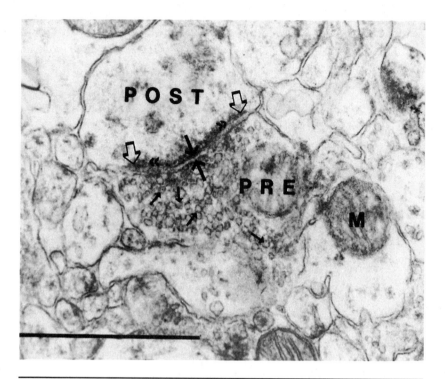

FIGURE 5–10.   Electron micrograph showing a synapse in the human brain. The presynaptic region (**PRE**) is an axon, which contains vesicles of neurotransmitters (**small arrows**). It is adjacent to the postsynaptic region (**POST**) of another neuron. The receptors embedded in the postsynaptic membrane can be visualized. **Open arrows** delineate the extent of the synapse identified by parallel pre- and postsynaptic membranes (**large arrows**). Synaptic vesicles and a postsynaptic density are marked by double brackets. **M** indicates mitochondria in a nearby location.
Source.   Courtesy of Carol Tamminga and Rosalinda C. Roberts.

On the other hand, if the synapse is very active, leading to depletion of neurotransmitters, then protein kinases stimulate phosphorylation of tyrosine hydroxylase, a process triggered by persistent membrane depolarization. Increased quantities of tyrosine hydroxylase also can be produced in the neuronal cell body under the supervision of nuclear DNA—a response that occurs as a result of long-term neuronal hyperactivity and synaptic depletion.

Finally, at least for neurons that possess presynaptic receptors, the release of neurotransmitters also can be downregulated through these presynaptic receptors. For example, noradrenergic neurons contain α_2 receptors at their terminals, which decrease the amount of norepinephrine released at the terminal when activated either by an increase in overall adrenergic activity or by exogenous α_2 agonists such as clonidine. The presynaptic receptors work principally to decrease the firing rate of the neuron and thereby the vesicular release of neurotransmitter. Thus, the regulation of neurotransmitter synthesis and release is governed by a complex set of interactive mechanisms that can adapt neuronal responsiveness to rapidly varying conditions.

After a neurotransmitter is released, it can experience a variety of fates. In the free-floating world of intersynaptic connections, enzymes such as catechol-O-methyltransferase (COMT) hover at the synapse and can lead to inactivation or breakdown of the neurotransmitter. It may saturate presynaptic receptors, thereby telling the transmitter neuron that it is time to slow down. It may cross the synapse and occupy a postsynaptic receptor, thereby actually succeeding in sending a message to another neuron. Finally, because nature often loves efficiency and abhors waste, it may be returned to the original transmitter neuron and again stored in the vesicles, eventually to be released again.

The receptor sites to which neurotransmitters complex are large protein molecules embedded in the neuronal membrane that recognize specific neurotransmitters in a highly selective way, which is related to the chemical structure of the receptor. The two main superfamilies of receptors are G-protein coupled (metabotropic) and ion channel (ionotropic). The messages produced by G-protein receptors occur more slowly, whereas the ion-channel receptors produce rapid changes in neuronal excitability. The G-protein receptors work principally by activating enzymes (e.g., adenylate cyclase, inositol phosphate, phospholipase A), which in turn aid in the amplification of the signal by a second messenger (e.g., cyclic adenosine monophosphate [cAMP]).

Knowledge of the structure and the working mechanisms of G-protein receptors has been increasing steadily. These receptors are of considerable interest in psychiatry because many of the major neuroreceptors thought to be involved in mental illnesses and/or modulated by the drugs used to treat them are in this superfamily (e.g., serotonergic, dopaminergic, α and β adrenergic, and muscarinic cholinergic). GABAergic, nicotinic, and some glutamatergic receptors are ionotropic, however. Many of these receptors have now been cloned, providing us with information about their specific DNA-driven amino acid sequences and opening up the possibility that specific drugs can be designed to interact with receptors in key chemical systems or brain regions involved in specific illnesses.

All receptors in the G-protein superfamily have a similar structure. A schematic diagram of a G-protein receptor is shown in Figure 5–11. The receptor itself is composed of seven helical loops embedded in the membrane that are composed of a specific sequence of amino acids. The various types of receptors—for example, dopamine D_1, D_2, D_3, D_4, and D_5 and serotonin type 2 (5-HT_2)—differ in amino acid sequence, which determines their affinity for specific drugs or neurotransmitters. Each receptor has a long tail on the extracellular side, which also determines drug affinity. Three loops of variable length are also present on the intracellular side, as well as an intracellular tail. These intracellular components provide the mechanism for passing the message on to the G protein and the effector protein.

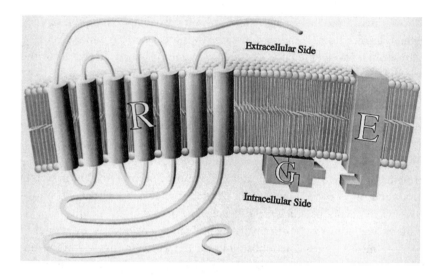

FIGURE 5–11. Schematic diagram of a G-protein receptor.
E = effector protein; G = G protein; R = receptor.
Source. Courtesy of Carol Tamminga.

Among the second messengers, the one coupled with cAMP is best understood; it appears to occur both at noradrenergic β receptors and at D_1 receptors. Within this system, the neurotransmitter-receptor interaction leads to a complexing of protein on the other side of the membrane, which then binds to adenylate cyclase and activates it, causing adenosine triphosphate (ATP) to convert to cAMP. cAMP then activates protein kinases, which in turn promote phosphorylation of key enzymes. Other second-messenger systems, associated with α_1-adrenergic receptors and muscarinic M_1 receptors, stimulate the breakdown of phospholipids, thereby increasing intracellular concentrations of phosphoinositides and diacylglycerol, which in turn leads to enzyme phosphorylation and activation.

Medications used to treat mental illness often exert their primary effects by acting on one of these aspects of neural communication. For example, the monoamine oxidase inhibitors (MAOIs), which prevent the breakdown of norepinephrine, enhance noradrenergic transmission by blocking the action of monoamine oxidase. The classic antidepressants, such as imipramine, also facilitate noradrenergic transmission by blocking the uptake mechanisms. Clonidine decreases anxiety by blocking presynaptic α_2 receptors, thereby producing downregulation. For many years, classic antipsychotics were thought to decrease the symptoms of psychosis by diminishing hyperdopaminergic activity through blocking postsynaptic D_2 receptors, a view that has been revised in light of the documented efficacy of the new atypical antipsychotics, which have a different pharmacological profile (see Chapter 27).

The Dopamine System

Dopamine, a catecholamine neurotransmitter, is the first product synthesized from tyrosine through the enzymatic activity of tyrosine hydroxylase. Its synthetic pathway, as well as the subsequent ones of norepinephrine and epinephrine, is shown in Figure 5–12.

Three subsystems within the brain use dopamine as their primary neurotransmitter. These all arise in the ventral tegmental area. One subsystem, arising in the substantia nigra, projects to the caudate and putamen and is referred to as the *nigrostriatal pathway*. Its terminations appear to be rich in D_1 and D_2 receptors. A second major subsystem, called the *mesocortical* or *mesolimbic* (or mesocorticolimbic) *tract*, projects to the prefrontal cortex and temporolimbic regions such as the amygdala and hippocampus. The concentration of D_2 receptors in these regions is minimal, whereas D_1 receptors predominate. The third component of the dopamine system originates in the arcuate nucleus of the hypothalamus and projects to the pituitary. These various dopamine subsystems are shown in Figure 5–13.

As Figure 5–13 indicates, the dopamine system is fairly specifically localized in the human brain. Because its projections include only a limited part of the cortex and focus primarily on brain regions important to cognition and emotion, it is considered one of the most important neurotransmitter systems for understanding these functions and potentially for understanding their disturbances in individuals with psychosis.

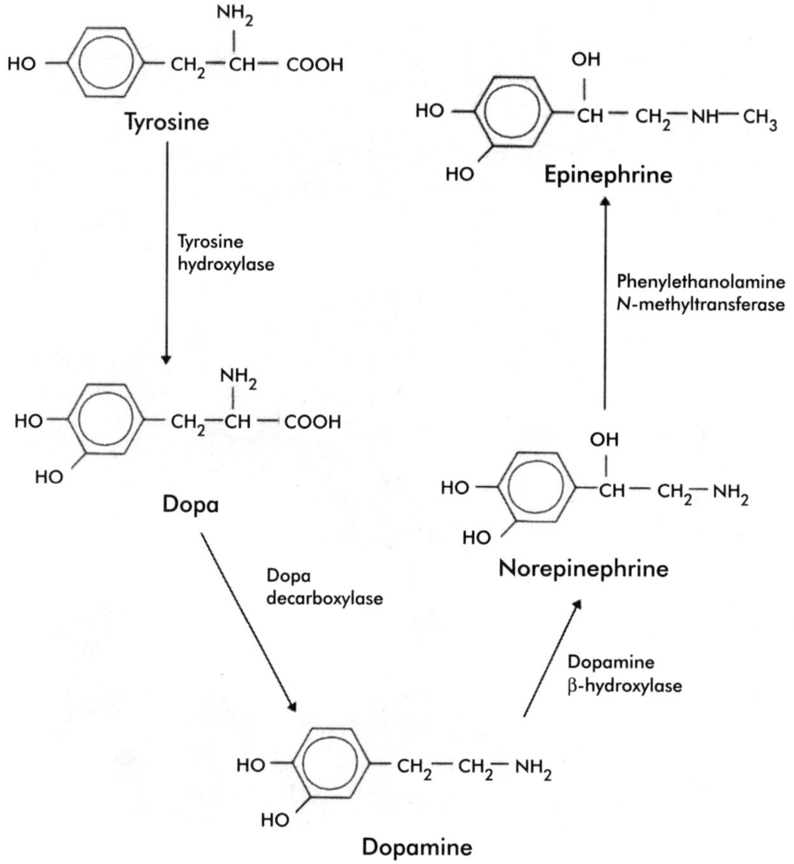

FIGURE 5–12.   Synthetic pathway of dopamine.

For many years, schizophrenia, the most important among the psychotic disorders, was explained by the *dopamine hypothesis*, which proposed that the symptoms of this illness were due to a functional excess of dopamine. Because the efficacy of many of the antipsychotic drugs used to treat psychosis is highly correlated with their ability to block D_2 receptors, as is shown in Figure 5–14, the dopamine hypothesis also suggested that the abnormality in this illness might be specifically in D_2 receptors. The efficacy of these drugs has a modest but much weaker correlation with their ability to block D_1 receptors (Figure 5–15). This hypothesis is currently being reappraised, however, in the light of several new lines of evidence that have emerged. First, the distribution of D_1 and D_2 receptors has been more specifically

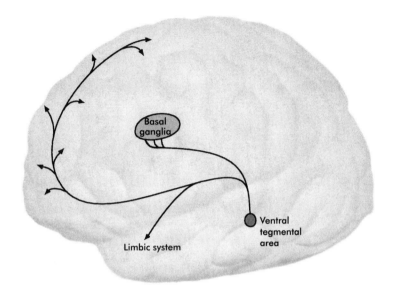

FIGURE 5–13. The dopamine system.
Source.   Andreasen 2001. Copyright 1984 Nancy C. Andreasen.

mapped during recent years, and there appears to be a rather sparse density of D_2 receptors in critical brain regions that mediate cognition and emotion, such as prefrontal cortex, amygdala, and hippocampus. These regions are, however, high in D_1 receptors, as well as in 5-HT_2 receptors. This latter observation, coupled with the prominent effects on serotonin and D_1 receptors by the new atypical antipsychotics, suggests that the traditional dopamine hypothesis must be revised.

Understanding the projections of the dopamine system, as well as the differential localization of D_1 and D_2 receptors, clarifies some of the other actions of antipsychotic drugs. Most of these drugs tend to have potent extrapyramidal effects as a consequence of blocking D_2 receptors in the nigrostriatal pathway. Drugs that have a weak D_2 effect (e.g., clozapine and risperidone) are more likely to have fewer extrapyramidal side effects as a consequence of their weak D_2 blockade. If only we understood more specifically the brain regions from which the symptoms of psychosis arise, then we could design a rational psychopharmacology that might target drugs to specific regions on the basis of what we know about the chemical anatomy of the brain. Such a rational psychopharmacology could capitalize on knowledge about the neurotransmitters involved, the brain regions in-

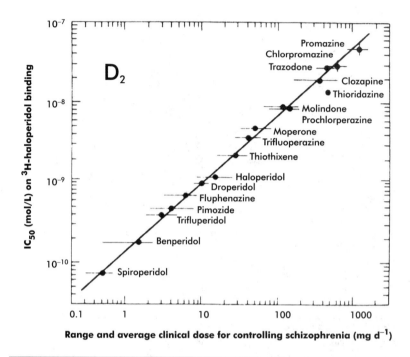

FIGURE 5–14.   Correlation between drug potency and dopamine D$_2$ receptor blockade.

Source.   Reprinted from Seeman P: "Dopamine Receptors and the Dopamine Hypothesis of Schizophrenia." *Synapse* 1:133–152, 1987. Used with permission.

volved, and the chemical structure of the relevant receptors, as revealed through receptor cloning.

The Norepinephrine System

The norepinephrine system arises in the locus coeruleus and sends projections diffusely throughout the entire brain. These projections are summarized in Figure 5–16. As that figure illustrates, norepinephrine appears to exert effects on almost every brain region in the human brain, including the entire cortex, the hypothalamus, the cerebellum, and the brain stem. This distribution suggests that it may have a diffuse modulatory or regulatory effect within the CNS.

Some evidence indicates that norepinephrine may play a major role in mediating symptoms of major mental illnesses, especially mood disorders. Soon after they were developed, tricyclic antidepressants were shown to inhibit norepinephrine reuptake, thereby enhancing the amount of norepi-

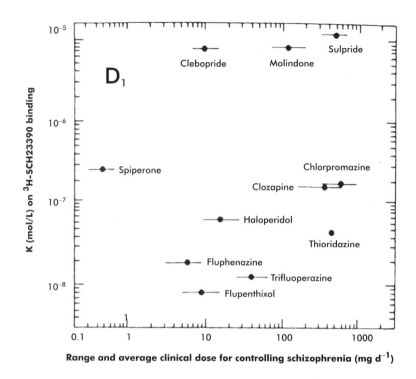

FIGURE 5–15. Correlation between neuroleptic potency and dopamine D_1 receptor blockade.
Source. Reprinted from Seeman P: "Dopamine Receptors and the Dopamine Hypothesis of Schizophrenia." *Synapse* 1:133–152, 1987. Used with permission.

nephrine available for stimulating postsynaptic receptors. Likewise, the MAOIs also enhance noradrenergic transmission by inhibiting neurotransmitter breakdown. As is described below, however, it is also clear that many antidepressants have mixed noradrenergic and serotonergic activities or purely serotonergic effects (i.e., the serotonin reuptake inhibitors). Thus, the original catecholamine hypothesis of affective illness, which suggested that depression was due to a functional deficit of norepinephrine at crucial nerve terminals and mania was due to a functional excess, is clearly an oversimplification.

The Serotonin System

Serotonergic neurons have a distribution strikingly similar to that of norepinephrine neurons (Figure 5–17). Serotonergic neurons arise in the raphe

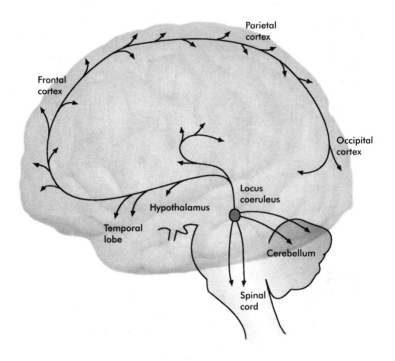

FIGURE 5–16.   The norepinephrine system.
Source.   Andreasen 2001. Copyright 1984 Nancy C. Andreasen.

nuclei, localized around the aqueduct in the midbrain. They project to a similar wide range of CNS regions, including the entire neocortex, the basal ganglia, temporolimbic regions, the hypothalamus, the cerebellum, and the brain stem. As is the case with the norepinephrine system, the serotonin system appears to be a general modulator.

A serotonin hypothesis of depression also has been proposed, largely because some antidepressant medications (e.g., fluoxetine) facilitate serotonergic transmission by blocking reuptake. As discussed above, serotonin is probably also involved in schizophrenia and other psychotic disorders. Thus, there are probably no simple single neurotransmitter–single illness relationships.

The Cholinergic System

Like dopamine, acetylcholine has a relatively more specific localization in the human brain. This is shown schematically in Figure 5–18. The cell bodies of a major group of acetylcholine neurons are located in the nucleus basa-

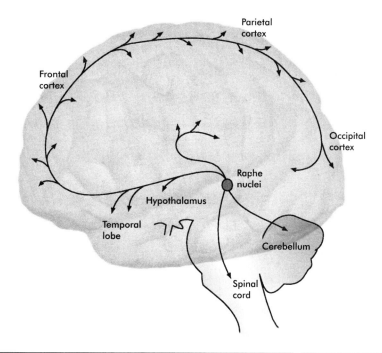

FIGURE 5–17. The serotonin system.
Source. Andreasen 2001. Copyright 1984 Nancy C. Andreasen.

lis of Meynert, which lies in the ventral and medial regions of the globus pallidus. Neurons from the nucleus basalis of Meynert project throughout the cortex. The second group of acetylcholine neurons, originating in the diagonal band of Broca and the septal nucleus, projects to the hippocampus and cingulate gyrus. A third group of cholinergic neurons are local circuit neurons that enter main structures within the basal ganglia.

The acetylcholine system plays a major role in the encoding of memory, although the precise mechanisms are not understood. Patients with Alzheimer's disease show losses of acetylcholine projections both to the cortex and to the hippocampus, and blockade of muscarinic receptors produces memory impairment. Dopamine and acetylcholine share heavy concentrations of activity within the basal ganglia, and the drugs used to block the extrapyramidal side effects of antipsychotics are cholinergic antagonists, suggesting a possible reciprocal relationship between dopamine and acetylcholine in the modulation of motor activity and possibly of psychosis as well. Patients taking anticholinergic medications also may have impaired cognitive functions such as learning and memory.

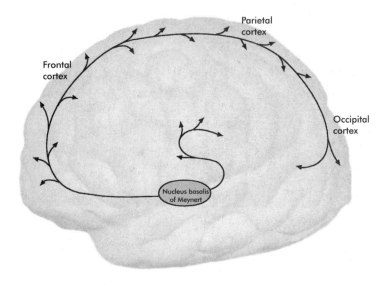

FIGURE 5–18.　The acetylcholine system.
Source.　Andreasen 2001. Copyright 1984 Nancy C. Andreasen.

The GABA System

GABA is an amino acid neurotransmitter, as is glutamate. These two major amino acid neurotransmitters appear to serve complementary functions, with GABA playing an inhibitory role and glutamate playing an excitatory role.

GABAergic neurons are a mix of local-circuit and long-tract systems. Within the cerebral cortex and the limbic system, GABAergic neurons are predominantly local circuit. The cell bodies of GABAergic neurons in the caudate and putamen project to the globus pallidus and substantia nigra, making them relatively long tract, and long-tract GABA neurons also occur in the cerebellum.

The GABA system has substantial importance for understanding the neurochemistry of mental illness. Many of the anxiolytic drugs (e.g., diazepam) act as GABA agonists, thereby increasing the inhibitory tone within the CNS. Loss of the long-tract GABA neurons connecting the caudate to the globus pallidus releases the latter structure from inhibitory control, thereby permitting the globus pallidus to "run free" and produce the choreiform movements that characterize Huntington's disease.

The Glutamate System

Glutamate, an excitatory amino acid neurotransmitter, is produced by pyramidal cells throughout the cerebral cortex and hippocampus. It has already been noted, for example, that the projections from the prefrontal cortex to the basal ganglia are glutamatergic.

It has been observed for many years that glutamate, in addition to being a neurotransmitter, is potentially a neurotoxin when present in amounts that produce excessive neuronal excitation. Recently, this observation was coupled with observations about the psychological and biochemical effects of phencyclidine (PCP) to suggest a possible role for glutamate in either psychosis or neurodegenerative diseases such as Huntington's disease. PCP blocks the effects of activating one subgroup of glutamate receptors, the N-methyl-D-aspartate (NMDA) receptors, probably by blocking the cation channel that the NMDA receptor activates. PCP intoxication produces a psychosis characterized by withdrawal, stupor, disorganized thinking and speech, and hallucinations. The possible relation between PCP, its characteristic psychosis, and its effects on the glutamate system suggest that glutamate may play some role in producing (or protecting against) the symptoms of psychosis. Such diseases could be produced by excessive glutamatergic activity, which might produce neuronal degeneration through excessive excitation.

The Genetics of Mental Illness

It has been recognized for many years that mental illnesses tend to run in families. Evidence that disorders are familial is sometimes said to imply that they are genetic as well, but this is not necessarily the case. Genetic disorders are precisely that: coded in the segments of DNA that constitute our genes. The history of research on the familial aggregation of mental illnesses has been one of an increasing ability to determine more specifically the degree to which mental illnesses are genetic in the literal sense. The era of molecular biology and molecular genetics has arrived. This era has been supported by a long history of research on the familial aggregation of mental illnesses, which has established that the study of familial transmission is relevant to understanding the mechanisms of mental illness.

Studies of Familial Aggregation

Studies of familial aggregation provided the first line of evidence for the familiality of major mental illnesses, as well as some indication that many mental illnesses may have a genetic component. The solid and increasingly methodologically rigorous studies of the prevalence of mental illnesses in families should not be minimized as we enter the era of molecular genetics; they have provided a major contribution. Such studies usually are divided into three broad groups: family studies, twin studies, and adoption studies. Each of these types of studies offers different perspectives on the genetics of disorders.

Family studies typically begin with the *proband method*. That is, individuals, or probands, are identified and used as the index cases because they have a particular disorder of interest, such as bipolar disorder or schizophrenia. Thereafter, all available first-degree relatives are typically evaluated. Early genetic studies used the *family history method*. This method involves interviewing the proband and one or two additional family members about whether other members of the family have any history of mental illness. This method is quick and simple but less methodologically rigorous.

Gradually, the family history method has nearly been supplanted by the *family study method,* which involves directly interviewing all available first-degree relatives. The introduction of structured interviews and diagnostic criteria has presumably produced a steady increase in the accuracy of such family studies. In family studies, the prevalence of the specific disorder under investigation is also evaluated in some appropriately selected control group. For example, patients entering the hospital for hernia repair might represent the control group for the probands, and all first-degree relatives of the hernia patients would serve as the control group for the first-degree relatives of the mentally ill probands. If an increased rate of the specific mental illness under study is observed in the first-degree relatives of the mentally ill probands, then investigators would conclude that a disorder is familial and possibly genetic.

Such studies do not exclude the possibility that the disorder is purely familial, however, and not due to a specifically genetic cause. Disorders could run in families because of learned behavior, role modeling, or predisposing social environments. For example, depression tends to run in families, and this tendency could represent either genetic transmission or social learning; responding to stressful life events with a depressive coping style could easily be a learned adaptive mechanism passed on from parents to children through role modeling. Likewise, antisocial behavior tends to run in families; although possibly genetic in origin, antisocial behavior also could be an adaptive response to social deprivation, nurtured by peer pressure from gangs, which tend to cluster in impoverished inner cities.

As is discussed in more detail in the chapters on the specific disorders (see Section 2), many major mental illnesses have been shown through family studies to be familial. Alzheimer's disease, schizophrenia, bipolar and unipolar mood disorders, anxiety disorders, and antisocial personality disorder all tend to have increased rates in first-degree relatives of probands with these disorders. The test for the geneticist, however, is to determine whether these disorders are truly genetic.

Thus, investigators have turned to other methods in addition to family studies to identify a more purely genetic component. Before techniques were available to look directly at genes, the best methods were *twin studies* and *adoption studies.*

Twin Studies

Twin studies typically began with ascertainment of whether a proband twin (monozygotic or dizygotic) has the disorder of interest. The co-twin is then evaluated to determine whether he also has the illness (i.e., is concordant). The concordance rate in monozygotic (identical) twins can then be compared with that in dizygotic twins (using only same-sex twins among the dizygotic (nonidentical) pairs to help control for random cultural and genetic "noise"). The higher the rate of concordance in monozygotic twins compared with dizygotic twins, the greater the degree of genetic influence.

The rationale behind twin studies is based on the fact that monozygotic twins have identical genetic material, whereas dizygotic twins theoretically share an average of 50% of their genetic material. (The percentage can actually run from 0% to 100%, but it should average to 50% across large numbers of twin pairs). Thus, if a disorder were totally genetic and fully penetrant, the concordance rate in monozygotic twins would theoretically be 100%, whereas that in dizygotic twins would be 50%. In fact, actual rates for both groups are lower for most major mental illnesses that have been studied with the twin method. Table 5–2 shows the concordance rates for schizophrenia in twin studies.

Although powerful, twin studies do not provide a perfect method for examining the genetics of major mental illnesses. Because twins are reared together, role modeling again could be an influential factor, particularly for milder disorders, such as depression, that have a potentially prominent psychological component. This psychological component could theoretically be greater in monozygotic than in dizygotic twins because monozygotic twins are often treated as identical by their parents and peers. The development of major mental illness in one's identical co-twin is clearly a serious psychological stressor that could be influential in the development of a disorder in the unaffected twin. If the unaffected twin is led to believe that he or she is in-

TABLE 5–2. Concordance rates in identical and nonidentical twins for various psychiatric conditions, coronary heart disease, and breast cancer

Type of illness	Identical twins	Nonidentical twins
Autism, schizophrenia, bipolar disorder	60%	5%
Coronary artery disease	40%	10%
Depression	50%	15%
Breast cancer	30%	10%

deed identical to his or her co-twin, the unaffected twin might develop a mental illness as part of a self-fulfilling prophecy. Alternatively, the unaffected twin might develop it out of sympathetic identification with a co-twin with whom he or she has been intimately nurtured for most of his or her life. Thus, environmental factors are not completely disentangled from genetic factors through the use of the twin method.

Adoption Studies

Adoption studies represent the most refined technique for disentangling environmental and genetic influences. In adoption studies, the population targeted for study is children who were born to parents with a major mental illness then adopted at birth and reared by parents without the disorder. These children can be compared with a control group consisting of children born to psychiatrically normal mothers, similarly adopted at birth, and reared by psychiatrically normal parents. To whatever extent the rate of illness is higher in the adopted children of the mothers with the specific mental illness, that mental illness can be considered to be transmitted genetically rather than environmentally. In this model, learned behavior and role modeling of parents with mental illness are excluded because the child is reared apart from the ill parent.

Like all paradigms, however, this one has inherent limitations and problems. Accurate diagnosis in the father is sometimes difficult, often relying on case registries and historical information rather than direct interview. Of even more concern is that information about the biological father of the child may not be available, and the mother may not even be able to identify the specific biological father because she has had multiple sex partners. An additional problem with adoption studies (and of family studies in general) is *assortative mating*. Assortative mating refers to the tendency of individuals with a specific mental illness to mate with, or marry, a person who has a similar illness. This may occur because of a "like attracts like" phenomenon or as a consequence of simple social convenience, because the partners often meet each other in mental hospitals and sometimes have few friends who are not mentally ill because of the social handicaps produced by some mental illnesses. Whatever the mechanism, assortative mating produces problems for family and genetic studies because it gives the offspring a double genetic loading.

Adoption studies are the most difficult to complete, largely because of problems in obtaining access to appropriate samples. Some major adoption studies have been done in Scandinavian countries, which have excellent epidemiological registries. Adoption data are available for schizophrenia, mood disorders, and antisocial personality disorder. In all cases, they add to the evidence for genetic factors in these disorders.

Studies of Genetic and Nongenetic Factors

Evidence from many sources indicates that major mental illness cannot be explained by purely genetic models. However, instead of creating a polarity between "genes" and "environment," we must begin to think about genetic and nongenetic factors because the word *environment* has misleading connotations. It suggests that the factors are psychological, social, and relatively recent. Environmental factors can be physical (e.g., birth injury, smaller size at birth, and a less developed brain secondary to less placental nutrition) and can affect the developing fetus before birth as well as at later stages of life. Therefore, it is more accurate to discuss as *nongenetic factors* all factors that are not a direct consequence of genes alone. Nongenetic factors influencing the development of mental illnesses may be as diverse as things that affect regulation of gene expression (e.g., maternal fever, maternal nutrition), exposure to toxins, radiation, birth injuries, head injuries, developmental processes such as onset of puberty (and their related endocrine effects), and psychological factors such as role modeling, personal loss, and exposure to an environmental stressor.

Twin and adoption data also indicate clearly that almost all major mental illnesses are multifactorial. That is, they occur as a consequence of or as an interaction between genetic and nongenetic factors. Apart from Huntington's disease, which is purely genetic as a result of a fully penetrant autosomal dominant gene, no mental illness can be explained on a purely genetic basis. The concordance rates for monozygotic and dizygotic twins make it clear that genetic factors can account for at most 40%–50% of the variance for major mental illnesses. Furthermore, transmission within families does not follow simple mendelian patterns. Like cancer, diabetes, and heart disease, mental illnesses are etiologically complex and multifactorial.

As is the case with cancer and other complex illnesses, most mental illnesses are now conceptualized within the context of a "multiple hit theory." A genetic predisposition may be necessary but not sufficient, or a genetic predisposition may be sufficient but not necessary. In the former case, a person may carry a gene or group of genes that predisposes, but the diathesis may not be released because an inadequate number of environmental factors accumulates. For example, a person may carry the apolipoprotein E (APOE) ε4 allele and yet never develop Alzheimer's disease because that person has not been exposed to other releasing environmental or nongenetic influences, such as insufficient exercise, poor diet, or one or more experiences with general anesthesia. However, a person may not carry any germ-line genes that predispose to an illness and yet develop a disease as a result of sufficient nongenetic factors. The most striking example is the occurrence of mutations in somatic genes that occur as a consequence of exposure to ionizing radiation and that may ultimately lead to the development of cancer, perhaps within the context of other nongenetic factors such as the effects of stress on the immune system.

Molecular Genetics

The tools of molecular genetics have been applied to the study of mental illnesses with mixed success so far. The identification of a polymorphic DNA marker linked to chromosome 4 in Huntington's disease in 1983 raised many hopes for rapid progress in treatment and prevention. As progress continued, a highly accurate premorbid test was developed within 2 years so that individuals could determine whether they carried this fully penetrant gene, would ultimately develop the disease, and could avoid passing it on to others by choosing not to have children. Furthermore, the gene was sequenced and the nature of the mutation was identified. We now know that Huntington's disease is a consequence of multiple trinucleotide repeats. In general, the more repeats, the earlier the age at onset and the more severe the illness. But despite all this knowledge, we still do not have a means to either treat or prevent Huntington's disease. This illness continues to exact its inexorable toll on those unlucky individuals who carry too many trinucleotide repeats on their fourth chromosome.

We can learn several lessons from the case of Huntington's disease. First, the process of solving the problems of mental illnesses (or any other biomedical illnesses) with the tools of molecular biology is not easy. Second, finding the gene is not enough. The process of understanding the molecular biology of biomedical disorders and using this information for the purposes of treatment and prevention involves multiple steps, which are summarized in Table 5–3.

TABLE 5–3.   Steps required for a complete understanding of the role of genes in mental illnesses

1. Finding or locating the gene
2. Cloning the gene
3. Sequencing the gene
4. Identifying the gene's product
5. Identifying the gene's function

Locating the gene that is associated with a particular disease is the initial, and often very difficult, step. We are still in this process for most mental illnesses, as well as for most other biomedical illnesses such as cancer, diabetes, and cardiovascular disease. The difficulty in finding genes arises not only because most common diseases are multifactorial but also because most are probably polygenic. The quick success with Huntington's disease was, in a sense, misleading because it is a classic mendelian single-gene disorder that is fully penetrant. It appears likely that most disorders are not classically mendelian, are not due to single genes, and involve genes that are not fully expressed or fully penetrant. Therefore, finding the genes has not been, and will not be, easy. However, the burgeoning technology and information of the Human Genome Project will certainly make this easier during the next several decades.

Once a gene has been found, cloning and sequencing are relatively simple and straightforward steps. When the fourth and fifth steps are reached, however, the joint efforts of clinicians and molecular biologists again become difficult. Simply knowing the sequence of amino acids after the gene has been sequenced does not necessarily explain what the gene product actually does. The product can be predicted by computers, but it must be verified by biological techniques, such as showing that it reacts with the antiserum of a known protein. Attesting to the difficulty of this step is the fact that we still do not know what enzyme or structural protein the Huntington's gene produces.

The fifth step, identifying the function of the abnormal allele (also known as *functional genomics*), is a difficult but necessary step. Even if one has identified a protein, one does not necessarily know how and when it acts to make the biological mischief that leads to disease. Even if we know that a particular gene has a disease-associated allele, and even if we know which enzyme is created through that gene, we do not necessarily know how and why an excess or a deficiency of that enzyme could cause a disease. Many enzymes are widely distributed in the brain, and human brain development and degeneration are prolonged processes that occur over many decades. Once we enter the domain of functional genomics and proteomics (understanding how changes in protein structure affect function), we must continually move up and down the cascade of events portrayed in Figure 5–1. We must traverse the range from genes to molecules to cells to circuits to functional systems of the mind/brain, ultimately understanding how aberrations in those functional systems lead to the illnesses that we recognize as Huntington's disease, Alzheimer's disease, schizophrenia, mood disorders, and anxiety disorders.

During the next several decades, multiple strategies will be used to study the molecular genetics and molecular biology of mental illnesses. These are summarized in Table 5–4.

TABLE 5–4.   Approaches to locating genes for mental illnesses

---

Linkage studies

Candidate genes and association studies

Genome scans

Snips and chips

Linkage studies were the earliest approaches to be applied to the search for genes in mental illnesses. Linkage techniques not only located the gene for Huntington's disease on chromosome 4 but also identified other linkages: much of this early work used the tools of restriction fragment length polymorphisms (RFLPs). This approach led to early reports of a linkage between bipolar illness and chromosome 11 and the X chromosome or linkages between schizophrenia and chromosomes 6, 8, and 22. Because linkage studies are cumbersome and prone to both false-positive and false-negative results, they have been largely abandoned in favor of other approaches.

Linkage studies are, in a sense, a blind search with no particular gene in mind, whereas candidate gene studies start with a theory that a particular gene may be involved in causing a mental illness. Genes used in the candidate gene approach must be polymorphic, and typically they involve a protein that could have some effect leading to mental illness. Examples of candidate genes include proteins regulating brain development such as brain-derived neurotrophic factor, neurotransmitters or neuroreceptors such as dopamine or the D_2 receptor, enzymes that affect neurotransmitter synthesis such as monoamine oxidase, and hormones that regulate brain activity such as neuropeptide Y. The strength of the candidate gene approach is that it directly permits investigators to determine whether a particular protein has any relevance to the production of a major mental illness. However, literally thousands of proteins might be investigated, so applying the candidate gene strategy is a bit like looking for a needle in a haystack. To date, this approach has not yielded many significant and consistently reproducible positive results.

Association studies are a related approach. In this instance, as in candidate gene studies, a case-control design is used to compare DNA from two groups of people: those who have diagnoses of a given illness and those who do not have the illness. (Refinements of this approach also may include family members.) One of the most successful examples of association studies was the discovery of the role of APOE in Alzheimer's disease. Association studies do not require a candidate gene but instead can use any DNA markers as long as they are reasonably closely spaced. Alan Roses and his colleagues studied a group of patients with Alzheimer's disease and found that the ε4 allele was significantly higher in the patients than in the control subjects (36% vs. 16%). This finding has now been replicated many times and has led to further studies of the role of APOE in Alzheimer's disease. This cholesterol-carrying protein may help form the senile plaques that occur in Alzheimer's disease. Whether the occurrence of plaques is a cause or a consequence of the illness is still hotly debated.

As Francis Collins, Craig Venter, and others progress steadily toward an increasingly refined map of the human genome, more elegant technologies will be applied to the study of mental illnesses. Scanning the entire genome of people with a given illness, as compared with healthy control subjects, is a logical step in the search for the genes that produce mental illness. This step has been held back by several factors, such as a lack of sufficient closely spaced markers and the inherent statistical problems of examining such a large volume of information. The risk of false-positive and false-negative results is always great when there is an excess of information. As of this writing, several scans of the entire genome have been done for major mental illnesses, and many more are likely to come. The results so far have been minimally useful, but this approach will almost certainly be fruitful in the future.

The search for genes in mental illness also will rely heavily on the techniques referred to as *snips and chips*. Snips is an abbreviation for SNPs, which refers to single nucleotide polymorphisms. These are point mutations that can be detected through the use of a powerful new microarray technology, the chip reader. Chip readers permit scientists to scan all 23 chromosomes from a given individual or group of individuals and to determine their allelic variations. As this technology matures and suitable samples from affected individuals or families are obtained, this technology will be used for case-control comparisons and association studies. These studies also must confront rigorous statistical challenges. However, the power of these techniques is indeed very exciting.

Bibliography

Andreasen NC: Brain imaging: applications in psychiatry. Science 239:1381–1388, 1988

Andreasen NC (ed): Brain Imaging: Applications in Psychiatry. Washington, DC, American Psychiatric Press, 1989

Andreasen NC: Brave New Brain. New York, Oxford University Press, 2001

Baron M, Risch N, Hamburger R, et al: Genetic linkage between X-chromosome markers and bipolar affective illness. Nature 326:289–292, 1987

Cooper JR, Bloom FE, Roth RA: The Biochemical Basis of Neuropharmacology, 7th Edition. New York, Oxford University Press, 1996

Creese I, Burt DR, Snyder SH: Dopamine receptor binding predicts clinical and pharmacological potencies of anti-schizophrenic drugs. Science 192:481–483, 1972

Davis M: The role of the amygdala in fear and anxiety. Ann Rev Neurosci 15:353–375, 1992

Doane BK, Livingston KF: The Limbic System: Functional Organization and Clinical Disorders. New York, Raven, 1986

Egeland JA, Gerhard DS, Pauls DL, et al: Bipolar affective disorders linked to DNA markers on chromosome 11. Nature 323:646–650, 1987

Faraone SV, Tsuang MT, Tsuang DW: Genetics of Mental Disorders. New York, Guilford, 1999

Fuster JM: The Prefrontal Cortex: Anatomy, Physiology, and Neuropsychology of the Frontal Lobe, 4th Edition. New York, Raven, 1997

Gazzaniga MS (ed): The New Cognitive Neurosciences, 2nd Edition. Cambridge, MA, MIT Press, 2000

Gershon ES, Cloninger CR: Genetic Approaches to Mental Disorders. Washington, DC, American Psychiatric Press, 1994

Gottesman II, Schields J: Schizophrenia: The Epigenetic Puzzle. New York, Cambridge University Press, 1982

Griffiths AJF, Miller JH, Suzuki DT, et al: An Introduction to Genetic Analysis, 6th Edition. New York, WH Freeman, 1996

Gusella JF, Wexler NS, Conneally PM, et al: A polymorphic DNA marker genetically linked to Huntington's disease. Nature 306:234–238, 1983

Hammond C: Cellular and Molecular Neurobiology. San Diego, CA, Academic Press, 1996

Heimer L: The Human Brain and Spinal Cord, 2nd Edition. New York, Springer-Verlag, 1995

Heston LL: The genetics of schizophrenic and schizoid disease. Science 167:249–256, 1970

Hyman SE, Nestler EJ: The Molecular Foundations of Psychiatry. Washington, DC, American Psychiatric Press, 1993

Isaacson RL: The Limbic System, 2nd Edition. New York, Plenum, 1982

Kallman FJ: The genetic theory of schizophrenia: an analysis of 691 schizophrenic twin index families. Am J Psychiatry 103:309–322, 1946

Kandel ER, Schwartz JH, Jessell TM: Principles of Neural Science, 4th Edition. New York, McGraw-Hill, 2000

Kelsoe JR, Ginns EI, Egeland JA, et al: Re-evaluation of the linkage relationship between chromosome 11p loci and the gene for bipolar affective disorder in the Old Order Amish. Nature 342:238–243, 1989

Kety SS, Rosenthal D, Wender PH, et al: Mental illness in the biological and adoptive families of adopted schizophrenics. Am J Psychiatry 128:302–306, 1971

LeDoux J: The Emotional Brain. New York, Simon & Schuster, 1996

Mesulam MM: Principles of Behavioral and Cognitive Neurology. New York, Oxford University Press, 2000

Nauta WJH, Feirtag M: Fundamental Neuroanatomy. New York, WH Freeman, 1986

Nurnberger JI, Berrettini W: Psychiatric Genetics. New York, Oxford University Press, 1997

Schatzberg AF, Nemeroff CB: The American Psychiatric Press Textbook of Psychopharmacology, 2nd Edition. Washington, DC, American Psychiatric Press, 1998

Seeman P, Lee T, Chau-Wong M, et al: Antipsychotic drug doses and neuroleptic-dopamine receptors. Nature 261:717–719, 1976

Slater E, Cowie V: The Genetics of Mental Disorders. London, Oxford University Press, 1971

Squire LR: Memory and Brain. Oxford, UK, Oxford University Press, 1987

Stuss DT, Benson DF: The Frontal Lobes. New York, Raven, 1986

Tulving E (ed): Memory, Consciousness, and the Brain. Philadelphia, PA, Psychology Press, 1999

Yudofsky SC, Hales RE: The American Psychiatric Press Textbook of Neuropsychiatry. Washington, DC, American Psychiatric Press, 1992

Self-Assessment Questions

1. What is the standard anatomical definition of the prefrontal cortex? Describe the functions performed by the prefrontal cortex. Contrast the euphoric syndrome with the apathetic syndrome.

2. Describe the limbic system, listing at least four of the structures included in it. What role does the limbic system play in emotion and memory?

3. Discuss possible relations between abnormalities in the frontal system, the memory system, and the language system in relation to the symptoms of psychosis.

4. Define a classic neurotransmitter and give five examples.

5. Describe the two receptor "superfamilies."

6. Discuss the ways that knowledge of receptor structure can influence the development of drugs used to treat mental illnesses.

7. Describe the location of cell bodies and projections for the dopamine system, the norepinephrine system, the serotonin system, and the acetylcholine system.

8. Describe the mechanisms by which abnormalities in GABA neurons may produce Huntington's disease. Describe the functions of glutamate and its possible relation to the symptoms of psychosis, using PCP as a model.

9. Describe the relative strengths of family studies, twin studies, and adoption studies as methods for determining the familiality of mental illnesses and the degree to which purely genetic factors play a causal role.

10. List the five steps involved in identifying disease genes, and summarize the progress made to date with Huntington's disease.

11. Discuss the possible interaction between genes and environmental factors in producing mental illness.

12. Describe the association studies of the APOE ε4 allele in Alzheimer's disease. Describe linkage methods, candidate gene strategies, association studies, and "snips and chips."

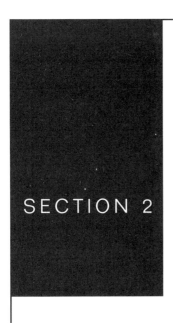

SECTION 2

Psychiatric Disorders

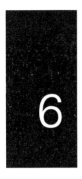

6 Cognitive Disorders

When age has crushed the body with its might, the
limbs collapse with weakness and decay, the judgment
limps, and mind and speech give way.

Lucretius

Mental disorders resulting from brain dysfunction have
been recognized for centuries. In the seventeenth century, the Italian anato-
mist Morgagni correlated clinical symptoms in patients with abnormal brain
findings identified on postmortem examination. Bayle, a Frenchman,
published the first systematic study of paresis in 1822 and linked changes in
brain parenchyma with progressive dementia. In Russia, Korsakoff described
an extreme form of amnesia thought to be due to brain stem lesions found
exclusively in chronic alcoholism—a condition frequently referred to as
Korsakoff's psychosis. In the late nineteenth century, the pioneering work of
the great neuropathologist-psychiatrists Alzheimer, Pick, Nissl, and Brodmann established conclusively that changes in brain structure and histology
underlay the dementing illnesses. Even Freud, the father of psychoanalysis,
understood the importance of neuroanatomical studies. He made the observation that most mental disorders would eventually be found to have a structural basis.

What historically have been referred to as *organic mental disorders* are
now classified in DSM-IV and DSM-IV-TR as cognitive disorders, mental dis-

orders due to a general medical condition, or substance-related disorders. Delirium, dementia, and amnestic disorder are the three major *cognitive disorders*. Each disturbance involves impaired memory, abstract thinking, or judgment and produces a clinically significant change from a previous level of functioning. All of the disorders discussed in this chapter result from medical illness (even though a specific condition may not be identified) or a substance (e.g., a drug of abuse, a medication), or a combination of factors. Mental disorders characterized by dysphoric mood, anxiety, psychosis, catatonia, or personality change that are substance related or due to a medical condition are also presented. In DSM-IV-TR, these latter conditions are included within the diagnostic category with which they share syndromal features; for instance, mania induced by psychostimulants is included with the mood disorders. The cognitive disorders are listed in Table 6–1, and other specific mental disorders that are substance induced or due to a general medical condition are in Table 6–2.

Cognitive Disorders

Delirium

Delirium is a syndrome characterized by a disturbance of consciousness, impaired attention, and a change in cognition. Its defining feature is a reduced awareness of the environment that is a consequence of a medical condition as evidenced by history, physical examination, or laboratory findings. Delirium develops quickly over hours or days and tends to fluctuate during the course of the day (see Table 6–3). Its symptoms are generally alarming and are considered a medical emergency.

Delirium is surprisingly common; in hospital settings, an estimated 10%–15% of medical patients develop a delirium. Delirium is particularly common among postsurgical and elderly patients, especially those older than 80 years. Other risk factors for delirium include a preexisting dementia, bone fractures, systemic infections, and use of narcotics or antipsychotics. Delirium is associated with high mortality—an estimated 40%–50% of the patients with delirium die within 1 year of developing the disturbance.

Clinical Findings

The hallmark of delirium is the rapid development of disorientation, confusion, and global cognitive impairment. Although the presentation of delirium differs among patients, several features are characteristic: disturbance of consciousness evidenced by a reduced clarity of awareness of the environment; difficulty focusing, sustaining, or shifting attention; impaired cogni-

TABLE 6–1.   Cognitive disorders

Delirium

    Due to a general medical condition

    Substance-induced

    Due to multiple etiologies

    Not otherwise specified

Dementia

    Of the Alzheimer type

        With early onset (age 65 years or below)

        With late onset (after age 65 years)

    Vascular

    Due to other general medical conditions

        HIV disease

        Head trauma

        Parkinson's disease

        Huntington's disease

        Pick's disease

        Creutzfeld-Jacob disease

        Other (e.g., normal pressure hydrocephalus, brain tumor, vitamin B12 deficiency)

    Substance-induced persisting dementia

    Due to multiple etiologies

    Not otherwise specified

Amnestic Disorder

    Due to a general medical condition

    Substance-induced persisting amnestic disorder

    Not other wise specified

Cognitive disorder not otherwise specified

tion; and perceptual disturbances (e.g., illusions). At times, the patient may appear normal but later in the day may be disoriented and hallucinating. Other symptoms typical of delirium include sleep-wake cycle disturbances with worsening at night (sundowning); disorientation to place, date, or person; incoherence; restlessness; and agitation or excessive somnolence.

TABLE 6–2.   Other specific mental disorders that are substance induced or due to a general medical condition

Psychotic disorder

    Substance induced

    Due to a general medical condition

Mood disorder

    Substance induced

    Due to a general medical condition

Anxiety disorder

    Substance induced

    Due to a general medical condition

Catatonic disorder due to a general medical condition

Personality change due to a general medical condition

Mental disorder not otherwise specified due to a general medical condition

TABLE 6–3.   DSM-IV-TR criteria for delirium due to a general medical condition

A. Disturbance of consciousness (i.e., reduced clarity of awareness of the environment) with reduced ability to focus, sustain, or shift attention.

B. A change in cognition (such as memory deficit, disorientation, language disturbance) or the development of a perceptual disturbance that is not better accounted for by a preexisting, established, or evolving dementia.

C. The disturbance develops over a short period of time (usually hours to days) and tends to fluctuate during the course of the day.

D. There is evidence from the history, physical examination, or laboratory findings that the disturbance is caused by the direct physiological consequences of a general medical condition.

    Coding note: If delirium is superimposed on a preexisting Vascular Dementia, indicate the delirium by coding 290.41 Vascular Dementia, With Delirium.

    Coding note: Include the name of the general medical condition on Axis I, e.g., 293.0 Delirium Due to Hepatic Encephalopathy; also code the general medical condition on Axis III.

The following vignette illustrates a relatively typical case of delirium seen in our hospital:

> An 84-year-old retired police chief was brought to the emergency room by his family because of a 4- to 5-day history of lassitude, lower-extremity weakness, bladder incontinence, and intermittent confusion and memory loss. The patient had fallen 4 weeks earlier and had sustained a scalp laceration that required suturing. He had no history of recent alcohol use.
>
> The patient was cooperative but drowsy and easily distracted. He was oriented to person but was disoriented to date and situation. His memory for recent events was extremely poor, and he was unable to recall three objects either immediately or at 3 minutes. He thought that Franklin Roosevelt was the current president. Interestingly, the patient had known the paternal grandfather of one of the authors (D.W.B.) and was able to speak at length of this remote relationship.
>
> A presumptive diagnosis of delirium was made, and a medical workup was begun. A computed tomography (CT) scan showed the presence of bilateral chronic subdural hematomas. The patient was transferred to the neurosurgery service, where burr hole evacuation was performed. The delirium cleared, but the patient had a residual dementia. He was transferred to a long-term nursing facility.

Etiology

Delirium most commonly occurs in persons who have serious medical, surgical, or neurological illness or who are in a state of drug intoxication or withdrawal. Because the development of a delirium can be the first manifestation of an underlying physical disorder, the presence of a delirium always should lead to an immediate search for a medical explanation. Because delirium is a syndrome and not a disease, it is best seen as the final common pathway of many potential causes. Metabolic disturbances, such as those caused by infection, febrile illness, hypoxia, hypoglycemia, drug intoxication or withdrawal states, or hepatic encephalopathy, commonly cause delirium. Common causes of delirium that lie within the central nervous system (CNS) include brain abscesses, stroke, traumatic injuries, and postictal states. Other causes seen frequently in the elderly are new-onset arrhythmias such as atrial fibrillation and cardiac ischemia. Delirium can be influenced by environmental events, but these events do not cause delirium. For example, before delirium was well understood, patients who became delirious postsurgery were thought to have an "ICU psychosis," presumably caused by the psychological reaction to the strange environment.

Assessment

The medical evaluation should be thorough, begin with a careful history, and include a complete physical examination. Informants should be interviewed because the patient may not be able to provide information. Close attention should be given to the presence of focal neurological signs, including weakness or sensory loss, papilledema, and frontal lobe release signs (e.g., suck, snout, palmomental, rooting reflexes), that indicate global deficit states. Laboratory tests should include routine blood and urine studies (e.g., complete blood count, urinalysis), chest X ray, a CT scan or magnetic resonance imaging (MRI) scan of the brain, an electrocardiogram (ECG), lumbar puncture (in selected patients), toxic screen, blood gases, and an electroencephalogram (EEG). Laboratory test results will vary depending on the underlying cause of the delirium. Delirious patients frequently have temperature elevations that probably represent autonomic instability or underlying infections. EEG findings are often abnormal and show generalized diffuse slowing.

The major problem in differential diagnosis is distinguishing delirium from a functional confusional state, which occasionally occurs in patients with schizophrenia or a mood disorder. Delirious patients tend to have a more acute presentation, are globally confused, and have greater impairment in attention. Hallucinations, when present, are fragmentary and disorganized and tend to be visual or tactile as opposed to the auditory hallucinations seen in patients with psychotic disorders. Delirious patients are less likely to have a personal or family history of psychiatric illness. However, the presence of a prior psychiatric illness does not preclude the possibility of developing a delirium.

Clinical Management

First, the underlying medical condition must be corrected whenever possible. Until the condition is corrected, measures must be taken to maintain the patient's health and safety, including constant observation, consistent nursing care, and frequent reassurance with repeated simple explanations. Restraints may be necessary in highly agitated patients, although experience has shown that they may actually increase agitation in a few patients. External stimulation should be minimized. Because shadows or darkness may be frightening, delirious patients tend to do better in quiet, well-lighted rooms. Delirious patients are exquisitely sensitive to drug side effects, so unnecessary medication should be discontinued, including sedatives or hypnotics (e.g., benzodiazepines). Highly agitated patients may be calmed with low doses of high-potency antipsychotic medication (e.g., haloperidol, thiothixene). Drugs with significant anticholinergic effects (e.g., chlorpromazine, thioridazine) should be avoided because they can worsen or prolong the delirium. In fact, plasma anticholinergic levels have been found to correlate with delirium in surgical patients. When sedation is necessary, low doses of short-acting benzodiazepines (e.g., oxazepam, lorazepam) can be helpful. Because unrecognized alcohol withdrawal can manifest as delirium, particularly in the postsurgical patient, benzodiazepines may be helpful because they will treat the withdrawal state. In this scenario, benzodiazepines should be continued over 3–5 days. (See Chapter 14 for the treatment of alcohol withdrawal.) Treatment recommendations are summarized in the box below.

Recommendations for management of delirium

In the hospital, a quiet, restful setting that is well lighted is best for the confused patient.

1. Consistency of personnel is less likely to upset the delirious patient.

2. Reminders of day, date, time, place, and situation should be prominently displayed in the patient's room.

3. Medication for behavioral management should be limited to those cases in which behavioral interventions have failed.

   - Only essential drugs should be prescribed, and polypharmacy should be avoided.
   - Sedative-hypnotics and anxiolytics should be avoided.
   - Unmanageable behavior also may require low-dose neuroleptics or, alternatively, benzodiazepines with short half-lives (e.g., lorazepam, 0.5 mg twice daily).

Dementia

Dementia is a syndrome of impaired memory and cognition accompanied by a decline in social and occupational functioning. Consciousness or level of alertness (i.e., sensorium) is generally not disturbed. Cognitive impairment can involve the four *A*'s:

1. Aphasia (language disturbance)
2. Amnesia
3. Apraxia (inability to carry out complex motor activities)
4. Agnosia (failure to recognize or identify objects despite intact sensory function)

Unlike mental retardation (which can be associated with these symptoms), dementias are acquired. The impairment created by dementia distinguishes it from the mild memory change ("benign senescent forgetfulness") that occurs during normal aging. Most dementias are irreversible, but some can be controlled by therapeutic interventions. A small number of dementias are potentially reversible, but only 3% fully resolve. A search for treatable causes is mandatory in the patient with dementia.

Dementia is relatively uncommon in persons younger than 65 years. About 10% of persons between ages 65 and 75 have dementia. Between ages 75 and 85, 25% or more have dementia; by age 90, the rate is 50%. The rates of dementia are even higher among elderly hospitalized patients and physically ill persons. Because the growth in the United States population of those older than 65 is outstripping the growth in the general population, it is projected that the problem of dementia will be even greater in the future.

Clinical Findings

Dementia usually develops insidiously, and preliminary signs may be overlooked or misattributed to normal aging. (Some forms of dementia, however, can develop fairly abruptly, such as a vascular dementia due to a stroke.) In its earliest stages, the only symptom may be a subtle change in the patient's personality, a decrease in the range of the patient's interests, the development of apathy, or the development of labile or shallow emotions. Intellectual skills are gradually affected and may be noticed initially in work settings where high performance is required. At this point, the patient may be unaware of the loss of intellectual sharpness or may deny the loss. Characteristics that help to separate delirium from dementia are highlighted in Table 6–4.

TABLE 6–4.   Clinical features differentiating dementia from delirium

Dementia	Delirium
Chronic or insidious onset	Acute or rapid onset
Level of consciousness unimpaired early on	Level of consciousness clouded
Normal level of arousal	Agitation or stupor
Usually progressive and deteriorating	Often reversible
Common in nursing homes and psychiatric hospitals	Common on medical, surgical, and neurological wards

As the dementia advances, cognitive impairment becomes more pronounced, the changes in mood and personality become more exaggerated, social skills are lost (whereas in earlier stages, they may have helped to preserve the patient's image of health), and psychotic symptoms may arise.

When the dementia is advanced, the patient may be unable to perform basic tasks such as self-feeding or caring for personal hygiene, may become incontinent, and may develop extreme emotional lability. Patients frequently forget names of friends and are sometimes unable to recognize close relatives. In the end stages of dementia, a patient may become mute and unresponsive. At this stage, death usually follows within a year.

It is important to separate dementia from *pseudodementia,* a condition that sometimes accompanies depressive illness. In this disturbance, the depressed patient appears to have dementia. He or she is unable to remember correctly, cannot calculate well, and complains, often bitterly, of lost cognitive abilities and skills. Features that are helpful in differentiating dementia from pseudodementia are presented in Table 6–5. The importance of this distinction is obvious; the patient with pseudodementia has a treatable illness (depression) and does not have a dementia. The dementia is an artifact of the patient's underlying mood disorder. Of course, the patient with dementia may develop a co-occurring major depression, which will likely intensify the cognitive and memory disturbance.

TABLE 6–5.   Clinical features differentiating pseudodementia from dementia

Pseudodementia	Dementia
Short duration	Long duration
Complaints of cognitive loss	Few complaints of cognitive loss
Complaints of cognitive dysfunction usually detailed	Complaints of cognitive dysfunction, usually imprecise
Communications of distress	Often appear unconcerned
Memory gaps for specific periods or events	Memory gaps for specific periods unusual
Attention and concentration usually well preserved	Attention and concentration faulty
"Don't know" answer typical	Near-miss answers frequent
Little effort to perform simple tasks	Patients struggle to perform tasks
Patients highlight failures	Patients delight in trivial accomplishments
Early loss of social skills	Social skills often retained
Mood change pervasive	Affect shallow and labile
History of psychiatric illness common	History of psychiatric illness uncommon

The noncognitive symptoms of dementia are often the most troublesome, especially from the family member's viewpoint (see Table 6–6). In some forms of dementia, such as Alzheimer's disease, up to half of the patients develop hallucinations and/or delusions. Nearly 20% develop clinical depression, although perhaps an equal number have milder depressive symptoms. Depression is even more common in patients with vascular dementia. Because symptoms of dementia and depression overlap, the distinction between dementia and depression may be difficult to determine. Clues to the diagnosis of depression include recent weight loss (in the absence of cancer or apraxia in swallowing), worsening sleep, frequent crying spells, self-deprecating comments ("I can't do anything!"), and recent behavior changes such as social withdrawal, psychomotor agitation, and extreme negativism.

Diagnosis

The best tools in the physician's armamentarium to detect dementia are the oldest: a thorough history, a careful physical examination, and a detailed mental status examination (MSE). To supplement a formal MSE, the Mini-Mental State Exam, a quick, at-the-bedside test, can be used to obtain a rough index of cognitive impairment. (This test is included in the Appendix.) The test assesses orientation, memory, constructional ability, and the ability to read, write, and calculate and can be administered quickly. Thirty points are possible: a score of less than 25 is suggestive of impairment, and a score of less than 20 usually indicates definite impairment.

Laboratory testing is an important part of the evaluation to exclude irreversible medical sources of cognitive impairment. All patients with a new onset of dementia should have a complete blood count; liver, thyroid, and renal function tests; serologic tests for syphilis and human immunodeficiency virus (HIV); urinalysis; ECG; and chest X ray. Serum electrolytes, serum glucose, and vitamin B_{12} and folate levels should be measured. Most of the readily reversible metabolic, endocrine, vitamin deficiency, and infectious states, whether causal or complicating, will be uncovered with these simple tests when combined with the history and physical examination findings. Other laboratory tests are helpful in carefully selected patients; for example, a CT or an MRI brain scan is appropriate in the presence of a history suggestive of a mass lesion, focal neurological signs, or a very brief dementia. EEGs are appropriate for patients with altered consciousness or suspected seizures. Arterial blood gases are indicated when compromised respiratory function is evident. Cerebral blood flow as measured by single photon emission computed tomography (SPECT) or positron-emission tomography

TABLE 6–6. Behavior problems of 55 patients cited by family members

Behavior	Families reporting problems, %
Memory disturbance	100
Temper outbursts	87
Demanding or critical behavior	71
Night awakening	69
Hiding things	69
Communication difficulties	68
Suspiciousness	63
Making accusations	60
Poor mealtime behavior	60
Daytime wandering	59
Poor hygiene	53
Hallucinations	49
Delusions	47
Physical violence	47
Incontinence	40
Difficulty with cooking	33
Hitting or assaults	32
Problems driving	20
Problems smoking	11
Inappropriate sexual behavior	2

Source. Adapted from Rabins et al. 1982b.

(PET) imaging can help to distinguish Alzheimer's dementia from other forms of dementia because these patients have a relatively characteristic bilateral decrease in posterior temporoparietal blood flow. The medical workup for dementia is summarized in Table 6–7.

Neuropsychological testing can be very helpful in the evaluation of dementia. Testing can be done to obtain baseline data by which to measure change both before and after treatment. Testing can be helpful in evaluating highly educated individuals suspected of developing an early dementia when brain imaging or other test results are ambiguous. Testing also may help distinguish delirium from dementia and depression.

Although most patients with dementia can be evaluated on an outpa-

TABLE 6–7. Medical workup for dementia

1. Complete history
2. Thorough physical examination, including neurological examination
3. Mental status examination
4. Laboratory studies
   - Complete blood count, with differential
   - Serum electrolytes
   - Serum glucose
   - Blood urea nitrogen
   - Creatinine
   - Liver function tests
   - Serology for syphilis and HIV
   - Thyroid function tests
   - Serum vitamin B_{12}
   - Folate
   - Urinalysis and urine drug screen
   - Electrocardiogram
   - Chest X ray
   - Brain computed tomography or magnetic resonance imaging
5. Neuropsychological testing
6. Optional tests
   - Cerebral blood flow (i.e., single photon emission computed tomography)
   - Lumbar puncture

tient basis, some patients will need to be hospitalized. In practice, most hospital admissions involving dementia patients are for the evaluation and treatment of behavioral and psychological complications such as aggression, violence, wandering, psychosis, or depression. Other reasons for hospitalization include suicidal threats or behaviors, rapid weight loss, or acute deterioration without an apparent cause.

Irreversible Causes of Dementia

Alzheimer's disease. Alzheimer's disease is the most common cause of degenerative dementias and accounts for 50%–60% of all cases of dementia.

It affects approximately 2.5 million Americans. In DSM-IV-TR, Alzheimer's dementia is divided into early (age 65 and younger) and late (older than 65 years) onset types. Most of the early-onset cases of Alzheimer's disease are classified as familial Alzheimer's disease. These patients often have an onset in the fifth decade, and the disorder has been linked to mutations on chromosomes 1, 14, and 21. (See Table 6–8 for the DSM-IV-TR diagnostic criteria for dementia of the Alzheimer's type.)

Alzheimer's disease usually begins insidiously, leading to death 8–10 years after its symptoms are recognized. Estimates of the prevalence of Alzheimer's disease range from 5% at age 65 to 20% by age 90. Symptoms begin to gradually and progressively worsen over many years, resulting in near collapse of intellectual functioning. Physical findings are generally absent, or they are present only in later stages: hyperactive deep tendon reflexes, Babinski's sign, and frontal lobe release signs. The presence of illusions, hallucinations, or delusions is associated with accelerated cognitive deterioration. Cortical atrophy and enlarged cerebral ventricles are typically seen on CT scan or MRI.

The case of composer Maurice Ravel illustrates the tragedy of dementia of the Alzheimer's type:

> Ravel, a leader of the French musical impressionist movement, excelled at piano composition and orchestration. At age 56, after completing his most famous work, Concerto in G Minor, he began to complain of fatigue and lassitude, symptoms that were in keeping with his chronic insomnia and lifelong hypochondriasis. His symptoms continued to progress, and his creative energy waned.
>
> The following year, after a minor automobile accident, Ravel's cognitive abilities began to erode. His capacity to remember names, to speak spontaneously, and to write became impaired. An eminent French neurologist noted that Ravel's ability to understand verbal speech was superior to his ability to speak or to write. Tragically, Ravel also developed amusia, the inability to comprehend musical sounds. His last public performance occurred shortly thereafter. He was no longer capable of the coordination, cognition, and speech necessary to lead an orchestra.
>
> Ravel's friends made futile attempts to help him, trying to stimulate him intellectually any way they could. But gradually his speech and intellectual functions declined further. Within 4 years of the onset of dementia, Ravel was mute and incapable of recognizing his own music.
>
> Ravel died at age 62 years, after a neurosurgical procedure, the indications for which remain unclear. No autopsy was done, but his neurologist had suspected a cerebral degenerative disease. Syphilis, a common illness of the day, had been ruled out. (Dalessio 1984)

TABLE 6–8. DSM-IV-TR criteria for dementia of the Alzheimer's type

---

A. The development of multiple cognitive deficits manifested by both

   (1) memory impairment (impaired ability to learn new information or to recall previously learned information)

   (2) one (or more) of the following cognitive disturbances:

       (a) aphasia (language disturbance)

       (b) apraxia (impaired ability to carry out motor activities despite intact motor function)

       (c) agnosia (failure to recognize or identify objects despite intact sensory function)

       (d) disturbance in executive functioning (i.e., planning, organizing, sequencing, abstracting)

B. The cognitive deficits in Criteria A1 and A2 each cause significant impairment in social or occupational functioning and represent a significant decline from a previous level of functioning.

C. The course is characterized by gradual onset and continuing cognitive decline.

D. The cognitive deficits in Criteria A1 and A2 are not due to any of the following:

   (1) other central nervous system conditions that cause progressive deficits in memory and cognition (e.g., cerebrovascular disease, Parkinson's disease, Huntington's disease, subdural hematoma, normal-pressure hydrocephalus, brain tumor)

   (2) systemic conditions that are known to cause dementia (e.g., hypothyroidism, vitamin B_{12} or folic acid deficiency, niacin deficiency, hypercalcemia, neurosyphilis, HIV infection)

   (3) substance-induced conditions

E. The deficits do not occur exclusively during the course of a delirium.

F. The disturbance is not better accounted for by another Axis I disorder (e.g., Major Depressive Disorder, Schizophrenia).

Code based on presence or absence of a clinically significant behavioral disturbance:

   294.10 Without Behavioral Disturbance: if the cognitive disturbance is not accompanied by any clinically significant behavioral disturbance.

   294.11 With Behavioral Disturbance: if the cognitive disturbance is accompanied by a clinically significant behavioral disturbance (e.g., wandering, agitation).

Specify subtype:

   With Early Onset: if onset is at age 65 years or below

   With Late Onset: if onset is after age 65 years

   Coding note: Also code 331.0 Alzheimer's disease on Axis III. Indicate other prominent clinical features related to the Alzheimer's disease on Axis I (e.g., 293.83 Mood Disorder Due to Alzheimer's Disease, With Depressive Features, and 310.1 Personality Change Due to Alzheimer's Disease, Aggressive Type).

Although Alzheimer's disease is not definitely diagnosable during life, characteristic brain pathology is found at autopsy, including senile plaques (degenerating neurons tangled around an amyloid core), neurofibrillary tangles (helical filaments tangled within neurons), neuronal granulovacuolar degeneration of nerve cell bodies, and Hirano bodies (elongated red structures often found in the hippocampus). Research has shown that loss of cholinergic neurons in basal forebrain pathways is a consistent biochemical feature of the disease.

Risk factors for Alzheimer's disease include a history of head injury, Down's syndrome, low educational and occupational level, and having a first-degree relative with Alzheimer's disease. In fact, up to 50% of the first-degree relatives of persons with dementia of the Alzheimer's type are affected with the disorder by age 90 years. A gene on chromosome 19, apolipoprotein E (APOE), has been found to influence the risk of Alzheimer's disease. The APOE ε4 allele increases risk and decreases age at onset of Alzheimer's disease, and the APOE ε2 allele has a protective effect. Alzheimer's disease susceptibility from APOE occurs worldwide.

Dementia with Lewy bodies. Dementia with Lewy bodies is progressive and irreversible and has clinical features similar to those of Alzheimer's disease. Prominent visual hallucinations and parkinsonian features tend to occur starting early in the illness. The course is often slightly more rapid than in Alzheimer's disease. In addition to changes in the brain parenchyma typical for Alzheimer's disease, Lewy bodies—eosinophilic inclusion bodies—are seen in the cerebral cortex and brain stem. Recent research suggests that dementia with Lewy bodies may account for up to one-quarter of dementia cases. Patients with this form of dementia are very sensitive to extrapyramidal side effects of conventional antipsychotics, which are contraindicated.

Pick's disease. Pick's disease accounts for about 5% of irreversible dementias. It tends to begin with personality changes, bizarre behavior, and social disinhibition. Once cognitive impairment becomes severe, it is clinically indistinguishable from Alzheimer's disease and can be definitively diagnosed only after death. At autopsy, the brain shows distinctive frontotemporal atrophy and ventricular dilatation. Microscopic examination shows neuronal loss with gliosis and the presence of Pick's bodies in the neurons. Pick's bodies contain masses of cytoskeletal elements that bind polyclonal antibodies against neurotubules and a monoclonal antibody against neurofilaments. The disorder is more common in men and in first-degree relatives of persons with Pick's disease.

Huntington's disease. Huntington's disease is a neuropsychiatric disorder with autosomal-dominant inheritance. Its gene has been located on the short arm of chromosome 4. Psychiatric manifestations range from mild depression, anxiety, and irritability to frank hallucinations and delusions, which may precede the onset of choreiform movements. Dementia occurs in the terminal phase of the illness and is characterized by impaired cognition without a language disorder.

Creutzfeldt-Jakob disease. Creutzfeldt-Jakob disease (CJD) is a virulent and irreversible cause of dementia. It is caused by prions, which are small proteinaceous particles that cause spongiform changes in the brain. In the past, CJD and other spongiform encephalopathies were thought to be due to "slow viruses." CJD is rare, has a peak incidence between 50 and 70 years, and is characterized by a rapidly progressive dementing illness that causes death, usually within a few months. The incubation period can be months to years. Severe cerebellar and/or extrapyramidal signs, along with myoclonus, are present; akinetic mutism and cortical blindness can occur. Triphasic complexes are found on EEGs in about 80% of the cases. Histopathology shows spongiform changes, which consist of fine vacuolation of the neuropil of the gray matter, associated with astrocytosis and neuronal loss. CJD occurs sporadically and may be inherited or transmitted by intracerebral electrodes, grafts of dura mater, corneal transplants, and human-derived growth hormone and gonadotropin. The disease is invariably fatal, and there are no known treatments. A new variant of CJD recently has been described that has an earlier onset (average age of 27 vs. 60), more psychiatric symptoms, a longer course (14 months vs. 4 months), and an absence of triphasic complexes on EEG.

Other irreversible causes of dementia. Other irreversible forms of dementia include diseases of the basal ganglia (Parkinson's disease), cerebellum (cerebellar, spinocerebellar, and olivopontocerebellar degeneration), and motor neuron (amyotrophic lateral sclerosis); the Parkinson-dementia complex of Guam; herpes simplex encephalitis; and the dementia of multiple sclerosis. Numerous hereditary metabolic diseases are associated with irreversible dementia, including Wilson's disease (hepatolenticular degeneration), metachromatic leukodystrophy, the adrenoleukodystrophies, and the neuronal storage diseases (e.g., Tay-Sachs disease).

Clinical Management

Cholinergic therapies address the well-known deficit of acetylcholine in Alzheimer's disease. Three drugs have been approved by the U.S. Food and Drug Administration: tacrine, donepezil, and rivastigmine. Tacrine is started at a dose of 10 mg four times a day and increased slowly to a total of 160 mg/day. Liver enzyme elevations occur in 40% of patients and require monitoring every other week during the dose escalation. Donepezil is started at a dose of 5 mg/day and increased to a dose of 10 mg/day after 4 weeks. Rivastigmine is started at 1.5 mg/day and increased every 2 weeks to a maximum of 6 mg/day. Neither donepezil nor rivastigmine are associated with hepatotoxicity. The drugs are equally effective and work to slow the rate of cognitive decline. There is a marked variation in response—some patients show tremendous improvement, whereas others show very little improvement. These drugs do not alter the course of the disease and work best in persons in the earliest stages of the disease.

Other medications are used for the symptomatic treatment of associated anxiety, psychosis, or depression, including the anxiolytics, antipsychotics, and antidepressants, respectively. The physician must find the lowest effective dose because patients with dementia often poorly tolerate drug side effects. In treating depression in patients with dementia, physicians should avoid tricyclic antidepressants and use the better-tolerated serotonin reuptake inhibitors (e.g., fluoxetine, paroxetine). Whatever drug is used, patients with dementia require lower doses than do persons without dementia.

Irritability, hostility, aggression, uncooperativeness, and assaultiveness are the most difficult and vexing problems to manage in patients with dementia. These disturbing and disruptive symptoms may make it difficult to keep the patient within his or her family or social situation and can lead to institutionalization. Antipsychotics are frequently prescribed to control behavior problems in dementia patients. High-potency antipsychotic medications (e.g., haloperidol 1–2 mg/day) are effective but can induce extrapyramidal side effects. Atypical antipsychotics (e.g., risperidone 0.5–2 mg/day) also appear effective and are better tolerated. Trazodone, given as a bedtime dose (25–100 mg), may be particularly effective in relieving nighttime agitation or sundowning. Anticonvulsants, including carbamazepine and valproate, also have been used to reduce agitation and are generally well tolerated. Buspirone, a nonbenzodiazepine anxiolytic, is of benefit to some patients with anxious symptoms, although its onset of action may take 2–3 weeks. Benzodiazepines should be avoided except for the treatment of occasional episodes of acute agitation in persons who otherwise have no need for ongoing antiagitation medication. In these situations, low doses of lorazepam (0.25–1 mg) may be useful.

The behavioral goals of treatment should be the maintenance of the patient's socialization and provision of support for the family. Reality orientation may be worthwhile; reminiscence group therapy may help patients to maintain their social skills. Even severely affected patients can react to familiar social activities and to music. Self-help groups for family members provide educational and psychological support. Day-care centers may provide needed relief for caregivers. A useful manual is *The 36-Hour Day* (Mace and Rabins 1999).

Treatment recommendations are summarized in the box below.

Recommendations for the management of dementia

1. Both at home and in care facilities, patients usually respond better to low-stimulus environments than to high-stimulus situations.

   • Patients with dementia have difficulty interpreting sensory input and easily become overwhelmed.

2. Consistency and routine are important for reducing confusion and agitation.

3. Families are often overwhelmed by caring for a cognitively impaired relative.

   • The clinician should recommend that family members attend support groups available in most communities.
   • The clinician should provide appropriate reading material.

4. Families should be given psychological support if the patient requires institutionalization, to lessen the guilt they almost inevitably feel.

5. Cholinergic therapies may slow the rate of cognitive decline. Tacrine, donepezil, and rivastigmine are effective, but the latter two are better tolerated. Nonetheless, accompanying depression generally responds to antidepressants, and acute agitation or psychosis may respond to antipsychotic medication.

   • Serotonin reuptake inhibitors are better tolerated than other antidepressants (e.g., fluoxetine, 5–20 mg/day).
   • Low-potency antipsychotics should be avoided because of their anticholinergic side effects; atypical antipsychotics are well tolerated and may be effective for the patient (e.g., risperidone, 0.5–2.0 mg/day).
   • For long-term behavioral management, lithium carbonate, propranolol, valproate, carbamazepine, and other agents have been tried, but benefit is inconsistent.
   • Trazodone given as a bedtime dose (e.g., 25–100 mg) is effective in relieving nighttime agitation.

Treatable Forms of Dementia

Vascular disorders

Vascular dementia is the second most common cause of dementia after Alzheimer's disease, accounting for about 15%–30% of dementia cases. In many cases, vascular dementia is combined with dementia of the Alzheimer's type. Vascular dementia can vary widely, depending on the specific etiology (e.g., multiple infarcts, strategic single vessel infarct, small vessel disease, hemorrhage). Dementia caused by multiple infarcts probably accounts for the bulk of the cases and results from accumulation of cerebral infarcts in persons with atherosclerotic disease of major vessels or heart valves. It is sometimes accompanied by focal neurological deficits. A history of rapid onset and a stepwise deterioration occurring in patients in their 50s or 60s help to distinguish dementia caused by multiple infarcts from the degenerative dementias. Patients with vascular dementia frequently have high blood pressure or diabetes and often have had prior strokes, many of them "silent." Atherosclerosis in major arteries may be surgically correctable, but because atherosclerosis occurs diffusely among smaller intracranial vessels, it is not amenable to any specific intervention. Hypertension can be controlled, and early treatment of asymptomatic patients can help prevent or arrest the development of vascular dementia. The administration of anticoagulants or aspirin, which can help prevent thrombus formation, decreases the risk of myocardial infarction and stroke.

Subdural hematoma may produce a dementia or may complicate other forms of dementia. Subdural hematomas are caused by a disruption of the veins that bridge the brain parenchyma and the meninges and usually are attributable to trauma, as in the vignette earlier in this chapter. Risk factors for subdural hematoma include being older than 60 years and having a history of alcoholism, epilepsy, or renal dialysis. The disorder is treated by evacuation of the hematoma through a burr hole in the skull.

Normal-pressure hydrocephalus

Normal-pressure hydrocephalus is caused by excessive accumulation of cerebrospinal fluid (CSF), which gradually dilates the ventricles of the brain in the presence of normal CSF pressure. The flow of CSF from the ventricles to its usual site of absorption becomes obstructed so that fluid collects within the ventricles, resulting in the triad of dementia, gait disturbance, and urinary incontinence. Normal-pressure hydrocephalus can result from brain trauma, but the cause usually is unknown. Some patients respond dramatically to shunting of the ventriculosubarachnoid reservoir.

Infections

Any infection that involves the brain is capable of producing a dementing illness. Many cases of dementia are prevented by the effective treatment of meningitis and encephalitis, whether caused by bacteria, fungi, protozoa, or viruses. Chronic infectious processes—for example, those caused by bacteria (e.g., Whipple's disease), fungi (e.g., *Cryptococcus*), or other microorganisms (e.g., syphilis)—may affect the brain in such a way that the process is reversible and arrestable, at least to some extent. A postinfectious encephalomyelitis occurring after a viral exanthem may produce sufficient brain damage to result in a dementia.

Dementia may occur in patients with acquired immunodeficiency syndrome (AIDS). The dementia can be caused by direct HIV infection of the nervous system, intracranial tumors, infections (e.g., toxoplasmosis, cryptococcosis), or the indirect effects of systemic disease (e.g., septicemia, hypoxia, electrolyte imbalance). Because dementia may occur in the early stages of HIV infection, evaluation for HIV seropositivity is indicated for persons at high risk for infection (e.g., homosexual men, drug-addicted persons) who develop cognitive, mood, or behavioral changes. (See Chapter 22 for a more complete discussion of the psychiatric aspects of HIV disease.)

Metabolic disorders

Chronic diseases of the thyroid, parathyroid, adrenal, and pituitary glands can cause reversible dementias and usually are readily identified. Pulmonary diseases can produce dementia as a result of hypoxia or hypercapnia. Chronic or acute renal failure may cause a reversible dementia, as can liver failure (i.e., hepatic encephalopathy). Dementia is common in diabetic patients as a result of either hypoglycemia or hyperosmolar coma.

Nutritional disorders

Chronic alcoholism may contribute to global dementia, and thiamine deficiency may lead to Wernicke's encephalopathy, an amnestic disorder. (Both disorders are discussed later in the chapter.) There are different mechanisms by which pernicious anemia can produce dementia, not all of which are reversible. Folate deficiency is potentially reversible if recognized early. Pellagra (niacin deficiency), a major problem in underdeveloped countries, shows a dramatic response to niacin, even when mental changes have been present for a long time.

Treatable causes of dementia are summarized in Table 6–9.

TABLE 6–9. Treatable causes of dementia

Vascular	Toxicity
Multiple infarcts	Bromides
Subacute bacterial endocarditis	Mercury
Decreased cardiac output	Others
Myocardial infarction, heart failure	Infections
Collagen vascular diseases (e.g., lupus, polyarteritis)	General paresis
	Cryptococcal meningitis
Metabolic and endocrine	Encephalitis
Hypothyroidism	Sarcoid
Hyperparathyroidism	Postinfectious
Pituitary insufficiency	encephalomyelitis
Repeated hypoglycemia	Mass Effect
Respiratory acidosis	Lymphoma and leukemia (with or without pathologic change)
Uremia	Intracranial tumor (e.g., subfrontal meningioma)
Hepatic encephalopathy	
Porphyria	Subdural hematoma
Wilson's disease	Subclinical seizures
Nutrition	Demyelinating disease
Pernicious anemia	Normal pressure hydrocephalus
Alcoholics and thiamine deficiency	
Pellagra	

Amnestic Disorder

The main feature of amnestic disorder is an inability to learn new information or to recall previously learned information, leading to significant impairment in social and occupational functioning. (The DSM-IV-TR criteria are shown in Table 6–10.) Patients with amnestic disorder may be oriented and alert but cannot remember what happened a few hours earlier. This disorder may be caused by trauma, tumor, infection, infarction, seizures, or drugs, but the most common cause is severe alcohol abuse. Alcohol-related amnesia is probably caused by chronic thiamine deficiency; this syndrome may occur in association with Wernicke's encephalopathy, characterized by ophthalmoplegia, ataxic gait, nystagmus, and mental confusion. This syndrome requires emergency treatment with thiamine. This condition may not improve despite abstinence from alcohol and maintenance on thiamine. The term *Wernicke-Korsakoff syndrome* is used when cognitive and memory impairment endures. Autopsies of patients with this syndrome show hemorrhage and sclerosis of the hypothalamic mamillary bodies and nuclei of the thalamus, as well as more diffuse lesions in the brain stem, cerebellum, and limbic system.

TABLE 6–10. DSM-IV-TR criteria for amnestic disorder due to a general medical condition

A. The development of memory impairment as manifested by impairment in the ability to learn new information or the inability to recall previously learned information.

B. The memory disturbance causes significant impairment in social or occupational functioning and represents a significant decline from a previous level of functioning.

C. The memory disturbance does not occur exclusively during the course of a delirium or a dementia.

D. There is evidence from the history, physical examination, or laboratory findings that the disturbance is the direct physiological consequence of a general medical condition (including physical trauma).

Specify if:

    Transient: if memory impairment lasts for 1 month or less

    Chronic: if memory impairment lasts for more than 1 month

    Coding note: Include the name of the general medical condition on Axis I, e.g., 294.0 Amnestic Disorder Due to Head Trauma; also code the general medical condition on Axis III.

Specific Mental Disorders That Are Substance Induced or Due to a General Medical Condition

DSM-IV-TR defines other specific syndromes that may be substance induced or due to a general medical condition: psychotic, mood, anxiety, and catatonic disorders and personality change. Cognitive or intellectual impairment usually is not prominent in these disorders but may be present. Mental disorder not otherwise specified due to a general medical condition is a residual category for patients whose disturbance does not meet criteria for a specific disorder (e.g., a dissociative disorder due to partial complex seizures).

Psychotic Disorders

Psychotic disorders may result from the effects of medical illness or a drug. Ingestion of psychostimulants (e.g., cocaine, amphetamines) may cause a syndrome indistinguishable from paranoid schizophrenia. It has been suggested that Hitler developed persecutory delusions and delusions of grandeur from his excessive and well-documented abuse of psychostimulants. Leonard and Renate Heston (1979) described the personality change observed in Hitler, which they believe was due to the daily amphetamine injections that he was documented to have received from 1942 to his suicide in 1945. He was observed to become increasingly suspicious, rigid, distractible, and irritable:

> He became unrestrained and reckless. He would lose his temper, flush deeply and in a rapid, loud voice breaking with excitement, denounce the incompetence and mendacious cowardice of the General Staff. After such an outburst he would have to pace the room furiously for a long time, wordlessly snapping his fingers until his agitation subsided somewhat. (p. 12)

In addition to behavioral changes, Hitler developed other signs of amphetamine toxicity, including chronic insomnia, tremors, and stereotypic behaviors such as biting the skin around his fingernails.

Although delusions usually are self-limited, they may persist for months or years after the chronic abuse of psychostimulants has ceased. Psychotic disorders also have been associated with traumatic, metabolic, infectious, and other causes. The psychosis associated with temporal lobe epilepsy is often chronic and may not develop until 15 years or more have elapsed after the onset of psychomotor seizures.

Mood Disorders

A mood disturbance that is substance induced or due to a medical condition is characterized by depressed mood, markedly diminished interest or pleasure, or elevated, expansive, or irritable mood. Depression is a more common induced symptom than mania, although the latter has been attributed to causes such as head trauma, physical illness, or medication (e.g., zidovudine in patients with AIDS). In typical cases of induced mood disorder, patients tend to be older and are less likely to have a family history of mood disturbance than are persons with a primary mood disorder.

The following patient with an induced mood disorder was seen in our inpatient unit:

Renee, a 29-year-old woman, was transferred to our hospital for evaluation of depression and suicidal ideations. Although Renee had a long history of reclusiveness and undue social anxiety, she was otherwise psychiatrically well until 4 months before admission, when she developed depression. One year earlier, she had been given a diagnosis of multiple sclerosis on the basis of slurred speech, gait ataxia, and multiple sclerotic plaques visualized by MRI.

Renee admitted to low mood, appetite loss, poor energy, and low self-esteem, and she had psychomotor retardation. Before admission, she had written a suicide note and had been found in her room with insecticide sprays with which she had been planning to kill herself.

Renee's mood disorder was believed to be caused by her multiple sclerosis. She was treated with eight bilateral electroconvulsive treatments after her symptoms did not respond to antidepressant medication. Her mood normalized, but she remained odd and reclusive.

As many as one-third of the patients who have a cerebrovascular stroke will experience depression in the 6- to 12-month period after the event. Left hemisphere strokes appear to result in more depression than do right hemisphere or brain stem strokes. Within the left hemisphere, the closer the lesion is to the frontal pole, the more likely it is to produce depression. These depressions are probably due to the direct structural and biochemical effects of the stroke, not the psychological reaction to a medical disorder. These patients appear to respond to antidepressant medication.

Anxiety Disorders

Anxiety disorders can result from medical conditions, the effects of a substance, or withdrawal from a substance. Prominent anxiety, panic attacks, or obsessions and compulsions may be seen. Examples commonly seen by clinicians include generalized anxiety or panic attacks caused by hyperthyroidism or the jitteriness caused by excessive caffeine intake. Withdrawal of a substance to which a person has become habituated (e.g., alcohol, benzodiazepines) may cause intense but transient anxiety.

Personality Change Due to a General Medical Condition

The personality change due to a general medical condition diagnosis recognizes that personality change can result from medical conditions (e.g., temporal lobe epilepsy). Resulting changes in attitudes and behavior often represent an exaggeration of preexisting personality traits. By definition, the personality disturbance represents a change from the patient's previous personality pattern and is not better accounted for by another mental disorder, such as major depression. (See Table 6–11 for the DSM-IV-TR criteria and subtypes for personality change due to a general medical condition.)

TABLE 6–11. DSM-IV-TR criteria for personality change due to a general medical condition

A. A persistent personality disturbance that represents a change from the individual's previous characteristic personality pattern. (In children, the disturbance involves a marked deviation from normal development or a significant change in the child's usual behavior patterns lasting at least 1 year.)

B. There is evidence from the history, physical examination, or laboratory findings that the disturbance is the direct physiological consequence of a general medical condition.

C. The disturbance is not better accounted for by another mental disorder (including other Mental Disorders Due to a General Medical Condition).

D. The disturbance does not occur exclusively during the course of a delirium.

E. The disturbance causes clinically significant distress or impairment in social, occupational, or other important areas of functioning.

Specify type:

Labile Type: if the predominant feature is affective lability

Disinhibited Type: if the predominant feature is poor impulse control as evidenced by sexual indiscretions, etc.

Aggressive Type: if the predominant feature is aggressive behavior

Apathetic Type: if the predominant feature is marked apathy and indifference

Paranoid Type: if the predominant feature is suspiciousness or paranoid ideation

Other Type: if the presentation is not characterized by any of the above subtypes

Combined Type: if more than one feature predominates in the clinical picture

Unspecified Type

Coding note: Include the name of the general medical condition on Axis I, e.g., 310.1 Personality Change Due to Temporal Lobe Epilepsy; also code the general medical condition on Axis III.

A remarkable example of an induced personality change is that of Phineas Gage, whose case is further discussed in Chapter 5. The case illustrates the frontal lobe syndrome typically associated with impaired judgment, disinhibition, amotivation, and witzelsucht (silly humor and punning), with relatively little intellectual impairment. Before the injury that destroyed his frontal lobes, Gage was a sober, responsible family man; afterward, he became loud, obnoxious, and foul-mouthed and was unable to keep a job.

The diagnosis is often used to describe the personality profile of some patients with temporal lobe epilepsy. These patients are described as *viscous,* a term that reflects their tendency to become fixated on philosophical concerns and talk endlessly, unaware that the listener may not share their enthusiasm. Patients may have hypergraphia, hyperreligiosity, and either hyper- or hyposexuality. Several historical figures appear to fit this description, including Dostoyevsky and Rasputin. Aggressive behavior also may occur as an interictal phenomenon but is rarely a manifestation of a seizure. Anticonvulsants such as carbamazepine and valproate have been used to treat these interictal changes in the belief that when the seizure disorder is better controlled, the personality changes will stabilize or reverse. These drugs also have been used to reduce aggressive tendencies in these patients. Although case reports suggest benefit, controlled trials are needed.

Catatonic Disorder Due to a General Medical Condition

Catatonic disorder due to a general medical condition is diagnosed when catatonic symptoms, such as motoric immobility, excessive motor activity, extreme negativism, mutism, peculiar voluntary movement, echolalia, or echopraxia, are judged to be related to a general medical condition. Conditions associated with catatonic features have included viral encephalitis, brain trauma, status epilepticus, Wernicke's encephalopathy, and tuberous sclerosis. Metabolic conditions have included diabetic ketoacidosis, acute intermittent porphyria, and hepatic encephalopathy.

Bibliography

American Psychiatric Association: Diagnostic and Statistical Manual of Mental Disorders, 4th Edition. Washington, DC, American Psychiatric Association, 1994

American Psychiatric Association: Diagnostic and Statistical Manual of Mental Disorders, 4th Edition Text Revision. Washington, DC, American Psychiatric Association, 2000

American Psychiatric Association: Practice guidelines for the treatment of patients with Alzheimer's disease and other dementias of late life. Am J Psychiatry 154 (suppl 5):1–39, 1997

American Psychiatric Association: Practice guidelines for the treatment of patients with delirium. Am J Psychiatry 156 (suppl 5):1–20, 1999

Ballard C, Holmes C, McKeith I, et al: Psychiatric morbidity in dementia with Lewy bodies: a prospective clinical and neuropathological comparative study with Alzheimer's disease. Am J Psychiatry 156:1039–1045, 1999

Caine ED, Shoulson I: Psychiatric syndromes in Huntington's disease. Am J Psychiatry 140:728–733, 1983

Clarfield AM: The reversible dementias: do they reverse? Ann Intern Med 109:476–486, 1988

Coccaro EF, Kramer E, Zemishlany Z, et al: Pharmacologic treatment of non-cognitive behavioral disturbances of elderly demented patients. Am J Psychiatry 147:1640–1645, 1990

Consensus Conference: Differential diagnosis of dementing diseases. JAMA 258:3411–3416, 1987

Dalessio DJ: Maurice Ravel and Alzheimer's disease. JAMA 252:3412–3413, 1984

Devanand DP, Marder K, Michaels KS, et al: A randomized, placebo-controlled dose-comparison trial of haloperidol for psychosis and disruptive behaviors in Alzheimer's disease. Am J Psychiatry 155:1512–1520, 1988

Drevets WC, Rubin EH: Psychotic symptoms and the longitudinal course of senile dementia of the Alzheimer type. Biol Psychiatry 25:35–48, 1989

Francis J, Martin D, Kapoor WN: A prospective study of delirium in hospitalized elderly. JAMA 263:1097–1101, 1990

Golinger RC, Peet T, Tune LE: Association of elevated plasma anticholinergic activity with delirium in surgical patients. Am J Psychiatry 144:1218–1220, 1987

Greendyke RM, Kanter DR, Schuster DB, et al: Propranolol treatment of assaultive patients with organic brain disease: double-blind, cross-over, placebo-controlled study. J Nerv Ment Dis 174:290–294, 1986

Heston LL, White JA, Mastri AR: Pick's disease: clinical genetics and natural history. Arch Gen Psychiatry 44:409–411, 1987

Johnson RT, Gibbs CJ: Creutzfeldt-Jakob disease and related transmissible spongiform encephalopathies. N Engl J Med 339:1994–2003, 1998

Katz IR, Jeste DV, Mintzer JE, et al: Comparison of risperidone and placebo for psychosis and behavioral disturbances associated with dementia: a randomized, double-blind trial. J Clin Psychiatry 60:107–115, 1999

Knapp MJ, Knopman DS, Solomon PR, et al: A 30-week randomized controlled trial of high-dose tacrine in patients with Alzheimer's disease. JAMA 271:985–991, 1994

Levine AM: Case report: buspirone and agitation in head injury. Brain Inj 2:165–167, 1988

Mace NL, Rabins PV: The 36-Hour Day, 3rd Edition. Baltimore, MD, Johns Hopkins University Press, 1999

Mayeux R, Stern Y, Williams JBW, et al: Clinical and biochemical features of depression in Parkinson's disease. Am J Psychiatry 143:756–759, 1986

McAllister TW: Overview: pseudodementia. Am J Psychiatry 140:528–533, 1983

Medalia A, Scheinberg IH: Psychopathology in patients with Wilson's disease. Am J Psychiatry 146:662–664, 1989

Pinner C, Rich CL: Effects of trazodone on aggressive behavior in seven patients with organic mental disorders. Am J Psychiatry 145:1295–1296, 1988

Rabins PV, Folstein MF: Delirium and dementia: diagnostic criteria and fatality rates. Br J Psychiatry 140:149–153, 1982a

Rabins PV, Mace NC, Lucas MJ: The impact of dementia on the family. JAMA 248:333–335, 1982b

Robinson RG, Kubose KL, Star LB, et al: Mood changes in stroke patients: relationship to lesion location. Compr Psychiatry 24:555–566, 1983

Schor JD, Levkoff SE, Lipsitz LA, et al: Risk factor for delirium in hospitalized elderly. JAMA 267:827–831, 1992

Small GW, Leiter F: Neuroimaging for the diagnosis of dementia. J Clin Psychiatry 59 (suppl 11):4–7, 1998

Stern Y, Gurland B, Tatemichi TK, et al: Influence of education and occupation on the incidence of Alzheimer's disease. JAMA 271:1004–1010, 1994

Walker Z, Allen RL, Shergill S, et al: Neuropsychological performance in Lewy body dementia and Alzheimer's disease. Br J Psychiatry 170:156–158, 1997

Weiner MF, Risser RC, Cullum CM, et al: Alzheimer's disease and its Lewy body variant: a clinical analysis of postmortem verified cases. Am J Psychiatry 153:1269–1273, 1996

Self-Assessment Questions

1. What are the differences between delirium and dementia?
2. What does the medical workup for delirium and dementia consist of?
3. Describe Alzheimer's disease. What are its histopathological findings?
4. What is the pathognomonic finding in Pick's disease?
5. What triad of symptoms cluster in normal-pressure hydrocephalus?
6. List the different causes of dementia.
7. What is pseudodementia? What are its typical signs?
8. How are dementia patients clinically managed?
9. What general medical conditions have been associated with catatonia?
10. Describe the frontal lobe syndrome.

Schizophrenia

> The psychopathology of schizophrenia is one of the
> most intriguing, since it permits a many-sided insight
> into the workings of the diseased as well as the healthy
> psyche.
>
> Eugen Bleuler

Schizophrenia is probably the most devastating illness that psychiatrists treat. An estimated 1% of the population has schizophrenia, which typically begins in the teens or early 20s, leaving most of those affected unable to return to normal young adult lives—to go to school, to find a job, or to marry and have children. Schizophrenia also creates an enormous economic burden, calculated in 1991 at $65 billion annually in direct and indirect costs. According to *The Global Burden of Disease,* a World Health Organization (WHO)–sponsored study of the cost of medical illnesses world-wide, schizophrenia is among the 10 leading causes of disability in the world among people in the 15–44 age range. Schizophrenia strikes people just when they should be achieving their greatest growth and productivity.

This chapter is adapted from Black DW, Andreasen NC: "Schizophrenia, Schizophreni-form Disorder, and Delusional (Paranoid) Disorders," in *The American Psychiatric Press Textbook of Psychiatry,* 3rd Edition. Edited by Hales RE, Yudofsky SC, Talbott JA. Washington, DC, American Psychiatric Press, 1999, pp. 425–477. Copyright 1999 American Psychiatric Press, Inc. Used with permission.

History

Schizophrenia and other psychotic disorders have been recognized in almost all cultures and described throughout much of recorded time. Its modern history dates to Emil Kraepelin, who is credited with identifying schizophrenia. His original term for schizophrenia, *dementia praecox,* was based on his observations that these patients developed their illness at a relatively early age (praecox) and were likely to have a chronic and deteriorating course (dementia). Kraepelin also was instrumental in separating dementia praecox from manic-depressive (bipolar) illness, which had its onset distributed throughout life and a more episodic course.

Dementia praecox was eventually renamed *schizophrenia,* a term coined by Eugen Bleuler to emphasize the cognitive impairment that occurs, which he conceptualized as a splitting of the psychic processes. Bleuler believed that certain symptoms were fundamental to the illness, including affective blunting, disturbance of association (i.e., fragmented thinking), autism, and ambivalence (i.e., fragmented emotional responses). He regarded other symptoms such as delusions and hallucinations as accessory to the illness because they could occur in other disorders, including manic-depressive illness.

Bleuler's ideas enjoyed wide acceptance throughout the United States, and generations of psychiatrists were taught the importance of his fundamental symptoms (the four *A*'s). Unlike hallucinations and delusions, these symptoms are on a continuum with normality. As Bleuler's original ideas were applied within the widely used psychodynamic tradition that prevailed during 1950s to 1980s, the conceptualization of schizophrenia in the United States became increasingly broad. The ideas of German psychiatrist Kurt Schneider, who emphasized specific "first-rank" psychotic symptoms, were introduced in DSM-III in an effort to narrow an overly broad conceptualization by defining schizophrenia on the basis of the presence of psychotic symptoms. Psychotic symptoms such as delusions and hallucinations lend themselves to narrow and objective definitions, but they do not capture the full clinical picture of schizophrenia. Therefore, the DSM-IV definition represented an attempt to synthesize many points of view: a Kraepelinian emphasis on course, inclusion of Schneiderian delusions and hallucinations, and acknowledgment of the importance of Bleuler's fundamental symptoms (reconceptualized as negative symptoms).

Definition

Schizophrenia is a disease characterized by a very broad range of mental symptoms. In fact, the symptoms are so diverse that they cover the entire spectrum of human thought, emotion, and behavior. This breadth of symptoms, with its corresponding challenge to explain the diversity on a neural level, is what makes schizophrenia a medically fascinating disorder.

In DSM-IV and DSM-IV-TR, schizophrenia is defined by a group of characteristic positive or negative symptoms; deterioration in social, occupational, or interpersonal relationships; and continuous signs of the disturbance for at least 6 months. In addition, schizoaffective disorder and mood disorder with psychotic features have been ruled out, and the disturbance is not due to the direct physiological effects of a substance or a general medical condition. (See Table 7–1 for the DSM-IV-TR diagnostic criteria for schizophrenia.)

Clinical Findings

Various methods have been developed to describe and classify the symptoms in schizophrenia. Traditionally, schizophrenia is considered a type of "psychosis," yet the definition of psychosis has been elusive. Older definitions stressed the subjective and internal psychological experience and defined psychosis as an "impairment in reality testing." At the opposite extreme, psychosis has been defined objectively and operationally as the occurrence of hallucinations and delusions.

Because schizophrenia is characterized by so many different types of symptoms, clinical investigators have tried to simplify the conceptualization of the disorder by exploring whether the manifestations fall into natural groups of interrelated symptoms. One of the authors (N.C.A.) developed the Scale for the Assessment of Positive Symptoms (SAPS) and the Scale for the Assessment of Negative Symptoms (SANS), which have become widely used clinical and research instruments to evaluate these symptoms. Table 7–2 shows the frequency of various positive and negative symptoms in a series of 111 patients with schizophrenia, based on the use of these scales, which are both included in the Appendix. Factor analytic studies that used these scales have repeatedly found three dimensions of psychopathology in schizophrenia: psychoticism, disorganization, and negative symptoms.

The Psychotic Dimension

The psychotic dimension refers to two classic "psychotic" symptoms that reflect a patient's confusion about the loss of boundaries between himself or herself and the external world: hallucinations and delusions. Both symptoms reflect a "loss of ego boundaries": the patient is unable to distinguish

TABLE 7–1.   DSM-IV-TR criteria for schizophrenia

A. *Characteristic symptoms:*   Two (or more) of the following, each present for a sig-
    nificant portion of time during a 1-month period (or less if successfully treated):
    (1) delusions
    (2) hallucinations
    (3) disorganized speech (e.g., frequent derailment or incoherence)
    (4) grossly disorganized or catatonic behavior
    (5) negative symptoms, i.e., affective flattening, alogia, or avolition
    Note: Only one Criterion A symptom is required if delusions are bizarre or
       hallucinations consist of a voice keeping up a running commentary on the
       person's behavior or thoughts, or two or more voices conversing with each other.

B. *Social/occupational dysfunction:*   For a significant portion of the time since the
    onset of the disturbance, one or more major areas of functioning such as work,
    interpersonal relations, or self-care are markedly below the level achieved prior
    to the onset (or when the onset is in childhood or adolescence, failure to achieve
    expected level of interpersonal, academic, or occupational achievement).

C. *Duration:*   Continuous signs of the disturbance persist for at least 6 months. This
    6-month period must include at least 1 month of symptoms (or less if successfully
    treated) that meet Criterion A (i.e., active-phase symptoms) and may include
    periods of prodromal or residual symptoms. During these prodromal or residual
    periods, the signs of the disturbance may be manifested by only negative symptoms
    or two or more symptoms listed in Criterion A present in an attenuated form (e.g.,
    odd beliefs, unusual perceptual experiences).

D. *Schizoaffective and Mood Disorder exclusion:*   Schizoaffective Disorder and Mood
    Disorder With Psychotic Features have been ruled out because either (1) no Major
    Depressive, Manic, or Mixed Episodes have occurred concurrently with the active-
    phase symptoms; or (2) if mood episodes have occurred during active-phase symp-
    toms, their total duration has been brief relative to the duration of the active and
    residual periods.

E. *Substance/general medical condition exclusion:*   The disturbance is not due to the
    direct physiological effects of a substance (e.g., a drug of abuse, a medication) or
    a general medical condition.

F. *Relationship to a Pervasive Developmental Disorder:*   If there is a history of Autistic
    Disorder or another Pervasive Developmental Disorder, the additional diagnosis
    of Schizophrenia is made only if prominent delusions or hallucinations are also
    present for at least a month (or less if successfully treated).

Classification of longitudinal course (can be applied only after at least 1 year has elapsed
since the initial onset of active-phase symptoms):

   Episodic With Interepisode Residual Symptoms (episodes are defined by the
       reemergence of prominent psychotic symptoms); *also specify if:*   **With Prom-
       inent Negative Symptoms**

TABLE 7–1. DSM-IV-TR criteria for schizophrenia *(continued)*

Episodic With No Interepisode Residual Symptoms

Continuous (prominent psychotic symptoms are present throughout the period of observation); *also specify if:* With Prominent Negative Symptoms

Single Episode In Partial Remission; *also specify if:* With Prominent Negative Symptoms

Single Episode In Full Remission

Other or Unspecified Pattern

between his or her own thoughts and perceptions and those that he or she obtains by observing the external world.

Hallucinations have sometimes been considered the hallmark of schizophrenia, although they may occur in other disorders, including mood disorders and disorders induced by medical illness or the effects of various substances. *Hallucinations* are perceptions experienced without an external stimulus to the sense organs and have a quality similar to a true perception. Schizophrenic patients commonly report auditory, visual, tactile, gustatory, or olfactory hallucinations or a combination of these hallucinations. Auditory hallucinations are the most frequent; they are commonly experienced as noises, music, or, more typically, voices. The voices may be mumbled or heard clearly, and they may speak words, phrases, or sentences. Visual hallucinations may be simple or complex and include flashes of light, persons, animals, or objects. Olfactory and gustatory hallucinations are often experienced together, especially as unpleasant tastes or odors. Tactile hallucinations may be experienced as sensations of being touched or pricked, electrical sensations, or the sensation of insects crawling under the skin, which is called *formication.*

Delusions involve disturbance in thought rather than perception; they are firmly held beliefs that are untrue as well as contrary to a person's educational and cultural background. Delusions occurring in schizophrenic patients may have somatic, grandiose, religious, nihilistic, sexual, or persecutory themes (Table 7–3). The type and frequency of the delusions tend to differ according to one's culture. For example, in the United States, a patient might worry about being spied on by the FBI or CIA; in sub-Saharan Africa, a Bantu or Zulu patient would more likely worry about persecution by demons or spirits.

Certain types of hallucinations and delusions were considered "first rank" by Schneider. These hallucinations include clearly audible voices commenting on a person's actions, arguing with one another about a patient,

TABLE 7–2.   Frequency of symptoms in 111 schizophrenic patients

Negative symptoms	%	Positive symptoms	%
Affective flattening		**Hallucinations**	
Unchanging facial expression	96	Auditory	75
Decreased spontaneous movements	66	Voices commenting	58
Paucity of expressive gestures	81	Voices conversing	57
Poor eye contact	71	Somatic-tactile	20
Affective nonresponsivity	64	Olfactory	6
Inappropriate affect	63	Visual	49
Lack of vocal inflections	73	**Delusions**	
Alogia		Persecutory	81
Poverty of speech	53	Jealous	4
Poverty of content of speech	51	Guilt, sin	26
Blocking	23	Grandiose	39
Increased response latency	31	Religious	31
Avolition-apathy		Somatic	28
Impaired grooming and hygiene	87	Delusions of reference	49
Lack of persistence at work or school	95	Delusions of being controlled	46
Physical anergia	82	Delusions of mind reading	48
Anhedonia-asociality		Thought broadcasting	23
Few recreational interests/activities	95	Thought insertion	31
Little sexual interest/activity	69	Thought withdrawal	27
Impaired intimacy/closeness	84	**Bizarre behavior**	
Few relationships with friends/peers	96	Clothing, appearance	20
Attention		Social, sexual behavior	33
Social inattentiveness	78	Aggressive-agitated	27
Inattentiveness during testing	64	Repetitive-stereotyped	28
		Positive formal thought disorder	
		Derailment	45
		Tangentiality	50
		Incoherence	23
		Illogicality	23
		Circumstantiality	35
		Pressure of speech	24
		Distractible speech	23
		Clanging	3

Source.   Adapted from Andreasen 1987.

TABLE 7–3. Varied content in delusions

Delusions	Foci of preoccupation
Grandiose	Possessing wealth or great beauty or having a special ability (e.g., extrasensory perception); having influential friends; being an important figure (e.g., Napoleon, Hitler)
Nihilistic	Believing that one is dead or dying; believing that one does not exist or that the world does not exist
Persecutory	Being persecuted by friends, neighbors, or spouse; being followed, monitored, or spied on by the government (e.g., FBI, CIA) or other important organizations (e.g., the Catholic church)
Somatic	Believing that one's organs have stopped functioning (e.g., that the heart is no longer beating) or are rotting away; believing that the nose or other body part is terribly misshapen or disfigured
Sexual	Believing that one's sexual behavior is commonly known; that one is a prostitute, pedophile, or rapist; that masturbation has led to illness or insanity
Religious	Believing that one has sinned against God, that one has a special relationship to God or some other deity, that one has a special religious mission, or that one is the Devil or is condemned to burn in Hell

or repeating aloud the patient's thoughts. The delusions include thought broadcasting, thought withdrawal, thought insertion, or being controlled (passivity). These symptoms commonly occur in schizophrenic patients but are also found in patients with psychoses due to mood or brain disorders, medical illness, or the effects of substances. (See Table 7–4 for a description of Schneider's first-rank symptoms.)

The Disorganization Dimension

The disorganization dimension includes disorganized speech, disorganized or bizarre behavior, and incongruous affect.

Disorganized speech, or *thought disorder*, was regarded as the most important symptom of schizophrenia by Bleuler. Historically, types of thought disorder have included associative loosening, illogical thinking, overinclusive thinking, and loss of ability to engage in abstract thinking. Standard definitions for various types of thought disorders have been developed that stress objective aspects of language and communication (which are empiri-

TABLE 7–4.   Schneider's first-rank symptoms

Hallucination of one's thoughts being spoken aloud

Hallucination of voices in the form of a running commentary about the patient

Hallucination of voices conversing about the patient ("third person" hallucination) or arguing

Somatic hallucination attributed to outside forces (e.g., X rays, hypnosis)

Delusions of thoughts being withdrawn from or inserted into the patient's mind by an outside person or force

Delusions of thoughts being broadcast so that the patient's private thoughts are known to others

Delusional perceptions in which highly personal meanings are attributed to perceptions

Delusions of being influenced or forced to do things or want things the patient does not wish to do and does not want

Delusions of being made to feel emotions or sensations (often sexual) that are not the patient's own

cal indicators of "thought"), such as derailment (loose associations), poverty of speech, poverty of content of speech, and tangential replies, and all have been found to occur frequently in both schizophrenia and mood disorders. Manic patients often have a thought disorder characterized by tangentiality, derailment, and illogicality. Depressed patients manifest thought disorder less frequently than do manic patients but often have poverty of speech, tangentiality, or circumstantiality. Other types of formal thought disorder include perseveration, distractibility, clanging, neologisms, echolalia, and blocking; with the possible exception of clanging in mania, none appears to be disorder specific.

An example of speech from a schizophrenic patient with a prominent thought disorder, especially derailment, follows:

> Let's see, there was one I would have liked if it wasn't for the instructor, well I go along with his, he was always wanted me to do the worse in the class, it seemed like, and I'd always get bad, the grade, in my grading, and he tried to make other people like they were good enough to be in Hollywood or something, you know I's be the last one down the ladder. That, that's the way they wanted the grading to be in the first place according to whose, theirs, they, they have all different reasons that I, I, I think that they use that they want one, won't come out. (Andreasen, *The Broken Brain,* p. 61)

Many schizophrenic patients have various types of disorganized motor and social behavior, another aspect of this dimension. Abnormal motor behaviors range from catatonic stupor to excitement. In a *catatonic stupor,* the patient may be immobile, mute, and unresponsive, yet fully conscious. In *catatonic excitement,* the patient may show uncontrolled and aimless motor activity. Patients sometimes assume bizarre or uncomfortable postures, such as squatting, and maintain them for long periods. Patients may have a *stereotypy,* which is a repeated movement that is not goal directed, such as back-and-forth rocking. They also may have *mannerisms,* which are normal goal-directed activities but are either odd in appearance or out of context, such as grimacing. Other common symptoms are *echopraxia,* or imitating the movements and gestures of another person; *automatic obedience,* or carrying out simple commands in a robotlike fashion; and *negativism,* or refusing to cooperate with simple requests for no apparent reason.

Deterioration of social behavior often occurs along with social withdrawal. Patients may neglect themselves, become messy or unkempt, and wear dirty or inappropriate clothing. They may ignore their surroundings so that they become cluttered and untidy. Patients may develop other odd behaviors that break social conventions, such as masturbating in public, foraging through garbage bins, or shouting obscenities. Many of today's street people are schizophrenic.

Incongruity of affect is the third component of the disorganized dimension. Patients may smile inappropriately when speaking of neutral or sad topics or giggle for no apparent reason. This symptom should not be confused with the nervous smiling or giggling that sometimes occurs in anxious patients.

The Negative Dimension

DSM-IV-TR lists three negative symptoms as characteristic of schizophrenia: alogia, affective blunting, and avolition. Other negative symptoms that are common in schizophrenia include anhedonia and attentional impairment. Negative symptoms reflect a deficiency of mental functioning that is normally present.

Alogia is characterized by a diminution in the amount of spontaneous speech or a tendency to produce speech that is empty or impoverished in content when the amount is adequate. It is the external expression in language of the impoverishment of thought that occurs in many patients with schizophrenia. Patients may have great difficulty producing fluent responses to questions.

Affective flattening or *blunting* is a reduced intensity of emotional expression and response. It is manifested by unchanging facial expression, decreased spontaneous movements, poverty of expressive gestures, poor eye contact, lack of voice inflections, and slowed speech.

Avolition is a loss of the ability to initiate goal-directed behavior and carry it through to completion. Patients seem to have lost their will or drive. They may initiate a project and then abandon it for a few days or weeks and then fail to appear or wander aimlessly away while at work. This symptom is sometimes interpreted as laziness, but in fact it represents the loss or diminution of basic drives and the capacity to formulate and pursue long-range plans.

Anhedonia is the inability to experience pleasure. Many patients describe themselves as feeling emotionally empty. They are no longer able to enjoy activities that previously gave them pleasure, such as playing sports or seeing family or friends. Their awareness that they have lost the capacity to enjoy themselves may be a source of great psychological pain.

Attentional impairment is reflected in the inability to concentrate or by stimuli that patients cannot process or filter, which makes them feel confused or experience fragmented thoughts.

Another aspect of the negative dimension is a *reduced intensity of emotional response* that leaves schizophrenic patients indifferent, apathetic, and anhedonic. Significant depressive symptoms occur in up to 60% of schizophrenic patients. Depression is often difficult to diagnose because symptoms of schizophrenia and depression frequently overlap. Antipsychotics also may cause what appears to be a depression but is actually a drug-induced akinesia. According to DSM-IV-TR, major depression that develops in a patient with well-established schizophrenia is diagnosed as *depressive disorder not otherwise specified.*

The following case vignette of a patient seen in our hospital illustrates many of the symptoms found in schizophrenia:

> Jane, a 55-year-old woman, was admitted to the hospital for evaluation of agitation and paranoia. A former schoolteacher, Jane had lived in a series of rooming houses and had held only temporary jobs in the past 10 years. She was socially isolated and interacted with others only at her church.
>
> Jane was born with a cleft palate that was surgically corrected at age 4 years. She was teased unmercifully as a child because of her appearance, despite good cosmetic results from the surgery. She was shy and socially awkward but was an avid reader and a model student. Jane had little interest in boys, never dated, and after graduating from high school, briefly joined a convent before attending college. She eventually obtained her teaching certificate after graduating from college but continued to live with her mother.
>
> She was first hospitalized at age 25 after developing the belief that her neighbors were harassing her. Over the next 20 years, she developed the

delusion that she was at the center of a government cabal to change her identity. The FBI, the judicial system, the Roman Catholic church, hospital personnel, and, it seems, most of her neighbors were involved. She believed that her neighbors were recruited to spy on her, harass her, and generally make her life miserable. She would often overhear them plotting to assault or rape her. At age 49, Jane was hospitalized after her landlord reported that she was pounding on the ceiling and walls of her apartment with a broom and yelling as she attempted to stop the perceived harassment by her neighbors.

Because of her delusional beliefs, Jane moved about every 6 months. However, she discovered, to her dismay, that wherever she went, her new neighbors also were involved in the plot. Still, she continued working, although she was gradually relegated to substitute teaching positions until even these opportunities dried up. A doctor had suggested that she obtain government disability benefits, but because she denied having any mental illness, Jane refused to apply. At the time of admission, Jane was working as a telemarketer.

At the time of her present hospitalization, Jane's landlord had complained about her yelling and screaming. She reported that she was simply responding to the discomfort her landlord and neighbors had caused by "zapping" her with electronic beams in an effort to harass her. She believed that electromagnetic waves were being used to control her actions and thoughts and described a bizarre sensation of electricity moving around her body when the landlord was nearby.

Jane cooperated well with her physicians and had no evidence of depressed mood, but she was clearly upset about her hospitalization, which she thought was unnecessary. Her speech was markedly circumstantial, although she spoke in a clear, strong voice that one might expect after years of teaching. She cooperated with her treatment plans. However, after 1 month of antipsychotic therapy, Jane remained delusional but was less concerned about her perceived harassment. Because of her poor insight and history of medication noncompliance, Jane was given an intramuscular antipsychotic before discharge.

Other Symptoms

Lack of insight is common in schizophrenia. A patient may not believe that he or she is ill or abnormal in any way. The hallucinations and delusions are real—not imagined—to the patient. Poor insight is one of the most difficult symptoms to treat, and it may persist even when other symptoms, such as hallucinations or delusions, respond to treatment. Orientation and memory usually are normal, unless they are impaired by the patient's psychotic symptoms, inattention, or distractibility. Some patients have difficulty giving their correct age ("age disorientation").

Nonlocalizing neurological soft signs occur in a substantial proportion of patients and include abnormalities in stereognosis, graphesthesia, balance, and proprioception. A disorder of the visual tracking of smoothly moving targets (i.e., smooth pursuit eye movement) has been observed in both schizophrenic patients and their relatives. Other ocular abnormalities commonly include the absence and avoidance of eye contact and staring for long periods. Decreased or rapid blink rates and bouts of rapid blinking may occur. Some patients have disturbances of sleep, sexual interest, and other bodily functions. A variety of disrupted sleep measures have been reported, but decreased delta sleep with diminished Stage IV sleep is the most consistent finding. Many schizophrenic patients have inactive sex drives and derive little or no pleasure from sexual activity. Many patients develop chronic constipation, and rare cases of megacolon have been reported.

Premorbid Personality

Several early writers, including Kraepelin and Bleuler, observed that patients with schizophrenia often had abnormal premorbid personalities. A review of early studies of personality and schizophrenia showed that premorbid schizoid traits were present in one-fourth of schizophrenic patients, but one-sixth had a range of other personality disturbances. Poor premorbid adjustment has been shown to correlate with early disease onset, poor overall prognosis, negative symptoms, cognitive deficits, and poor social functioning.

Alcohol and Drug Abuse

Alcohol and drug abuse are especially common in patients with schizophrenia. Drug-using patients tend to be young, male, and poorly compliant with treatment; they also tend to have frequent hospitalizations. It is believed that many abuse drugs in an attempt to treat their depression or their medication side effects (e.g., akinesia) or to ameliorate their lack of motivation and pleasure.

Subtypes of Schizophrenia

Five DSM-IV-TR subtypes of schizophrenia are recognized: paranoid, disorganized, catatonic, undifferentiated, and residual (see Table 7–5). Their usefulness is primarily descriptive because their reliability and validity are not established. As a practical matter, many patients seem to fit several of these subtypes during the course of their illness.

The *paranoid* subtype involves preoccupation with one or more systematized delusions or frequently auditory hallucinations; disorganized speech and behavior, catatonic behavior, and flat or inappropriate affect are not prominent. Compared with patients who have the disorganized subtype, paranoid patients tend to be an older age at onset and are more likely to be married, to have children, and to be employed; both their premorbid functioning and their outcome tend to be better.

Disorganized (hebephrenic) schizophrenic patients have disorganized speech and behavior and flat or inappropriate affect; they do not meet criteria for catatonic schizophrenia. Delusions and hallucinations, if present, tend to be fragmentary, unlike the often well-systematized delusions of the paranoid schizophrenic patient. The onset of this subtype occurs at an early age with the development of nonparanoid symptoms such as avolition, flat affect, deterioration of habits, and cognitive impairment. These patients often seem silly and childlike and occasionally grimace, giggle inappropriately, and appear self-absorbed; mirror gazing is frequently described.

Catatonic schizophrenia is a subtype dominated by at least two of the following: motoric immobility (e.g., catalepsy, stupor), excessive motor activity, extreme negativism, peculiarities of voluntary movement (e.g., stereotypies, mannerisms, grimacing), and echolalia or echopraxia. This subtype of schizophrenia is reported to be less common than it was in the past, which may be a benefit of the modern treatment era.

The *undifferentiated* subtype is a residual category for patients meeting criteria for schizophrenia but not criteria for the paranoid, disorganized, or catatonic subtypes.

Residual schizophrenia, as described in DSM-IV-TR, is a diagnosis for patients who no longer have prominent psychotic symptoms but who once met criteria for schizophrenia and have continuing evidence of illness such as blunted affect or eccentric behavior.

Course of Illness

Schizophrenia is typically viewed as a chronic disorder that begins early in life and has a poor long-term outcome. Its onset generally begins with a *prodromal phase* characterized by social withdrawal and other subtle changes in behavior and emotional responsiveness, peculiar behavior, deterioration in personal hygiene and grooming, and strange ideation. The prodrome varies in length but typically lasts from months to years.

The prodrome is followed by an *active phase* in which psychotic symptoms first appear. At this point, clinical disorder becomes evident, and a diagnosis of schizophrenia can be made. This phase is characterized by hallucinations and delusions, which alarm both friends and family members

TABLE 7-5. DSM-IV subtypes of schizophrenia

Subtype	Criteria	Associated features
Paranoid	A. Preoccupation with one or more delusions or auditory hallucinations B. None of the following is prominent: disorganized speech, disorganized or catatonic behavior, or flat or inappropriate affect.	Often associated with unfocused anger, anxiety, argumentativeness, or violence Stilted, formal quality or extreme intensity of interpersonal interactions may be seen.
Catatonic	The clinical picture is dominated by at least two of the following: A. Motoric immobility as evidenced by catalepsy or stupor B. Excessive motor activity (that is apparently purposeless and not influenced by extreme stimuli) C. Extreme negativism (an apparently motiveless resistance to all instructions or maintenance of a rigid posture against attempts to be moved) or mutism D. Peculiarities of voluntary movements as evidenced by posturing, stereotyped movements, prominent mannerisms, or prominent grimacing E. Echolalia or echopraxia	Marked psychomotor disturbance present (stupor or agitation), and unusual motor disturbances may be present. May need medical supervision because of malnutrition, exhaustion, hyperpyrexia, or self-injury. Interviewing patient while he or she is under the influence of amobarbital sodium ("Amytal interview") may be helpful diagnostically.

TABLE 7–5. DSM-IV subtypes of schizophrenia (*continued*)

Subtype	Criteria	Associated features

Disorganized	A. All of the following are prominent:
	  1. Disorganized speech
	  2. Disorganized behavior
	  3. Flat or inappropriate affect
	B. Does not meet criteria for catatonic type.
		Silly and childlike behavior is common.
		Associated with extreme social impairment, poor premorbid functioning, and poor long-term functioning

Undifferentiated	Symptoms meeting criterion A[a] are present, but the criteria are not met for paranoid, catatonic, or disorganized types.	Probably the most common presentation in clinical practice
Residual	A. Absence of prominent delusions, hallucinations, disorganized speech, and grossly disorganized or catatonic behavior B. There is continuing evidence of the disturbance as indicated by the presence of negative symptoms or two or more symptoms listed in criterion A for schizophrenia present in an attenuated form.	Active-phase symptoms (i.e., psychotic symptoms) are not present, but patient still shows emotional blunting, eccentric behavior, illogical thinking, and mild loosening of associations.

[a]For definition of criterion A, see Table 7–1.

and often lead to medical intervention. A *residual phase* follows the resolution of the active phase and is similar to the prodromal phase. Psychotic symptoms may persist during this phase, but at a lower level of intensity, and they may not be as troublesome to the patient. During the residual phase, active-phase symptoms may occur episodically (acute exacerbations), with variable levels of remission between episodes. The frequency and timing of these episodes are unpredictable, although stressful situations or, in some instances, drug abuse may precede these relapses. Relapses are often preceded by changes in thought, feeling, or behavior noticed by the patient and family members. Symptoms preceding relapse include dysphoria, seclusiveness, sleep disturbance, anxiety, and ideas of reference. The stages of schizophrenia are described in Table 7–6.

TABLE 7–6.   Typical stages of schizophrenia

Stage	Typical features
Prodromal phase	Insidious onset occurs over months or years; subtle behavior changes include social withdrawal, work impairment, inappropriate affect, avolition, and strange ideation.
Active phase	Psychotic symptoms develop, including hallucinations, delusions, or disorganized speech and behavior. These florid symptoms are alarming and lead to medical intervention. Acute-phase symptoms may reemerge during the residual phase ("acute exacerbation").
Residual phase	Active-phase symptoms are absent or no longer prominent. There is role impairment, negative symptoms, or attenuated positive symptoms.

Patients gradually accrue increased levels of morbidity in the form of residual or persistent symptoms and decrements in function from their premorbid status. Relatively severe psychosis is continuous and unrelenting in some patients. Schizophrenia may reach a plateau of severity at about 5 years without further deterioration. The course of schizophrenia is illustrated in Figure 7–1.

The clinical course and outcome in schizophrenia have been studied and debated, but a recent summary of the outcome of 51,800 schizophrenic patients from 320 studies showed that 40% of the patients were considered improved. Improvement was essentially defined as recovery, remission, or having minimal symptoms.

Several long-term follow-up studies that used contemporary definitions of schizophrenia have been published. One of the best known is the "Iowa

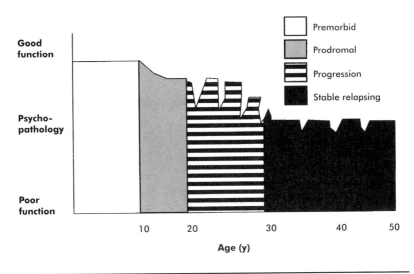

FIGURE 7-1. Natural history of schizophrenia.
Source. Lieberman JA: "Atypical Antipsychotic Drugs as a First-Line Treatment of Schizophrenia: A Rationale and Hypothesis." *The Journal of Clinical Psychiatry* 57(suppl 11):68–71, 1996. Reprinted by permission of Physicians Postgraduate Press.

500," in which 186 schizophrenic patients admitted to the University of Iowa Psychiatric Hospital between 1934 and 1944 were followed up. Twenty percent were reported to be psychiatrically well at follow-up, but 54% had incapacitating psychiatric symptoms; 21% were married or widowed, but 67% had never married; 34% lived in their own home or with a relative, but 18% were in mental institutions; and 35% were economically productive, but 58% had never worked. The group experienced excessive mortality from both natural and unnatural causes, and more than 10% committed suicide. In a recent reanalysis of this study, only two of the schizophrenic patients followed up were found to be completely free of symptoms (i.e., had "zero symptoms").

In summary, outcome studies show that schizophrenia is a devastating illness that affects every aspect of the patient's life. Many patients with schizophrenia will have a relatively good outcome and do not experience the severe deterioration considered by some to be a hallmark of the disorder.

Outcome Predictors

It is difficult to predict outcome in individual patients based on these studies. However, features associated with a good outcome include acute onset, short duration of illness, lack of psychiatric history, presence of affective symptoms or confusion, good premorbid functioning, steady work history, marriage, and older age at onset. Poor prognostic features include insidious onset, long duration of symptoms, history of psychiatric problems, affective blunting, obsessive-compulsive symptoms, assaultiveness, poor premorbid personality, poor work history, celibacy, and young age at onset. Prognostic features in schizophrenia are summarized in Table 7–7.

TABLE 7–7.   Features associated with good and poor outcome in schizophrenia

Feature	Good outcome	Poor outcome
Onset	Acute	Insidious
Duration	Short	Chronic
Psychiatry history	Absent	Present
Mood symptoms	Present	Absent
Sensorium	Clouded	Clear
Obsession/compulsions	Absent	Present
Assaultiveness	Absent	Present
Premorbid functioning	Good	Poor
Marital status	Married	Never married
Psychosexual functioning	Good	Poor
Neurological functioning	Normal	Soft signs present
Structural brain abnormalities	None	Present
Social class	High	Low
Family history of schizophrenia	Negative	Positive

Schizophrenic patients are more likely to experience a good outcome now than they were 100 years ago for several reasons: 1) the illness has changed, 2) antipsychotic medication and other treatments have altered the natural history of the illness, and 3) our definitions of good outcome have changed. For example, good outcome now may include patients living in care facilities or nursing homes who have minimal symptoms but are clearly not well.

For reasons that are not well understood, cross-cultural studies have shown that patients in less-developed countries tend to have better outcomes than those in more-developed countries. It may be that the schizophrenic patient is better accepted in less-developed societies, has fewer external demands, and is more likely to be taken care of by family members. Women, in general, tend to have a better outcome than men in their response to medication and in their long-term course.

Differential Diagnosis

Schizophrenia should be thought of as a diagnosis of exclusion because the consequences of the diagnosis are severe and limit therapeutic options. Because no definitive tests for schizophrenia are available, the diagnosis rests on historical and clinical information.

A thorough physical examination and history must rule out medical causes of schizophrenic symptoms. Atypical presentations should be carefully investigated. Psychotic symptoms are found in many other illnesses, including substance abuse (e.g., hallucinogens, phencyclidine [PCP], amphetamines, cocaine, alcohol), intoxication due to commonly prescribed medications (e.g., corticosteroids, anticholinergics, levodopa), infections, metabolic and endocrine disorders, tumors and mass lesions, and temporal lobe epilepsy of many years' duration. Routine laboratory tests may be helpful in ruling out medical etiologies. Testing may include a complete blood count, urinalysis, liver enzymes, serum creatinine, blood urea nitrogen, thyroid function tests, and serologic tests for evidence of an infection with syphilis or human immunodeficiency virus. Computed tomography (CT) or magnetic resonance imaging (MRI) may be useful in selected patients to rule out alternative diagnoses or during the initial workup for new-onset cases.

The major differential diagnosis involves separating schizophrenia from schizoaffective disorder, mood disorder, delusional disorder, and personality disorders (Table 7–8). The chief distinction from schizoaffective disorder and psychotic mood disorders is that in schizophrenia, a full depressive or manic syndrome either is absent, develops after the psychotic symptoms, or is brief relative to the duration of psychotic symptoms. Unlike delusional disorder, schizophrenia is characterized by bizarre delusions, and hallucinations are common. Patients with personality disorders, particularly those disorders within the eccentric cluster (e.g., schizoid, schizotypal, and paranoid), may be characterized by indifference to social relationships and have a restricted affect, bizarre ideation, or odd speech, but they are not psychotic.

Other psychiatric disorders also must be ruled out, including schizophreniform disorder, brief psychotic disorder, factitious disorder with psychological symptoms, and malingering. If symptoms persist for more than 6 months, schizophreniform disorder can be ruled out. The history of how the illness presents will help to rule out a brief psychotic disorder because

TABLE 7–8.   Differential diagnosis of schizophrenia

Psychiatric illness	Medical illness
Bipolar disorder with psychotic features	Temporal lobe epilepsy
Major depression with psychotic features	Tumor, stroke, brain trauma
	Endocrine/metabolic disorders (e.g., porphyria)
Schizoaffective disorder	Vitamin deficiency (e.g., B_{12})
Brief psychotic disorder	Infectious disease (e.g., neurosyphilis)
Schizophreniform disorder	Autoimmune disorder (e.g., systemic lupus erythematosus)
Delusional disorder	
Shared psychotic disorder	Toxic illness (e.g., heavy metal poisoning)
Panic disorder	
Depersonalization disorder	**Drugs**
Obsessive-compulsive disorder	Stimulants (e.g., amphetamine, cocaine)
Personality disorders (e.g., "eccentric cluster")	Hallucinogens (e.g., phencyclidine [PCP])
	Anticholinergics (e.g., belladonna alkaloids)
	Alcohol withdrawal
	Barbiturate withdrawal

schizophrenia generally has an insidious onset and no precipitating stressors. (See Chapter 8 for a discussion of both schizophreniform disorder and brief psychotic disorder.) Factitious disorder may be difficult to distinguish from schizophrenia, especially when the patient is knowledgeable about mental illness or is medically trained, but careful observation should enable the clinician to make the distinction between real and feigned psychosis. Likewise, a malingerer could attempt to simulate schizophrenia, but careful observation will help to distinguish the disorders. With the malingerer, obvious secondary gain, such as avoiding incarceration, will be evident, and the history may suggest antisocial personality disorder.

Epidemiology

The worldwide prevalence of schizophrenia has been estimated at between 0.5% and 1%. Pockets of high prevalence have been reported in areas of Croatia, Sweden, and Ireland; among Canadian Catholics; and among the Tamils in southern India. Low prevalence rates have been reported among the American Old Order Amish and aboriginal tribes in Taiwan and Ghana.

Schizophrenia can develop at any age, but the mean age at the first psychotic episode is about 21 years for men and 27 years for women. Of persons with schizophrenia, 9 of 10 men—but only 2 of 3 women—develop the illness by age 30 years. Age at onset is probably under both genetic and environmental control, but it is unknown why women develop the illness later than men. Patients with schizophrenia tend not to marry and are less likely to have children than persons in the general population. These facts are probably a result of the illness itself, which impairs motivation, creates social isolation, and is associated with low sex drive. Schizophrenic patients also tend to be concentrated in low social classes, a finding most likely due to the downward drift resulting from impaired social and occupational functioning.

Schizophrenic persons are at high risk for committing suicidal acts. About one-third will attempt suicide, and 1 in 10 will eventually complete suicide. Risk factors for suicide include male gender, age under 30 years, unemployment, chronic course, prior depression, past treatment for depression, history of substance abuse, and recent hospital discharge.

Recent research shows that patients with schizophrenia and other severe mental disorders have relatively high rates of violent behavior and criminality. In the Epidemiologic Catchment Area study, schizophrenic patients had rates of violent behavior five times higher than persons without mental illness, although the rate was about one-half that seen in persons with alcohol abuse or dependence. Schizophrenic patients with coexisting alcoholism are even more likely to commit violent acts.

Etiology and Pathophysiology

Models of Neural Mechanisms

Contemporary models of schizophrenia conceptualize it as a neurocognitive disorder, with the various signs and symptoms reflecting the downstream effects of a more fundamental cognitive deficit. Schizophrenia poses special challenges to the development of cognitive and neural models because of its breadth and diversity of symptoms. The symptoms include nearly all domains of function: perception (hallucinations), inferential thinking (delusions), fluency of thought and speech (alogia), clarity and organization of thought and speech (formal thought disorder), motor activity (catatonia), emotional expression (affective blunting), ability to initiate and complete goal-directed behavior (avolition), and ability to seek out and experience emotional gratification (anhedonia). In the absence of visible lesions and known pathogens, investigators have turned to the exploration of models that could explain the diversity of symptoms through a single cognitive mechanism. The convergent conclusions of these different models are striking.

One approach has been to divide the symptoms into three broad groups, which are similar to the three dimensions described earlier in this chapter: 1) disorders of willed action (which lead to symptoms such as alogia and avolition), 2) disorders of self-monitoring (which lead to symptoms such as auditory hallucinations of alien control), and 3) disorders in monitoring the intentions of others ("mentalizing") (which lead to symptoms such as formal thought disorder and delusions of persecution). These could represent a more general underlying mechanism: a disorder of consciousness or self-awareness that impairs the ability to think with "metarepresentations" (higher-order abstract concepts that are representations of mental states).

Another model suggests that the fundamental impairment in schizophrenia is an inability to guide behavior by representations, often referred to as a defect in working memory. *Working memory* involves the ability to hold a representation "on-line" and perform cognitive operations in a flexible manner, to formulate and modify plans, and to base behavior on internally held ideas and thoughts rather than being driven by external stimuli. A defect in this ability can explain various symptoms in schizophrenia. For example, the inability to hold a discourse plan in mind and monitor speech output leads to disorganized speech and thought disorder, the inability to maintain a plan for behavioral activities could lead to negative symptoms such as avolition or alogia, and the inability to reference a specific external or internal experience against associative memories (mediated by cortical and subcortical circuitry involving frontal, parietal, and temporal regions and the thalamus) could lead to an altered consciousness of sensory experience that would be expressed as delusions or hallucinations. The model also explains the perseverative behavior observed in studies that used the Wisconsin Card Sorting Test and is consistent with the compromised blood flow to the prefrontal cortex in these patients, which is discussed later in the chapter. Overall, this model suggests a major role for prefrontal regions and their multiple distributed cortical, thalamic, and striatal connections in a fundamental cognitive function—representationally guided behavior—that permits organisms to adapt flexibly to a changing environment and to achieve temporal and spatial continuity between past experiences and present and future actions.

One of the authors (N.C.A.) has used the clinical presentation of schizophrenia as a point of departure, postulating that the symptoms arise from "cognitive dysmetria." This refers to impaired connectivity between frontal, cerebellar, and thalamic regions as a consequence of one or more neurodevelopmental defects. Motor dysmetria has been observed in schizophrenia since its original description by Kraepelin, and soft signs of poor coordination are reported in more contemporary studies. More injurious, however, is the related "cognitive dysmetria," which produces "poor coordination" of mental activities. The word *metron* literally means "measure": a person with schizophrenia has a fundamental deficit in taking measure of time and space and in making inferences about interrelationships between himself or herself and others or between past, present, and future. He or she cannot accurately time input and output and therefore cannot coordinate the perception, prioritization, retrieval, and expression of experiences and ideas. This model has received extensive support from work with MRI and positron-emission tomography (PET).

The common thread in these observations is that schizophrenia reflects a disruption in a fundamental cognitive process that affects a specific circuitry in the brain. Various research teams may use different terminology and somewhat different concepts—metarepresentations, representationally guided behavior, information processing/attention, and cognitive dysmetria—but they convey a common theme. The cognitive dysfunction in schizophrenia is an inefficient temporal and spatial referencing of information and experience as the person attempts to determine boundaries between self and nonself and to formulate effective decisions or plans that will guide him or her through the small-scale (speaking a sentence) or large-scale (finding a job) maneuvers of daily living. This capacity is sometimes referred to as *consciousness.*

Investigators also converge on similar conclusions about the neuroanatomical substrates of the cognitive dysfunction. All agree that it must involve distributed circuits rather than a single specific "localization," and all suggest a key role for interrelations among prefrontal cortex, other interconnected cortical regions, and subcortical regions, particularly the thalamus and striatum.

A consensus now exists among many investigators that schizophrenia is best conceptualized as a "multiple-hit" illness similar to cancer. Individuals may carry a genetic predisposition, but this vulnerability is not "released" unless other factors also intervene. Although most of these factors are considered environmental, in the sense that they are not encoded in DNA and could potentially produce mutations or influence gene expression, most are also biological rather than psychological and include factors such as birth injuries or nutrition. Current studies of the neurobiology of schizophrenia examine a multiplicity of factors, including genetics, anatomy (primarily through structural neuroimaging), functional circuitry (through functional neuroimaging), neuropathology, electrophysiology, neurochemistry and neuropharmacology, and neurodevelopment.

Genetics

Evidence for a genetic contribution to schizophrenia is based on family studies, twin studies, and studies of adoptees. Summaries of individual family studies have shown that siblings of schizophrenic patients have about a 10% chance of developing schizophrenia, whereas children who have one parent with schizophrenia have a 5%–6% chance. The risk of family members developing schizophrenia increases markedly when two or more family members have the illness. The risk of developing schizophrenia is 17% for persons with one sibling and one parent with schizophrenia and 46% for the children of two schizophrenic parents. Twin studies have been remarkably consistent in demonstrating high concordance rates for identical twins—an average of 46% compared with 14% concordance in nonidentical twins. Adoption studies show that the risk for schizophrenia is greater in the biological relatives of index adoptees who had schizophrenia than in the biological relatives of mentally healthy control adoptees.

Investigators are now working actively to extend these observations with the multiple tools of molecular biology and molecular genetics. Multiple linkages have been reported for schizophrenia, including chromosomes 3, 5, 6, 8, 13, and 18. Furthermore, multiple candidate gene studies have been completed, examining genes that code for neuroreceptors and genes that regulate brain development. Based on observation of anticipation (increasingly younger age at onset in sequential generations of a family with the illness), investigators also have found large trinucleotide repeats (CAG/CTG) on chromosomes 17 and 18. Current genetic models of schizophrenia assume that it is likely to be polygenic and multifactorial, making the genetic search challenging.

Neuroanatomy and Structural Neuroimaging

Since the early work of Kraepelin, Alzheimer, and Nissl in the late nineteenth and early twentieth centuries, many psychiatrists have been convinced that patients with schizophrenia have some type of structural brain abnormality. Early pneumoencephalographic and neuropathological studies provided partial support for this hypothesis, but in recent years new technology has been able to support it more fully. Early work with CT, conducted during the 1980s, firmly established that schizophrenia is a brain disorder with a measurable structural component that can be observed at the gross anatomical level when groups of patients are pooled together, averaged, and compared with healthy volunteer control subjects.

Cerebral ventricular enlargement is the most consistently replicated finding, but sulcal enlargement and cerebellar atrophy also are reported. Examination of ventricular size in schizophrenic and nonschizophrenic subjects over a broad age range suggests that enlargement does not progress over time at a greater rate in schizophrenic patients than normally and that structural brain abnormalities are present from the outset. Ventricular enlargement is associated with poor premorbid functioning, negative symptoms, poor response to treatment, and cognitive impairment.

The earliest MRI study reported a selective decrease in the frontal lobe size in addition to smaller cerebral and intracranial size, and it suggested that this combination of findings was consistent with a neurodevelopmental process in which the brain failed to grow normally rather than with a neurodegenerative process. Many subsequent studies examined the issue of brain size; a recent meta-analysis confirmed a small but highly statistically significant difference between patients and control subjects in both brain and intracranial volume. The decrease in frontal lobe size has been less consistently replicated, although hypotheses about a dysfunction of the frontal cortex continue to be widely discussed. Three of the four recent studies that used relatively sophisticated measurement techniques have shown decreased frontal lobe size in both chronic and first episode patients. When all studies are pooled, however, negative studies are as frequent as positive ones.

MRI also has been used to explore possible abnormalities in other specific brain subregions such as the thalamus, amygdala/hippocampus, temporal lobes, and basal ganglia. Several studies indicated that the size of temporal regions was decreased in schizophrenia and that there may even be a relatively specific abnormality in the superior temporal gyrus or planum temporale that is correlated with the presence of hallucinations or formal thought disorder.

Although the thalamus is relatively difficult to measure reliably with MRI, several studies have reported a decreased size in schizophrenic patients. Like the prefrontal cortex, the thalamus is an interesting candidate region for schizophrenia; although the precise functions of the various thalamic nuclei are still being mapped, it is a major relay station that could serve functions such as gating or filtering or even generating input and output because it receives afferent input from and sends efferent output to widely distributed cortical and primary sensory and motor regions.

Sophisticated image analysis techniques have been developed to measure the total volume of gray matter, white matter, and cerebrospinal fluid (CSF), and these techniques also have been applied to the study of schizophrenia. Most studies consistently show a decrease in total brain tissue volume in schizophrenia and an increase in CSF in the ventricles and on the brain surface. Most studies that have evaluated the relative changes in gray and white matter have found a selective decrease in cortical gray matter, although some have found white matter decreases as well.

A variety of developmental anomalies are seen by MRI in some patients with schizophrenia. The most consistently reported is an increased frequency of large cavum septi pellucidi, a midline anomaly reflecting a fusion failure of the septal leaflets. In addition, partial callosal agenesis (a severe midline anomaly) appears to be modestly increased in schizophrenia. Finally, findings that reflect abnormalities in neuronal migration (e.g., gray matter heterotopias) are seen with increased incidence, although only in a few patients.

Functional Circuitry and Functional Neuroimaging

Studies of regional cerebral blood flow have been used to explore the possibility of functional or metabolic abnormalities in schizophrenia. Early work suggested that schizophrenic patients had a relative "hypofrontality," which was associated with prominent negative symptoms. Functional imaging studies have become more sophisticated, and it is now clear that PET can be used to explore the functional circuitry used by healthy individuals while they perform a variety of mental tasks and to identify circuits that are dysfunctional in schizophrenia. Although no single group of regions has definitely emerged as the "schizophrenia circuit," a consensus is developing about some of the nodes that may be involved, including a variety of subregions within the frontal cortex (orbital, dorsolateral, medial), the anterior cingulate gyrus, the thalamus, several temporal lobe subregions, and the cerebellum.

Some of these regions have been examined by testing *willed action* (which is analogous to negative symptoms) by giving subjects tasks for which the correct response is not evident from context, such as verbal fluency or choosing a finger movement. Nonschizophrenic subjects activate a frontal circuit during such tasks, whereas patients with schizophrenia show relative decreases in frontal regions and decreases in temporal regions. When the pace of the verbal fluency task is slowed, however, frontal function is similar to that in nonschizophrenic subjects, and only the temporal abnormalities remain. Examination of the correlations between flow in these regions suggests that the normal relation between them has broken down and that functional connectivity is abnormal.

In examining hallucinations, researchers have developed a task to potentially mimic hallucinations; subjects are asked to perform a sentence completion task and imagine that the response was spoken in another person's voice. The researchers found that this task led to activation of speech production and perception regions, such as Broca's area, the supplementary motor area, and the left superior and middle temporal regions. When they applied the same task to patients with schizophrenia and compared hallucinations with nonhallucinations, they found that the hallucinations led to decreased flow in the areas used to monitor speech, such as the left middle temporal gyrus and supplementary motor area. They also examined flow in patients who were experiencing auditory hallucinations and found activations primarily in subcortical regions (thalamus, striatum) and limbic and paralimbic regions (anterior cingulate, parahippocampal gyrus, and cerebellum); they speculated that activity in subcortical regions may generate or moderate hallucinations, whereas the content (e.g., auditory, tactile) may be determined by the specific neocortical regions that are engaged.

Work by one of the authors (N.C.A.) also has provided support for abnormalities in multiple frontal subregions, the thalamus, and the cerebellum. In a study comparing schizophrenic patients with healthy volunteers during random episodic silent thought, blood flow abnormalities were observed in medial, orbital, and dorsolateral frontal regions, as well as in temporal, cingulate, thalamic, and cerebellar areas. In another study of practiced and novel recall of complex narrative material, abnormalities were found in multiple brain regions, including frontal, thalamic, and cerebellar sites.

These findings are consistent with the theory that schizophrenia is a disease of multiple distributed circuits in the brain. The disease is characterized by a cognitive dysmetria caused by a disruption in the pontine-cerebellar-thalamic-frontal feedback loop. The thalamus is a crucial way station in the brain that has complex interconnections to many other regions. Various parts of the prefrontal cortex (i.e., dorsolateral, orbital, and medial) are connected to it, as are other regions such as the basal ganglia and anterior cingulate. Furthermore, various thalamic nuclei have relay connections to virtually all other parts of the cerebral cortex, including sensory, motor, and association regions. Finally, the cerebellum also projects to multiple cortical regions via thalamic relay nuclei.

Neuropathology

A better understanding of neurodevelopment has helped shape contemporary postmortem studies. During the second trimester, neurons in the fetal brain must migrate to the appropriate layers of the cortex and then connect with other groups of neurons to form functional networks. Other developmental processes include excessive proliferation of cells and dendrites, followed by pruning and programmed cell death (apoptosis) of subplate neurons; surviving cells remain as interstitial neurons (or interneurons) of the white matter. The resulting network of neurons and cytoplasmic processes is called the *neuropil*. Research suggests that schizophrenia could be related to disturbances in any of these phases of brain maturation, ranging from migration to apoptosis. Failure of the cells to migrate to their proper position may show up as ectopic gray matter or neuronal disarray in specific regions of the hippocampus.

Displacement of neurons and a paucity of neurons in the superficial layers in the rostral and intermediate portions of the entorhinal cortex of the parahippocampal gyrus also have been reported and have been attributed to faulty neuronal migration. More recently, researchers have observed displacement of interneurons in the frontal lobe cortex, including decreased cell density in the superficial white matter and increased cell density in the deeper white matter, findings also thought to be consistent with an alteration in the migration of subplate neurons or in the pattern of programmed cell death.

Neuropathology also has been used to explore whether abnormalities exist in key candidate regions such as the thalamus or prefrontal cortex. Decreased cell density in the medial dorsal nucleus of the thalamus, a crucial nucleus that projects to the prefrontal cortex, thalamic abnormalities, and increased cell packing density in the prefrontal cortex have been described. The latter finding is consistent with a loss of the surrounding neuropil and consequent shrinkage of the interneuronal space. A convergence of findings is beginning to emerge from the variable perspectives of structural and functional neuroimaging and neuropathology. These perspectives are all consistent with neurodevelopmental mechanisms and with abnormalities in frontal, temporal, and thalamic regions.

Neurodevelopmental Influences

Several lines of evidence have supported speculation that schizophrenia is a neurodevelopmental disorder that results from brain injury occurring early in life. For example, schizophrenic patients are more likely than nonschizophrenic control subjects to have a history of birth injury and perinatal complications, which could result in a subtle brain injury, setting the stage for the development of schizophrenia. Seasonality of birth in schizophrenic patients also has suggested to some a neurodevelopmental etiology. Throughout the temperate northern latitudes, more people with schizophrenia are born in the winter than in any other season. This suggests that some schizophrenic persons could have sustained central nervous system damage in the womb from a viral illness.

Neurochemistry and Neuropharmacology

Schizophrenia is widely believed to have a neurobiological basis. The most popular pathophysiological explanation for schizophrenia is the *dopamine hypothesis,* which suggests that the symptoms of schizophrenia are due primarily to a functional hyperactivity in the dopamine system. Much of the support for the dopamine hypothesis arose from the observation that the efficacy of many of the antipsychotic drugs used to treat schizophrenia was highly correlated with their ability to block dopamine (D_2) receptors. Conversely, drugs that enhance dopamine transmission, such as the amphetamines, tend to worsen the symptoms of schizophrenia. Therefore, the dopamine hypothesis suggested that the abnormality in this illness might lie specifically in the D_2 receptors.

Recent work in neuropharmacology and chemical anatomy has identified five types of dopamine receptors, which differ in their cerebral distribution. The D_1 receptor is linked to adenylate cyclase and is located in the cortex and basal ganglia. The D_2 receptor is not linked to adenylate cyclase and is prominent in the striatum. The D_3 and D_4 receptors have a higher distribution in limbic regions. This distribution raises questions about the classic dopamine hypothesis because limbic regions (or, alternatively, frontal or temporal regions) have been the presumed target for neuroleptic drug action, yet D_2 receptors are not densely concentrated in these target regions. D_5 receptors are limited to the thalamus, hippocampus, and hypothalamus.

Postmortem brain research has documented increased dopamine or homovanillic acid (a metabolite of dopamine) in these limbic regions and in the left amygdala in schizophrenic patients. There is a concern, however, that these findings may be an artifact of treatment with antipsychotics. Animal work has shown that antipsychotic drugs produce receptor supersensitivity in response to receptor blockage by increasing the number of D_2 receptors available. Thus, an increase in D_2 receptors in postmortem brains could be a direct consequence of treatment with antipsychotic medication.

PET has provided another way to assess neurochemical transmission in schizophrenia. Early work appeared to confirm the presence of increased D_2 receptors in schizophrenia, but the finding was not verified by later research.

These results also have lessened confidence that D_2 receptors alone could explain the symptoms of schizophrenia.

PET also has been used to measure receptor occupancy, providing an in vivo method for directly observing the mechanisms of pharmacological action. This work, taken together with the development of the highly effective atypical antipsychotics, has shed further doubt on a simple D_2 theory of schizophrenia. As described in the next section, the new atypical antipsychotic drugs have a very broad pharmacological profile, blocking serotonin type 2 (5-HT_2) receptors, dopamine D_1 receptors, and some subtypes of adrenergic receptors. One study showed that typical antipsychotics have prominent D_2 occupancy (78%) and no obvious D_1 occupancy, whereas atypical antipsychotics showed a 48% occupancy of D_2 receptors and a 38%–52% occupancy of D_1 receptors. This may help to explain why atypical antipsychotics are much less likely to induce extrapyramidal side effects; patients with these effects have a higher D_2 receptor occupancy than do those without such effects.

Clinical Management

The mainstay of treatment for schizophrenia is antipsychotic medication. The putative mechanism of action of antipsychotics is their ability to block postsynaptic dopamine D_2 receptors in the limbic forebrain. This blockade is thought to initiate a series of events responsible for both acute and chronic therapeutic actions. These drugs also block noradrenergic, cholinergic, and histaminic receptors to differing degrees, accounting for the unique side effect profile of each agent. Recommendations for the treatment of schizophrenia are listed in the box below.

Recently, several atypical antipsychotics have been introduced that represent an important advance in the treatment of schizophrenia. Clozapine, risperidone, olanzapine, and quetiapine are the first in this new generation of drugs and soon will be joined by other atypical antipsychotics. They appear more effective than the older conventional antipsychotics, such as chlorpromazine or haloperidol, and are less likely to induce extrapyramidal side effects. They do not appear to increase prolactin levels, making them potentially useful for women who develop galactorrhea or irregular menses while taking conventional antibiotics. In addition to their D_2 receptor blockade, these agents block 5-HT_2 receptors in the frontal cortex and striatal system, which may help to minimize extrapyramidal side effects. The rational use of these drugs is also discussed in Chapter 27.

Recommendations for management of schizophrenia

1. Psychotic symptoms should be treated aggressively with medication.

   - Atypical antipsychotics are the first-line therapy because they are effective and well tolerated.
   - Intramuscular medication is useful in uncooperative or poorly compliant patients.

2. The clinician should engage the patient in an empathic relationship.

   - This task may be particularly challenging because many schizophrenic patients are unemotional, aloof, and withdrawn.
   - The clinician should be practical and help the patient with problems that matter to him or her, such as finding adequate housing.

3. The clinician should help the patient find a daily routine that he or she can manage to help improve socialization and reduce boredom.

   - Partial hospitalization or day treatment programs are available in many areas.
   - Sheltered workshops that provide simple, repetitive chores may be helpful.

4. The clinician should develop a close working relationship with local social services.

   - Patients tend to be poor and disabled; finding adequate housing and food takes the skills of a social worker.
   - The clinician should help the patient obtain disability benefits.

5. Family therapy is important for the patient who lives at home or who still has close family ties.

   - As a result of the illness, many patients will have broken their family ties.
   - Families desperately need education about schizophrenia and need to learn how to reduce their expressed emotion.
   - The clinician should help family members find a support group through referral to a local chapter of the Alliance for the Mentally Ill (AMI).

Treatment of Acute Psychosis

Most acutely psychotic schizophrenic patients will respond to antipsychotic medication. The newer atypical antipsychotics have become first-line therapy because of their low side-effect profile. The target dosages are 10–20 mg/day for olanzapine, 4–6 mg/day for risperidone, and 150–800 mg/day for quetiapine. Higher dosages may be needed in some patients but will increase the likelihood of adverse side effects. Clozapine is a second-line choice because of its expense and propensity to cause agranulocytosis. Typical antipsychotics provide another alternative (e.g., haloperidol, in doses ranging from 2 to 10 mg/day). The monitoring of plasma levels of antipsychotic drugs can be helpful in selected cases. Levels of haloperidol between 5 and 18 ng/mL appear to be effective for most patients, as are levels of clozapine greater than 350 ng/mL.

Agitation can be controlled with equally spaced doses of an antipsychotic drug. The atypical antipsychotics are just becoming available in liquid or intramuscular forms that are suitable for administration to agitated or potentially noncompliant patients. High-potency antipsychotic medications (e.g., haloperidol) also can be given every 30–120 minutes orally or intramuscularly until agitation is under control. More than 20–30 mg of haloperidol in a 24-hour period should be avoided. A combination of a lower dose of antipsychotic medication and a benzodiazepine may work even better to rapidly control agitated psychotic patients (e.g., haloperidol 5 mg/lorazepam 4 mg). Rapid sedation also may be achieved with droperidol (5–10 mg im).

Maintenance Therapy

Patients benefiting from short-term treatment with antipsychotic medications are candidates for long-term prophylactic treatment, which has as its goal the sustained control of psychotic symptoms. At least 1–2 years of treatment are recommended after the initial psychotic episode because of the high risk of relapse and the possibility of social deterioration from further relapses. At least 5 years of treatment for multiple episodes is recommended because a high risk of relapse remains. Beyond this, data are incomplete, but indefinite (perhaps lifelong) treatment is recommended for patients who pose a danger to themselves or others.

A reliable dose-response curve has not been established for maintenance medication, but recent literature supports the use of lower and more conservative doses for conventional antipsychotics. Generally, doses between 50 and 150 mg of chlorpromazine or its equivalent are probably adequate for most patients. Atypical antipsychotics also appear effective for long-term maintenance, but dosing recommendations are less certain.

Adjunctive Treatments

Electroconvulsive therapy is rarely useful in treating schizophrenia, unless a catatonic syndrome is present or the patient has developed a severe depression. Psychosurgery has no role in the treatment of schizophrenia.

Adjunctive psychotropic medications are occasionally useful in the schizophrenic patient, but their role has not been clearly defined. Many patients benefit from anxiolytics (e.g., benzodiazepines) if anxiety is prominent. Lithium carbonate, valproate, and carbamazepine have been used to reduce impulsive and aggressive behaviors, hyperactivity, or excitation or to stabilize mood, although their effectiveness in schizophrenic patients has not been adequately determined. Antidepressants have been used to treat depression in schizophrenic patients. Early studies suggested that antidepressants were not helpful in treating depressed schizophrenic patients and could cause a worsening of thought disorder, but more recent studies have shown that they can be effective adjunctive therapies.

Noncompliance

Noncompliance with antipsychotic medication is a significant problem in the care of schizophrenic patients and should be carefully assessed. There are many contributing factors, but denial of illness resulting from poor insight and discomfort from adverse medication side effects are among the most common. Strategies to minimize drug side effects (e.g., lowering the dosage, prescribing adjunctive medication, or switching to a better-tolerated drug such as an atypical antipsychotic) may work to enhance compliance. In general, the newer atypical antipsychotics have helped reduce noncompliance because of their favorable side-effect profile. In some cases, long-acting intramuscular antipsychotics may be necessary.

Psychosocial Interventions

Psychosocial interventions play an important role in the management of schizophrenia and should be integrated with pharmacotherapy. Like antipsychotic medication, psychosocial treatments should be tailored to fit the schizophrenic patient's needs. The fit will depend on the individual, the phase of illness, and the living situation. For example, patients living with their families might benefit from family therapy, whereas patients living alone might benefit from the social stimulation provided in a day hospital program or contact with a visiting home nurse. Clinicians must work actively to ensure that schizophrenic patients receive adequate mental health care and community benefits and are encouraged to develop a close working relationship with their local social service agencies.

As hospitalizations have become briefer in the past decade, the locus of treatment has shifted to outpatient settings and to the community. Hospitalization now is reserved for schizophrenic patients who pose a danger to themselves or others; who refuse to properly care for themselves (e.g., refuse food or fluids); and who require special medical observation, tests, or treatment. (See Table 7–9 for the reasons to hospitalize schizophrenic patients.)

TABLE 7–9.   Reasons to hospitalize the schizophrenic patient

1.   When the illness is new, to rule out alternative diagnoses, and to stabilize the dose of antipsychotic medication

2.   For special medical procedures such as electroconvulsive therapy

3.   When aggressive or assaultive behavior presents a danger to the patient or others

4.   When the patient becomes suicidal

5.   When the patient is unable to properly care for himself or herself (e.g., refuses to eat or take fluids)

6.   When medication side effects become disabling or potentially life threatening (e.g., severe pseudoparkinsonism, severe tardive dyskinesia, neuroleptic malignant syndrome)

Partial Hospitalization/Day Treatment

Schizophrenic patients who do not need the supervision provided in the hospital may still benefit from the structure provided in partial-hospital (or day treatment) programs, especially patients with substantial symptoms that have not responded adequately to medication. These programs generally operate on weekdays, and patients return home on evenings and weekends. Psychopharmacological management is provided along with psychosocial rehabilitation. With most programs, the services provided and frequency of attendance will be individualized to fit the needs of the patient.

Outpatient Care

The outpatient clinic is the locus of treatment for most schizophrenic patients and the most appropriate setting in which to coordinate care. A well-equipped clinic should be able to provide close monitoring of patients for relapse detection and prevention through careful medication management, to provide both individual or group counseling and psychoeducation, to arrange family intervention, and to arrange special programmatic interventions such as social skills training and cognitive rehabilitation.

Family Interventions

Family therapy, combined with antipsychotic medication, has been shown to reduce relapse rates in schizophrenia. Family therapy may gain some of its effect through enhanced medication compliance but also may help to protect the schizophrenic patient from the demands of the "real world" by providing improved social support, structure, and guidance.

Although the exact mechanism of improvement in family therapy is unknown, several recommendations can be made. First, families can benefit from education about schizophrenia itself. This should include information about the chronic nature of the disorder and the need for long-term care based on realistic expectations. Education will improve cooperation and compliance of both patient and family. However, education must be combined with other family interventions aimed at improving communication while learning to minimize criticism and emotional overinvolvement ("high expressed emotion"), which will help to decrease the schizophrenic patient's level of stress and reduce risk of relapse.

Self-Help Organizations

In addition to more formal family interventions, self-help organizations for family members can be enormously beneficial. They provide a forum for family members to learn about schizophrenia, to gain encouragement from others, and to learn how to cope with schizophrenia's manifestations. The best known group in the United States is the Alliance for the Mentally Ill (AMI), and local chapters can be found in many communities. Many other countries have similar national organizations.

Cognitive Therapy Techniques

Cognitive rehabilitation has as its goal the remediation of abnormal thought processes known to occur in schizophrenia and uses techniques pioneered in the treatment of brain-injured persons. Work with schizophrenic patients is focused on improving information-processing skills such as attention, memory, vigilance, and conceptual abilities.

Cognitive content approaches focus on changing the schizophrenic patient's abnormal thoughts (e.g., delusions) or his or her responses to them and his or her abnormal experiences (e.g., hallucinations). Patients learn various coping strategies such as listening to music to mask auditory hallucinations or reality testing of delusional beliefs.

Social Skills Training

Because social and interpersonal skills are generally deficient in schizophrenic patients, social skills training aims to help patients develop more appropriate behavior. This training is accompanied by modeling and social reinforcement and by providing opportunities, both individual and group, to practice the new behaviors. This could be as simple as helping the patient learn to maintain eye contact or as complicated as helping him or her learn conversational skills. Research has shown that social skills training can significantly enhance social functioning but probably has little effect on risk of relapse. The best results appear to occur in patients whose social development would have been disrupted by the emergence of illness and in persons who persist in a training program for more than 1 year.

Psychosocial Rehabilitation

Psychosocial rehabilitation is a term used to describe services that aim to restore the patient's ability to function in the community. This may involve the medical and psychosocial treatments described above in addition to ways to foster social interaction, to promote independent living, and to encourage vocational performance. Patients are encouraged to become involved in developing and implementing their rehabilitation plan, which focuses on enhancing the patient's talents and skills. The goal of psychosocial rehabilitation is to integrate the patient back into his or her community rather than segregating the patient in separate facilities, as has occurred in the past. In many locations, patient clubhouses are available to promote psychosocial rehabilitation, such as Fountain House, a program in New York that patients help to manage.

Appropriate and affordable housing is a major concern for many patients, and, depending on the community, options may range from supervised shelters and group homes (halfway houses) to boarding homes to supervised apartment living. Group homes provide peer support and companionship, along with on-site staff supervision. Supervised apartments provide greater independence and offer the availability and backup of trained staff. Persons with greater levels of impairment may need around-the-clock supervision in a nursing home.

Vocational training and support can be of enormous benefit to schizophrenic patients in helping to mainstream them back into the community. Research shows that vocational interventions can help patients find and maintain paid jobs. Vocational rehabilitation may involve supported employment, competitive work in integrated settings, and more formal job training programs. A simple, repetitive job environment offering both interpersonal distance and on-site supervision may be the best initial setting, such as that found in a sheltered workshop. Although some patients will not be employable in any setting because of apathy, amotivation, or chronic psychosis, employment should be encouraged in able patients. A job will serve to improve self-esteem, provide additional income, and provide a social outlet for the patient.

In some areas, assertive community treatment (ACT) is available, which consists of the careful monitoring of patients, the availability of mobile mental health teams, and aggressive programming individually tailored to each patient. ACT programs operate 24 hours a day and have been shown to reduce hospital admission rates and to improve the quality of life for many schizophrenic patients. ACT involves teaching patients basic living skills, helping patients work with community agencies, and helping patients develop a social support network. Voluntary job placement and supported work settings (i.e., sheltered workshops) are an important part of the program.

Bibliography

American Psychiatric Association: Diagnostic and Statistical Manual of Mental Disorders, 3rd Edition. Washington, DC, American Psychiatric Association, 1980

American Psychiatric Association: Diagnostic and Statistical Manual of Mental Disorders, 4th Edition. Washington, DC, American Psychiatric Association, 1994

American Psychiatric Association: Diagnostic and Statistical Manual of Mental Disorders, 4th Edition Text Revision. Washington, DC, American Psychiatric Association, 2000

American Psychiatric Association: Practice Guidelines for the treatment of patients with schizophrenia. Am J Psychiatry 154:1–63, 1997

Andreasen NC: Negative symptoms in schizophrenia: definition and reliability. Arch Gen Psychiatry 39:784–788, 1982

Andreasen NC: The Broken Brain: The Biologic Revolution in Psychiatry. New York, Harper & Row, 1984

Andreasen NC: The diagnosis of schizophrenia. Schizophr Bull 13:9–22, 1987

Andreasen NC: Understanding the causes of schizophrenia. N Engl J Med 340:645–647, 1999

Andreasen NC, Olson S: Negative versus positive schizophrenia: definition and validation. Arch Gen Psychiatry 39:789–794, 1982

Andreasen NC, Arndt S, Swayze V, et al: Thalamic abnormalities in schizophrenia visualized through magnetic resonance image averaging. Science 266:294–298, 1994

Andreasen NC, O'Leary DS, Cizadlo T, et al: Schizophrenia and cognitive dysmetria: a positron-emission tomography study of dysfunctional prefrontal-thalamic-cerebellar circuitry. Proc Natl Acad Sci U S A 93:9985–9990, 1996

Black DW, Boffeli TJ: Simple schizophrenia: past, present, and future. Am J Psychiatry 146:1267–1273, 1989

Breier A, Astrachan BM: Characterization of schizophrenic patients who commit suicide. Am J Psychiatry 141:206–209, 1984

Cook JA, Pickett SA, Rozzano L, et al: Rehabilitation services for persons with schizophrenia. Psychiatric Annals 26:97–104, 1996

Crow TJ: Positive and negative schizophrenic symptoms and the role of dopamine. Br J Psychiatry 137:383–386, 1980

Davies N, Russell A, Jones P, et al: Which characteristics of schizophrenia predate psychosis? J Psychiatr Res 32:121–131, 1998

Farde L, Wiesel FA, Stone-Elander S, et al: D2 dopamine receptors in neuroleptic-naive schizophrenic patients: a positron emission tomography study with raclopride. Arch Gen Psychiatry 47:213–219, 1990

Flashman LA, Flaum M, Gupta S, et al: Soft signs and neuropsychological performance in schizophrenia. Am J Psychiatry 153:526–532, 1996

Frith CD: The Cognitive Neuropsychology of Schizophrenia. East Sussex, UK, Lawrence Erlbaum, 1992

Garza-Trevino ES, Hollister LE, Overall JE, et al: Efficacy of combinations of intramuscular antipsychotics and sedative-hypnotics for control of psychotic agitation. Am J Psychiatry 146:1598–1601, 1989

Goldman-Rakic PS: Working memory dysfunction in schizophrenia. J Neuropsychiatry Clin Neurosci 6:348–357, 1994

Hirsh SR, Weinberger DR: Schizophrenia. Oxford, UK, Blackwell Science, 1995

Holzman PS, Levy DL, Proctor LR: Smooth pursuit eye movements, attention, and schizophrenia. Arch Gen Psychiatry 45:641–647, 1976

Huxley NA, Rendall M, Sederer L: Psychosocial treatments in schizophrenia: a review of the past 20 years. J Nerv Ment Dis 188:187–201, 2000

Kane J, Honigfeld G, Singer J, et al: Clozapine for the treatment of resistant schizophrenia. Arch Gen Psychiatry 45:789–796, 1988

Levinson DF, Mahtani MM, Nancarrow DJ, et al: Genome scan of schizophrenia. Am J Psychiatry 155:741–750, 1998

Marder SR, Wirshing WC, Mintz J, et al: Two-year outcome of social skills training and group psychotherapy for outpatients with schizophrenia. Am J Psychiatry 153:1585–1592, 1996

McGlashan TH: The Chestnut Lodge follow-up study, II: long-term outcome in schizophrenia and the affective disorders. Arch Gen Psychiatry 41:586–601, 1984

McGuire PK, Frith CD: Disordered functional connectivity in schizophrenia. Psychol Med 26:663–667, 1996

McNeil TF, Cantor-Graae E, Weinberger DR: Relationship of obstetric complications and differences in size of brain structure in monozygotic twin pairs discordant for schizophrenia. Am J Psychiatry 157:203–212, 2000

Murray CJL, Lopez AD: The Global Burden of Disease. Boston, MA, Harvard University Press, 1996

Nicholson R, Lenane M, Singaracharlu S, et al: Premorbid speech and language impairment in childhood-onset schizophrenia—associated with risk factors. Am J Psychiatry 157:794–800, 2000

Penn DL, Mueser KT: Research update on the psychosocial treatment of schizophrenia. Am J Psychiatry 153:607–617, 1996

Sedvall G, Terenius L: Schizophrenia: Pathophysiological Mechanisms. Amsterdam, The Netherlands, Elsevier, 2000

Selemon LD, Rajkowska G, Goldman-Rakic S: Abnormally high neuronal density in the schizophrenic cortex. Arch Gen Psychiatry 52:805–818, 1995

Sensky T, Turkington D, Kingdom D, et al: A randomized, controlled trial of cognitive-behavioral therapy for persistent symptoms in schizophrenia resistant to medication. Arch Gen Psychiatry 57:165–172, 2000

Shenton ME, Wible CG, McCarley RW: A review of magnetic resonance imaging studies of brain anomalies in schizophrenia, in Brain Imaging in Clinical Psychiatry. Edited by Krishnan KRR, Doraiswamy PM. New York, Marcel Dekker, 1997, pp 297–380

Siris SG, Bermanzohn PC, Mason SE, et al: Maintenance imipramine therapy for secondary depression in schizophrenia: a controlled trial. Arch Gen Psychiatry 51:109–115, 1994

Staal W, Hulshoff HE, Schnack HG, et al: Structural brain abnormalities in patients with schizophrenia and their healthy siblings. Am J Psychiatry 157:416–421, 2000

Winokur G, Tsuang MT: The Natural History of Mania, Depression, and Schizophrenia. Washington, DC, American Psychiatric Press, 1996

Wright IC, Rabe-Hesketh S, Woodruff P, et al: Meta-analysis of regional brain volumes in schizophrenia. Am J Psychiatry 157:16–25, 2000

Self-Assessment Questions

1. What were Bleuler's four *A*'s? What were his fundamental and accessory symptoms?
2. How is schizophrenia diagnosed? What is its differential diagnosis?
3. What are typical signs and symptoms of schizophrenia?
4. What are the subtypes of schizophrenia?
5. What is the prevalence and sex distribution of schizophrenia? What is its age at onset?
6. What recent developments have occurred in the study of the genetics of schizophrenia?

7. What evidence supports a neurobiological basis for schizophrenia?
8. What is the natural history of schizophrenia?
9. How is schizophrenia managed, both pharmacologically and psychosocially?
10. When should the schizophrenic patient be hospitalized?

8 Delusional Disorder and Other Psychotic Disorders

In a sense, the paranoiac's behavior is justified; he perceives something that escapes the normal person; he sees clearer than one of normal intellectual capacity, but his knowledge becomes worthless when he imputes to others the state of affairs he thus recognizes.

Sigmund Freud

Although schizophrenia is clearly the most significant psychotic disorder, and mood disorder with psychotic features is the most common, several less-well-known psychotic disorders are seen by psychiatrists and are briefly reviewed here. These disturbances include delusional disorder, schizoaffective disorder, schizophreniform disorder, brief psychotic disorder, shared psychotic disorder, and psychotic disorder not otherwise specified (see Table 8–1). Psychotic disorders thought to be due to the effects of a substance or a general medical condition are discussed in Chapter 6.

Delusional Disorders

Delusional disorders constitute a small but important group of disturbances characterized by the presence of well-systematized, nonbizarre delusions accompanied by affect appropriate to the delusion and occurring in the presence of a relatively well-preserved personality.

TABLE 8–1.   Delusional disorder and other DSM-IV-TR psychotic disorders

Delusional disorder

    Erotomanic type

    Grandiose type

    Jealous type

    Persecutory type

    Somatic type

    Mixed type

    Unspecified type

Schizoaffective disorder

Schizophreniform disorder

Brief psychotic disorder

Shared psychotic disorder

Psychotic disorder not otherwise specified

History

Delusional disorders have a long history. In the past, they were called paranoid disorders, which translated from the Greek *para nous* as a "mind beside itself," a phrase originally used to describe insanity. The term *paranoia* was revived in the nineteenth century by German psychiatrists interested in disorders characterized by delusions of persecution and grandeur. Kraepelin, best known for separating manic depression from dementia praecox (schizophrenia), used the term to describe persons with systematized delusions, an absence of hallucinations, and a prolonged course without recovery but not leading to mental deterioration.

Epidemiology, Etiology, and Course

Delusional disorder has an estimated prevalence in the community of between 24 and 30 per 100,000 persons and is rare in psychiatric hospitals. In one study, only 0.14% of the hospitalized patients admitted over a 55-year period had a delusional disorder. It is generally considered a disorder of middle to late adult life, and it affects more women than men. Most patients with delusional disorders seen in hospitals are married, poorly educated, and from lower socioeconomic classes.

Family studies have generally shown that delusional disorder is unrelated to schizophrenia and mood disorders, but delusional disorder is so uncommon that it is difficult to show that it runs in families. Nonetheless, paranoid personality traits have been found in relatives of delusional disorder probands, suggesting that the disorder may have a genetic basis.

Psychosocial stressors have long been thought to cause delusional disorder in some persons. For example, persons migrating from one country to another have been observed to be at risk for developing a *migration psychosis,* which is generally persecutory in nature. Solitary confinement in prison is another example of a stressor thought to induce a persecutory psychosis in some persons.

Delusional disorder tends to have a chronic, unremitting course, but unlike patients with schizophrenia, patients with delusional disorder are generally self-supporting and employed. The disorder is diagnostically stable, and it is unlikely that these patients will develop schizophrenia.

Diagnosis

Delusional disorder is diagnosed when nonbizarre delusions are present, have lasted at least 1 month, and involve situations that occur in real life (see Table 8–2). The patient's behavior is generally not odd or bizarre apart from the delusion or its ramifications, and functioning is not markedly impaired. In addition, bizarre delusions like those that occur in schizophrenia (i.e., impossible delusions, such as being controlled by Martians), grossly disorganized behavior, prominent hallucinations, and negative symptoms such as apathy or avolition are not present. Mood disorders, if present, are brief relative to the duration of the delusions, and the effects of drugs (e.g., amphetamines) and medical illness (e.g., acquired immunodeficiency syndrome [AIDS]) have been ruled out as causing the symptoms.

The core feature of delusional disorder is the presence of a well-systematized, encapsulated, nonbizarre delusion. The term *systematized* indicates that the delusion and its ramifications fit into a complex, all-encompassing scheme that makes logical sense to the patient. The term *encapsulated* indicates that, apart from the delusion or its ramifications, the patient generally behaves normally, or at least is not obviously odd or bizarre.

Clinical Findings

Patients with delusional disorder tend to be socially isolated, seclusive, and chronically suspicious. Those with persecutory or jealous delusions some-

TABLE 8–2.   DSM-IV-TR diagnostic criteria for delusional disorder

A. Nonbizarre delusions (i.e., involving situations that occur in real life, such as being followed, poisoned, infected, loved at a distance, or deceived by spouse or lover, or having a disease) of at least 1 month's duration.

B. Criterion A for Schizophrenia has never been met.   **Note:** Tactile and olfactory hallucinations may be present in Delusional Disorder if they are related to the delusional theme.

C. Apart from the impact of the delusion(s) or its ramifications, functioning is not markedly impaired and behavior is not obviously odd or bizarre.

D. If mood episodes have occurred concurrently with delusions, their total duration has been brief relative to the duration of the delusional periods.

E. The disturbance is not due to the direct physiological effects of a substance (e.g., a drug of abuse, a medication) or a general medical condition.

Specify type (the following types are assigned based on the predominant delusional theme):

> **Erotomanic Type:**   delusions that another person, usually of higher status, is in love with the individual
>
> **Grandiose Type:**   delusions of inflated worth, power, knowledge, identity, or special relationship to a deity or famous person
>
> **Jealous Type:**   delusions that the individual's sexual partner is unfaithful
>
> **Persecutory Type:**   delusions that the person (or someone to whom the person is close) is being malevolently treated in some way
>
> **Somatic Type:**   delusions that the person has some physical defect or general medical condition
>
> **Mixed Type:**   delusions characteristic of more than one of the above types but no one theme predominates
>
> **Unspecified Type**

times become angry and hostile, emotions that can lead to violent outbursts. Many patients become litigious and end up as lawyers' clients rather than as psychiatrists' patients. Sexual problems and depressive symptoms are common, and patients are often overtalkative and circumstantial, especially when discussing their delusions. Comorbid major depressive episodes are frequent complications. Common symptoms in a series of patients are shown in Table 8–3.

The following subtypes are based on the predominant delusional theme:

- *Persecutory type:* the belief that one is being treated badly in some way
- *Erotomanic type* (De Clérembault's syndrome): the belief that a person, usually of higher status, is in love with the patient

TABLE 8–3. Common symptoms in 29 patients with delusional disorder

Symptoms	%
Delusions of persecution	83
Delusions of reference	76
Chronic suspiciousness	66
Sexual problems or dysfunction	55
Delusional jealousy	48
Manic symptoms	48
Depressive symptoms	45
Overtalkativeness/circumstantiality	30
Suicide attempts	14
Somatic delusions	10
Suicide threats	7
Delusions of grandeur	7
Significant drinking history	3

Source. Adapted from Winokur 1977.

- *Grandiose type:* the belief that one is of inflated worth, power, knowledge, or identity or that one has a special relationship to a deity or famous person
- *Jealous type:* the belief that one's sexual partner is unfaithful
- *Somatic type:* the belief that one has some physical defect, disorder, or disease, such as AIDS

The residual category *unspecified type* is for patients who do not fit the previous categories (e.g., those who have been ill less than 1 month), and the category *mixed type* is for those with delusions characteristic of more than one subtype but without any single theme predominating.

The following vignette illustrates the erotomanic subtype:

Doug, a 33-year-old restaurant manager, was brought to the hospital under court order. It was alleged that he had harassed and threatened a young woman.

The patient had had an uneventful childhood in a small midwestern town. Although quiet and bookish, he had had many friends. He had excelled in school and graduated from college with honors. He had later obtained a master's degree.

After admission, the following story unfolded. Doug had had a 4½-year fantasy relationship with a comely young shop clerk who had recently married. He had become convinced that the young woman was in love with him, although they had never met. He took as evidence of her affection glances and smiles that they had exchanged when they occasionally crossed paths in their small town. After becoming convinced of her love, he mailed a "sexual business letter" to her after learning her name and address. Doug continued to send love letters over the next few years and kept careful track of her whereabouts. There were no other communications, but the letters indicated his belief that she was infatuated with him and his desire that she act on it. In one letter, he wrote: "What do you think I am? A can of vegetables that can just sit on your shelf to open or throw away whenever it suits you?"

The young woman became concerned and complained to the police, who warned Doug not to call or write to her. The warning had little effect. (Interestingly, Doug himself complained to the police about his imagined harassment by her.) The woman and her husband eventually sought a court order for Doug's hospitalization when the letters to her developed a more threatening tone and a restraining order had failed to keep him away from the shop where she worked. Doug felt jilted by the woman's relationship and subsequent marriage, and he suggested in recent letters that the three get together to "work things out."

In the hospital, Doug dressed neatly and was well groomed. He was articulate and intelligent and indignant about his hospitalization. Although he was notably circumstantial in describing his fantasy relationship, no evidence of a mood disorder, hallucinations, or bizarre delusions was seen. He reported a history of a similar relationship 10 years earlier, consisting mostly of letters, which ended only when the girl moved out of town. Although Doug was a loner with few friends, he was highly functional in his position at work and was active in several community organizations.

At his hearing, Doug denied that his behavior was inappropriate, but he agreed to undergo outpatient psychiatric treatment. The young woman eventually moved out of town.

Two unusual syndromes have been described in some patients with delusional disorder: *Capgras' syndrome,* in which a patient believes that a person closely related to him or her has been replaced by a double (this belief was the theme of the 1950s horror movie *Invasion of the Body Snatchers*), and *Fregoli syndrome,* in which the patient identifies a familiar person in various other people he or she encounters. The patient may maintain that although there is no physical resemblance between the familiar person and others, they are nonetheless psychologically identical.

Differential Diagnosis

A careful diagnostic evaluation is necessary to rule out other psychiatric or medical disorders that could have caused the delusions. The workup should include a physical examination to rule out alcoholism; drug-induced states; dementia; and infectious, metabolic, and endocrine disorders. Routine laboratory tests may be indicated, depending on the results of the history and physical examination. A computed tomography or magnetic resonance imaging scan of the brain may be helpful in selected cases, especially when mass lesions are suspected and need to be ruled out.

The major differential diagnosis involves separating delusional disorder from mood disorders with psychotic features, schizophrenia, and paranoid personality. The chief distinction from psychotic mood disorders is that in delusional disorder, a depressive or manic syndrome is absent, develops after the psychotic symptoms, or is brief in relation to the psychotic symptoms. Unlike schizophrenia, delusional disorders are characterized by nonbizarre delusions and generally either no hallucinations or hallucinations that are not prominent or are very brief. (Tactile and olfactory hallucinations may be present when they are related to the delusional theme.) Furthermore, patients with delusional disorders do not develop other symptoms typically associated with schizophrenia, such as incoherence or grossly disorganized behavior, and personality is generally preserved. Persons with paranoid personality may be suspicious and hypervigilant, but they are not delusional.

Clinical Management

Treatment recommendations are based on clinical observation, not empirical evidence, because no systematic studies have compared treatments in patients with delusional disorder. Because most patients have little insight about their illness and refuse to acknowledge their disorder, the initial obstacle often is getting the patient to the physician. The patient's reluctance to seek care may account for the low frequency of cases reported by physicians.

The physician should make an effort to develop a trusting relationship with the patient, after which he or she may gently challenge the patient's beliefs by showing how they interfere with the patient's life. The patient should be assured of the confidential nature of the doctor-patient relationship. Tact and skill are necessary to persuade a patient to accept treatment, and the physician must neither condemn nor collude in the beliefs. Group therapy is not recommended because patients with delusional disorder tend to be suspicious and hypervigilant and are prone to misinterpret situations that may arise in the course of the therapy.

For reasons that are not understood, delusional disorder has a relatively poor response to antipsychotic medication, although these drugs should be tried. They may help relieve the agitation and anxiety that sometimes accompany the delusions but leave the core delusion intact. Any of the standard antipsychotics may be used. The newer atypical antipsychotics may be preferred because of their more favorable side effect profile (e.g., risperidone, 2–6 mg/day; olanzapine, 5–20 mg/day). The use of depot antipsychotics (e.g., haloperidol decanoate) may help to prevent noncompliance in particularly suspicious patients. *Monohypochondriacal paranoia* (i.e., delusional disorder, somatic subtype) has been specifically reported to respond to the antipsychotic pimozide at doses of 4–8 mg/day. Serotonin reuptake inhibitors (e.g., fluoxetine, paroxetine) also have been reported to be helpful in reducing delusional beliefs. Electroconvulsive therapy (ECT) has no role in the treatment of delusional disorder, unless it is used to treat a superimposed major depression.

Recommendations for the management of delusional disorder

1. Because the patient with delusional disorder is so suspicious, it may be very difficult to establish a therapeutic relationship.

   - Building a relationship will take time and patience.
   - The therapist must neither condemn nor collude in the delusional beliefs of the patient.
   - The patient must be assured of complete confidentiality.

2. Once rapport is established, the patient's delusional beliefs may be gently challenged by pointing out how they interfere with his or her functioning.

   - Tact and skill are needed to convince the patient to accept treatment.

3. A patient with delusional disorder may be more accepting of medication if it is explained as a treatment for the anxiety, dysphoria, and stress that the patient invariably experiences as a result of his or her delusions.

   - Antipsychotic medication should be tried, although results are unpredictable. Atypical antipsychotics may be preferred because they are better tolerated (e.g., risperidone, 2–6 mg/day; olanzapine, 5–20 mg/day).
   - Patients with the somatic subtype may preferentially respond to pimozide (1–6 mg/day).

4. Treatment for the jealous subtype may include separation and divorce. Delusional beliefs of infidelity may transfer to future lovers or spouses.

Anxiolytic and antidepressant medications can be used to treat accompanying anxiety or depressive syndromes, respectively, although they have not been systematically evaluated in patients with delusional disorder.

Schizoaffective Disorder

The term *schizoaffective* was first used in 1933 by Kasanin to describe a group of patients with concurrent schizophrenic and mood symptoms, a history of a precipitating stressor, acute onset, and a family history of mood disorder. Kasanin believed that these patients had a subtype of schizophrenia, even though they recovered from their symptoms. After his initial description, patients with this mixture of symptoms tended to receive a variety of diagnoses, such as schizophrenia, good prognosis schizophrenia, cycloid psychosis, and reactive schizophrenia, because there was little agreement about definition or the relation of these disorders to schizophrenia or mood disorders. In all likelihood, patients with schizoaffective disorders constitute two groups: 1) patients with mood disorders and 2) patients with schizophrenia. Although some experts have argued that schizoaffective patients have both disorders, schizoaffective disorder probably does not represent an independent psychosis.

Schizoaffective disorder is thought to have a prevalence of less than 1% and occurs more often in women. The diagnosis is common in psychiatric hospitals and clinics but is primarily a diagnosis of exclusion. Its hallmark is the presence of either a depressive or a manic episode concurrent with symptoms characteristic of schizophrenia, such as bizarre delusions (see Table 8–4). During the illness, hallucinations or delusions must be present for 2 weeks or more in the absence of prominent mood symptoms, but mood symptoms must be present for a substantial portion of the total duration of the illness. (Some experts consider a "substantial portion" to be 30% or more of the total duration.) Finally, the effects of medical illness and drugs have been excluded as having caused the symptoms. There are two subtypes: the bipolar type, marked by a current or previous manic syndrome; and the depressive type, marked by the absence of any manic syndromes.

The differential diagnosis for schizoaffective disorder consists primarily of schizophrenia, psychotic mood disorders, and disorders induced by medical illness or drugs. In schizophrenia, the duration of all episodes of a mood syndrome is brief relative to the total duration of the psychotic disturbance. Although psychotic symptoms may occur in persons with mood disorders, they are generally not present in the absence of depression or mania, helping to set the boundary between schizoaffective disorder and psychotic mania or depression. It is usually clear from the history, physical examination, or laboratory tests when a drug or medical illness has initiated and maintained the disorder.

Family studies have shown an increased prevalence of both schizophrenia and mood disorders in relatives of schizoaffective patients. In general,

TABLE 8–4.   DSM-IV-TR diagnostic criteria for schizoaffective disorder

A. An uninterrupted period of illness during which, at some time, there is either a Major Depressive Episode, a Manic Episode, or a Mixed Episode concurrent with symptoms that meet Criterion A for Schizophrenia.

    Note: The Major Depressive Episode must include Criterion A1: depressed mood.

B. During the same period of illness, there have been delusions or hallucinations for at least 2 weeks in the absence of prominent mood symptoms.

C. Symptoms that meet criteria for a mood episode are present for a substantial portion of the total duration of the active and residual periods of the illness.

D. The disturbance is not due to the direct physiological effects of a substance (e.g., a drug of abuse, a medication) or a general medical condition.

Specify type:

   Bipolar Type: if the disturbance includes a Manic or a Mixed Episode (or a Manic or a Mixed Episode and Major Depressive Episodes)

   Depressive Type: if the disturbance only includes Major Depressive Episodes

schizoaffective patients have higher rates of schizophrenia and lower rates of mood disorders in their families than do patients with mood disorder but higher rates of mood disorder and lower rates of schizophrenia in their families than do patients with schizophrenia. Other research also suggests that patients with schizoaffective disorder are a mixture of schizophrenic patients with severe mood symptoms and mood disorder patients with severe psychoses.

The signs and symptoms of schizoaffective disorder include those seen in schizophrenia and the mood disorders. The symptoms may present together or in an alternating fashion, and psychotic symptoms may be mood congruent or mood incongruent. The course and prognosis of schizoaffective disorder are variable and represent a middle ground between outcome in schizophrenia and outcome in mood disorders. Some studies indicate that the bipolar type of schizoaffective disorder has an outcome similar to that of bipolar disorder and that the depressed type of schizoaffective disorder has a prognosis similar to that of schizophrenia. A worse outcome is associated with poor premorbid adjustment, insidious onset, lack of a precipitating stressor, predominance of psychotic symptoms, early onset, unremitting course, and a family history of schizophrenia.

The treatment of schizoaffective disorder should target both psychotic and mood symptoms. Most patients will benefit from antipsychotic medication. As a general rule, when conventional antipsychotics are used, a mood stabilizer or an antidepressant medication should be prescribed as well, depending on whether the patient is manic or depressed. When an atypical antipsychotic is used, the single drug may adequately target both psychotic and mood symptoms. Thus, these new drugs (e.g., olanzapine, risperidone) may represent an ideal first-line treatment for schizoaffective disorder. Patients not responding to medication often will respond to ECT, although medication is typically reinstituted for long-term prophylaxis.

Schizoaffective patients who are a danger to themselves or others or who are unable to properly care for themselves should be hospitalized.

Schizophreniform Disorder

Langfeldt used the term *schizophreniform* in 1939 to describe acute, reactive psychoses that occurred in persons with normal personalities. The definition of schizophreniform disorder requires 1) that the patient has psychotic symptoms characteristic of schizophrenia, 2) that the symptoms are not due to a substance or general medical condition, 3) that schizoaffective disorder and mood disorder with psychotic features have been ruled out, and 4) that the duration is at least 1 month but less than 6 months (see Table 8–5).

TABLE 8–5.   DSM-IV-TR diagnostic criteria for schizophreniform disorder

A. Criteria A, D, and E of Schizophrenia are met.

B. An episode of the disorder (including prodromal, active, and residual phases) lasts at least 1 month but less than 6 months. (When the diagnosis must be made without waiting for recovery, it should be qualified as "Provisional.")

Specify if:

Without Good Prognostic Features

With Good Prognostic Features: as evidenced by two (or more) of the following:

   (1) onset of prominent psychotic symptoms within 4 weeks of the first noticeable change in usual behavior or functioning

   (2) confusion or perplexity at the height of the psychotic episode

   (3) good premorbid social and occupational functioning

   (4) absence of blunted or flat affect

The diagnosis changes to schizophrenia once the symptoms have extended past 6 months, even if the only symptoms remaining are residual ones. The diagnosis is considered provisional in patients who have not recovered because many persons who meet criteria for schizophreniform disorder will eventually meet criteria for schizophrenia. In the past, patients with schizophreniform disorder would have received a diagnosis of *acute schizophrenia.*

This relatively new diagnosis has little empirical support, and the relevant research has yielded conflicting data. For example, one study found that schizophreniform and schizophrenic patients have similar structural brain abnormalities, but another investigator concluded that at least a portion of schizophreniform patients have a mood disorder, based on family history, treatment response, and neuroendocrine testing.

Research shows that patients with schizophreniform disorder have widely varying outcomes. Outcome measures used in one study (e.g., living situation, marital status, psychiatric symptoms) showed that outcome in schizophreniform patients was more similar to that in patients with schizophrenia than to that in patients with mood disorders. This finding implies that some patients with schizophreniform disorder actually have a mood disorder and that the others, probably the majority, later develop schizophrenia. The study also found that the morbidity risk for mood disorders among first-degree relatives of schizophreniform patients was no different from that observed among relatives of schizophrenic patients but was significantly lower than that observed among relatives of mood disorder patients. In a more recent study, one-quarter of the schizophreniform patients developed a remitting psychotic illness, and the rest developed schizophrenia. Clearly, the proper boundaries of this disorder remain in question. Its main use is to guard against premature diagnosis of schizophrenia.

Treatment of schizophreniform disorder has not been systematically evaluated. The principles for its management are similar to those for an acute exacerbation of schizophrenia, which is described in Chapter 7.

Brief Psychotic Disorder

A patient with a brief psychotic disorder has psychotic symptoms that last at least 1 day but no more than 1 month, with gradual recovery. Psychotic mood disorders, schizophrenia, and the effects of drugs or medical illness have been ruled out as causing the symptoms. Signs and symptoms are similar to those seen in schizophrenia, including hallucinations, delusions, and grossly disorganized behavior (see Table 8–6). The three subtypes are 1) with marked stressor(s), 2) without marked stressor(s), and 3) with postpartum onset. In the past, patients with marked stressors would have received a diagnosis of a reactive, hysterical, or psychogenic psychosis. This disorder is similar to what Scandinavian psychiatrists regard as *reactive psychoses,* which arise in psychologically vulnerable persons subjected to stress.

TABLE 8–6.   DSM-IV-TR diagnostic criteria for brief psychotic disorder

A.   Presence of one (or more) of the following symptoms:
   (1) delusions
   (2) hallucinations
   (3) disorganized speech (e.g., frequent derailment or incoherence)
   (4) grossly disorganized or catatonic behavior
   Note: Do not include a symptom if it is a culturally sanctioned response pattern.
B.   Duration of an episode of the disturbance is at least 1 day but less than 1 month, with eventual full return to premorbid level of functioning.
C.   The disturbance is not better accounted for by a Mood Disorder With Psychotic Features, Schizoaffective Disorder, or Schizophrenia and is not due to the direct physiological effects of a substance (e.g., a drug of abuse, a medication) or a general medical condition.

Specify if:

   With Marked Stressor(s) (brief reactive psychosis):   if symptoms occur shortly after and apparently in response to events that, singly or together, would be markedly stressful to almost anyone in similar circumstances in the person's culture

   Without Marked Stressor(s):   if psychotic symptoms do *not* occur shortly after, or are not apparently in response to events that, singly or together, would be markedly stressful to almost anyone in similar circumstances in the person's culture

   With Postpartum Onset: if onset within 4 weeks postpartum

Patients with postpartum onset generally develop symptoms within 1–2 weeks after delivery. Symptoms include disorganized speech, misperceptions, labile mood, confusion, and hallucinations. *Postpartum psychosis*, as it is often called, tends to arise in otherwise normal individuals and resolves within 2–3 months. The disorder should be distinguished from *postpartum blues*, which occurs in up to 80% of new mothers, lasts for a few days after delivery, and is considered normal.

The prevalence and gender ratio of brief psychotic disorder are unknown. The disorder is thought to occur more commonly in the lower socioeconomic classes and among individuals with personality disorders, especially borderline and schizotypal personality disorders.

The differential diagnosis of brief psychotic disorder includes schizophrenia, psychotic mood disorders, factitious disorder with psychological symptoms, malingering, and disorders induced by medical illness or drugs. In schizophrenia, the onset is usually insidious, and the duration is at least 4 weeks. In mood disorders, psychotic symptoms occur in the context of a full depressive or manic episode. In factitious disorder with psychological symptoms, there is evidence of intentional production of the symptoms coupled with the need to assume a sick role that may bring secondary gain (e.g., more attention from family members). In malingering, the symptoms are voluntarily produced in response to an obvious external motivation (e.g., escaping from military duties). In some cases, the differential between brief psychotic disorder, factitious disorder, and malingering is difficult, and observation may be needed to help clarify the diagnosis. In cases induced by medical illness or drugs, evidence from the history, laboratory tests, or physical examination indicates that a general medical condition or a substance (e.g., amphetamines) initiated and maintained the disturbance.

As in any acute psychosis, hospitalization may be necessary for the safety of the patient or others. Because a brief psychotic disorder is probably self-limiting, no specific treatment is indicated, and the hospital milieu itself may be sufficient to help the patient recover. Antipsychotic medications (e.g., risperidone, 2–6 mg/day) may be helpful early on, especially when the patient is highly agitated or experiencing great emotional turmoil. Once the patient has sufficiently recovered, the therapist can help him or her explore the meaning of the psychotic reaction and of the triggering stressor. Supportive psychotherapy may help restore morale and self-esteem.

Shared Psychotic Disorder

The essence of shared psychotic disorder is the transmission of delusional beliefs from one person to another. It was called *shared paranoid disorder* in DSM-III to highlight the possibility that several persons may share a similar delusion. In the past, this disorder also was called *folie à deux*, a French term meaning "double insanity." The disorder is apparently rare, and information is limited to case reports. See Table 8–7 for the DSM-IV-TR criteria.

TABLE 8–7. DSM-IV-TR diagnostic criteria for shared psychotic disorder

A. A delusion develops in an individual in the context of a close relationship with another person(s), who has an already-established delusion.

B. The delusion is similar in content to that of the person who already has the established delusion.

C. The disturbance is not better accounted for by another Psychotic Disorder (e.g., Schizophrenia) or a Mood Disorder With Psychotic Features and is not due to the direct physiological effects of a substance (e.g., a drug of abuse, a medication) or a general medical condition.

Most cases of shared psychotic disorder involve two members of the same family, most commonly siblings, a parent and child, or a husband and wife. Its development requires the presence of a dominant person with an established delusion and a more submissive and suggestible person who gains the acceptance of the more dominant individual by adopting his or her delusional beliefs. Clinical lore suggests that separation may result in rapid improvement of the submissive person.

Psychotic Disorder Not Otherwise Specified

Psychotic disorder not otherwise specified is a residual category for persons with psychotic symptoms such as hallucinations, delusions, or grossly disorganized behavior who do not clearly fit into any of the other better-defined categories. For example, a person with persistent auditory hallucinations who is otherwise well adjusted, employed, and socially competent would fit this category. The category also should be used to classify psychoses for which information is inadequate to make a specific diagnosis.

Certain culture-bound syndromes may fit this category, including an interesting condition known as *koro*. This condition is indigenous to China and other parts of the Far East. An individual develops the belief that his or her genitals are retracting into the body. Typically, a man believes that his penis is retracting, whereas a woman believes that her breasts are retracting. Persons with this condition usually have no history of mental illness, and the disorder remits spontaneously. Folk remedies include having the relatives pull on the person's genitals (or breasts) to prevent them from retracting. Epidemics of koro have been documented to occur in remote parts of China.

Bibliography

American Psychiatric Association: Diagnostic and Statistical Manual of Mental Disorders, 3rd Edition. Washington, DC, American Psychiatric Association, 1980

American Psychiatric Association: Diagnostic and Statistical Manual of Mental Disorders, 4th Edition. Washington, DC, American Psychiatric Association, 1994

American Psychiatric Association: Diagnostic and Statistical Manual of Mental Disorders, 4th Edition Text Revision. Washington, DC, American Psychiatric Association, 2000

Coryell WH, Tsuang MT: Outcome after 40 years in DSM-III schizophreniform disorder. Arch Gen Psychiatry 43:324–328, 1986

Evans JD, Heaton RK, Paulsen JS, et al: Schizoaffective disorder: a form of schizophrenia or affective disorder? J Clin Psychiatry 60:874–882, 1999

Harding JJ: Postpartum psychiatric disorders: a review. Compr Psychiatry 30:109–112, 1989

Kasanin J: The acute schizoaffective psychoses. Am J Psychiatry 90:97–126, 1933

Kendler KS: Demography of paranoid psychoses (delusional disorder). Arch Gen Psychiatry 39:890–902, 1982

Kendler KS, Spitzer RL, Williams JBW: Psychotic disorders in DSM-III-R. Am J Psychiatry 146:953–962, 1989

Kendler KS, McGuire M, Gruenberg AM, et al: Examining the validity of DSM-III-R schizoaffective disorder and its putative subtypes in the Roscommon family study. Am J Psychiatry 152:755–764, 1995

Langfeldt G: Schizophreniform States. Copenhagen, Denmark, E Munksgard, 1939

Levitt JJ, Tsuang MT: The heterogeneity of schizoaffective disorder: implications for treatment. Am J Psychiatry 145:926–936, 1988

Maj M: Lithium prophylaxis in schizoaffective disorder: a prospective study. J Affect Disord 14:129–135, 1988

McElroy SL, Keck PE Jr, Strakowski SM: An overview of the treatment of schizoaffective disorder. J Clin Psychiatry 60 (suppl 5):16–21, 1999

Munoz RA, Amado H, Hyatt S: Brief reactive psychosis. J Clin Psychiatry 48:324–327, 1987

Munro A: Psychiatric disorders characterized by delusions: treatment in relation to specific types. Psychiatric Annals 22:232–240, 1992

Opjordsmoen S: Long-term course and outcome in delusional disorder. Acta Psychiatr Scand 78:556–586, 1988

Pope HG, Lipinski JF, Cohen BM: Schizoaffective disorder: an invalid diagnosis? A comparison of schizoaffective disorder, schizophrenia, and affective disorder. Am J Psychiatry 137:921–927, 1980

Sacks MH: Folie à deux. Compr Psychiatry 29:270–277, 1988

Targum SD: Neuroendocrine dysfunction in schizophreniform disorder: correlation with six-month clinic outcome. Am J Psychiatry 140:309–313, 1983

Tran PV, Tollefson GD, Sanger TM, et al: Olanzapine versus haloperidol in the treatment of schizoaffective disorder: acute and long-term therapy. Br J Psychiatry 174:15–22, 1999

Tseng WS, Kan-Ming M, Hsu J, et al: A sociocultural study of koro epidemics in Guangdong, China. Am J Psychiatry 145:1538–1543, 1988

Watt JAG: The relationship of paranoid states to schizophrenia. Am J Psychiatry 142:1456–1458, 1985

Winokur G: Delusional disorder (paranoia). Compr Psychiatry 18:453–479, 1977

Winokur G: Familial psychopathology and delusional disorder. Compr Psychiatry 26:241–248, 1985

Zhang-Wong J, Beiser M, Bean M, et al: Five-year course of schizophreniform disorder. Psychiatry Res 59:109–117, 1995

Self-Assessment Questions

1. How does delusional disorder differ from schizophrenia?
2. What are systematized and encapsulated delusions?
3. What are the subtypes of delusional disorder?
4. How does schizoaffective disorder differ diagnostically from both schizophrenia and psychotic mood disorders?
5. Why is schizoaffective disorder a controversial diagnosis?
6. What evidence is there to link schizophreniform disorder to either schizophrenia or the mood disorders?
7. What is the differential diagnosis of a brief psychotic disorder?
8. How is a brief psychotic disorder managed?
9. What is the commonly accepted treatment in shared psychotic disorder for the patient who develops a delusion in the context of a close relationship with another person?
10. Give an example of a situation in which the diagnosis *psychotic disorder not otherwise specified* is used.
11. What is koro?

 **9 Mood
Disorders**

I see the lost are like this, and their curse
To be, as I am mine, their sweating selves. But worse.

Gerard Manley Hopkins

If a physician chooses to know only one group of mental illnesses very well, he or she should choose mood disorders. Masked as complaints about insomnia, fatigue, or unexplained aches and pains, mood disorders are a common reason that a patient decides to visit the doctor's office. The patient usually is unaware that these problems are due to depression and may need to be convinced to accept treatment for it. As public awareness of mood disorders has improved, however, and as the power of newer antidepressant medications such as fluoxetine have become more widely known, patients also may self-diagnose and arrive at an office requesting treatment for depression.

Whatever the case, mood disorders are very common. Furthermore, they have a very high level of both morbidity and mortality. For people aged 15–45 years, depression has the highest cost to society, accounting for an astounding 10.3% of all costs of biomedical illnesses worldwide. Furthermore, bipolar disorder (manic-depressive illness), the severe form of mood disorder characterized by extreme mood swings, ranks sixth. Yet these substantial costs to society, documented in *The Global Burden of Disease,* may be unnecessary. When correctly diagnosed and treated, mood disorders usually respond well. Learning to diagnose and treat mood disorders should be as basic and fundamental a skill in medicine as the diagnosis and management of myocardial infarction or streptococcal pharyngitis.

History

The recognition that some human beings develop an abnormal syndrome characterized by a disorder in mood has been present for many millennia. Perhaps the oldest medical document available to us is from ancient Egypt, the Eber papyrus, and it describes a medical condition characterized by severe despondency that is equivalent to modern concepts of depression. In the Old Testament, the case of Saul is described in the Book of Samuel during the eighth century B.C. Saul, King of Israel, developed periods of severe depression, guilt, and incapacity. Several different treatments were attempted, including placing a young woman in his bed and having the young shepherd David play soothing music for him. He responded to the music of David for a time and even accepted David as a member of the royal household. Later, however, he relapsed again, became severely psychotic, and even attempted to kill David and his own son Jonathan.

The original name for this disorder, *melancholy*, appears in Hippocratic writings of the fourth century; the term *melancholy* literally means "black bile," and it reflects the belief that this disorder was caused by a chemical imbalance of the humors of the body. Clear and explicit references to disorders of mood continue from classical times to the present. Saint Augustine, Saint John of the Cross, Shakespeare's Hamlet, John Keats, William James, and Leo Tolstoy are only a few of the many notable figures who have described their personal struggles with periods of depression or despondency.

Mood disorders are thus historically among the oldest psychiatric syndromes that have been recognized. They are also psychologically understandable. We have all experienced mild periods of despondency after some personal loss or failure, and it is therefore very easy to identify with people who have the more severe forms of the illness. As later portions of this chapter indicate, effective treatments for these illnesses have become available during the past few decades, making these among the most treatment-responsive disorders in psychiatry and in medicine generally. As a result, working with patients with mood disorders tends to be very gratifying.

An additional aspect of mood disorders that makes them quite intriguing is their association with giftedness or creativity. As early as the fourth century B.C., Aristotle commented that "those who have become eminent in philosophy, politics, poetry, and the arts have all had tendencies toward melancholia." People with mood disorders may, as a group, be somewhat more creative or gifted than the general population. For example, in a group of successful creative writers selected from the rotating faculty at The University of Iowa Writers' Workshop, the rate of mood disorder was nearly three times greater than that of a socioeconomically and educationally equivalent control group. This finding, first reported in the 1970s, has been repeatedly replicated in subsequent studies by several different investigators. The list of notable writers who clearly have had a mood disorder is long, including Robert Lowell, Ernest Hemingway, Sylvia Plath, John Berryman, William Styron, and Anne Sexton.

Many eminent philosophers, scientists, and politicians have had mood disorders as well. Aristotle cites both Plato and Alexander the Great as examples. Oliver Cromwell, Martin Luther, Abraham Lincoln, and Winston Churchill are probably examples as well. It is a sad commentary on the stigma attached to mental illness in our society that American presidential candidates are screened for a history of psychiatric illness, and even the untrue attribution of such a history is considered to be an effective form of mudslinging. Many of our great leaders of the past would have been prevented from accomplishing their missions had a history of mood disorder been considered grounds for disqualification.

These disorders are variously referred to as either *mood* or *affective disorders.* DSM-IV and DSM-IV-TR use the term *mood disorders,* but DSM-III and much of the older clinical and research literature used the alternative term. Although more traditional and more widely used, the concept of an abnormality of affect as a unifying principle for these disorders is somewhat problematic on several grounds. The term *affect* is sometimes used to refer to the external expression of an internal state (i.e., mood). The distinction between mood and affect also sometimes turns on transient versus sustained states, with affect being more transient and mood being more sustained (affect is to weather as mood is to climate). According to this distinction, the abnormality in affective or mood disorders is more often one of mood because the change in emotion lends a constant and pervasive coloring to the individual's perception of reality during the period of illness. Furthermore, patients with schizophrenia often have pronounced abnormalities in affect that are fundamental to the illness. Thus, the term *mood disorders* is preferable to refer to this group of disorders.

Diagnostic Criteria and Clinical Findings

The mood disorders fall into two broad syndromes: depression and mania.

Major Depressive Episode

Because feelings of sadness and despondency are very much part of normal human experience, having diagnostic criteria to demarcate pathological sadness from normal responses to stress and injury is particularly important. The DSM-IV-TR criteria for an episode of major depression appear in Table 9–1. These criteria specify that the patient must have at least five of nine symptoms of depression (and one of them must be depressed mood or loss of interest or pleasure). These characteristic symptoms define major depression, and they must be present for at least 2 weeks to rule out transient mood fluctuations. Criteria B, D, and E serve to rule out other conditions, such as a bipolar disorder (e.g., presence of a mixed episode), abnormalities in mood due to abuse of a substance (e.g., amphetamines) or to a general medical condition (e.g., myxedema), or a disturbance in mood due to bereavement. Criterion C specifies that the symptoms must cause distress or impairment in order to differentiate a disorder from normal fluctuations in mood.

Because major depression is perhaps the most common psychiatric illness that clinicians in any branch of medicine are likely to encounter, it is worthwhile to commit the nine characteristic symptoms to memory. In interviewing patients to determine whether they are depressed, the clinician will repeatedly mentally run through this list of symptoms. Consequently, it is convenient to have it stored in an accessible memory bank so that the evaluation can be done fluently and smoothly. This can be facilitated through the use of a simple mnemonic: "Depression Is Worth Studiously Memorizing Extremely Grueling Criteria. Sorry." (DIWSMEGCS). The initials stand for Depressed mood, Interest, Weight, Sleep, Motor activity, Energy, Guilt, Concentration, Suicide.

As the DSM-IV-TR criteria imply, the basic abnormality in depression is an alteration in mood: a person who is depressed feels sad, despondent, down in the dumps, or full of despair. Although the dysphoric mood is most frequently expressed as a complaint of feeling sad, occasionally patients will complain of feeling tense or irritable, with only a small component of sadness, or of having lost their ability to feel pleasure or to experience interest in things they normally enjoy.

The depressive syndrome is frequently accompanied by a group of vegetative symptoms, such as decreased appetite or insomnia. Decreased appetite often leads to some weight loss, although some depressed persons will force themselves to eat despite decreased appetite, or they may be urged to eat by a parent or spouse so that the weight loss is minimal. Less frequently, depression expresses itself as a desire to eat excessively and is accompanied by weight gain.

TABLE 9–1. DSM-IV-TR diagnostic criteria for major depressive episode

A. Five (or more) of the following symptoms have been present during the same 2-week period and represent a change from previous functioning; at least one of the symptoms is either (1) depressed mood or (2) loss of interest or pleasure.

Note: Do not include symptoms that are clearly due to a general medical condition, or mood-incongruent delusions or hallucinations.

  (1) depressed mood most of the day, nearly every day, as indicated by either subjective report (e.g., feels sad or empty) or observation made by others (e.g., appears tearful).   Note: In children and adolescents, can be irritable mood.

  (2) markedly diminished interest or pleasure in all, or almost all, activities most of the day, nearly every day (as indicated by either subjective account or observation made by others)

  (3) significant weight loss when not dieting or weight gain (e.g., a change of more than 5% of body weight in a month), or decrease or increase in appetite nearly every day.   Note: In children, consider failure to make expected weight gains.

  (4) insomnia or hypersomnia nearly every day

  (5) psychomotor agitation or retardation nearly every day (observable by others, not merely subjective feelings of restlessness or being slowed down)

  (6) fatigue or loss of energy nearly every day

  (7) feelings of worthlessness or excessive or inappropriate guilt (which may be delusional) nearly every day (not merely self-reproach or guilt about being sick)

  (8) diminished ability to think or concentrate, or indecisiveness, nearly every day (either by subjective account or as observed by others)

  (9) recurrent thoughts of death (not just fear of dying), recurrent suicidal ideation without a specific plan, or a suicide attempt or a specific plan for committing suicide

B. The symptoms do not meet criteria for a Mixed Episode.

C. The symptoms cause clinically significant distress or impairment in social, occupational, or other important areas of functioning.

D. The symptoms are not due to the direct physiological effects of a substance (e.g., a drug of abuse, a medication) or a general medical condition (e.g., hypothyroidism).

E. The symptoms are not better accounted for by Bereavement, i.e., after the loss of a loved one, the symptoms persist for longer than 2 months or are characterized by marked functional impairment, morbid preoccupation with worthlessness, suicidal ideation, psychotic symptoms, or psychomotor retardation.

Insomnia may be initial, middle, or terminal. *Initial insomnia* means that the patient has difficulty falling asleep, often tossing or turning for several hours before dozing off. *Middle insomnia* refers to awakening in the middle of the night, remaining awake for an hour or two, and finally falling asleep again. *Terminal insomnia* refers to awakening early in the morning and being unable to return to sleep. Patients with insomnia will often worry and ruminate while they are lying awake. Patients who have terminal insomnia may have more severe depressive syndromes. Depressed patients also may complain of restless sleep, indicating that they have awakened so frequently throughout the night that they scarcely got any sleep at all. These various types of sleep disturbance have been well documented by electroencephalography (EEG) research in sleep laboratories. Occasionally, the sleep difficulty may involve a need to sleep excessively: the patient may complain of feeling chronically tired and needing to spend 10–14 hours each day in bed.

Motor activity is often altered in depression. Patients may subjectively complain of feeling either slowed down or agitated, but objective evidence is required as well to ensure that the symptom is truly present. Patients with *psychomotor retardation* may sit quietly in a chair for hours without speaking to anyone, simply staring into space. When these patients get up and move about, they walk at a snail's pace, their speech is slow, and their replies are brief and laconic. If asked about their thinking, they may complain that it is markedly slowed down. Conversely, patients with *psychomotor agitation* are restless and seem extremely nervous. Agitated patients may complain more of irritability or tenseness than of depression. They are unable to sit in a chair and frequently pace about. They may wring their hands or perform some other stereotyped and repetitive nervous gesture such as drumming their fingers on a table, pulling on their hair or clothing, or playing with objects in their hands. Their speech usually is somewhat rapid, and they may complain in a high-pitched and staccato whine about the various miseries from which they are suffering.

Depressed patients also complain frequently of fatiguing too easily or lacking energy or pep. In a general medical setting, this may be one of the most common presenting complaints of depression, and the clinician will need to probe to determine whether the easy fatigability is due to a depressive syndrome.

Feelings of worthlessness and guilt are also very common in depression. Depressed persons may lose confidence in themselves so that they are fearful of going to work, taking examinations, or assuming responsibility for household tasks. They may not answer the telephone or return telephone calls to avoid responsibilities or social relationships that they feel unable to handle. They may become completely hopeless and full of despair, believing that their situation can never be improved or even that they do not deserve to feel better. Depressed patients may feel quite guilty over actual or fantasized misdeeds they have committed in the past. Usually the misdeed is seen as more terrible than it actually was, so that depressed persons believe that they should be social pariahs because of a lie told as a child or sent to prison for a long term because of a questionable deduction taken on an income tax return.

Complaints of difficulty in concentrating or thinking clearly are also common in depression. Depressed patients feel that they function less well at work, are unable to study, or (in severe cases) are even unable to perform simple cognitive tasks such as watching a football game on television or reading.

Depressed patients may think a great deal about death or suicide. This may be seen either as an escape from their suffering or as a deserved punishment for their various misdeeds. The suicidal patient often expresses the notion that "everyone would be better off without me." Suicide risk is high in depressed patients and should always be assessed carefully. (See Chapter 21 for more detail on evaluation and management of the suicidal patient).

In addition to the nine core symptoms summarized in the diagnostic criteria, other symptoms may occur in patients with depression. *Diurnal variation,* another vegetative symptom, is a fluctuation in mood during the course of a 24-hour day; it may reflect some type of neuroendocrine abnormality in depression. Most typically, patients state that their mood is worse in the morning but that it improves as the day progresses, so that they feel best in the evening. Less frequently, this problem is reversed, with the patient stating that he or she feels best in the morning.

Sex drive may decrease markedly, so that the patient has no interest in sex or even begins to experience impotence or anorgasmia. The depressed patient also may complain of other physical symptoms such as constipation or dry mouth.

Occasionally, patients experience *masked depression.* This term means that the full depressive syndrome is not immediately obvious because the patient does not report a depressed mood. With the introduction of diagnostic criteria, however, the diagnosis is unmasked because a thorough and systematic interview that runs through the various criteria will identify the presence of decreased interest and a substantial clustering of symptoms. Masked depression may be especially important in primary care settings. For example, an older person may come in complaining primarily of many physical symptoms so troubling that he or she is unable to concentrate, work, and sleep. This patient will deny being in a despondent or irritable mood, stating that he or she is indeed upset but would feel fine if only the physical symptoms were corrected. These symptoms are often pain or gastrointestinal problems, such as piercing headache, burning pains in the rectum, or persistent heartburn. Although a careful medical workup reveals no physical abnormalities, the patient continues to insist on the troubling nature of the various somatic and depressive symptoms. When the masked depression clears with appropriate treatment, however, the physical complaints tend to disappear, making it clear that they were secondary to a depressive syndrome.

Patients who are severely depressed may experience psychotic symptoms such as delusions or hallucinations. These are usually consistent with the depressed mood; for example, people who are depressed may hear the voice of the Devil telling them that they have fallen so far from God's ways that their souls are forever lost and that they will be tormented in Hell throughout eternity. They may begin to believe that the world is coming to an end and that they have seen various signs as indicators of its impending demise. They may develop the delusion that the FBI or police are following them and bugging their house or office to catch them in the various misdeeds that their excessive guilt makes them believe they have committed. They may think that a fatal disease is consuming their bodies and rotting away their internal organs. Less frequently, the delusions will not be consistent with depressed mood. For example, patients may report that they are being spied on because they are on the verge of developing some great invention that others are attempting to steal—a persecutory delusion that is not directly related to depressed mood.

The following case history is relatively typical of a major depressive episode:

> Wilma was brought to the hospital at the request of her family, and of her husband in particular. She described herself as being despondent and demoralized because her husband was having an affair with a woman who had been his secretary, but her husband adamantly denied this and indicated that this belief was a delusion resulting from his wife's depressed condition.
>
> Wilma admitted to having a depressed mood plus a full constellation of depressive symptoms, including feelings of worthlessness, suicidal thoughts, hypersomnia, increased appetite and weight gain, decreased interest in and enjoyment of activities she normally found pleasurable (such as following the many activities of her four teenage children), and decreased energy.
>
> When interviewed alone, she indicated that she was absolutely convinced that her husband, a successful local insurance agent, was secretly involved with another woman. She attributed most of her depressive symptoms to this situation, which she believed had been going on for at least 6 months (as had her depression). She had no specific evidence to

support the occurrence of the affair, but she said that her husband had been away more in the evenings, had a marked decrease in sexual interests, and had talked frequently about Lydia's secretarial skills until Wilma became jealous and angry. Because of pressure from Wilma, her husband eventually urged Lydia to seek another position, but Wilma believed that her husband was continuing to see Lydia secretly. Both in the presence of his wife and when interviewed alone, Bill adamantly denied the affair. He indicated that he was a devout Catholic (as was Wilma) and that such behavior was strongly discordant with his religious beliefs, as well as risky to his community position. Bill indicated that his sexual interest had decreased because Wilma had become increasingly overweight and less attractive. Wilma had had one prior episode of depression that had been successfully treated with antidepressants approximately 5 years earlier.

Depression was therefore diagnosed again, and Wilma was given imipramine, with the dosage gradually increased to 150 mg/day. She showed some improvement on this medication, and both Bill and Wilma also were seen for marital counseling. Their relationship improved somewhat, but Wilma continued to be suspicious.

Wilma continued taking antidepressants for the next 3 months and saw a psychotherapist at weekly intervals to learn techniques to decrease her chronic negative mind-set, her suspicious attitude toward her husband, and her tendency to use food as a way of raising her spirits.

After 3 months of psychotherapy, she came in one day with a new firmness of step and her eyes flashing with anger. While cleaning out the pockets of one of her husband's suits in preparation for sending it to the cleaners, she found a love letter from Lydia. She did not confront Bill immediately but instead followed him the next night when he indicated that he was going back to the office to get caught up on some dictation. Ten minutes after his departure, Wilma left, drove past Lydia's house, and found Bill's car parked in her garage. Thereafter, she confronted him, and he finally confessed to an affair that had been going on for nearly 2 years.

The direction of marital counseling changed sharply, and Bill was urged to seek individual psychotherapy himself. Wilma continued to take antidepressant medication for another 6 months, and she gradually came to terms with the fact of her husband's infidelity (which was actually more painful than having her suspicions discounted by both her husband and the medical community). Eventually, however, the couple was able to work through this situation, to remain married, and eventually to establish a reasonably good relationship with each other.

Manic Episode

The DSM-IV-TR criteria for a manic episode (Table 9–2) require the presence of an abnormally elevated, expansive, or irritable mood lasting at least 1 week plus three of seven characteristic symptoms. The criteria are similar to those used to define depression, in that the mood disturbance

TABLE 9–2. DSM-IV-TR diagnostic criteria for manic episode

A. A distinct period of abnormally and persistently elevated, expansive, or irritable mood, lasting at least 1 week (or any duration if hospitalization is necessary).

B. During the period of mood disturbance, three (or more) of the following symptoms have persisted (four if the mood is only irritable) and have been present to a significant degree:

    (1) inflated self-esteem or grandiosity

    (2) decreased need for sleep (e.g., feels rested after only 3 hours of sleep)

    (3) more talkative than usual or pressure to keep talking

    (4) flight of ideas or subjective experience that thoughts are racing

    (5) distractibility (i.e., attention too easily drawn to unimportant or irrelevant external stimuli)

    (6) increase in goal-directed activity (either socially, at work or school, or sexually) or psychomotor agitation

    (7) excessive involvement in pleasurable activities that have a high potential for painful consequences (e.g., engaging in unrestrained buying sprees, sexual indiscretions, or foolish business investments)

C. The symptoms do not meet criteria for a Mixed Episode.

D. The mood disturbance is sufficiently severe to cause marked impairment in occupational functioning or in usual social activities or relationships with others, or to necessitate hospitalization to prevent harm to self or others, or there are psychotic features.

E. The symptoms are not due to the direct physiological effects of a substance (e.g., a drug of abuse, a medication, or other treatment) or a general medical condition (e.g., hyperthyroidism).

    Note: Manic-like episodes that are clearly caused by somatic antidepressant treatment (e.g., medication, electroconvulsive therapy, light therapy) should not count toward a diagnosis of Bipolar I Disorder.

must be sufficiently severe to cause marked impairment or to require hospitalization. As in the case of depression, the symptoms cannot be due to the physiological effects of drugs of abuse, medications, or a general medical condition.

The manic patient's mood is typically cheerful, enthusiastic, and expansive. The cheerfulness often has an infectious quality, making interviewing an enjoyable and sometimes amusing experience. Sometimes, however, the patient's mood is simply irritable, particularly when he or she is thwarted, and such irritable manic patients can be quite difficult to manage. Because of their euphoria, manic patients usually have very little insight into their problems. In fact, they may deny that anything is wrong with them and instead blame friends or family for attributing an abnormality to them that is in fact not present. Because mania is characterized by other symptoms that are clearly pathological, such as poor judgment and extreme grandiosity, it is usually not difficult for the clinician to differentiate manic euphoria from a normal good mood.

Manic patients typically have inflated self-esteem and grandiosity, which may reach delusional proportions. Manic patients may believe that they have special abilities or powers that clearly are outside the normal range for their educational background or intellectual achievement. They may develop plans to write books, record compact discs, lead religious movements, or undertake expansive business ventures. When the grandiosity reaches delusional proportions, patients may report that they are rock stars, famous athletes or politicians, or even religious figures such as the Messiah.

The euphoria and grandiosity are typically accompanied by increased energy, activity levels, and cognitive speed. Patients with mania usually require less sleep than usual, often getting by on only 2 or 3 hours per night. Unlike the patient with depression, the manic patient does not feel tired and does not complain about his or her inability to sleep. Patients may become more social and gregarious, going to bars, planning parties, or calling friends at all hours of the night. Interest in sex is often increased, leading the manic patient to exhaust his or her partner or to make inappropriate overtures to casual acquaintances or strangers. Patients with mania are usually physically restless and unable to sit still. The increased level of activity is often accompanied by poor judgment. Patients with mania tend to overextend themselves in ways that lead them into serious trouble after the manic episode is over. They spend money excessively, commit themselves to projects that they are unable to complete, become involved in extramarital affairs, or engage in quarrels with business associates or family members who disagree with them or try to slow them down.

Manic patients tend to talk excessively and to manifest *pressured speech*. Thus, they answer questions at great length, continue to talk even when interrupted, and sometimes talk when no one is listening. Their speech usually is rapid, loud, and emphatic. Underlying the pressured speech is probably a rapid flow of thought, sometimes referred to as *flight of ideas*. This increased speed in cognitive functioning is inferred by listening to the patient's speech, which manifests derailment, incoherence, and distractibility. Manic patients tend to skip from one topic to another as they describe their experiences, ideas, or symptoms. Thus, positive formal thought disorder is quite common in mania. Distractibility is observed in both their speech and their social behavior. While speaking, they may shift their topic in response to some stimulus in the environment, and they manifest the same pattern of distractibility when trying to perform tasks or complete activities. Unfortunately, the increased energy and cognitive productivity are usually not sufficiently well organized to produce the magnificent goals that are projected in the patients' grandiose plans.

As in the case of depression, manic patients may manifest symptoms of psychosis. Indeed, psychotic symptoms are almost more the norm than the exception in mania. Approximately one-half of manic patients have psychotic symptoms, compared with only about one-fifth of depressed patients. Psychotic symptoms may include either delusions or hallucinations and typically express themes consistent with the mood, such as delusions about special abilities or powers. Less commonly, the delusions may be mood incongruent and express themes that are not related to the euphoric and grandiose mood.

The following case history illustrates a relatively typical manic episode:

> Charles was brought to the emergency room by the local police after he had jumped from his seat in the middle of a performance of *Les Miserables,* run onto the stage, and begun yelling that the injustices of the Reagan administration were as extensive and profound as those portrayed in the performance. He had begun conversing with Jean Valjean, urging him to leave the performance, to join the Democratic party, and to assist in the effort to place a Democrat in the White House. This speech was accompanied by an extensive speech on the injustice of packing the Supreme Court with a group of extreme conservatives.
>
> In the emergency room, Charles indicated that he did not live in Iowa City but had come from Des Moines (100 miles away) to attend the performance and to consult with friends and colleagues at the law school. He described himself as a prominent lawyer, a graduate of Harvard Law School who had edited the *Law Review,* a close friend of the Kennedy family and other prominent Democrats, and a dedicated crusader against social injustice. He described the Reagan administration as a rerun of the industrial-totalitarian axis that had been created in Nazi Germany, complained about a conspiracy that he believed was under way to destroy the Democratic party by either persecution or assassination of key figures, and indicated that one of the purposes of his trip to Iowa City was to warn his colleagues at the law school about these dangerous circumstances. He was organizing a campaign to assist a little-known Arkansas politician in his effort to run for president in the next election, believing that this person would be a reincarnation of John Kennedy.
>
> His appearance was somewhat unkempt and disheveled, not consistent with his description of his prominent status. Although he was attired in an expensive-appearing pinstripe suit, his hair was uncombed, his eyes were red, and he was unshaven. Charles talked excitedly in a rapid manner, and his voice rose to a shout at times. His speech was disjointed and diffi-

cult to follow, as his topic changed from his own special importance and abilities to the various conspiracies that he thought were under way in the Reagan government. He described a complex internal structure in the Reagan administration that he believed would "lead to another Watergate," and he marshaled evidence to support this position by referring to special implications in recent television programs such as *Dynasty* and the *Late Show.*

When admission to the hospital was proposed, he became physically agitated and tried to run away. He became physically combative at attempts to restrain him, asserting in a threatening manner that he was a former state wrestling champion who was also a finalist for the Olympic team in his weight class.

Because of his agitation, a decision was made to obtain an emergency hospitalization order. His claims of special importance and abilities were discounted and attributed to his manic state. Later, as more history was obtained, it became evident that Charles was indeed a prominent attorney with many important national connections and also had been a star wrestler. The conspiracy against the Democratic party, although potentially bearing some credence, contained enough implausible elaborations to qualify as delusional thinking. (The beliefs about the Arkansas politician also were thought to be delusional!) Interviews with his family members revealed that he had had one prior hospitalization for mania and had been treated for depression as an outpatient. He had been taking maintenance lithium but had decided to discontinue it abruptly approximately 3 days before coming to Iowa City to attend the performance of *Les Misérables*. Within a day after discontinuing the lithium, he became increasingly euphoric, irritable, and grandiose. His wife had been reluctant to let him go alone, but he had insisted that he would be fine and left against her wishes.

Charles was given a therapeutic dose of lithium, and his symptoms cleared rapidly over the course of 4–5 days. He was able to leave the hospital and to return to work within 1 week. His second episode of mania helped him appreciate the importance of maintenance lithium because his insight about his illness increased, and he has been able to prevent subsequent relapses and to function effectively.

Mixed and Hypomanic Episodes

A small number of patients present with a mixture of both manic and depressive symptoms within a single episode of illness. When this occurs, it is referred to as a *mixed* episode. The clinical presentation of mixed episodes can be quite confusing because the patient's mood and symptom picture tend to alternate rapidly. At one moment, the patient will be talkative, energetic, and expansive and minutes later may burst into tears and complain of feeling hopeless and suicidal. DSM-IV-TR requires that full criteria for both a manic episode and a depressive episode be met within a 1-week period to diagnose the presence of a mixed episode. Patients with a mixed episode are difficult to treat because medications must target both poles of mood disorder.

Hypomania is another important form of mood disorder that may be more common than full-blown mania. The syndrome is similar to mania, but it is milder, briefer, and less florid. During a hypomanic episode, the patient experiences the elevated mood and other classic symptoms that define mania, but they are not accompanied by delusional beliefs or hallucinations, and they are not severe enough to require hospitalization or to markedly impair social and occupational functioning. (The criteria for a hypomanic episode appear in Table 9–3.) Many patients with hypomania also have chronic mild depression, so it can sometimes be difficult to determine whether they are "back to their usual selves" or "just feeling good for a change." Obtaining information from family and friends usually is helpful in determining whether the presence of a good mood is indeed pathological rather than a patch of normal happiness in the midst of feeling chronically blue. Examining the level and quality of social and occupational functioning can provide a clue as to whether the episode is hypomania; the hypomanic person is clearly somewhat impaired and suboptimal in these functions, despite subjectively feeling good or even great. Subtle clues, such as tactlessness in a usually sensitive person or flirtatious behavior in a typically discreet person, indicate that the hypomanic episode reflects a real and pathological change from the normal baseline level of functioning.

Dysthymia and Cyclothymia

DSM-IV-TR also recognizes two somewhat milder forms of mood disorder: *dysthymic disorder* and *cyclothymic disorder.*

Dysthymic disorder (sometimes referred to as *depressive neurosis*) is a chronic and persistent disturbance in mood that has been present for at least 2 years and is characterized by relatively typical depressive symptoms, such as anorexia, insomnia, decreased energy, low self-esteem, difficulty concentrating, and feelings of hopelessness (see Table 9–4). Because dysthymic disorder is a mild chronic disorder, only two of these symptoms are necessary, but they must have persisted more or less continuously for at least a 2-year period.

Patients with dysthymia are chronically unhappy and miserable. Some of them also develop the relatively more severe major depressive syndrome; when the major depressive episode clears, these patients subsequently return to their chronic state of dysthymia. The coexistence of these mild and severe forms of depression is sometimes referred to as *double depression.*

TABLE 9–3. DSM-IV-TR diagnostic criteria for hypomanic episode

A. A distinct period of persistently elevated, expansive, or irritable mood, lasting throughout at least 4 days, that is clearly different from the usual nondepressed mood.

B. During the period of mood disturbance, three (or more) of the following symptoms have persisted (four if the mood is only irritable) and have been present to a significant degree:

   (1) inflated self-esteem or grandiosity

   (2) decreased need for sleep (e.g., feels rested after only 3 hours of sleep)

   (3) more talkative than usual or pressure to keep talking

   (4) flight of ideas or subjective experience that thoughts are racing

   (5) distractibility (i.e., attention too easily drawn to unimportant or irrelevant external stimuli)

   (6) increase in goal-directed activity (either socially, at work or school, or sexually) or psychomotor agitation

   (7) excessive involvement in pleasurable activities that have a high potential for painful consequences (e.g., the person engages in unrestrained buying sprees, sexual indiscretions, or foolish business investments)

C. The episode is associated with an unequivocal change in functioning that is uncharacteristic of the person when not symptomatic.

D. The disturbance in mood and the change in functioning are observable by others.

E. The episode is not severe enough to cause marked impairment in social or occupational functioning, or to necessitate hospitalization, and there are no psychotic features.

F. The symptoms are not due to the direct physiological effects of a substance (e.g., a drug of abuse, a medication, or other treatment) or a general medical condition (e.g., hyperthyroidism).

   Note: Hypomanic-like episodes that are clearly caused by somatic antidepressant treatment (e.g., medication, electroconvulsive therapy, light therapy) should not count toward a diagnosis of Bipolar II Disorder.

A second mild mood syndrome is cyclothymic disorder, a condition in which the patient has mild swings between the two poles of depression and hypomania (see Table 9–5). While in the manic phase, the person appears to be high but not so high as to be socially or professionally incapacitated. During the depressed phase, the individual has some symptoms of depression, but these are not severe enough to meet criteria for a full major depressive episode (i.e., five symptoms persisting for 2 weeks). Thus, the individual with cyclothymic disorder tends to swing from high to low with a chronic mild instability of mood.

TABLE 9–4. DSM-IV-TR diagnostic criteria for dysthymic disorder

A. Depressed mood for most of the day, for more days than not, as indicated either by subjective account or observation by others, for at least 2 years. Note: In children and adolescents, mood can be irritable and duration must be at least 1 year.

B. Presence, while depressed, of two (or more) of the following:

   (1) poor appetite or overeating

   (2) insomnia or hypersomnia

   (3) low energy or fatigue

   (4) low self-esteem

   (5) poor concentration or difficulty making decisions

   (6) feelings of hopelessness

C. During the 2-year period (1 year for children or adolescents) of the disturbance, the person has never been without the symptoms in Criteria A and B for more than 2 months at a time.

D. No Major Depressive Episode has been present during the first 2 years of the disturbance (1 year for children and adolescents); i.e., the disturbance is not better accounted for by chronic Major Depressive Disorder, or Major Depressive Disorder, In Partial Remission.

   Note: There may have been a previous Major Depressive Episode provided there was a full remission (no significant signs or symptoms for 2 months) before development of the Dysthymic Disorder. In addition, after the initial 2 years (1 year in children or adolescents) of Dysthymic Disorder, there may be superimposed episodes of Major Depressive Disorder, in which case both diagnoses may be given when the criteria are met for a Major Depressive Episode.

E. There has never been a Manic Episode, a Mixed Episode, or a Hypomanic Episode, and criteria have never been met for Cyclothymic Disorder.

F. The disturbance does not occur exclusively during the course of a chronic Psychotic Disorder, such as Schizophrenia or Delusional Disorder.

G. The symptoms are not due to the direct physiological effects of a substance (e.g., a drug of abuse, a medication) or a general medical condition (e.g., hypothyroidism).

H. The symptoms cause clinically significant distress or impairment in social, occupational, or other important areas of functioning.

Specify if:

   Early Onset: if onset is before age 21 years

   Late Onset: if onset is age 21 years or older

Specify (for most recent 2 years of Dysthymic Disorder):

   With Atypical Features

TABLE 9–5. DSM-IV-TR diagnostic criteria for cyclothymic disorder

A. For at least 2 years, the presence of numerous periods with hypomanic symptoms and numerous periods with depressive symptoms that do not meet criteria for a Major Depressive Episode. **Note:** In children and adolescents, the duration must be at least 1 year.

B. During the above 2-year period (1 year in children and adolescents), the person has not been without the symptoms in Criterion A for more than 2 months at a time.

C. No Major Depressive Episode, Manic Episode, or Mixed Episode has been present during the first 2 years of the disturbance.

   Note: After the initial 2 years (1 year in children and adolescents) of Cyclothymic Disorder, there may be superimposed Manic or Mixed Episodes (in which case both Bipolar I Disorder and Cyclothymic Disorder may be diagnosed) or Major Depressive Episodes (in which case both Bipolar II Disorder and Cyclothymic Disorder may be diagnosed).

D. The symptoms in Criterion A are not better accounted for by Schizoaffective Disorder and are not superimposed on Schizophrenia, Schizophreniform Disorder, Delusional Disorder, or Psychotic Disorder Not Otherwise Specified.

E. The symptoms are not due to the direct physiological effects of a substance (e.g., a drug of abuse, a medication) or a general medical condition (e.g., hyperthyroidism).

F. The symptoms cause clinically significant distress or impairment in social, occupational, or other important areas of functioning.

Classification and Subtypes

The mood disorders may be subdivided into two main groups: those that are characterized by depression only (i.e., have a major depressive episode or some milder mood disturbance) and those that are bipolar; the latter are characterized by mania (i.e., have a manic episode or a hypomanic episode) either alone or in combination with depression (see Table 9–6). Thus, this classification initially subdivides the types of mood disorders into unipolar and bipolar types.

The term *unipolar* is not included in DSM-IV-TR, but it is widely used by clinicians to refer to patients who have depression only. Thus, patients are subdivided in DSM-IV-TR on a syndromal basis: those who have had an episode of mania are always referred to as having bipolar disorder (even if they have never had a depression), whereas those who have had depression only are classified as having depressive disorder. This subdivision is based on its predictive power. These two subtypes of mood disorder typically have different familial patterns, require different treatments, and perhaps have a different pathophysiology and etiology.

TABLE 9–6.   DSM-IV-TR classification of mood disorders

Bipolar disorders	Depressive disorders
Bipolar disorder, manic	Major depression, single episode
Bipolar disorder, depressed	Major depression, recurrent
Bipolar disorder, mixed	Dysthymic disorder
Cyclothymic disorder	Depressive disorder not otherwise specified
Bipolar disorder not otherwise specified	

The depressive disorders include major depressive disorder and dysthymic disorder as well as a residual category (*depressive disorder not otherwise
specified*). Major depressive disorder is defined by the presence of at least one
episode of major depression. The disorder can be further characterized by a
variety of specifiers, as described below. Dysthymic disorder is defined on
the basis of the criteria enumerated above. The residual category is used for
the occasional odd case that does not fit any of the criteria but does seem to
fit the overall syndrome.

The bipolar disorders include bipolar I disorder, bipolar II disorder, cyclothymic disorder, and bipolar disorder not otherwise specified.

Bipolar I disorder is defined by the occurrence of at least one manic or
mixed episode. Typically, bipolar I disorder is characterized by recurrent episodes of both mania and depression, which may be separated by intervals of
months to years. Although the episodes may lead to psychosocial morbidity
because of the effect of a severe recurrent illness on interpersonal relationships or work functioning, interepisode functioning may be good or even excellent. When well, individuals with bipolar disorder can be high achievers.
As described below, both the most recent episode and the longitudinal
course can be characterized by a variety of specifiers.

Bipolar II disorder is characterized by periods of hypomania that typically occur either before or after periods of depression but also may occur
independently. These mild manic episodes are not sufficiently severe to require hospitalization, although they may lead to personal, social, or work
difficulties. During the mild bipolar phase, the patient is upbeat, shows signs
of poor judgment, and has other indices of mania such as increased energy
or insomnia, but the symptoms do not meet full criteria for a manic episode.
Bipolar II disorder appears to breed true within families, in that relatives of
bipolar II patients themselves have higher rates of bipolar II disorder than
either bipolar I (i.e., criteria are met for a full manic episode) or unipolar
major depression. Bipolar II patients also tend to have a high rate of

comorbidity with other disorders, such as substance abuse.

As previously defined, cyclothymic disorder is the mildest form of bipolar disorder, whereas bipolar disorder not otherwise specified is a residual category.

The nature of the mood disorder is further characterized in a variety of ways. Because mood disorders tend to be recurrent, the various additional specifiers give the clinician a way of characterizing the most recent episode (for which the patient is currently in treatment) and the overall lifetime course of the disorder.

It is very useful to characterize the most recent manic or depressive episode in terms of its severity. This way of subdividing depression is summarized in Table 9–7. The subdivision for manic or mixed episodes is very similar. The episode is classified as mild, moderate, severe, or in partial or full remission. This classification recognizes the continuum of severity within the mood disorders and permits the clinician to indicate where a particular patient falls on that continuum. The most severe form is psychotic mania or depression, which is characterized by psychotic symptoms such as delusions or hallucinations. When the psychotic symptoms are consistent with the patient's mood, they are referred to as *mood congruent*. When the psychotic symptoms are inconsistent with the patient's mood, they are referred to as *mood incongruent*. Mood-incongruent delusions or hallucinations are a relatively worse prognostic feature, and so this form of psychotic mood disorder is delineated as a separate category.

Several additional descriptors of the depressive episode are also used: chronic, with catatonic features, with melancholic features, with atypical features, and with postpartum onset.

Melancholia

Among these various specifiers, *melancholic features* is perhaps the most important (see Table 9–8). The concept of *melancholia* is thought to identify a relatively severe form of depression that is more likely to respond to somatic therapy. The concept is based on an older historic distinction between endogenous and reactive depression, a distinction that was based on both presumed etiology and a characteristic clustering of symptoms. In the original definition of *endogenous depression,* it had no precipitating factors (endogenous means "grows from within"), whereas a *reactive depression* occurred in reaction to some stressful life event such as a divorce or loss of a job. The term *endogenous* is no longer used because increasing evidence has suggested that severe depressions also may be triggered by various physiological or psychological stressors.

TABLE 9–7.   Types of major depressive episode

Mild: Few, if any, symptoms in excess of those required to make the diagnosis, and symptoms result in only minor impairment in occupational functioning or in usual social activities or relationships with others.

Moderate: Symptoms or functional impairment between "mild" and "severe."

Severe, Without Psychotic Features: Several symptoms in excess of those required to make the diagnosis, and symptoms markedly interfere with occupational functioning or with usual social activities or relationships with others.

Severe, With Psychotic Features: Delusions or hallucinations. If possible, specify whether the psychotic features are mood congruent or mood incongruent.

Mood-congruent psychotic features: Delusions or hallucinations whose content is entirely consistent with the typical depressive themes of personal inadequacy, guilt, disease, nihilism, or deserved punishment.

Mood-incongruent psychotic features: Delusions or hallucinations whose content does not involve typical depressive themes of personal inadequacy, guilt, disease, death, nihilism or deserved punishment. Included are symptoms such as persecutory delusions (not directly related to depressive themes), thought insertion, thought broadcasting, and delusions of control.

TABLE 9–8.   DSM-IV-TR diagnostic criteria for melancholic features specifier

Specify if:

 With Melancholic Features (can be applied to the current or most recent Major Depressive Episode in Major Depressive Disorder and to a Major Depressive Episode in Bipolar I or Bipolar II Disorder only if it is the most recent type of mood episode)

A. Either of the following, occurring during the most severe period of the current episode:
    (1) loss of pleasure in all, or almost all, activities
    (2) lack of reactivity to usually pleasurable stimuli (does not feel much better, even temporarily, when something good happens)
B. Three (or more) of the following:
    (1) distinct quality of depressed mood (i.e., the depressed mood is experienced as distinctly different from the kind of feeling experienced after the death of a loved one)
    (2) depression regularly worse in the morning
    (3) early morning awakening (at least 2 hours before usual time of awakening)
    (4) marked psychomotor retardation or agitation
    (5) significant anorexia or weight loss
    (6) excessive or inappropriate guilt

Melancholia requires the presence of two specific characteristic features: pervasive loss of interest or pleasure and inability to respond to pleasurable stimuli. Three from a list of six additional features also are required: distinct quality of depressed mood, diurnal variation, terminal insomnia, severe psychomotor retardation or agitation, anorexia or weight loss, and excessive guilt. Many of these symptoms are predominantly somatic or vegetative, and sometimes this form of depression is referred to as *vegetative*. A substantial body of research has suggested that this clustering of symptoms predicts a good response to antidepressant medication or electroconvulsive therapy (ECT).

Atypical Features

Additional specifiers highlight other aspects of the most recent episode that also may be clinically useful and guide decisions about management. The *atypical features* specifier identifies a group of patients who are diametrically opposed to those with melancholic features; they do not present with the classic vegetative symptoms such as insomnia, weight loss, or anorexia but instead have weight gain and hypersomnia (see Table 9–9). In addition, instead of having a nonreactive mood, they are quite responsive to their life situation, and they are particularly sensitive to slights or rejections. This rejection sensitivity often leads to difficulties in interpersonal relationships, with a stormy personal life characterized by being easily hurt, having many partners, and experiencing frequent breakups. Subjectively, these patients often express their somatic state by complaining of "leaden paralysis," the feeling that their arms and legs weigh them down and make activities difficult for them. Patients with atypical features are difficult to treat and may require a mixture of psychotherapy and medications. Monoamine oxidase inhibitors (MAOIs) have proved particularly useful with this group of patients, and serotonin reuptake inhibitors (SRIs) also may be effective.

Chronic, Postpartum, and Catatonic Specifiers

Other specifiers identify other aspects of the recent episode that also may be clinically important. The *chronic* specifier simply indicates that the full criteria for a major depressive episode have been present for 2 years; patients in this group are refractory to treatment and clinically challenging. The *postpartum onset* specifier identifies those patients who experience a depressive, manic, or mixed episode within the first 4 weeks postpartum. Although feeling a bit depressed after delivery is common (referred to as the postpartum blues), some women develop a full mood syndrome that requires medical at-

TABLE 9–9.   DSM-IV-TR diagnostic criteria for atypical features specifier

Specify if:

With Atypical Features (can be applied when these features predominate during the most recent 2 weeks of a current Major Depressive Episode in Major Depressive Disorder or in Bipolar I or Bipolar II Disorder when a current Major Depressive Episode is the most recent type of mood episode, or when these features predominate during the most recent 2 years of Dysthymic Disorder; if the Major Depressive Episode is not current, it applies if the feature predominates during any 2-week period)

A. Mood reactivity (i.e., mood brightens in response to actual or potential positive events)

B. Two (or more) of the following features:

  (1) significant weight gain or increase in appetite

  (2) hypersomnia

  (3) leaden paralysis (i.e., heavy, leaden feelings in arms or legs)

  (4) long-standing pattern of interpersonal rejection sensitivity (not limited to episodes of mood disturbance) that results in significant social or occupational impairment

C. Criteria are not met for With Melancholic Features or With Catatonic Features during the same episode.

tention with either somatic therapy or psychotherapy or both. At its most severe, the mood episode may become psychotic and/or life-threatening to the mother or child; such severe abnormalities have been estimated to occur in 1 of 500 to 1 of 1,000 deliveries, and the risk of recurrence in subsequent deliveries is great—between 30% and 50% of cases. The *catatonic features* specifier identifies a subgroup of patients who have catatonic features similar to those that historically have been observed primarily in schizophrenia (e.g., posturing, waxy flexibility, catalepsy, negativism, and mutism). The presence of this specifier serves to remind the clinician that such symptoms also may occur in other disorders and that they are not pathognomonic of schizophrenia. These types of symptoms tend to occur primarily in the mood disorders at the severe and psychotic end of the continuum.

Longitudinal Course Specifiers

DSM-IV-TR also provides a system for specifying the longitudinal course of the disorder as well as the clinical characteristics of the most recent episode. The clinician usually is asked to specify whether the disorder involves only a single episode (usually the first episode, for which the patient is currently being treated) or whether the condition is recurrent. If recurrent, the clinician is reminded that closer follow-up is needed and that the prognosis may be more guarded. The need for prophylactic long-term medications to prevent relapse is substantially increased.

Because the various specifiers permit description of many different permutations and combinations of features, the classification of mood disorders may appear quite complicated. A summary of the various combinations appears in Table 9–10. An example of some typical patterns of longitudinal course is shown in Figure 9–1, which displays the various combinations of major depression and dysthymia that may occur. Similar variations in pattern also are seen in the bipolar disorders. We often recommend to our students that they map out the longitudinal course of their patient's illness; this helps to pin down the course and give the student a better understanding of the patient.

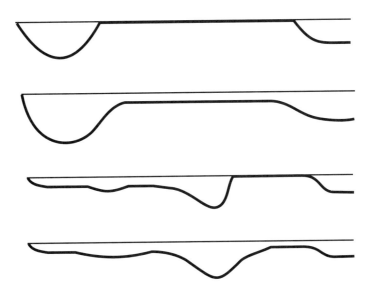

FIGURE 9–1. DSM-IV patterns of longitudinal course of mood disorders. **Top**: recurrent, with full interepisode recovery, with no dysthymic disorder. **Second**: recurrent, without full interepisode recovery, with no dysthymic disorder. **Third**: recurrent, with full interepisode recovery, superimposed on dysthymic disorder (also code 300.4). **Bottom**: recurrent, without full interepisode recovery, superimposed on dysthymic disorder (also code 300.4).

TABLE 9–10. DSM-IV-TR episode specifiers that apply to mood disorders

	Severity/psychotic/ remission	Chronic	With catatonic features	With melancholic features	With atypical features	With post-partum onset
Major depressive disorder, single episode	X	X	X	X	X	X
Major depressive disorder, recurrent	X	X	X	X	X	X
Dysthymic disorder					X	
Bipolar I disorder, single manic episode	X		X			X
Bipolar I disorder, most recent episode hypomanic						
Bipolar I disorder, most recent episode manic	X		X			X
Bipolar I disorder, most recent episode mixed	X		X			X
Bipolar I disorder, most recent episode depressed	X	X	X	X	X	X
Bipolar I disorder, most recent episode unspecified						
Bipolar II disorder, hypomanic						
Bipolar II disorder, depressed	X	X	X	X	X	X
Cyclothymic disorder						

The various longitudinal descriptors also permit identification of two other facets of long-term course: *with seasonal pattern* and *with rapid cycling*. (The criteria for the seasonal pattern specifier are summarized in Table 9–11.) Clinicians have recognized for many decades that some individuals have a characteristic onset of mood symptoms in relation to changes of season, with depression typically occurring more frequently during the winter months and remissions or changes from depression to mania occurring during the spring. This seasonal pattern also has important implications for prevention and treatment, in that medications can be adjusted appropriately once the pattern is recognized. The rapid-cycling specifier identifies those patients who have had at least four episodes of a major depressive, manic, hypomanic, or mixed episode during the past 12 months. This specifier also warns the clinician of the need for close follow-up and careful medication management. Rapid cyclers are clearly at high risk for relapse and also have a high suicide risk.

TABLE 9–11. DSM-IV-TR diagnostic criteria for seasonal pattern specifier

---

Specify if:

With Seasonal Pattern (can be applied to the pattern of Major Depressive Episodes in Bipolar I Disorder, Bipolar II Disorder, or Major Depressive Disorder, Recurrent)

A. There has been a regular temporal relationship between the onset of Major Depressive Episodes in Bipolar I or Bipolar II Disorder or Major Depressive Disorder, Recurrent, and a particular time of the year (e.g., regular appearance of the Major Depressive Episode in the fall or winter).

   Note: Do not include cases in which there is an obvious effect of seasonal-related psychosocial stressors (e.g., regularly being unemployed every winter).

B. Full remissions (or a change from depression to mania or hypomania) also occur at a characteristic time of the year (e.g., depression disappears in the spring).

C. In the last 2 years, two Major Depressive Episodes have occurred that demonstrate the temporal seasonal relationships defined in Criteria A and B, and no nonseasonal Major Depressive Episodes have occurred during that same period.

D. Seasonal Major Depressive Episodes (as described above) substantially outnumber the nonseasonal Major Depressive Episodes that may have occurred over the individual's lifetime.

Epidemiology

Because epidemiological surveys of the prevalence or incidence of mood disorder have not used identical criteria to define mood disorders, the prevalence and incidence are uncertain. One study done in New Haven, Connecticut, that used diagnostic criteria closely equivalent to those in DSM-IV, indicated that approximately 4.3% of the population has depression at any given time. Investigators in Iceland reported a current rate of 3.8%, and investigators in Denmark reported 3.4%. Estimates of lifetime prevalence vary, but it seems likely that somewhere between 8% and 20% of the population will experience a significant depression at some time, depending on how narrowly or broadly *significant depression* is defined.

Depression is more common in women than in men. The current ratio in the United States is approximately 2:1. Bipolar disorder is much less common than unipolar major depression. The lifetime prevalence for bipolar disorder is between 0.5% and 1%. Bipolar disorder also is more common in women than in men, with a ratio of approximately 3:2.

Data from the Epidemiologic Catchment Area (ECA) study showed that dysthymic disorder has a lifetime prevalence of approximately 3%, and it is more common in women younger than 65, unmarried persons, and persons with low income. A recent study indicated that dysthymic disorder also may be quite common in elderly persons. There are no comparable figures for cyclothymic disorder.

The age at onset for major depression appears to be getting steadily lower, a phenomenon referred to as the *cohort effect*. That is, a proportionately larger number of individuals in the baby boom generation have had episodes of major depression compared with older individuals. Among the baby boomers—people born after 1940—the age at onset is reported to be earlier than in older individuals. This cohort effect was observed in a major project, the Collaborative Study of Depression, which evaluated more than 1,000 patients with mood disorders and more than 3,000 other family members. To determine the relation between age at onset and long-term outcome, the subjects were divided into cohorts, based on their birth date: before 1910, 1910–1919, 1920–1929, 1930–1939, 1940–1949, and after 1950. The groups also were divided into men and women to examine gender differences. The results of this analysis appear in Figure 9–2, which shows a striking difference in age cohorts. The curves show cumulative risk, or the likelihood that people will become seriously depressed at some time in their lives. These curves plateau for people born before 1930, but they continue to climb for later cohorts. Baby boomers have curves that point nearly straight up, suggesting that most baby boomers may become depressed at some time during their lives. The prospects for women are worse than for men. These epidemiological data provide strong support for the likelihood that nongenetic psychosocial factors play a role in the etiology of depression.

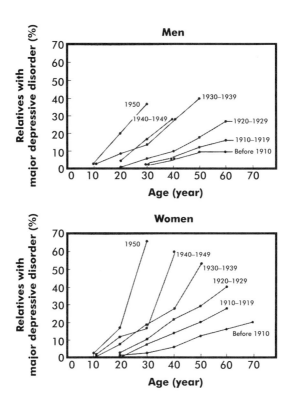

FIGURE 9–2. Cohort effect demonstrated in the Collaborative Study of Depression. These graphs show that the age of onset for major depression is getting steadily lower with each successive birth cohort in men and women.

Etiology and Pathophysiology

Many different ideas have been proposed to explain the etiology and pathophysiology of mood disorders. These explanations encompass the domains of genetics, social and environmental factors, and neurobiological factors.

Genetics

It has been recognized for many years that mood disorders tend to run in families. As discussed in Chapter 5, however, familiality does not necessarily indicate genetic transmission because role modeling, learned behavior, social environmental factors such as economic deprivation, and physical environmental factors such as prenatal and perinatal birth complications all may provide nongenetic contributions to the development of a disorder, and these contributions could themselves be familial. (For example, before the advent of antibiotics, tuberculosis tended to run in families for environmental rather than genetic reasons.)

Studies of familial aggregation in mood disorders have provided empirical evidence that these disorders run in families. Data from family studies are summarized in Figures 9–3 and 9–4. Figure 9–3 summarizes data based on studies that used bipolar patients as the index case. Figure 9–4 shows the rates of bipolar illness in the first-degree relatives of unipolar patients. Nearly all studies show significantly increased rates of mood disorder, especially bipolar disorder, in the first-degree relatives of bipolar patients compared with psychiatrically normal control subjects. Unipolar patients tend to have much less bipolar illness among their first-degree relatives but a high rate of unipolar illness. Control rates vary from study to study but typically are around 1% in the psychiatrically normal population for bipolar disorder and between 5% and 15% for unipolar disorder; rates vary depending on the methods of definition. As these figures indicate, the first-degree relatives of bipolar patients tend to have a higher rate of bipolar illness than unipolar illness, although unipolar illness is also quite common in the first-degree relatives of bipolar patients. The opposite effect is seen in the first-degree relatives of unipolar patients. Thus, these disorders not only are familial but also tend to breed true. The fact that they do not breed perfectly true (i.e., bipolar illness *only* in the relatives of bipolar patients and unipolar illness *only* in the relatives of unipolar patients) also suggests that these two forms of mood disorder may not be totally distinct from each other.

Twin and adoption studies have complemented these family studies and have provided evidence that mood disorders are genetic in addition to familial. The twin studies are summarized in Table 9–12. The total number of available twin pairs was less than 500; the overall monozygotic-to-dizygotic ratio in this entire sample was approximately 4:1 (65:14). Within individual studies, the monozygotic-to-dizygotic ratio ranged from 75:0 to 57:23. These data are certainly sufficient to indicate that mood disorders must have a strong genetic component. Adoption studies also support this conclusion.

Mood disorders were the first among the major mental illnesses to be studied with the techniques of molecular biology using the linkage method. Several types of linkage have been reported. In a study of the Old Order Amish, linkage to the short arm of chromosome 11 was reported for bipolar disorder, a finding not supported by a subsequent reanalysis. Several other studies have reported X linkage for bipolar disorder. Linkage to other genes also has been reported, including loci on chromosome 21, chromosome 6,

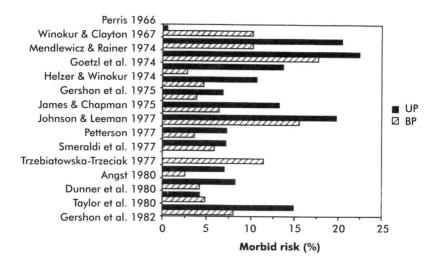

FIGURE 9–3. Morbid risk for bipolar (BP) and unipolar (UP) illness in first-degree relatives of bipolar probands.

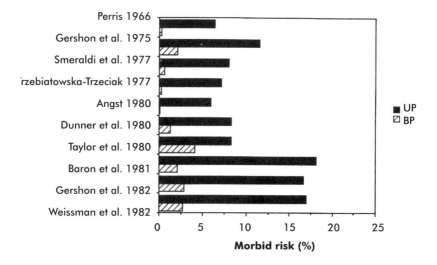

FIGURE 9–4. Morbid risk for bipolar (BP) and unipolar (UP) illness in first-degree relatives of unipolar probands.

TABLE 9–12.   Concordance rates for mood disorders in monozygotic and dizygotic twins

Study	Monozygotic twins		Dizygotic twins	
	Concordant pairs/total pairs	Concordance (%)	Concordant pairs/total pairs	Concordance (%)
Luxenberger 1930	3/4	75.0	0/13	0.0
Rosanoff et al. 1935	16/23	69.6	11/67	16.4
Slater 1953	4/7	57.1	4/17	23.5
Kallmann 1954	25/27	92.6	13/55	23.6
Harvald and Hauge 1965	10/15	66.7	2/40	5.0
Allen et al. 1974	5/15	33.3	0/34	0.0
Bertelsen 1979	32/55	58.2	9/52	17.3
Totals	95/146	65.1	39/278	14.0

chromosome 18 (several different loci), chromosome 4, and the X chromosome. Candidate genes also have been examined, with some positive results, focusing primarily on dopamine and serotonin receptors.

There is now nearly universal consensus that single gene models for mood disorders are unlikely to be either valid or useful for most, or perhaps all, cases. A central problem in the application of molecular genetics and molecular biology to the study of mood disorders is the definition of the *phenotype*. This problem has several facets. First, mood disorders do not breed true. Families that are ascertained through a bipolar proband frequently turn out to have other family members who have unipolar illness, as is evident in Figures 9–3 and 9–4. These results suggest that bipolar and unipolar mood disorders may represent a continuum of severity and that the "mood phenotype" may include both bipolar and unipolar depressive forms. However, environmental phenocopies are a potentially serious problem in the case of depression. As discussed below, at least some individuals who experience an episode of major depression may be developing their symptoms in response to psychosocial stressors, in the absence of any genetic diathesis at all. Definition of the phenotype is perhaps the central problem in the application of the tools of molecular genetics and molecular biology to the study of mood disorders.

Social and Environmental Factors

One of the fundamental questions about the nature of depression is how to draw the line between a normal response to a painful personal life experience and a clinically significant depression. Everyone experiences transient episodes of sadness after breaking up with a girlfriend or boyfriend, getting a divorce, performing badly on an examination, or losing a loved one. Diagnostic criteria were developed to assist in drawing this line, suggesting that the sadness must persist for more than 2 months after a bereavement (i.e., loss of a loved one). However, the criteria do not help with disentangling the effects of less serious life experiences.

People who experience a loss or disappointment often develop symptoms similar to those of major depression: feelings of sadness, difficulties with sleep or appetite, indecisiveness, poor concentration, or guilt or self-criticism. We all know people who continue to have these symptoms for more than a few weeks after a personal loss or other psychosocial stressor. When the symptoms persist long enough, then the person who experienced the stressor does in fact meet criteria for major depression, and this person may respond well to treatment with an antidepressant. Therefore, it is intuitively obvious that psychosocial stressors may play a role in the etiology of depression. The crucial question is not "Do psychosocial and environmental factors play a role in precipitating depression?" but rather "What is the nature of the role that psychosocial and environmental factors play? Do they tip a predisposed person over the edge, or are they sufficient in and of themselves?"

We do not know the answer to this question. Many investigators have attempted to examine the role that life events play in the development of mood disorders, and the results are conflicting. Some studies have indicated that stressful life events are both necessary and sufficient, whereas others have found no relation. Most of the studies are problematic because they treated genetics versus the environment as an either/or situation instead of looking for cumulative or additive risks.

A plausible model for the role of stressful life events is that they do induce a biological reaction (e.g., an outpouring of cortisol). Once this biological reaction is initiated, it is difficult to stop and may trigger or exacerbate a depressive syndrome, particularly in individuals who have been previously primed because of either a genetic diathesis or experiences that made them particularly vulnerable to stress. In fact, a tendency to be neurobiologically oversensitive to the effects of psychosocial stress could be one of the genetic factors that is transmitted within families. Likewise, early life events, such as harsh or abusive parenting during childhood, could create a diathesis by making a person more psychologically sensitive to rejection and more biologically sensitive to stress.

This conceptualization has been supported by animal research. Investigators have examined factors such as maternal deprivation in monkeys or the effects of repeated electric shocks in rats placed in a situation in which they were unable to escape the shocks. These studies used careful, well-controlled designs. They showed that maternal deprivation and "learned helplessness" can induce an animal syndrome of depression that closely mimics that observed in humans.

Finally, the cohort effect for mood disorders, described earlier in this chapter, also provides evidence that psychosocial factors may have a role in the development of mood disorders. Various explanations for the cohort effect have been explored. The baby boom generation has had an early onset of mood disorders and higher rates of illness. This group of people may have experienced more economic and social stresses than their predecessors. Because of the large numbers of individuals in this cohort, they have had more intensive competition with one another in most aspects of life than any generation in recent history. They have had to compete with one another for college admission and jobs in an economy that has been steadily downsizing its workforce. The concurrent rise of technology favors the minority of individuals who are educated and technically skilled but leaves the majority in a "have-not" status. Extended families are dispersed throughout the country, reducing the base of supportive individuals, and divorce and separation in both parents and the baby boomers themselves also have taken a toll. Value systems that older generations used for psychological consolation, such as the strong sense of moral and social responsibility that guided people born in the cohorts from 1910 to 1940, have been replaced by an emphasis on economic well being—an external support that can be difficult to sustain and perhaps is less psychologically rewarding.

Neurobiology

Neurobiological studies of mood disorders have pursued four major areas of investigation: abnormalities in neurotransmission, neuroimaging of brain structure and blood flow, abnormalities in neurophysiological function (especially sleep), and abnormalities in neuroendocrine function.

Abnormalities in Neurotransmission

The *catecholamine hypothesis* was the earliest formulation concerning the role of neurotransmitters in depression. As originally proposed, it suggested that depression was caused by a deficit of norepinephrine at crucial nerve terminals throughout the brain. This hypothesis received support from studies of the mechanism of action of antidepressant medications used during the 1970s and 1980s. Classic work by Julius Axelrod, which led to his Nobel Prize, demonstrated that antidepressants such as imipramine increase the amount of norepinephrine functionally available at nerve terminals by inhibiting reuptake. Other antidepressants, the MAOIs, also increase the amount of norepinephrine available by inhibiting breakdown of norepinephrine through monoamine oxidase. Reserpine, which depletes monoamines, worsens depression.

The development of other types of antidepressant medications during the past decade has indicated, however, that other neurotransmitters also may play a role in depression. The SRIs also are very effective treatments for depression, yet they do not act on the norepinephrine system. Instead, they appear to exert their therapeutic effect by increasing the amount of serotonin functionally available at nerve terminals. Furthermore, patients with severe depression have been found to have a decrease in a major serotonin metabolite, 5-hydroxyindoleacetic acid (5-HIAA), in their cerebrospinal fluid. In addition, numbers of serotonin type 2 ($5\text{-}HT_2$) receptors have been decreased in postmortem brains of persons who have committed suicide.

Either a catecholamine hypothesis or a serotonin hypothesis is an oversimplification, although these hypotheses have been heuristically useful. They have turned attention to examining the biological mechanisms of emotional and cognitive states and the role that these mental systems play in disease processes.

Neuroimaging Studies

Both structural and functional brain imaging techniques have been applied to study the mechanisms of mood disorders. Computed tomography studies of stroke patients have applied the lesion method to determine the possible anatomical substrates of mood abnormalities. These studies suggested that anterior left hemisphere strokes are likely to induce dysphoria, perhaps by disconnecting noradrenergic circuits projecting to the left prefrontal cortex; right hemisphere strokes are more likely to induce euphoria. Positron-emission tomography studies provide some additional support for these findings, in that mood induction of dysphoria in psychiatrically normal individuals appears to activate left frontal regions, and areas of decreased metabolic activity or perfusion also have been noted in these regions in individuals with depression. The most consistently noted abnormality to date based on magnetic resonance imaging has been an increased number of focal signal hyperintensities in white matter; the functional significance of this abnormality is unclear, but it has been noted in both bipolar and unipolar mood disorders.

Abnormalities in Neurophysiological Function

Neurophysiological abnormalities also have been extensively studied in mood disorders. The largest and most consistent body of data involves the use of sleep EEG. (Sleep EEG, or polysomnography, is further discussed in Chapter 24.) Studies have consistently found that patients with depression have a variety of abnormal EEG findings during sleep, including decreased slow-wave sleep (i.e., deep sleep), a shortened time before the onset of rapid eye movement (REM) sleep (the period when dreams and nightmares occur), and longer periods of REM sleep than do subjects without depression. These three types of abnormality are referred to as decreased delta sleep, decreased REM latency, and increased REM density, respectively. All of these abnormalities in sleep EEG are consistent with the subjective complaints of insomnia expressed by depressed patients. Depressed patients typically state that they do not sleep very deeply or very long; their decreased delta sleep indicates that their sleep is indeed not as deep as normal sleep, and the abnormalities in REM sleep are consistent with their complaints of light, fitful sleep.

Abnormalities in Neuroendocrine Function

Neuroendocrine abnormalities also have been extensively explored in patients with depression. Early research in this area suggested that depressed patients had larger quantities of cortisol metabolites in their urine than did psychiatrically normal subjects, as well as higher blood levels of cortisol and abnormal diurnal variation in cortisol production. The dexamethasone suppression test (DST) has been used extensively to explore the possibility of neuroendocrine dysregulation in depression and to attempt to determine the place on the hypothalamic-pituitary-adrenal axis where this abnormality might occur.

Accumulated evidence suggests that 30%–70% of the patients with severe depression do not show normal suppression of cortisol secretion after the administration of dexamethasone. For a time, an abnormal DST result was thought to provide a potential tool in the differential diagnosis of depression, but it has become clear that the test is quite nonspecific. Rates of DST nonsuppression in other psychiatric conditions, such as anorexia nervosa, dementia, and substance abuse, are also relatively high. (The DST is further discussed in Chapter 4.)

In addition to the hypothalamic-pituitary-adrenal axis, other aspects of the neuroendocrine system have been explored. Depressed patients have been shown to have a blunting of growth hormone output in response to insulin challenge, as well as a blunted production of thyroid-stimulating hormone in response to thyrotropin-releasing hormone. The abnormalities across a variety of neuroendocrine target organs (e.g., adrenals, pancreas, thyroid) indicate that the problem is not in these organs, and the patterns of abnormal response to challenge suggest that it is also not in the pituitary. More likely, the abnormality is at the level of the hypothalamus, a brain region regulated largely through monoamine neurotransmitters.

Course and Outcome

Depressive Episode

A depressive episode may begin either suddenly or gradually. The duration of an untreated episode may range from a few weeks to months or even years, although it is suspected that most depressive episodes clear spontaneously within approximately 6 months. The prognosis for any single depressive episode is quite good, particularly in view of the efficacy of the available antidepressant medications. Unfortunately, a substantial number of patients will have a recurrence of depression at some time in their lives, and about 20% develop a chronic form of depression.

Suicide is the most serious complication of depression. Approximately 10%–15% of all patients hospitalized with depression will eventually take their own lives. Several factors suggest an increase in suicidal risk: being divorced or living alone, having a history of alcohol or drug abuse, being older than 40, having a history of a prior suicide attempt, and expressing suicidal ideation (particularly when detailed plans have been formulated). Suicidal risks always should be carefully evaluated in any patient with depression, beginning with a direct inquiry as to whether the patient has considered taking his or her life. A patient considered to be at risk for suicide usually should be treated as an inpatient rather than as an outpatient to minimize the risk. Suicide is discussed in more detail in Chapter 21.

Although suicide is the most important serious complication of depression, other social and personal complications may occur. Decreased energy, poor concentration, and lack of interest may cause poor performance at school or work. Apathy and decreased sexual interest may lead to marital discord. Patients may attempt to treat depressive symptoms themselves with sedatives, alcohol, or stimulants, thereby initiating problems with drug and alcohol abuse.

Manic Episode

The onset of mania is frequently abrupt, although it may begin gradually over the course of a few weeks. The episodes usually last from a few days to months. They tend to be briefer and to have a more abrupt termination than depressive episodes. Although the prognosis for any particular episode is reasonably good, especially with the availability of effective treatments such as lithium and antipsychotics, the risk for recurrence is significant. Not uncommonly, an episode of mania is followed by an episode of depression. Some patients with bipolar disorder recover relatively fully, but a substantial subset continue to have chronic mild instability of mood, particularly recurrent episodes of mild depression.

The complications of mania are primarily social: marital discord, divorce, business difficulties, financial extravagance, and sexual indiscretions. Drug or alcohol abuse may occur during a manic episode. When mania is relatively severe, the patient may be almost completely incapacitated and require protection from the consequences of poor judgment or hyperactivity. In the past, mania sometimes resulted in death from physical exhaustion. The excessive activity level continues to be a significant risk in patients with cardiac problems. A manic syndrome can switch rapidly to depression, and the risk for suicide is heightened when the patient becomes remorsefully aware of inappropriate behavior that occurred during the manic episode. Patients rarely commit suicide while manic.

Differential Diagnosis

When evaluating a patient with a mood disorder, the physician always should consider that the illness may result from some specific extrinsic factor that can induce a manic or depressive syndrome, such as drugs of abuse, sedatives, tranquilizers, antihypertensives, oral contraceptives, and glucocorticoids. General medical conditions such as hypothyroidism and systemic lupus erythematosus also may present with prominent depressive symptoms. If the episode of mood disorder is judged to be the result of a specific drug or medical illness, the disorder is diagnosed as secondary to it. Treatment usually involves withdrawing or reducing the drug or treating the underlying general medical illness.

A depressive episode in elderly persons may be difficult to distinguish from the various dementias because both may be characterized by apathy, difficulty concentrating, and complaints of poor memory. If the features suggesting a depressive episode are at least as prominent as those suggesting a dementia, then it is usually best to treat such patients for depressive symptoms because a successful treatment will result in the disappearance of symptoms, suggesting a possible dementia. Neuroimaging techniques such as single photon emission computed tomography and neuropsychological testing may assist in the differential diagnosis. (See Chapter 4 for more details on laboratory assessment and Chapter 6 for a discussion of pseudodementia.)

Dysphoric mood is a common symptom in schizophrenia. In schizophrenia, the dysphoric mood is more typically apathetic or empty, whereas in depression, the dysphoric mood usually is experienced as intensely painful. The onset of schizophrenia usually is more gradual, but patients with schizophrenia also typically have a more severe deterioration in function than do patients with depression. Patients with schizophrenia and patients with major depression may both have psychotic symptoms; thus, severe psychotic depression is often very difficult to distinguish from schizophrenia with acute onset. In this relatively difficult case, it is often best to treat the depression and to observe the course of illness over time. If psychotic symptoms tend to persist after mood symptoms remit, then the diagnosis of schizophrenia or schizoaffective disorder is more likely.

The differential diagnosis between mania and schizophrenia is also quite important. Several features are useful in making this distinction. Personality and general functioning are usually satisfactory before and after a manic episode, even though mild disturbances in mood may occur. Although manic episodes may present with disorganized speech that is indistinguishable from the speech sometimes observed in schizophrenia, speech abnormalities in mania are always accompanied by a disturbance in mood and usually by overactivity and physical agitation. Manic patients may experience delusions or hallucinations, but these typically reflect the underlying disturbance in mood. (Mood-incongruent psychotic symptoms occur occasionally, making the differential diagnosis more difficult.) It may be particularly difficult to distinguish an irritable and angry manic patient from an excited patient with paranoid schizophrenia, based on a simple cross-sectional evaluation. As in the case of a difficult differential diagnosis of depression, it is usually best to defer definitive diagnosis and to treat the mania because mania has a better prognosis. Additional guidelines that make the diagnosis of manic episode more likely include a family history of a mood disorder, good premorbid adjustment, and a previous episode of a mood disorder from which the patient completely or substantially recovered. However, when psychotic symptoms persist in the absence of an abnormality in mood, the diagnosis of schizophrenia or schizoaffective disorder is more likely.

People with bereavement may have many depressive symptoms and experience them for a sufficient duration to meet criteria for a depressive episode. Nevertheless, such patients are not given the diagnosis of depressive disorder because the presence of the symptoms is considered a normal reaction. The symptoms are usually self-limiting, clear spontaneously over time, have a different cause and prognosis than major depression, and usually do not respond to antidepressant medication. When bereavement is accompanied by psychomotor retardation, suicidal ideation, or psychotic symptoms, a diagnosis of major depression may be appropriate.

Clinical Management

Good psychopharmacological management is fundamental to the treatment of mood disorders. Both depression and mania usually respond remarkably well to the wide array of available medications. A more detailed discussion of antidepressant and antimanic medications, as well as ECT, appears in Chapter 27.

Treatment of Depression

Various medications are available to treat depression: tricyclics and other related compounds, MAOIs, SRIs, and newer antidepressants that do not fit neatly into the other categories, such as bupropion and venlafaxine. These drugs are all thought to work by altering levels of various neurotransmitters at crucial nerve terminals in the central nervous system. They are largely similar in their overall effectiveness, and from 65% to 70% of persons who receive antidepressants will markedly improve. The side effect profiles, basic pharmacokinetics, and dosages of antidepressants are compared in Chapter 27.

We generally recommend that treatment begin with one of the SRIs because they are well tolerated and safe in overdose. Low dosages are generally effective, and frequent dosage adjustments are unnecessary. In particular, patients with cardiac conduction defects should receive an SRI (or one of the other new agents), and impulsive or suicidal patients should receive an SRI or one of the newer agents that are unlikely to be fatal in overdose.

Certain presenting complaints will help the clinician select a particular antidepressant. Patients with insomnia or anorexia may do better with more sedating medications, perhaps largely because they will begin to sleep better almost immediately, whereas patients with lethargy and lower levels of tension and anxiety may prefer the less sedating medications such as fluoxetine or bupropion. Fluoxetine, in particular, has a specific tendency to produce insomnia and weight loss, making it a useful drug for those patients with depression characterized by hypersomnia and weight gain. For an especially severe and worsening depression, ECT may be the better choice.

Drug trials should last from 4 to 8 weeks. If the patient fails to respond within 4 weeks of treatment, the dose should be increased or the patient should be switched to another drug, preferably from another class (e.g., providing a different balance of norepinephrine, serotonin, and acetylcholine).

One useful strategy to boost the effectiveness of antidepressants is to augment, or coadminister, another drug. Augmentation with lithium carbonate is the best supported approach. Other agents have been used for augmentation, including liothyronine, a thyroid preparation; psychostimulants such as methylphenidate; benzodiazepines; and antipsychotics. When the depressed patient is psychotic, we generally recommend coadministering an antipsychotic, such as one of the newer atypical agents (e.g., risperidone, 1–6 mg/day, or olanzapine, 5–20 mg/day). Benzodiazepines coadministered with the antidepressant may help calm the anxious or agitated depressed patient relatively quickly (e.g., lorazepam 0.5–1 mg twice daily, clonazepam 0.25–0.50 mg twice daily).

For patients who are experiencing their first episode of depression, the drug should be continued for another 16–20 weeks after the patient is thought to be well. Thereafter, the clinician may choose to attempt to discontinue the medication while monitoring the patient closely. Because some antidepressants produce undesirable side effects such as weight gain, and because conservative prescription of medications is always a good clinical guideline, discontinuance should almost always be attempted in patients who do not have a history of recurrent depression. The medication should be discontinued gradually because many patients experience some mild withdrawal effects when tricyclics or SRIs (except fluoxetine) are discontinued abruptly. Patients sometimes subjectively experience these withdrawal symptoms as a recurrence or relapse. Other symptoms that occur on abrupt withdrawal of antidepressants include insomnia and nervousness, nightmares, and gastrointestinal symptoms such as nausea or vomiting.

Patients with recurrent depressions often will need long-term maintenance, typically at the full treatment dose. Lithium prophylaxis to prevent depressive relapse is an option that may be particularly useful for those pa-

Recommendations for management of depression

1. A hopeful, optimistic tone should be established at the initial interview.

   - The severity of the depressive syndrome should be assessed, remembering that there may be individual and cultural differences in the way depression is experienced and expressed.

   - Extensive psychological probing should not be attempted when the patient is deeply depressed.

   - Suicidal risk should be determined initially and reassessed frequently.

2. Severe to moderate depression should be treated aggressively with somatic therapy.

   - Severely depressed or suicidal patients may require hospitalization.

   - Severely depressed outpatients may need frequent (e.g., twice-weekly) brief (e.g., 10- to 15-minute) contacts for support and medication management until their depression lifts.

   - Most patients will require at least 16–20 weeks of maintenance medication following an initial episode and thereafter should be given a trial of decreasing or discontinuing the medication. If symptoms reemerge, medication should be reinstituted.

3. The clinician should determine whether psychosocial stressors are present that are contributing to the depressed mood and should counsel the patient on ways to cope with them.

4. Depressed patients tend to "get down" on themselves because they have been depressed; the clinician should help the patient learn to abandon negative or self-deprecating attitudes toward his or her depression through cognitive-behavioral therapy or other psychotherapeutic techniques.

tients who have had three or four previous episodes of depression. Maintenance lithium dosages may range from 600 to 1,200 mg/day, and blood levels usually are maintained in the 0.6–0.8 mEq/L range.

MAOIs may be used to treat those patients whose symptoms do not respond to the first-line antidepressants or who are unable to tolerate their side effects. MAOIs should be used with caution because they have potentially more dangerous side effects and interactions than do the other antidepressants. Nevertheless, for a subset of patients, MAOIs may be useful. These patients tend to be those characterized by atypical depression, with symptoms such as hypersomnia, increased appetite, and personality difficulties such as rejection sensitivity.

ECT is the treatment of choice for some patients with severe depression. Methods for administering and monitoring ECT, as well as its side effects, are described in more detail in Chapter 27. In general, indications for ECT include very severe depression, high potential for suicide, cardiovascular disease (which may preclude use of some antidepressants), and pregnancy. ECT is highly effective in producing a rapid remission of depressive symptoms. Response occurs relatively consistently in approximately 80% of patients. Patients will need maintenance antidepressant treatment after the course of ECT is completed.

Treatment of Mania

The medications used to treat mania are referred to as *mood stabilizers*. They include lithium, carbamazepine, and valproate. More recently, gabapentin and lamotrigine, both anticonvulsants, also have been used. Lithium and valproate are considered first-line treatments for mania. Patients receiving lithium are typically given a dose of 1,200–2,400 mg/day, with a goal of achieving serum blood levels between 0.9 and 1.4 mEq/L. Valproate is given in doses ranging from 1,250 to 2,500 mg/day, with the goal of achieving a blood level of 50–125 g/mL. When the patient is severely agitated and psychotic, antipsychotics (and/or benzodiazepines) should be coadministered with the mood stabilizers to provide adequate behavioral control. As the psychotic symptoms or agitation clear, the antipsychotic medications (and/or benzodiazepines) can be gradually discontinued. Manic patients will almost always require maintenance medication.

Patients whose symptoms do not respond to lithium or valproate may be given a variety of alternative treatments. Carbamazepine, gabapentin, and lamotrigine are the most effective second-line treatments, often in combination with antipsychotics. ECT is also highly effective for mania. The treatment of mania is more fully explored in Chapter 27.

Other Treatments

Experiencing an episode of mood disorder is often a major blow to the patient's confidence and self-esteem. Consequently, most patients will require some supportive psychotherapy in addition to whatever medications are prescribed. During the acute episode, the clinician will typically let the depressive wound begin to heal, but as the patient recovers, the clinician may begin to review with him or her the various social and psychological factors that may be causing distress or that may have worsened as a consequence of depression. Work, school performance, and interpersonal relationships all may be impaired because of a mood disorder. It is important to help patients assess these problems, recognize that their illness is responsible rather than

Recommendations for management of mania
1. Somatic therapies should be used aggressively to treat manic symptoms as rapidly as possible.
2. The patient should be followed up closely as the mania "breaks" to determine whether a subsequent depression is emerging; if this occurs, antidepressants should be used as needed.
3. After an episode of mania, patients should receive maintenance medication; typically they will continue to take mood stabilizers for several years, and perhaps for the remainder of their lives, to prevent subsequent relapses.
4. Even when they are stable, patients should be followed up regularly to ensure continued compliance with medication and to monitor blood levels (if applicable).
5. Manic episodes can have devastating personal, social, and economic consequences; patients will usually require (at a minimum) supportive psychotherapy to help them cope with these consequences and maintain their self-esteem.
6. Family members should be provided with both psychological support, as needed, and educational materials to help them understand the disorder, its symptoms, and its need for continued treatment.
7. Patients with bipolar illness are often appreciative of being told about the "good side" of their illness: its association with creativity and high achievement.

feeling that they themselves are responsible, and instill confidence that they can now begin to restore and repair whatever injuries have occurred as a consequence of their episode of mood disorder.

Some patients will respond well to this type of brief supportive psychotherapy used as an adjunct to medications. Others may require more intensive psychotherapy depending on their personality structure, social situation, disability induced by the mood disorder, and environmental supports. These psychotherapies may include psychodynamic psychotherapy, cognitive-behavioral therapy, or behavior therapy. These various psychotherapies are described in more detail in Chapter 26.

Some patients may respond to psychotherapy alone. In particular, a patient with a brief, situation-based depression may respond well to crisis intervention. A person presenting with depressive symptoms who is attempting to cope with a stressful life event, such as separation or divorce, may have a relatively painful and persistent mood disorder for weeks to months yet not require the use of medications. These patients also may benefit substantially from supportive and psychodynamic therapy. Patients with chronic mild depression (e.g., dysthymia) also may be more likely to benefit from a treatment regimen that emphasizes psychotherapy as its primary tool. In particular, these patients are likely to benefit from cognitive-behavioral therapy, interpersonal therapy, behavior therapy, or long-term psychodynamic therapy.

Bibliography

Allen MG, Cohen S, Pollin W, et al: Affective illness in veteran twins: a diagnostic review. Am J Psychiatry 131:1234–1239, 1974

American Psychiatric Association: Diagnostic and Statistical Manual of Mental Disorders, 3rd Edition. Washington, DC, American Psychiatric Association, 1980

American Psychiatric Association: Diagnostic and Statistical Manual of Mental Disorders, 4th Edition. Washington, DC, American Psychiatric Association, 1994

American Psychiatric Association: Diagnostic and Statistical Manual of Mental Disorders, 4th Edition Text Revision. Washington, DC, American Psychiatric Association, 2000

Andreasen NC: Creativity and mental illness: prevalence rate in writers and their first-degree relatives. Am J Psychiatry 144:1288–1292, 1987

Andreasen NC, Rice J, Endicott J, et al: Familial rates of affective disorder: a report from the National Institute of Mental Health Collaborative Study. Arch Gen Psychiatry 44:461–469, 1987

Angst J, Frey R, Lohmeyer B, et al: Bipolar manic-depressive psychoses: results of a genetic investigation. Hum Genet 55:237–254, 1980

Baron M, Risch N, Hamburger R, et al: Genetic linkage between X-chromosome markers and bipolar affective illness. Nature 326:289–292, 1987

Baxter LR, Schwartz JM, Phelps ME, et al: Reduction of prefrontal cortex glucose metabolism common to three types of depression. Arch Gen Psychiatry 46:243–250, 1989

Bertelsen A: A Danish twin study of manic-depressive disorders, in Origin, Prevention and Treatment of Affective Disorders. Edited by Schou M, Stromgren E. London, Academic Press, 1979, pp 227–239

Black DW, Nasrallah A: Hallucinations and delusions in 1,715 patients with unipolar and bipolar affective disorders. Psychopathology 22:28–34, 1989

Cameron OC (ed): Adrenergic Dysfunction and Psychobiology. Washington, DC, American Psychiatric Press, 1994

Coppen AJ, Doogan DP: Serotonin and its place in the pathogenesis of depression. J Clin Psychiatry 49 (suppl 8):4–11, 1988

Davis JM, Koslow SH, Gibbons RD, et al: Cerebrospinal fluid and urinary biogenic amines in depressed patients and healthy controls. Arch Gen Psychiatry 45:705–717, 1988

Drevets WC, Videen TO, Price JL, et al: A functional anatomical study of unipolar depression. J Neurosci 12:3628–3641, 1992

Faraone SV, Tsuang MT, Tsuang DW: Genetics of Mental Disorders. New York, Guilford, 1999

Gershon ES, Cloninger CR: Genetic Approaches to Mental Disorders. Washington, DC, American Psychiatric Press, 1994

Gershon ES, Bunney WE, Leckman JF, et al: The inheritance of affective disorders: a review of data and hypotheses. Behav Genet 6:227–261, 1976

Gillin JC, Byerley WA: Sleep: a neurobiological window on affective disorders. Trends Neurosci 8:537–542, 1985

Gold PW, Goodwin FK, Chrousos GP: Clinical and biochemical manifestation of depression: relation to the neurobiology of stress (parts 1 and 2). N Engl J Med 319:348–353, 1988

Goodnick PJ (ed): Mania: Clinical and Research Perspectives. Washington, DC, American Psychiatric Press, 1998

Goodwin FK, Jamison KR: Manic-Depressive Illness. New York, Oxford University Press, 1990

Harvald B, Hauge M: Genetics and the epidemiology of chronic diseases (PHS Publ No 1163). Edited by Neal JV, Shaw W, Shull WJ. Washington, DC, Department of Health, Education and Welfare, 1965, pp 61–76

Kallmann FJ: Genetic principles in manic-depressive psychosis, in Depression: Proceedings of the American Psychopathologic Association. Edited by Zubin J, Hock P. New York, Grune & Stratton, 1954, pp 1–24

Kelsoe JR, Ginns EI, Egeland JA, et al: Re-evaluation of the linkage relationship between chromosome 11p loci and the gene for bipolar affective disorder in the Old Order Amish. Nature 342:238–243, 1989

Klein DN, Schwartz JE, Rose S, et al: Five-year course and outcome of dysthymic disorder: a prospective naturalistic follow-up study. Am J Psychiatry 157:931–939, 2000

Klerman GL, Lavori PW, Rice J, et al: Birth cohort trends in rates of major depressive disorder among relatives of patients with affective disorder. Arch Gen Psychiatry 42:689–693, 1985

Kraepelin E: Manic-Depressive Insanity and Paranoia. Edinburgh, Scotland, E & S Livingstone, 1921

Luxenberger H: Psychiatrisch-neurologische Zwillings-pathologie. Zentralblatt fur Diagesamte Neurologie und Psychiatrie 14:56–57, 145–180, 1930

Meltzer HY: Lithium mechanisms in bipolar illness and altered intracellular calcium functions. Biol Psychiatry 21:492–510, 1986

Murray CJL, Lopez AD: The Global Burden of Disease. Boston, MA, Harvard University Press, 1996

Nemeroff CB: The role of corticotropin-releasing factor in the pathogenesis of major depression. Pharmacopsychiatry 21:76–82, 1988

Paradiso S, Robinson RG, Andreasen NC, et al: Emotional activation of limbic circuitry in elderly normal subjects in a PET study. Am J Psychiatry 154:384–389, 1997

Paradiso S, Johnson DL, Andreasen NC, et al: Cerebral blood flow changes associated with attribution of emotional valence to pleasant, unpleasant, and neutral visual stimuli in a PET study of normal subjects. Am J Psychiatry 156:1618–1629, 1999

Paykel ES (ed): Handbook of Affective Disorders, 2nd Edition. New York, Guilford, 1992

Preisig M, Belliver F, Fenton BT, et al: Association between bipolar disorder and monoamine oxidase A gene polymorphisms: results of a multicenter study. Am J Psychiatry 157:948–955, 2000

Rice J, Reich T, Andreasen NC, et al: The familial transmission of bipolar illness. Arch Gen Psychiatry 44:441–444, 1987

Robinson RG, Szetela B: Mood change following left hemisphere brain injury. Ann Neurol 9:447–453, 1981

Rosanoff AJ, Handy L, Plesset IR: The etiology of manic-depressive symptoms with special reference to their occurrence in twins. Am J Psychiatry 91:725–762, 1935

Slater E: Psychotic and neurotic illness in twins (Medical Research Council Special Report Series No 278). London, Her Majesty's Stationery Office, 1953

Starkstein SE, Robinson RG (eds): Depression in Neurological Disease. Baltimore, MD, Johns Hopkins University Press, 1993

Swayze VW, Andreasen NC, Alliger RJ, et al: Structural brain abnormalities in bipolar affective disorder: ventricular enlargement and focal signal hyperintensities. Arch Gen Psychiatry 47:1054–1059, 1990

Watson SJ (ed): Biology of Schizophrenia and Affective Disease. Washington, DC, American Psychiatric Press, 1996

Weissman MM, Kidd KK, Prusoff BA: Variability in rates of affective disorders in relatives of depressed and normal probands. Arch Gen Psychiatry 39:1397–1403, 1982

Weissman MM, Leaf PJ, Bruce ML, et al: The epidemiology of dysthymia in five communities: rates, risks, comorbidity, and treatment. Am J Psychiatry 145:815–819, 1988

Winokur G, Tsuang MT: The Natural History of Mania, Depression, and Schizophrenia. Washington, DC, American Psychiatric Press, 1996

Self-Assessment Questions

1. What are the nine symptoms used to define a major depressive episode in DSM-IV?
2. What is the difference between delusions that are mood congruent and those that are mood incongruent?
3. What are some symptoms that typically predict a good response to antidepressants?
4. What is the lifetime prevalence for bipolar disorder and for (unipolar) major depressive disorder?
5. Why have variable rates been reported for depression?
6. What is the cohort effect?
7. Review the evidence that suggests that mood disorders are familial and may be genetic.
8. Which neurotransmitter systems have been proposed to be dysfunctional in mood disorders?
9. Which brain region has been found to be abnormal in both lesion and positron-emission tomography studies?
10. What is the evidence indicating that neuroendocrine abnormalities occur in patients with mood disorders?
11. What is the difference between bereavement and a depressive episode?
12. Describe the first-line treatments for depression, as well as the various alternative treatments and their indications.
13. Describe the appropriate program of treatment for a manic episode. What alternative treatments are available?

 **Anxiety Disorders**

I stood stunned, my hair rose, the voice stuck in my throat.

Virgil

Unlike depression, a syndrome recognized for centuries, the syndrome of anxiety has been recognized only in relatively recent times. DaCosta was first credited with describing anxiety as a disorder that he called *irritable heart* in the *American Journal of Medical Sciences* in 1871. Because chest pain, palpitations, and dizziness were the main symptoms of this syndrome, DaCosta thought the disorder resulted from a functional cardiac disturbance caused by an overreactive nervous system. Physicians frequently diagnosed this syndrome in patients undergoing significant stress, such as that encountered in warfare. In fact, DaCosta first described this syndrome in a soldier who developed the disorder during the Civil War. Shortly thereafter, the condition was identified in many other settings and was variously referred to as *soldier's heart,* the *effort syndrome,* or *neurocirculatory asthenia.*

While internists were emphasizing cardiovascular aspects of the anxiety syndrome, psychiatrists and neurologists became more concerned with its psychological aspects. Freud was responsible for recognizing anxiety as the core symptom of the syndrome and for introducing the term *anxiety neurosis.*

Freud's conceptualization of the syndrome brought the patient's inner subjective feelings to the forefront, emphasizing the sense of fearfulness, terror, panic, and impending doom.

The relation between the physical and the psychological symptoms of anxiety has remained a matter of debate. Early in the twentieth century, psychologist William James postulated that the psychological experience of anxiety is nothing more than an awareness of the physical symptoms of anxiety, thus implying that the physical experience is primary. Conversely, Freud believed that the psychological symptoms of anxiety were primary and led to the development of physical symptoms. Whichever is primary, the relation is probably interactive and the symptoms mutually reinforcing.

Nervousness and fear are common human emotions that nearly everyone has experienced at one time or another. For that reason, defining the diagnostic boundaries of the anxiety disorders is not always clear-cut. Physicians must recognize the difference between pathological anxiety and anxiety as a normal or adaptive response. Feeling anxious when being stalked by a grizzly bear is both normal and natural and prepares the individual for the classic flight-or-fight response. Feeling anxious before taking an examination or giving a talk is also normal and adaptive, as long as the alertness or tension is not excessive or inappropriate. Even classic phobias, such as fear of heights, may reflect some primitive adaptive response. The potentially adaptive mechanism of anxiety or arousal, so useful in helping human beings to cope with the stresses and threats of life, becomes a disorder only when the anxiety becomes crippling or disabling.

Until 1980, panic disorder and generalized anxiety were classified together as anxiety neurosis. In DSM-III, anxiety neurosis was divided because it had been learned that panic disorder and generalized anxiety disorder (GAD) were each associated with a different natural history, familial aggregation, and response to treatment. At the same time, a new diagnosis, posttraumatic stress disorder (PTSD), was introduced. Acute stress disorder was added in 1994. In this chapter, we review panic disorder, agoraphobia, specific and social phobias, generalized anxiety, and both PTSD and acute stress disorder. A residual category, anxiety disorder not otherwise specified, is used to diagnose conditions that do not meet criteria for a specific disorder, such as mixed symptoms of anxiety and depression. Anxiety disorders thought to result from the effects of a substance or a general medical condition are discussed in Chapter 6. Obsessive-compulsive disorder (OCD), discussed in Chapter 11, is classified as an anxiety disorder, but there is uncertainty about its true relation to the other anxiety disorders. The anxiety disorders are listed in Table 10–1.

TABLE 10–1. Anxiety disorders

Panic disorder

  With agoraphobia

  Without agoraphobia

Agoraphobia

Social phobia (social anxiety disorder)

Specific phobia

Obsessive-compulsive disorder (see Chapter 11)

Generalized anxiety disorder

Posttraumatic stress disorder

Acute stress disorder

Anxiety disorder due to a general medical condition (see Chapter 6)

Substance-induced anxiety disorder (see Chapter 6)

Anxiety disorder not otherwise specified

Panic Disorder and Agoraphobia

Panic disorder consists of recurrent, unexpected panic (or anxiety) attacks accompanied by at least 1 month or more of persistent concern about having another attack, worry about the implications of having an attack, or significant behavioral change related to the attacks. The requirement for unexpected attacks helps to distinguish panic disorder from normal anxiety. Being robbed at gunpoint, for example, might cause anxiety in most everyone. As a practical matter, patients with unexpected attacks generally have situational attacks as well. At least 4 of 13 characteristic symptoms, such as shortness of breath, dizziness, palpitations, and trembling or shaking, must occur during the attacks (see Table 10–2). Lastly, the clinician should determine that the attacks are not induced by a substance (e.g., caffeine) or a medical illness (e.g., hyperthyroidism) and that the anxiety is not better accounted for by another mental disorder, such as social phobia. Panic disorder is further classified as occurring with or without agoraphobia, a condition explained below. The DSM-IV-TR criteria for panic disorder without agoraphobia are shown in Table 10–3.

  Agoraphobia is a disabling complication of panic disorder (see Table 10–4). Although originally conceptualized as separate disorders, research suggests that panic disorder and agoraphobia actually represent a single ill-

318   Introductory Textbook of Psychiatry

TABLE 10–2. DSM-IV-TR criteria for a panic attack

Note: A Panic Attack is not a codable disorder. Code the specific diagnosis in which the Panic Attack occurs (e.g., 300.21 Panic Disorder With Agoraphobia).

A discrete period of intense fear or discomfort, in which four (or more) of the following symptoms developed abruptly and reached a peak within 10 minutes:

    (1) palpitations, pounding heart, or accelerated heart rate
    (2) sweating
    (3) trembling or shaking
    (4) sensations of shortness of breath or smothering
    (5) feeling of choking
    (6) chest pain or discomfort
    (7) nausea or abdominal distress
    (8) feeling dizzy, unsteady, lightheaded, or faint
    (9) derealization (feelings of unreality) or depersonalization (being detached from oneself)
    (10) fear of losing control or going crazy
    (11) fear of dying
    (12) paresthesias (numbness or tingling sensations)
    (13) chills or hot flushes

ness. In fact, agoraphobia in the absence of panic is unusual. The term *agoraphobia* translates literally from Greek as "fear of the marketplace." Although many patients with agoraphobia are uncomfortable in shops and markets, their true fear is to be separated from their source of security. Agoraphobic patients often fear having a panic attack in a public place and embarrassing themselves or having a panic attack and not being near their physician or medical clinic. They tend to avoid crowded places, such as shops, restaurants, theaters, and church, because they feel trapped. Many have difficulty driving long distances (i.e., because they fear being away from help should a panic attack occur), crossing bridges, and driving through tunnels. Many agoraphobic patients insist on being accompanied to places they might otherwise avoid. At its most severe, agoraphobia leads many patients to become housebound. Common situations that either provoke or relieve anxiety in people with agoraphobia are shown in Table 10–5.

The following case example illustrates how these common disorders affected one of our patients:

Susan, a 32-year-old housewife, came to the outpatient clinic for evaluation of anxiety. She reported the onset of panic attacks at age 13, which she remembered as terrifying. She vividly recalled her first attack, which oc-

---

TABLE 10–3. DSM-IV-TR diagnostic criteria for panic disorder without agoraphobia

---

A. Both (1) and (2):

    (1) recurrent unexpected Panic Attacks

    (2) at least one of the attacks has been followed by 1 month (or more) of one (or more) of the following:

        (a) persistent concern about having additional attacks

        (b) worry about the implications of the attack or its consequences (e.g., losing control, having a heart attack, "going crazy")

        (c) a significant change in behavior related to the attacks

B. Absence of Agoraphobia.

C. The Panic Attacks are not due to the direct physiological effects of a substance (e.g., a drug of abuse, a medication) or a general medical condition (e.g., hyperthyroidism).

D. The Panic Attacks are not better accounted for by another mental disorder, such as Social Phobia (e.g., occurring on exposure to feared social situations), Specific Phobia (e.g., on exposure to a specific phobic situation), Obsessive-Compulsive Disorder (e.g., on exposure to dirt in someone with an obsession about contamination), Posttraumatic Stress Disorder (e.g., in response to stimuli associated with a severe stressor), or Separation Anxiety Disorder (e.g., in response to being away from home or close relatives).

---

curred during a history class. "I was just sitting in class when my heart began to beat wildly, my skin began to tingle, and I began feeling shaky. There was no need for me to feel nervous," she observed. Over the following 19 years, attacks became chronic and unrelenting, occurring up to 10 times daily. To Susan, the panic was devastating: "I grew up all those years feeling that I wasn't quite normal." The panic attacks made her feel different from others and kept her from developing a normal social life.

Along with her fear of panic attacks, Susan began to avoid crowded places, particularly shopping centers, grocery stores, movie theaters, and restaurants. She was a religious person and attended church, but she would sit in a pew near an exit. Her phobic avoidance tended to wax and wane, and although she had never been housebound, she would insist on having her husband or a friend accompany her when she went shopping.

Susan had never sought treatment before and thought that no one could help her. At times, she had gone to emergency rooms for evaluation, but she had never received a diagnosis of panic disorder. Because Susan believed that to admit her symptoms was a sign of weakness, she had never told her husband of 15 years about her panic.

Susan was given fluvoxamine and within 1 month was free of panic attacks; within 3 months, she was no longer avoiding crowded places. At a 6-month follow-up, she remained free of all anxiety-related symptoms. Susan reported feeling like a new person and felt much better about herself.

TABLE 10–4.   DSM-IV-TR criteria for agoraphobia

Note: Agoraphobia is not a codable disorder. Code the specific disorder in which
the Agoraphobia occurs (e.g., 300.21 Panic Disorder With Agoraphobia or 300.22
Agoraphobia Without History of Panic Disorder).

A. Anxiety about being in places or situations from which escape might be difficult
(or embarrassing) or in which help may not be available in the event of having
an unexpected or situationally predisposed Panic Attack or panic-like symptoms.
Agoraphobic fears typically involve characteristic clusters of situations that include being outside the home alone; being in a crowd or standing in a line; being
on a bridge; and traveling in a bus, train, or automobile.

Note: Consider the diagnosis of Specific Phobia if the avoidance is limited to
one or only a few specific situations, or Social Phobia if the avoidance is limited
to social situations.

B. The situations are avoided (e.g., travel is restricted) or else are endured with
marked distress or with anxiety about having a Panic Attack or panic-like symptoms, or require the presence of a companion.

C. The anxiety or phobic avoidance is not better accounted for by another mental
disorder, such as Social Phobia (e.g., avoidance limited to social situations because
of fear of embarrassment), Specific Phobia (e.g., avoidance limited to a single
situation like elevators), Obsessive-Compulsive Disorder (e.g., avoidance of dirt
in someone with an obsession about contamination), Posttraumatic Stress Disorder (e.g., avoidance of stimuli associated with a severe stressor), or Separation
Anxiety Disorder (e.g., avoidance of leaving home or relatives).

TABLE 10–5.   Common situations that either provoked or relieved
anxiety in 100 agoraphobic patients

Situations that provoke anxiety	%	Situations that relieve anxiety	%
Standing in line at a store	96	Being accompanied by spouse	85
Having an appointment	91	Sitting near the door in church	76
Feeling trapped at hairdresser, etc.	89	Focusing thoughts on something else	63
Increasing distance from home	87	Taking the dog, baby carriage, etc., along	62
Being at particular places in neigh-borhood	66	Being accompanied by friend	60
Having cloudy, depressing weather	56	Reassuring self	52
		Wearing sunglasses	36

Source.   Adapted from Burns and Thorpe 1977.

Nine years later, Susan continued to be well, although she was now taking fluoxetine (20 mg/day). In the interim, she had divorced her husband, who, she felt, was unable to cope with a more confident and independent spouse. She eventually remarried, enrolled at a community college, and moved away from her small town.

Epidemiology and Clinical Findings

According to the Epidemiologic Catchment Area study, 2%–3% of women and 0.5%–1.5% of men have panic disorder. The prevalence of agoraphobia is slightly higher. Panic disorder and agoraphobia each typically have an onset in the mid-20s, although age at onset may vary; nearly 8 in 10 panic patients develop the disorder before age 30 years. Women are more likely than men to develop agoraphobia.

There are usually no precipitating stressors before the onset of either panic disorder or agoraphobia. Many patients, however, will report that panic attacks began after an illness, an accident, or the breakup of a relationship; developed postpartum; or occurred after taking mind-altering drugs such as lysergic diethylamide (LSD) or marijuana. The initial panic attack is generally alarming to people and may prompt a visit to an emergency room, where routine laboratory tests and electrocardiograms generally have normal results. The symptoms are often attributed to "nerves" or stress. Many patients undergo extensive, often unnecessary medical workups. Psychiatrists are typically consulted when no obvious physical cause for the anxiety is found. The psychiatrist's consultation is preceded by six or seven evaluations that focus on the target symptoms the patient reports (see Table 10–6).

Panic attacks generally have a sudden onset, peak within minutes, and last 5–30 minutes. Although many patients claim that their attacks last hours to days, it is likely that their continuing symptoms represent either a recurrence of panic or mild symptoms that persist after an attack. Symptoms reported by patients with panic disorder and agoraphobia are presented in Table 10–7.

Etiology and Pathophysiology

The biology of panic disorder is being intensively studied. Among the biological disturbances possibly underlying panic are increased catecholamine levels in the central nervous system, an abnormality in the locus coeruleus (an area of the brain stem regulating alertness), carbon dioxide (CO_2) hypersensitivity, a disturbance in lactate metabolism, and abnormalities of the γ-aminobutyric acid (GABA) neurotransmitter system. Some data support each of these possibilities, although none explains all of the symptoms of

TABLE 10–6. Specialists consulted depending on target symptoms of panic disorder

Specialist	Target symptoms
Pulmonologist	Shortness of breath, hyperventilation, smothering sensations
Dermatologist	Sweating, cold, clammy hands
Cardiologist	Palpitations, chest pain or discomfort
Neurologist	Tingling and numbness, imbalance, dizziness, derealization or depersonalization, tremulousness or jitteriness, light-headedness
Otolaryngologist	Choking sensation, dry mouth
Gynecologist	Hot flashes, sweating
Gastroenterologist	Nausea, diarrhea, abdominal pain or discomfort (i.e., "butterflies")
Urologist	Frequent urination

TABLE 10–7. Common symptoms reported by patients with panic disorder and agoraphobia

Symptoms	%	Symptoms	%
Fearfulness or worry	96	Restlessness	80
Nervousness	95	Trouble breathing	80
Palpitations	93	Easy fatigability	76
Muscle aching or tension	89	Trouble concentrating	76
Trembling or shaking	89	Irritability	74
Apprehension	83	Trouble sleeping	74
Dizziness or imbalance	82	Chest pain or discomfort	69
Fear of dying or going crazy	81	Numbness or tingling	65
Faintness/light-headedness	80	Tendency to startle	57
Hot or cold sensations	80	Choking or smothering sensations	54

Source. Adapted from Noyes et al. 1987b.

panic disorder. Many of the competing theories are based on the ability of different substances to induce panic attacks, such as isoproterenol (a β antagonist), yohimbine (an α_2 receptor blocker), CO_2, and sodium lactate. For example, the observation that exposure to 5% CO_2 induces panic attacks has led to the "false suffocation alarm" theory. The theory posits that patients with panic disorder are hypersensitive to CO_2 because they have an overly sensitive brain stem suffocation alarm system that produces respiratory distress, hyperventilation, and anxiety.

Family and twin studies strongly suggest that panic disorder is hereditary. When the results of family studies are pooled, the morbidity risk for panic disorder is nearly 20% among the relatives of patients with panic disorder compared with only 2% among the relatives of control subjects. Twin studies have shown a higher concordance rate for anxiety disorder among identical twins than among nonidentical twins, about 45% compared with 15%, a finding that indicates that genetic influences predominate over environmental influences. There have been no adoption studies specifically of panic disorder.

Psychoanalysts postulate that repression, a common defense mechanism, may somehow be involved with the development of panic. Freud believed that repression was the mental mechanism that holds all unacceptable sexual thoughts, impulses, or desires out of conscious reach. When the psychic energy attached to these unacceptable elements becomes too strong to be held back by repression, they are brought into consciousness in a distorted way, which causes anxiety and panic.

Meanwhile, learning theorists argue that anxiety attacks are a conditioned response to a fearful situation; a car accident might be paired with the experience of heart palpitations and anxiety. Long after the accident, palpitations alone, whether from vigorous exercise or emotional upset, become capable in themselves of provoking the *conditioned response* of a panic attack.

Course and Outcome

Panic disorder and agoraphobia generally are considered chronic and lifelong. Each tends to fluctuate in intensity and severity, and the course of these disorders usually runs in parallel. Although total remission is uncommon, research suggests that from 50% to 70% of patients with panic disorder will show some amount of improvement over time. Panic disorder patients are at increased risk for peptic ulcer disease and hypertension and have higher death rates than expected. Suicide rates are high even among panic patients who are not depressed.

The most common complications of panic disorder are depression and alcohol abuse. Major depression occurs in up to 50% of the patients with panic disorder or agoraphobia and may be severe, although it is often mild and reactive to situational circumstances. Alcohol abuse complicates these disorders in about 20% of the cases and may start in an attempt at self-medication. This complication is important to keep in mind when evaluating patients with substance abuse because their disorder may have begun with spontaneous panic attacks or chronic anxiety.

Differential Diagnosis

The clinician should rule out other medical and psychiatric disorders as a cause of anxiety when evaluating patients with panic disorder or agoraphobia (see Table 10–8). Medical illness is particularly important to rule out because the physical manifestations of panic are frequently suggestive of many different disorders, including hyperthyroidism, hyperparathyroidism, pheochromocytoma, diseases of the vestibular nerve, hypoglycemia, and supraventricular tachycardia. Until recently, many physicians have tended to overdiagnose mitral valve prolapse in patients with panic disorder. Mitral valve prolapse usually is a benign condition that occurs more frequently in panic disorder patients than in others, leading clinicians to regard panic symptoms as a manifestation of mitral valve prolapse. Research has shown, however, that panic patients with or without mitral valve prolapse have a similar course of illness and treatment response. The presence of mitral valve prolapse does not preclude a diagnosis of panic disorder.

Other psychiatric disorders also must be ruled out. Patients with major depression often have panic attacks and anxiety, which resolve when the depression is treated. Panic attacks also may occur in patients with GAD, schizophrenia, depersonalization disorder, somatization disorder, and borderline personality disorder. When anxiety symptoms occur in response to a recognizable stressor, the diagnosis of adjustment disorder with anxiety is often appropriate (see Chapter 19).

Clinical Management

Panic disorder generally is treated with a combination of medication and individual psychotherapy. Tricyclic antidepressants (TCAs), monoamine oxidase inhibitors (MAOIs), and serotonin reuptake inhibitors (SRIs) are effective in the treatment of panic and agoraphobia and will block panic attacks in up to 80% of patients. Because SRIs are safer and better tolerated than TCAs and MAOIs, they have become the drugs of choice. TCAs and

TABLE 10–8. Differential diagnosis of anxiety

Medical illness	Drugs
Angina	Caffeine
Cardiac arrhythmias	Aminophylline and related
Congestive heart failure	compounds
Hypoglycemia	Sympathomimetic agents (e.g., decongestants and diet pills)
Hypoxia	
Pulmonary embolism	Monosodium glutamate
Severe pain	Psychostimulants and hallucinogens
Thyrotoxicosis	Alcohol withdrawal
Carcinoid	Withdrawal from benzodiazepines and
Pheochromocytoma	other sedative-hypnotics
Menière's disease	Thyroid hormones
	Antipsychotic medication
Psychiatric illness	
Schizophrenia	
Mood disorders	
Personality disorders	
Adjustment disorder with anxious mood	

MAOIs are generally reserved for patients whose symptoms do not respond to the SRIs. Benzodiazepines also are effective in blocking panic attacks when prescribed in high doses, but they are potentially habit forming. β-Adrenergic-blocking drugs, such as propranolol, often are prescribed to patients with anxiety disorders but are much less effective than antidepressants or benzodiazepines. Drug treatment of panic disorder is discussed in more detail in Chapter 27.

In general, patients who respond well to treatment tend to have milder anxiety symptoms, an older age at onset, fewer panic attacks, and a relatively normal personality. The presence of a depressed mood is not a requirement for antidepressant medications to be effective in blocking panic attacks.

The antidepressant dosage depends on the specific medication but is usually similar to the dosage used to treat depression (e.g., fluoxetine, 20 mg/day; sertraline, 50 mg/day; or paroxetine, 20 mg/day). Once panic attacks have remitted, the patient should continue taking medication for 6 months to 1 year to prevent relapse. After this period, it is advisable to gradually taper and discontinue the medication. Although panic disorder tends to recur, up to two-thirds of patients will not relapse immediately after cessation of medication. When a patient relapses and panic attacks recur, the drug can be reintroduced. Some patients will need to take medication chronically.

Patients should avoid caffeine because it tends to induce anxiety. Patients often fail to realize how much caffeine they are ingesting with coffee (50–150 mg), tea (20–50 mg), cola drinks (30–60 mg), and even milk chocolate (1–15 mg).

Cognitive-behavioral therapy (CBT), a form of individual psychotherapy, also appears to be effective in the treatment of panic disorder; its combination with medication may be even more powerful. CBT usually involves distraction and breathing exercises, along with education to help the patient make more appropriate attributions for distressing somatic symptoms. For example, patients learn that panic-induced chest pain will not cause a heart attack. An effective therapist will help to boost the generally low morale and self-esteem of panic disorder patients. Therapists also can help patients to solve everyday problems and recommend books and other reading materials about panic disorder and agoraphobia.

Patients with agoraphobia, with or without panic attacks, should receive behavior therapy. Exposure in vivo is the most effective intervention and in its most basic form may consist of gentle encouragement for patients to enter feared situations, such as shopping in a grocery store. Some patients may require direct supervision by the therapist to expose themselves to different situations.

Generalized Anxiety Disorder

GAD is characterized by excessive anxiety and worry that is difficult to control, without the specific symptoms that characterize either phobic disorders, panic disorder, or OCD (i.e., phobias, panic attacks, obsessions, and compulsions). Patients with GAD worry excessively about life circumstances, including their health, finances, social acceptance, job performance, and marital adjustment. This worry is central to the diagnosis of GAD.

The diagnostic criteria require that GAD not be diagnosed when the symptoms occur exclusively during the course of another illness such as major depression or schizophrenia or when the generalized anxiety occurs in the context of panic disorder, social phobia, or OCD (Table 10–9). The anxiety or worry in GAD should not relate solely to anxiety about having a panic attack, being embarrassed in public, being contaminated, or gaining weight (as in anorexia nervosa). The criteria also require that the individual have at least three of six symptoms, which include feeling restless or keyed up, having poor concentration, being irritable, having muscle tension, or experiencing poor sleep. The symptoms must cause significant distress or impairment in social, occupational, or other important areas of functioning. Finally, the

TABLE 10–9. DSM-IV-TR diagnostic criteria for generalized anxiety disorder

A. Excessive anxiety and worry (apprehensive expectation), occurring more days than not for at least 6 months, about a number of events or activities (such as work or school performance).

B. The person finds it difficult to control the worry.

C. The anxiety and worry are associated with three (or more) of the following six symptoms (with at least some symptoms present for more days than not for the past 6 months).   **Note:** Only one item is required in children.

   (1) restlessness or feeling keyed up or on edge

   (2) being easily fatigued

   (3) difficulty concentrating or mind going blank

   (4) irritability

   (5) muscle tension

   (6) sleep disturbance (difficulty falling or staying asleep, or restless unsatisfying sleep)

D. The focus of the anxiety and worry is not confined to features of an Axis I disorder, e.g., the anxiety or worry is not about having a Panic Attack (as in Panic Disorder), being embarrassed in public (as in Social Phobia), being contaminated (as in Obsessive-Compulsive Disorder), being away from home or close relatives (as in Separation Anxiety Disorder), gaining weight (as in Anorexia Nervosa), having multiple physical complaints (as in Somatization Disorder), or having a serious illness (as in Hypochondriasis), and the anxiety and worry do not occur exclusively during Posttraumatic Stress Disorder.

E. The anxiety, worry, or physical symptoms cause clinically significant distress or impairment in social, occupational, or other important areas of functioning.

F. The disturbance is not due to the direct physiological effects of a substance (e.g., a drug of abuse, a medication) or a general medical condition (e.g., hyperthyroidism) and does not occur exclusively during a Mood Disorder, a Psychotic Disorder, or a Pervasive Developmental Disorder.

effects of a substance or a general medical condition should be ruled out as a cause of the symptoms. The condition must persist for 6 months or longer.

Epidemiology, Course, and Outcome

Community surveys indicate that GAD is relatively common and has a lifetime prevalence between 4% and 7% in the general population. Rates are higher in women, African Americans, and persons younger than 30 years. The disorder has an onset in the early 20s; persons at any age may develop the disorder. Few persons with GAD seek psychiatric treatment, although many seek evaluations from medical specialists for specific symptoms, such as palpitations or shortness of breath. The disorder appears to have a chronic course, with symptoms that fluctuate in severity over time. About one-quarter of the patients with GAD develop panic disorder.

The most frequent complications of GAD are major depression and substance abuse. Many patients experience one or more episodes of major depression over the course of the illness, and many meet criteria for social phobia or a specific phobia. Some patients use alcohol or drugs to control their symptoms, which can lead to substance abuse.

Etiology

The cause of GAD is unknown, although one family study showed that nearly 25% of the first-degree relatives of GAD patients are affected with GAD themselves, female relatives more often than male relatives; male relatives were at higher risk for alcoholism. The same study showed that life events also were important to the development of GAD. In a large twin study, genetic factors were found to play a role in the etiology of GAD, but nongenetic factors were thought to be even more important. Several different neurotransmitter systems have been implicated in the disorder, including the noradrenergic, GABA, and serotonergic systems in the frontal lobe and limbic system.

Differential Diagnosis

The differential diagnosis of GAD is the same as for panic disorder and agoraphobia. It is particularly important to rule out drug-induced conditions such as caffeine intoxication, stimulant abuse, alcohol withdrawal, and sedative-hypnotic withdrawal. The mental status examination and patient history should cover the diagnostic possibilities of panic disorder, specific phobias, social phobia, OCD, schizophrenia, and major depression.

Clinical Management

The treatment of GAD usually involves individual psychotherapy and medication. The patient should be educated about the chronic nature of the disorder and the tendency of symptoms to wax and wane, often along with external stressors that the patient may be experiencing. Behavior therapy may help the patient to recognize and control anxiety symptoms. Relaxation training, rebreathing exercises, and progressive muscle relaxation can be easily taught and may be effective, especially if the condition is mild.

The following case is of a patient seen in our outpatient clinic who benefited from behavior therapy.

Kelly, a 19-year-old college student, presented for evaluation of "nerves." He had been anxious for as long as he could remember but denied being sad or blue. The problem had been worse since he finished high school and moved away from home to attend college.

Kelly worried about everything—his physical appearance, his grades in school, whether he had the right kind of friends, the health of his parents, and even his sexual inexperience.

Kelly was mildly tremulous and swallowed frequently; sweat was beaded up on his brow. He acknowledged being tense and unable to relax and had recently been evaluated for stress headaches. He chewed gum to counter his chronically dry mouth. He often had clammy hands and a feeling of a lump in his throat.

There was no apparent explanation for his chronic anxiety, but stress made his condition worse. He requested tranquilizers but agreed to try rebreathing exercises and progressive muscle relaxation as an initial treatment. After learning to use these techniques, he remained anxious but no longer felt that he needed tranquilizers.

Buspirone, a nonbenzodiazepine anxiolytic, is the drug of choice for GAD. Buspirone is given in doses between 10 and 40 mg/day. Its onset of action takes several weeks, but the drug is well tolerated and has little abuse potential. An extended-release form of the antidepressant venlafaxine also has been effective in the treatment of GAD (e.g., 75–225 mg once daily). Like buspirone, venlafaxine has little abuse potential but takes several weeks to take effect. Benzodiazepines also are effective but have the potential complications of tolerance and dependence. They should be prescribed in a maintenance dose (e.g., diazepam, 5 mg three times daily or 5–10 mg at bedtime) for short periods (e.g., weeks or months) when the anxiety is particularly severe. Sedating TCAs, such as doxepin or amitriptyline, also may be useful when given in low doses (e.g., 25–100 mg at bedtime).

Phobic Disorders

A phobia is an irrational fear of specific objects, places or situations, or activities. Although fear itself is to some degree adaptive, the fear in phobias is irrational, excessive, and disproportionate to any actual danger. Three categories of phobia are listed in DSM-IV-TR: *agoraphobia*, which has already been described; *social phobia*, in which there is fear of humiliation or embarrassment in public places; and *specific phobia*, a category that includes isolated phobias such as the irrational and intense fear of snakes.

Persons with social phobia fear situations in which they might be observed by other people, which explains why the disturbance is also referred to as *social anxiety disorder.* These persons also commonly fear speaking in public, eating in public restaurants, writing in front of other persons, or using public rest rooms. Sometimes the fear becomes generalized, so that phobic persons avoid almost all social situations. Specific phobias are usually well circumscribed and involve objects that could conceivably cause harm such as snakes, heights, flying, or blood, but the person's reaction to them is excessive and inappropriate.

The DSM-IV-TR criteria for social and specific phobias are presented in Tables 10–10 and 10–11, respectively. Examples of common specific phobias are presented in Table 10–12.

Epidemiology and Clinical Findings

Phobias are surprisingly common in the general population. Social phobia is reported to affect 3%–5% of the population; specific phobias may affect more than one-third of the population at some point during their lives. Specific phobias are more prevalent among women, although social phobia affects men and women about equally. Specific phobias begin in childhood, most starting before age 12 years. Social phobia begins during adolescence; the onset is usually before age 25 years. Among specific phobias, the most commonly feared objects or situations are animals, storms, heights, illness, injury, and death.

Despite the frequency of phobias in the general population, few phobic persons seek treatment. Most individuals are likely to perceive their phobias as bothersome but not pathological. Fear of snakes, for instance, will hardly keep a person from succeeding socially or occupationally, unless the person is employed in a zoo. This may help to explain why patients with phobias constitute only 2%–3% of psychiatric outpatients.

Persons with social and specific phobias experience anxiety when exposed to feared objects or situations and manifest autonomic arousal and avoidance behavior. Initially, exposure leads to an unpleasant subjective state of anxiety. This state leads to the physiological manifestations typically associated with anxiety, such as rapid heartbeat, shortness of breath, and jitteriness. Socially phobic persons learn to avoid the situations that lead to overwhelming anxiety and the fear that others will recognize their anxiety. They may eventually avoid public speaking engagements, eating in public, riding public transportation, or using public toilets. In severe cases, the socially phobic person avoids almost all social encounters.

For the person with a specific phobia, distress varies with the exposure to whatever object or situation is feared. For example, a hospital employee

---

TABLE 10–10. DSM-IV-TR diagnostic criteria for social phobia

A. A marked and persistent fear of one or more social or performance situations in which the person is exposed to unfamiliar people or to possible scrutiny by others. The individual fears that he or she will act in a way (or show anxiety symptoms) that will be humiliating or embarrassing. **Note:** In children, there must be evidence of the capacity for age-appropriate social relationships with familiar people and the anxiety must occur in peer settings, not just in interactions with adults.

B. Exposure to the feared social situation almost invariably provokes anxiety, which may take the form of a situationally bound or situationally predisposed Panic Attack. **Note:** In children, the anxiety may be expressed by crying, tantrums, freezing, or shrinking from social situations with unfamiliar people.

C. The person recognizes that the fear is excessive or unreasonable. **Note:** In children, this feature may be absent.

D. The feared social or performance situations are avoided or else are endured with intense anxiety or distress.

E. The avoidance, anxious anticipation, or distress in the feared social or performance situation(s) interferes significantly with the person's normal routine, occupational (academic) functioning, or social activities or relationships, or there is marked distress about having the phobia.

F. In individuals under age 18 years, the duration is at least 6 months.

G. The fear or avoidance is not due to the direct physiological effects of a substance (e.g., a drug of abuse, a medication) or a general medical condition and is not better accounted for by another mental disorder (e.g., Panic Disorder With or Without Agoraphobia, Separation Anxiety Disorder, Body Dysmorphic Disorder, a Pervasive Developmental Disorder, or Schizoid Personality Disorder).

H. If a general medical condition or another mental disorder is present, the fear in Criterion A is unrelated to it, e.g., the fear is not of Stuttering, trembling in Parkinson's disease, or exhibiting abnormal eating behavior in Anorexia Nervosa or Bulimia Nervosa.

Specify if:

> **Generalized:** if the fears include most social situations (also consider the additional diagnosis of Avoidant Personality Disorder)

---

who fears blood might experience near constant distress because of the availability of blood at hospitals. Apart from contact with the feared stimulus, the phobic person is usually symptom-free.

The following case example is of a boy with a specific phobia and the problems the disorder caused for him.

> John, a 13-year-old boy, was brought to the clinic by his mother. His mother reported that John wouldn't wear shirts that had buttons on them and was worried that this peculiarity would cause problems for John when he was

---

TABLE 10–11.   DSM-IV-TR diagnostic criteria for specific phobia

---

A. Marked and persistent fear that is excessive or unreasonable, cued by the presence or anticipation of a specific object or situation (e.g., flying, heights, animals, receiving an injection, seeing blood).

B. Exposure to the phobic stimulus almost invariably provokes an immediate anxiety response, which may take the form of a situationally bound or situationally predisposed Panic Attack.   **Note:** In children, the anxiety may be expressed by crying, tantrums, freezing, or clinging.

C. The person recognizes that the fear is excessive or unreasonable.   **Note:** In children, this feature may be absent.

D. The phobic situation(s) is avoided or else is endured with intense anxiety or distress.

E. The avoidance, anxious anticipation, or distress in the feared situation(s) interferes significantly with the person's normal routine, occupational (or academic) functioning, or social activities or relationships, or there is marked distress about having the phobia.

F. In individuals under age 18 years, the duration is at least 6 months.

G. The anxiety, Panic Attacks, or phobic avoidance associated with the specific object or situation is not better accounted for by another mental disorder, such as Obsessive-Compulsive Disorder (e.g., fear of dirt in someone with an obsession about contamination), Posttraumatic Stress Disorder (e.g., avoidance of stimuli associated with a severe stressor), Separation Anxiety Disorder (e.g., avoidance of school), Social Phobia (e.g., avoidance of social situations because of fear of embarrassment), Panic Disorder With Agoraphobia, or Agoraphobia Without History of Panic Disorder.

Specify type:

        Animal Type

        Natural Environment Type (e.g., heights, storms, water)

        Blood-Injection-Injury Type

        Situational Type (e.g., airplanes, elevators, enclosed places)

        Other Type (e.g., fear of choking, vomiting, or contracting an illness; in children, fear of loud sounds or costumed characters)

---

older. Already, his mother pointed out, not being able to wear regular collared shirts had kept John out of scouting troops and the school orchestra because of the uniforms he would have to wear. Doctors had told John's mother in the past that he would outgrow this fear. John clearly was uncomfortable and appeared embarrassed by his mother's recitation of the story but admitted that it was true. John said that at about age 4, he had developed a fear of buttons but was not sure why. Since then, he had worn only T-necked shirts or sweaters and had refused to wear collared shirts. In fact, John said, just thinking about such shirts bothered him, and he even avoided touching his brother's shirts that hung in the closet they shared.

TABLE 10–12. Common specific phobias by type

Phobia	Focus of fear	Phobia	Focus of fear
Animal type		**Blood, injection, injury type**	
Ailurophobia	Cats	Hemophobia	Blood
Arachnophobia	Spiders	Odynophobia	Pain
Cynophobia	Dogs	Poinephobia	Punishment
Entomophobia	Insects		
Ophidiophobia	Snakes	**Situation type**	
		Apeirophobia	Infinity
Natural environment type		Claustrophobia	Closed spaces
Acrophobia	Heights	Topophobia	Stage fright
Amathophobia	Dust		
Frigophobia	Cold weather	**Other**	
Keraunophobia	Thunder	Gynophobia	Women
Nyctophobia	Night	Homophobia	Homosexuals
Phonophobia	Loud noises	Kakorrhaphiophobia	Failure
Photophobia	Light	Logophobia	Words
Pyrophobia	Fire	Theophobia	God
		Triskaidekaphobia	Number 13

Ten years later, John had finished college and had enrolled in graduate school. He had overcome the phobia by himself at age 16 and was able to wear regular collared shirts, but he still reported that he avoided wearing these shirts when possible.

Etiology

Phobic disorders tend to run in families. Recent studies of both specific and social phobias showed that relatives of phobic persons were significantly more likely to have phobias than those of nonphobic control subjects and that the disorders "breed true"; that is, the proband with social phobia is likely to have relatives with social phobia, not a specific phobia. A large population-based twin study of women also reported a heritable component to social phobia.

The biological underpinnings of the phobias are not well understood. Research has shown that serotonergic pathways may play a role in social phobia; this is suggested by the clinical effectiveness of SRIs and evidence of hypersensitive serotonin receptors in the central nervous system. An early positron-emission tomography study showed that socially anxious patients had increased blood flow in the anterior cingulate and insulae, areas that control emotions and autonomic activity.

Learning also may play an important role in the etiology of phobias. Behaviorists have pointed out that many phobias tend to arise in association with traumatic events, such as developing a fear of heights after sustaining a fall. Psychoanalysts have long held that phobias result from unresolved conflicts in childhood and attribute phobias to the use of displacement and avoidance as defense mechanisms.

Course and Outcome

Social phobias tend to develop slowly, are chronic, and have no obvious precipitating stressors. Whether the disorder is perceived as disabling depends on the nature and extent of the fear, as well as one's occupation and social position. A business executive whose job requires meeting with the public, for instance, would face much greater disability from a social phobia than would a lighthouse keeper.

Many patients with social phobia become dependent on alcohol or sedative drugs and use them to reduce their anxiety in feared situations; in some persons, this pattern of use can lead to alcohol dependence.

Specific phobias tend to remit spontaneously with age, as illustrated in the case of John. When they persist into adulthood, specific phobias often become chronic but rarely cause disability.

Differential Diagnosis

The differential diagnosis of phobic disorders includes other anxiety disorders (e.g., panic disorder, OCD, GAD), mood disorders, schizophrenia, and avoidant personality disorder. The irrational fear that characterizes phobias must be distinguished from a schizophrenic delusion, which involves a fixed false belief (e.g., "The people I'm avoiding are plotting to kill me"). The person with OCD has multiple fears and phobias, not merely an isolated, circumscribed fear. The differentiation between avoidant personality disorder and social phobia may be difficult, and, in fact, both disorders overlap. Generally, the person with avoidant personality does not fear specific social situations but feels insecure in social situations and requires reassurance.

Clinical Management

Medication and behavior therapy have become the mainstays for the treatment of social phobia. MAOIs, benzodiazepines, and SRIs are all effective. TCAs are probably less effective, and persons with social phobia may be overly sensitive to their activating side effects (e.g., jitteriness, irritability, insomnia) even with relatively low doses. The SRIs are considered the treatment of choice because they are well tolerated and have no abuse potential. Doses tend to be the same as those used to treat major depression (e.g., fluoxetine, 20 mg/day; sertraline, 50 mg/day). Other drugs, including nefazodone and valproate, are being studied for social phobia and may be effective; buspirone is ineffective. β-Blocking drugs are effective for the short-term treatment of performance anxiety but are ineffective with generalized forms of social phobia. Patients tend to relapse when the drugs are discontinued. Medication is generally ineffective in the treatment of specific phobias.

Behavior therapy is useful in the treatment of both social phobias and specific phobias and involves exposure through the techniques of systematic desensitization and flooding. In the former, patients are gradually exposed to their feared situations, beginning with the situation that they fear the least. With flooding, patients are instructed to enter situations that are generally associated with anxiety until the anxiety associated with the exposure (e.g., eating in restaurants) subsides. Patients tend not to improve unless they are willing to confront feared situations. (Commonly used behavioral techniques are discussed further in Chapter 26.)

CBT can be used to correct dysfunctional thoughts about fear of failure, humiliation, or embarrassment. For example, it may help to point out to the socially phobic person that others are scrutinizing him or her no more than they are scrutinizing others. Supportive psychotherapy can help to restore morale and self-confidence. Marriage or family counseling is indicated when disturbed marital or family situations contribute to or exacerbate the symptoms.

Posttraumatic Stress Disorder

PTSD occurs in persons who have experienced a trauma in which they experienced, witnessed, or were confronted with an event involving actual or threatened death, serious physical injury, or a threat to one's physical integrity. Examples include combat, physical assault, rape, and disasters such as home fires. The three major elements of PTSD include 1) reexperiencing the trauma through dreams or recurrent and intrusive thoughts, 2) showing emotional numbing such as feeling detached from others, and 3) having symptoms of autonomic hyperarousal such as irritability and exaggerated startle response. Two subtypes are specified: acute if the duration of symptoms is less than 3 months and chronic if symptoms last 3 months or longer. If onset is delayed more than 6 months after the stressor, that delay is specified. The DSM-IV-TR criteria for PTSD are included in Table 10–13.

The term *posttraumatic stress disorder* was introduced in 1980 in DSM-III, although the concept behind this disturbance has a long history. Much earlier, the disorder was recognized as *shell shock* or *war neurosis* because it was seen most commonly in wartime situations. It gradually became clear that many of its typical symptoms, such as intrusive thoughts and autonomic hyperarousal, also were seen in victims of other traumatic events, such as natural disasters and physical assaults. In DSM-I, the disorder was diagnosed as *gross stress reaction*.

Epidemiology and Clinical Findings

The prevalence of PTSD in the general population is estimated at about 0.5% in men and 1.2% in women. Most men with the disorder have experienced combat. For women, the most frequent precipitating stressor is a physical assault or rape. The disorder can occur at any age, and even young children have been observed to develop the disorder, such as after the Chowchilla school bus kidnapping incident in 1976 or several of the more recent school shooting incidents. The frequency of PTSD among survivors of catastrophes varies, but in one well-studied tragedy, the Cocoanut Grove nightclub fire in the 1940s, 57% of the patients still had an acute posttraumatic syndrome 1 year later.

We recently saw a woman in our psychiatric clinic who had developed PTSD after a sexual assault:

> Megan, a 21-year-old college student, presented for evaluation of depression and flashbacks. At a fraternity party 3 months earlier, Megan had become interested in one of the men. The man suggested they go elsewhere to have sexual relations. Although intoxicated, Megan objected, but the man persisted. He forced her into another room, tore off her clothing, and raped her. Later, feeling embarrassed and humiliated, Megan chose not to tell her friends, and she did not seek a medical evaluation. She thought that the police would ignore what they might consider consensual sex.
>
> Although she never missed a class or her part-time clerical job, Megan became depressed and anxious and began to experience episodes of anger and irritability. She ruminated about the rape, would recall its unpleasant details, and withdrew from her friends. Several concerned friends convinced her to seek help.

TABLE 10–13. DSM-IV-TR diagnostic criteria for posttraumatic stress disorder

---

A. The person has been exposed to a traumatic event in which both of the following were present:

(1) the person experienced, witnessed, or was confronted with an event or events that involved actual or threatened death or serious injury, or a threat to the physical integrity of self or others

(2) the person's response involved intense fear, helplessness, or horror. **Note:** In children, this may be expressed instead by disorganized or agitated behavior

B. The traumatic event is persistently reexperienced in one (or more) of the following ways:

(1) recurrent and intrusive distressing recollections of the event, including images, thoughts, or perceptions. **Note:** In young children, repetitive play may occur in which themes or aspects of the trauma are expressed.

(2) recurrent distressing dreams of the event. **Note:** In children, there may be frightening dreams without recognizable content.

(3) acting or feeling as if the traumatic event were recurring (includes a sense of reliving the experience, illusions, hallucinations, and dissociative flashback episodes, including those that occur on awakening or when intoxicated). **Note:** In young children, trauma-specific reenactment may occur.

(4) intense psychological distress at exposure to internal or external cues that symbolize or resemble an aspect of the traumatic event

(5) physiological reactivity on exposure to internal or external cues that symbolize or resemble an aspect of the traumatic event

C. Persistent avoidance of stimuli associated with the trauma and numbing of general responsiveness (not present before the trauma), as indicated by three (or more) of the following:

(1) efforts to avoid thoughts, feelings, or conversations associated with the trauma

(2) efforts to avoid activities, places, or people that arouse recollections of the trauma

(3) inability to recall an important aspect of the trauma

(4) markedly diminished interest or participation in significant activities

(5) feeling of detachment or estrangement from others

(6) restricted range of affect (e.g., unable to have loving feelings)

(7) sense of a foreshortened future (e.g., does not expect to have a career, marriage, children, or a normal life span)

TABLE 10–13.   DSM-IV-TR diagnostic criteria for posttraumatic stress disorder (*continued*)

D. Persistent symptoms of increased arousal (not present before the trauma), as indicated by two (or more) of the following:
   (1) difficulty falling or staying asleep
   (2) irritability or outbursts of anger
   (3) difficulty concentrating
   (4) hypervigilance
   (5) exaggerated startle response
E. Duration of the disturbance (symptoms in Criteria B, C, and D) is more than 1 month.
F. The disturbance causes clinically significant distress or impairment in social, occupational, or other important areas of functioning.

Specify if:
   Acute: if duration of symptoms is less than 3 months
   Chronic: if duration of symptoms is 3 months or more

Specify if:
   With Delayed Onset: if onset of symptoms is at least 6 months after the stressor

---

Based on the history and symptoms, PTSD was diagnosed and explained to Megan; she was referred for group therapy at a local rape crisis advocacy center. Fluoxetine (20 mg/day) was prescribed to treat symptoms of depression and anxiety.

Etiology and Pathophysiology

The major etiological event leading to PTSD is the stressor. Stressors of all types have been reported to cause PTSD but by definition must be severe enough to be outside the range of normal human experience. Business losses, marital conflicts, and the death of a loved one are not considered stressors that cause PTSD. In general, the more severe the stressor, the greater the likelihood of developing PTSD. In wartime situations, for example, certain experiences are highly linked to the development of PTSD: witnessing a friend being killed in action, witnessing wartime atrocities, or participating in atrocities.

A person's age, history of emotional disturbance, level of social support, and proximity to the stressor are all factors that affect the likelihood of developing PTSD. Eighty percent of young children who sustain a burn injury, for example, show symptoms of posttraumatic stress 1–2 years after the initial injury, but only 30% of adults who sustain a similar injury do so. Persons who have received prior psychiatric treatment are more likely to develop PTSD, presumably because the previous illness reflects the person's greater sensitivity to stress. Persons with adequate social support are less likely to develop the disorder than are persons with poor support. Certain biological abnormalities, such as decreased rapid eye movement latency in Stage IV sleep, have been found in persons with PTSD, and these abnormalities may play a role in its development. Recent research suggests that the sustained levels of high emotional arousal can lead to dysregulation of the hypothalamic-pituitary-adrenal axis. The noradrenergic and serotonergic pathways in the central nervous system also have been implicated in the genesis of PTSD.

Course and Outcome

PTSD may begin within hours or days of the stressor, but it may be delayed for months or years. The disorder is chronic for many and has been reported to last 40 years or more in some cases. Symptoms fluctuate but typically worsen during stressful periods. Rapid onset of symptoms, good premorbid functioning, strong social support, and the absence of psychiatric or medical comorbidity are factors associated with a good outcome.

Many patients with PTSD develop frank major depression, other anxiety disorders, alcohol and drug abuse, anger and irritability, and poor impulse control. PTSD often has been used as an excuse for misbehavior, but persons in whom such behavior develops probably had similar behavior before the onset of PTSD.

Differential Diagnosis

The differential diagnosis for PTSD includes major depression, adjustment disorder, panic disorder, GAD, acute stress disorder, OCD, depersonalization disorder, factitious disorder, or malingering. In some cases, a physical injury may have occurred during the stressful incident to induce the PTSD (e.g., motor vehicle accident), so a brain injury must be ruled out as well.

Clinical Management

Although there is no universally accepted pharmacological approach to PTSD, research indicates that antidepressant medication and the benzodiazepine tranquilizers are helpful. The drugs help to decrease depression, to reduce intrusive symptoms such as nightmares and flashbacks, and to normalize sleep. Other medications, including the mood stabilizers (e.g., carbamazepine, valproate) and the antipsychotics, have been the subject of case reports. Sertraline has recently been approved by the U.S. Food and Drug Administration for the treatment of PTSD, but the other SRIs are probably effective as well. The SRIs are the drugs of choice because of their safety, tolerability, and lack of abuse potential.

Psychotherapy also is important. Behavioral techniques employing direct therapeutic exposure (i.e., flooding) can be helpful in reducing the intrusive symptoms of PTSD. CBT also may help to reduce anxiety by providing patients with the skills to control anxiety and to counter dysfunctional thoughts (e.g., "I deserved to be raped"). Group therapy and family therapy are also useful and have been widely recommended for veterans of war. The Department of Veterans Affairs has organized groups for distressed veterans across the country.

Acute Stress Disorder

Acute stress disorder occurs in some individuals after a traumatic experience and is considered a precursor to PTSD. By definition, the individual must have at least three dissociative symptoms (e.g., emotional numbing, derealization, amnesia) and one or more intrusion, avoidance, and hyperarousal symptoms; the symptoms must cause clinically significant difficulties in functioning and last from 2 days to 4 weeks (see Table 10–14).

The diagnosis was introduced in DSM-IV because research had shown that dissociative symptoms occurring immediately after a traumatic event predicted the development of PTSD. For example, from 78% to 82% of motor vehicle accident survivors with acute stress disorder have PTSD 6 months posttrauma. The diagnosis permits clinicians to more accurately identify persons less likely to recover from their traumatic experience and to develop PTSD.

Because acute stress disorder was recently defined, there is little information about its prevalence, gender distribution, or risk factors. The differential diagnosis is between PTSD, brief psychotic disorder, a dissociative disorder, or an adjustment disorder. PTSD lasts more than 1 month, and although dissociative symptoms may be present, they are usually not prominent. Brief psychotic disorder lasts less than 1 month but is characterized by hallucinations, delusions, or bizarre behavior. Dissociative disorders do not necessarily occur in response to traumatic situations or involve emotional numbing, reexperiencing of the trauma, or signs of autonomic hyperarousal. An adjustment disorder occurs in response to stressful situations (e.g., personal bankruptcy) but not necessarily a traumatic event involving serious

TABLE 10–14. DSM-IV-TR diagnostic criteria for acute stress disorder

A. The person has been exposed to a traumatic event in which both of the following were present:

    (1) the person experienced, witnessed, or was confronted with an event or events that involved actual or threatened death or serious injury, or a threat to the physical integrity of self or others

    (2) the person's response involved intense fear, helplessness, or horror

B. Either while experiencing or after experiencing the distressing event, the individual has three (or more) of the following dissociative symptoms:

    (1) a subjective sense of numbing, detachment, or absence of emotional responsiveness

    (2) a reduction in awareness of his or her surroundings (e.g., "being in a daze")

    (3) derealization

    (4) depersonalization

    (5) dissociative amnesia (i.e., inability to recall an important aspect of the trauma)

C. The traumatic event is persistently reexperienced in at least one of the following ways: recurrent images, thoughts, dreams, illusions, flashback episodes, or a sense of reliving the experience; or distress on exposure to reminders of the traumatic event.

D. Marked avoidance of stimuli that arouse recollections of the trauma (e.g., thoughts, feelings, conversations, activities, places, people).

E. Marked symptoms of anxiety or increased arousal (e.g., difficulty sleeping, irritability, poor concentration, hypervigilance, exaggerated startle response, motor restlessness).

F. The disturbance causes clinically significant distress or impairment in social, occupational, or other important areas of functioning or impairs the individual's ability to pursue some necessary task, such as obtaining necessary assistance or mobilizing personal resources by telling family members about the traumatic experience.

G. The disturbance lasts for a minimum of 2 days and a maximum of 4 weeks and occurs within 4 weeks of the traumatic event.

H. The disturbance is not due to the direct physiological effects of a substance (e.g., a drug of abuse, a medication) or a general medical condition, is not better accounted for by Brief Psychotic Disorder, and is not merely an exacerbation of a preexisting Axis I or Axis II disorder.

personal threats; adjustment disorders may last up to 6 months, and the diagnosis is mainly used when criteria for other Axis I disorders are not met. A diagnosis of acute stress reaction would preempt a diagnosis of adjustment disorder.

Research shows that CBT involving exposure and anxiety management (e.g., relaxation training, rebreathing exercises) helps prevent the progression to full-blown PTSD. When anxiety is severe, a brief course of a benzo-diazepine may be helpful (e.g., lorazepam, 0.5–1.0 mg twice daily).

Management of Anxiety Disorders

Recommendations for the management of anxiety disorders appear in the box.

Recommendations for treatment of anxiety disorders

1. Mild cases of panic may respond to cognitive-behavioral therapy, but many patients will need medication.
   - Serotonin reuptake inhibitors are the drugs of first choice because of their effectiveness and tolerability.
2. The agoraphobic patient should be gently encouraged to get out and explore the world.
   - Progress will not occur unless the phobic patient confronts the feared places or situations.
3. Patients with anxiety disorders should minimize caffeine intake, a known anxiogenic.
4. Behavioral techniques (e.g., exposure, flooding, desensitization) will help most persons with social and specific phobias.
   - Some people with a social phobia respond well to medication. Serotonin reuptake inhibitors are the drugs of choice because of their effectiveness and tolerability. Tricyclic antidepressants are not effective.
5. Generalized anxiety disorder may respond to simple behavioral techniques (e.g., relaxation training), but many patients will need medication.
   - Buspirone (10–40 mg/day) is the drug of choice because it has no abuse potential; a slow-release form of venlafaxine has recently been approved for treatment of generalized anxiety disorder and is well tolerated at doses of 75–225 mg/day.
   - Benzodiazepines, when used, should be prescribed for a limited time (e.g., weeks or months).
6. Posttraumatic stress disorder tends to be chronic, but many patients will benefit from a combination of medication and therapeutic support.
   - Sertraline (50–200 mg/day) has been approved for the treatment of posttraumatic stress disorder. The other serotonin reuptake inhibitors are probably effective as well.
   - Many patients will benefit from the support available in group therapy. Group therapy has become especially popular with veterans. Most veteran organizations can offer help in finding a group.

Bibliography

American Psychiatric Association: Diagnostic and Statistical Manual of Mental Disorders, 3rd Edition. Washington, DC, American Psychiatric Association, 1980

American Psychiatric Association: Diagnostic and Statistical Manual of Mental Disorders, 4th Edition. Washington, DC, American Psychiatric Association, 1994

American Psychiatric Association: Diagnostic and Statistical Manual of Mental Disorders, 4th Edition Text Revision. Washington, DC, American Psychiatric Association, 2000

Baldwin D, Bobes J, Stein DJ, et al: Paroxetine in social phobia/social anxiety disorder: randomized, double-blind, placebo-controlled study. Br J Psychiatry 175:120–126, 1999

Ballenger JC, Burrows GD, DuPont RL, et al: Alprazolam in panic disorder and agoraphobia—results from a multicenter trial, I: efficacy in short-term treatment. Arch Gen Psychiatry 45:413–422, 1988

Black DW, Wesner R, Bowers W, et al: A comparison of fluvoxamine, cognitive therapy, and placebo in the treatment of panic disorder. Arch Gen Psychiatry 50:44–50, 1993

Brady K, Pearlstein T, Asnis GM, et al: Efficacy and safety of sertraline treatment of posttraumatic stress disorder: a randomized controlled trial. JAMA 283:1837–1844, 2000

Brawman-Mintzer O, Lydiard B, Emmanuel N, et al: Psychiatric comorbidity in patients with generalized anxiety disorder. Am J Psychiatry 150:1216–1218, 1993

Breslau N, Davis GC: Post-traumatic stress disorder: the etiologic specificity of wartime stressors. Am J Psychiatry 144:578–583, 1987

Bryant RA, Sackville T, Dang ST, et al: Treating acute stress disorder: an evaluation of cognitive behavior therapy and supportive counseling techniques. Am J Psychiatry 156:1780–1786, 1999

Burns LE, Thorpe GL: The epidemiology of fears and phobias (with particular reference to the National Survey of Agoraphobics). J Int Med Res 5(suppl):1–7, 1977

Classen C, Koopman C, Hales R, et al: Acute stress disorder as a predictor of posttraumatic stress symptoms. Am J Psychiatry 155:620–624, 1998

Connor KM, Sutherland SM, Tupler LA, et al: Fluoxetine in post-traumatic stress disorder: randomized, double-blind study. Br J Psychiatry 175:17–22, 1999

Davidson JRT, DuPont RL, Heges D, et al: Efficacy, safety, and tolerability of venlafaxine extended release and buspirone in outpatients with generalized anxiety disorder. J Clin Psychiatry 60:528–535, 1999

DeWitt DJ, Ogborne A, Oxford DR, et al: Antecedents of the risk of recovery from DSM-III-R social phobia. Psychol Med 29:569–582, 1999

Freed LA, Levy D, Levine RA, et al: Prevalence and clinical outcome of mitral-value prolapse. N Engl J Med 341:1–7, 1999

Fyer AJ, Mannuzza S, Gallops MS, et al: Familial transmission of simple phobias and fears—a preliminary report. Arch Gen Psychiatry 47:252–256, 1990

Heimberg RG, Liebowitz MR, Hope DA, et al: Cognitive behavioral group therapy vs. phenelzine therapy for social phobia: 12-week outcome. Arch Gen Psychiatry 55:1133–1141, 1998

Helzer JE, Robins LE, McEvoy L: Post-traumatic stress disorder in the general population: findings of the Epidemiologic Catchment Area survey. N Engl J Med 317:1630–1634, 1987

Katon WJ, Van Korff M, Lin E: Panic disorder: relationship to high medical utilization. Am J Med 92 (suppl 1A):7S–11S, 1992

Klein DF: False suffocation alarms, spontaneous panics, and related conditions: an integrative hypothesis. Arch Gen Psychiatry 50:306–317, 1993

Lee MA, Flegel P, Greden JF, et al: Anxiogenic effects of caffeine in panic and depressed patients. Am J Psychiatry 145:632–635, 1988

Marks I, Lovell K, Moshirvani H, et al: Treatment of posttraumatic stress disorder by exposure and/or cognitive restructuring: a controlled study. Arch Gen Psychiatry 55:317–325, 1998

Noyes R: Suicide and panic disorder: a review. J Affect Disord 22:1–11, 1991

Noyes R, Clarkson C, Crowe R, et al: A family study of generalized anxiety disorder. Am J Psychiatry 144:119–124, 1987a

Noyes R, Clancy J, Garvey MJ, et al: Is agoraphobia a variant of panic disorder or a separate illness? J Affect Disord 1:3–13, 1987b

Nutt DJ, Bell CJ, Malizia AC: Brain mechanisms of social anxiety disorder. J Clin Psychiatry 59 (suppl 17):4–9, 1998

Ross RJ, Ball WA, Sullivan KA, et al: Sleep disturbance as the hallmark of post-traumatic stress disorder. Am J Psychiatry 146:697–707, 1989

Shaw DM, Churchill CM, Noyes R, et al: Criminal behavior and post-traumatic stress disorder in Vietnam veterans. Compr Psychiatry 28:403–411, 1987

Smith EM, North CS, McCool RE, et al: Acute post-disaster psychiatric disorders: identification of persons at risk. Am J Psychiatry 147:202–206, 1990

Solomon SD, Gerrity ET, Muff AM: Efficacy of treatments for post-traumatic stress disorder: an empirical review. JAMA 268:633–638, 1992

Stein MB, Chartier MJ, Hazen AL: A direct interview family study of generalized social phobia. Am J Psychiatry 155:90–97, 1998

Terr LC: Chowchilla revisited: the effects of psychic trauma four years after a school bus kidnapping. Am J Psychiatry 140:1543–1550, 1983

Thyer BA, Parrish RT, Curtis GC, et al: Ages of onset of DSM-III anxiety disorder. Compr Psychiatry 26:113–122, 1985

Van Amerigan M, Mancini C, Oakman JM: Nefazodone in social phobia. J Clin Psychiatry 60:96–100, 1999

Yonkers KA, Warshaw MB, Massion AO, et al: Phenomenology and course of generalized anxiety disorder. Br J Psychiatry 168:308–313, 1996

Self-Assessment Questions

1. What is the relation between panic disorder and agoraphobia?
2. What is the irritable heart syndrome?
3. What are the findings in genetic studies of panic disorder?
4. What is the differential diagnosis of panic disorder?
5. What is the pharmacological treatment of panic disorder? Generalized anxiety disorder? Social phobia?
6. What are social and specific phobias? How do they differ?
7. What is the natural history of the different anxiety disorders?
8. When does PTSD develop? What factors predispose to its development?
9. What behavioral treatments are useful in the different anxiety disorders?
10. When is anxiety normal, and when is it abnormal?

11 Obsessive-Compulsive Disorder

He had another peculiarity—This was his anxious care
to go out or in at a door or passage by a certain number
of steps from a certain point...

James Boswell, *Life of Samuel Johnson*, 1791

S amuel Johnson, the noted eighteenth-century lexicographer so carefully observed by Boswell, probably had obsessive-compulsive disorder (OCD). Shakespeare, in describing the guilt-laden hand-washing rituals of Lady Macbeth, appears to have had some familiarity with the symptoms of the disorder. More recently, industrialist Howard Hughes developed crippling contamination obsessions in late adulthood that resulted in a fanatic preoccupation with germs and a bizarre life of filth and neglect. Like most mental illnesses, OCD has been recognized for centuries, but it was first formally described in 1838 by Esquirol, a French psychiatrist. Earlier, rituals were probably regarded as personal quirks or, worse, as evidence of possession by the Devil. One wonders how many luckless OCD patients were burned at the stake!

By the end of the nineteenth century, obsessions and compulsions were generally believed to be manifestations of depressive illness. Later, in part because of the influence of Freud, these symptoms were recognized as *obsessional neurosis,* a syndrome believed to result from intrapsychic conflicts. This view remained prominent until recently, when biologically oriented research supported the disease model of OCD, and behaviorally oriented clinicians began to reconceptualize OCD in terms of learning theory. Obsessional neurosis was renamed *obsessive-compulsive disorder* in 1980, reflecting these new etiological concepts. Although the cause of OCD is still unknown, its study has been reinvigorated by new research methods, as well as by the development of effective treatments that have altered its formerly poor prognosis.

Definition

Obsessions or compulsions, or more commonly both, are the hallmark of OCD. According to DSM-IV-TR (see Table 11–1), obsessions are recurrent and persistent ideas, thoughts, impulses, or images that are experienced as intrusive and inappropriate and that cause marked anxiety or distress. Common obsessions include fears of harming other persons or sinning against God. For example, a person may have an obsessional thought to kill a loved one, or a religious person may have blasphemous thoughts. (The content of typical obsessions is shown in Table 11–2.)

Compulsions are repetitive, purposeful, and intentional behaviors or mental acts performed in response to obsessions or according to certain rules that must be applied rigidly. Examples include repetitive hand washing or ritualistic checking. Compulsions are meant to neutralize or reduce discomfort or to prevent a dreaded event or situation. The rituals are not connected in a realistic way to the event or situation or are clearly excessive. For example, one may believe that failing to reread the directions on a box of detergent might cause harm to one's child. In short, obsessions create anxiety, which is relieved by compulsive rituals. The frequency of common obsessions and compulsions in a series of 250 patients is presented in Table 11–3.

To receive a diagnosis of OCD, a person must have either obsessions or compulsions that cause marked distress, are time-consuming (more than 1 hour daily), or significantly interfere with the person's normal routine, occupational functioning, or usual social activities and relationships. In addition, at some point the person must recognize that the obsessions and compulsions are unreasonable, and the clinician will have determined that the symptoms are not due to another Axis I disorder, such as major depression, and that they are not caused by the effects of a substance or general medical condition.

Many psychiatrically normal individuals—particularly children—have occasional obsessional thoughts or repetitive behaviors, but they tend not to cause distress or interfere with living. In fact, in many ways rituals add need-

---

TABLE 11–1. DSM-IV-TR criteria for obsessive-compulsive disorder

---

A. Either obsessions or compulsions:

Obsessions as defined by (1), (2), (3), and (4):

   (1) recurrent and persistent thoughts, impulses, or images that are experienced, at some time during the disturbance, as intrusive and inappropriate and that cause marked anxiety or distress

   (2) the thoughts, impulses, or images are not simply excessive worries about real-life problems

   (3) the person attempts to ignore or suppress such thoughts, impulses, or images, or to neutralize them with some other thought or action

   (4) the person recognizes that the obsessional thoughts, impulses, or images are a product of his or her own mind (not imposed from without as in thought insertion)

Compulsions as defined by (1) and (2):

   (1) repetitive behaviors (e.g., hand washing, ordering, checking) or mental acts (e.g., praying, counting, repeating words silently) that the person feels driven to perform in response to an obsession, or according to rules that must be applied rigidly

   (2) the behaviors or mental acts are aimed at preventing or reducing distress or preventing some dreaded event or situation; however, these behaviors or mental acts either are not connected in a realistic way with what they are designed to neutralize or prevent or are clearly excessive

B. At some point during the course of the disorder, the person has recognized that the obsessions or compulsions are excessive or unreasonable.   **Note:** This does not apply to children.

C. The obsessions or compulsions cause marked distress, are time consuming (take more than 1 hour a day), or significantly interfere with the person's normal routine, occupational (or academic) functioning, or usual social activities or relationships.

D. If another Axis I disorder is present, the content of the obsessions or compulsions is not restricted to it (e.g., preoccupation with food in the presence of an Eating Disorder; hair pulling in the presence of Trichotillomania; concern with appearance in the presence of Body Dysmorphic Disorder; preoccupation with drugs in the presence of a Substance Use Disorder; preoccupation with having a serious illness in the presence of Hypochondriasis; preoccupation with sexual urges or fantasies in the presence of a Paraphilia; or guilty ruminations in the presence of Major Depressive Disorder).

E. The disturbance is not due to the direct physiological effects of a substance (e.g., a drug of abuse, a medication) or a general medical condition.

Specify if:

   With Poor Insight: if, for most of the time during the current episode, the person does not recognize that the obsessions and compulsions are excessive or unreasonable

---

TABLE 11–2.   Varied content in obsessions

Obsession	Foci of preoccupation
Aggression	Physical or verbal assault on self or others (includes suicidal and homicidal thoughts); accidents; mishaps; wars and natural disasters; death
Contamination	Excreta, human or otherwise; dirt, dust; semen; menstrual blood; other bodily excretions; germs; illness, especially venereal diseases; AIDS
Symmetry	Orderliness in arrangements of any kind (e.g., books on the shelf, shirts in the dresser)
Sexual	Sexual advances toward self or others; incestuous impulses; genitalia of either gender; homosexuality; masturbation; competence in sexual performance
Hoarding	Collecting items of any kind, typically items with little or no intrinsic value (e.g., string, shopping bags); inability to throw things out
Religious	Existence of God; validity of religious stories, practices, or holidays; committing sinful acts
Somatic	Preoccupation with body parts (e.g., nose); concern with appearance; belief in having disease or illness (e.g., cancer)

Source. Adapted from Akhtar et al. 1975.

TABLE 11–3.   Frequency of common obsessions and compulsions in 560 patients with obsessive-compulsive disorder

Obsessions	%	Compulsions	%
Contamination	50	Checking‘	61
Pathological doubt	42	Washing	50
Somatic	33	Counting	36
Need for symmetry	32	Need to ask or confess	34
Aggressive impulse	31	Symmetry and precision	28
Sexual impulse	24	Hoarding	18
Multiple obsessions	72	Multiple compulsions	58

Source. Adapted from Rasmussen and Eisen 1990.

ed structure to our lives. Most of us have daily routines that have probably changed little in years (e.g., drinking coffee in the morning, eating lunch at noon, having dinner at 6:00 P.M., and retiring at 11:00 P.M.). Many of us double-check locks, avoid stepping on cracks, and say prayers before meals. Rituals also enhance the spiritual life of many. These daily rituals are viewed as acceptable and desirable and are easily adapted to changing circumstances. To the obsessive-compulsive person, however, rituals are a distressing and unavoidable way of life.

The following case history is of a patient treated in our clinic who endured the crippling effects of OCD:

> Todd, a 24-year-old man, was accompanied to the clinic by his mother for evaluation of obsessions and compulsive rituals. The rituals had begun in childhood and included touching objects a certain number of times and rereading prayers in church, but these symptoms were not disabling. After graduating from college, he moved to a large midwestern city to work as an accountant for a major firm. Soon after, he began to check the locks on his doors frequently and to check his automobile for signs of intruders. Eventually, he began to check other things around his apartment, such as appliances, water faucets, and electrical switches, fearing that they might be unsafe. Fearing contamination, he also developed extensive grooming and bathing rituals. Because of his time-consuming rituals, he was often late for work, and, in fact, his workload became too much for him. He would find himself adding columns of numbers over and over to make sure that he had "done it right." He eventually quit his accounting job.
>
> In addition to extensive rituals, Todd developed thoughts of losing control and assaulting others, yelling embarrassing words in public, becoming contaminated, and possibly contracting the human immunodeficiency virus. He also worried about the arrangement and symmetry of objects. Much of the time, his rituals consisted of debating whether he needed to actually conduct a ritual and, in fact, mentally rehearsing rituals. Todd knew that his rituals were irrational and excessive but felt powerless to control them.
>
> Todd moved back into his parents' home. His rituals became even more extensive and eventually took up nearly his entire day. The rituals mostly involved bathing (he showered for a half hour and had to wash his body in a specific order), dressing in a certain way, and repeating activities, such as walking in and out of doorways a certain number of times.
>
> Todd was a slender, unkempt young man with a scraggly beard, long hair, and unclipped fingernails. His shoelaces were untied, and he wore several layers of clothing. His rituals had become so time-consuming that he had found it easier not to shave or wash at all. He wore the same clothes every day for the same reason.
>
> Todd began treatment with fluoxetine (20 mg/day), and his daily dose was gradually increased to 80 mg. Within 2 months, his rituals were re-

duced to less than 1 hour per day, and his grooming had improved. After 6 months, Todd still had minor rituals but reported that he felt like his old self. He had obtained a job and was coaching track at a nearby high school.

Ten years later, Todd remained well. Attempts to stop the medication had always led to an increase in symptoms. In the interim, Todd had received a law degree, had married, and had developed a growing law practice.

Epidemiology

OCD typically begins in the late teens or early 20s; about one-third of patients develop the illness by age 15 and nearly three-quarters by age 30 years. Onset is generally gradual but may occur suddenly over a period of 1 month in the absence of any obvious stressor. It had been estimated that about 7½ years pass between the onset of obsessions and compulsions and the initiation of treatment. The delay now may be shorter because of the availability of effective treatments and the growing public awareness of OCD.

Data from the Epidemiologic Catchment Area study suggested that as many as 2%–3% of the general population meet criteria for OCD at some point during their lives. Men and women are equally likely to develop OCD, although men have an earlier onset. Patients with OCD have a normal range of intelligence, despite early reports (drawn from samples of persons seeking treatment) that they possess above-average intellect.

Etiology and Pathophysiology

Over the years, OCD has been explained in genetic, psychodynamic, behavioral, and neurobiological terms. No explanation accounts for the richness of OCD, and a combination of these explanations likely will account for the disturbance.

Some family studies have shown that up to 20% of the first-degree relatives of patients with OCD have obsessive-compulsive symptoms, whereas others have shown an increased prevalence of anxiety and mood disorders in relatives. Family studies also have linked OCD with Tourette's disorder, suggesting that the two disorders are genetically related. Twin studies generally have found a higher concordance of OCD among identical than among nonidentical twins, also suggesting an inherited predisposition to OCD.

Psychodynamically oriented clinicians have long explained OCD as stemming from a fixation at the genital stage of development and regression to the earlier anal stage, which involves a preoccupation with anger, dirt, magical thinking, and ambivalence. This leads to an overdeveloped superego and a variety of neurotic defense mechanisms, such as isolation, undoing, reaction formation, and displacement, to control these patients' internal anxious state. (Defense mechanisms are explained in Chapter 26.) Although obsessions and ritualistic behaviors often appear laden with symbolic meaning, psychodynamic approaches have not been helpful in treating this disorder and are primarily of historic interest.

Behaviorists have explained the development of OCD in terms of learning theory. They believe that anxiety, at least initially, becomes paired with specific environmental events (i.e., classical conditioning), for example, becoming dirty or contaminated. The person then engages in compulsive rituals, such as compulsive hand washing, to decrease the anxiety. When the rituals successfully reduce the anxiety, the compulsive behavior is believed more likely to be repeated in the future (i.e., operant conditioning). Although behavioral models of OCD have had little empirical support, behavioral techniques have become a mainstay in treating the disorder.

The neurobiological model of OCD has received widespread support in the past decade. Evidence supporting this model includes the fact that OCD occurs more often in persons who have various neurological disorders, including cases of head trauma, epilepsy, Sydenham's chorea, and Huntington's chorea. OCD also has been linked to birth injury, abnormal electroencephalogram findings, abnormal auditory evoked potentials, growth delays, and abnormalities in neuropsychological test results. Additional support for the biological basis of OCD comes from animal studies in which bilateral hippocampal lesions or chronic amphetamine administration led to stereotypic behaviors that resemble compulsive rituals. Recently, a type of OCD has been identified in children after a group A β-streptococcal infection. These children not only develop obsessions and compulsions but also have emotional lability, separation anxiety, and tics.

The most widely studied biochemical model has focused on the neurotransmitter serotonin because antidepressant drugs that block its reuptake are effective in treating the symptoms of OCD, whereas other antidepressant drugs are ineffective. Specifically, clomipramine and the serotonin reuptake inhibitors (SRIs) (e.g., citalopram, fluoxetine, fluvoxamine, paroxetine, and sertraline) are all potent serotonin reuptake blockers, and all are effective in treating OCD. Other evidence supporting the "serotonin hypothesis" is indirect and sometimes contradictory but is consistent with the view that either levels of the neurotransmitter or variations in the number or function of serotonin receptors are disturbed in patients with OCD.

Brain imaging techniques have provided some evidence of basal ganglia involvement in persons with OCD. Several groups of investigators who used positron-emission tomography (PET) or single photon emission computed tomography (SPECT) scanning showed increased glucose metabolism in the caudate nuclei and the orbital cortex of the frontal lobes, abnormalities that have been shown to partially normalize following successful treatment. One hypothesis is that basal ganglia dysfunction leads to the complex motor programs involved in OCD, whereas the prefrontal hyperactivity may be related to the tendency to worry and plan excessively. As discussed in Chapter 5, the prefrontal cortex has important connections with the basal ganglia.

Relation Between Obsessive-Compulsive Disorder and Obsessive-Compulsive Personality Disorder

Obsessive-compulsive personality disorder and OCD should not be confused, despite their similar name. Obsessive-compulsive personality—which is characterized by perfectionism, orderliness, and obstinacy—was once thought to lead to OCD; however, research shows that this rarely happens. In fact, most persons with OCD do not have obsessive-compulsive personality disorder and are more likely to have dependent, avoidant, or passive-aggressive character traits.

Admittedly, the distinction between the two disorders sometimes can be difficult. For example, we recently saw a 45-year-old man whose wife was "sick and tired" of his book collecting, which had "taken over" their house. He saw nothing wrong with his hobby, which he enjoyed. He pointed out that many of the books were quite valuable. In this case, the patient viewed his obsessive-compulsive traits as desirable and had not resisted them. Based on his history of a rigid and aloof demeanor, miserliness, and perfectionism, in addition to the collecting, he received a diagnosis of obsessive-compulsive personality disorder. (A further discussion of this personality disorder is found in Chapter 16.)

Course and Outcome

In a study of 250 patients, 85% were reported to have a chronic course, 10% a progressive or deteriorating course, and 2% an episodic course with periods of remission. Because these and other data were collected before effective treatments were available, future outcome studies may yield more favorable results. One recent study of children and adolescents with OCD seems to bear this trend out. At a 5-year follow-up, most still had obsessive-compulsive symptoms, but they were less severe, and 6% of the youth had achieved full remission.

Mild or typical symptoms and good premorbid adjustment have been associated with good outcome; early onset and the presence of a severe personality disorder have been associated with poor outcome. Obsessive-compulsive symptoms are usually worsened by depressed mood and stressful events. In fact, it is often depression that leads the OCD patient to seek help, not the obsessions or compulsions. Recurrent episodes of major depression occur in up to 80% of patients with OCD. Although suicidal thoughts often figure prominently in obsessional thinking, the rate of suicide among persons with OCD is probably not increased.

Differential Diagnosis

The diagnosis of OCD rests on the patient's history and the mental status examination, not laboratory or psychological tests. The disorder overlaps with many other psychiatric syndromes (see Table 11–4), which must be ruled out. Schizophrenia is the most important disorder to exclude, and several features are common to both conditions. Both OCD and schizophrenia have a relatively early onset and are chronic. Severe obsessional thoughts can resemble delusional thinking. This was illustrated for us by Earl, a 38-year-old disabled truck driver who had extensive cleaning and checking rituals and felt compelled to describe the rituals in a loud voice as he was performing them—so loudly, in fact, that neighbors complained. Earl firmly believed that harm would come to his family if he did not announce his rituals in this fashion. Although we tried, we were unable to reassure him that his belief was unreasonable. Earl aside, in most patients the distinction between obsessions and delusions is usually clear-cut. Obsessions are unwanted, resisted, and recognized by the patient as having an internal origin, whereas delusions are typically not resisted and are looked on as being of external origin. Obsessive-compulsive patients may occasionally develop hallucinations or delusions, particularly in the context of severe depression, but follow-up studies show that these patients are not at increased risk for developing schizophrenia.

Patients with well-established OCD who develop recurrent major depression (often called a *secondary depression*) should be distinguished from patients with primary major depression in which obsessional thinking develops, usually in the form of morbid preoccupations and guilty ruminations (e.g., "I have sinned!"). In these situations, the ruminations are viewed by the patient as reasonable, although perhaps exaggerated, and are seldom resisted. Whereas the depressed patient tends to focus on past events, the obsessional patient focuses on the prevention of future events. In general,

TABLE 11–4.   Differential diagnosis of obsessive-compulsive disorder

Disorder	Similarities and differences
Anorexia nervosa	Both involve rituals and tend to be chronic; with anorexia, symptoms are generally not resisted or thought unreasonable; anorexia mainly affects women
Autistic disorder	Stereotypies in autism resemble rituals, but they are not resisted; autism mainly affects males, and many autistic patients are mentally retarded
Hypochondriasis	Both may involve recurrent thoughts about physical illness, but this is the main symptom in hypochondriasis; hypochondriacal symptoms are rarely resisted or thought unreasonable
Major depression	Depressed patients may develop transient obsessions or compulsions, but the disorder is episodic and mainly affects women; depressive ruminations often resemble obsessions but are generally considered appropriate
Posttraumatic stress disorder	Both involve intrusive, unwanted thoughts, which cause physiological arousal and anxiety; precipitating stressors are rare in OCD, and many symptoms in posttraumatic stress disorder, such as emotional numbing and depersonalization, tend to be uncommon in OCD
Schizophrenia	Both tend to be chronic and develop in the late teens or early 20s; schizophrenia tends to be severely disabling and is associated with psychotic symptoms
Specific phobia	Both involve fears and avoidance, but the fear is well circumscribed in phobias; phobias tend to begin in childhood and are rarely resisted
Tourette's disorder	Both tend to be chronic, and many Tourette's patients have rituals; Tourette's disorder mainly affects males and usually has a childhood onset
Trichotillomania	Both involve excessive, unreasonable behaviors and may respond to similar treatments; trichotillomania mainly affects women and has a childhood onset; obsessional thoughts are uncommon

obsessive-compulsive symptoms arising in the context of depression will fully resolve when the depression is treated.

OCD also has a close association with phobias or other anxiety disorders. Both OCD and anxiety disorder patients have intense anxiety, have both subjective and autonomic responses to certain objects or situations, and respond to behavioral interventions. Many persons with OCD do in fact have specific phobias, such as a fear of snakes, which may be unrelated to the content of their obsessions. Social phobia also is relatively common in patients with OCD who worry excessively about public scrutiny and embarrassment.

Other disorders need to be ruled out as well. Tourette's disorder, characterized by vocal and motor tics, may coexist with OCD. Autistic disorder, a childhood condition characterized by repetitive or stereotyped behaviors, may resemble OCD. Posttraumatic stress disorder is characterized by recurrent, intrusive thoughts that may suggest obsessional thinking. Trichotillomania, or compulsive hair pulling, is classified as an impulse-control disorder, but it has many features in common with OCD, such as an irresistible urge to pull. Anorexia nervosa also resembles OCD because both disorders involve ritualistic behavior; however, the patient with anorexia views the behavior as desirable and rarely resists it. Some patients with anorexia nervosa also meet criteria for OCD and, in addition to their food-related rituals, will have symptoms typical of OCD, such as frequent hand washing and checking.

Clinical Management

The treatment of OCD has traditionally been viewed as difficult and unsatisfactory. Recent developments in the treatment of OCD have changed this picture dramatically and have instilled a greater sense of optimism. The mainstays of treatment are pharmacotherapy and behavior therapy (see box). Behavior therapies, which tend to be more successful for ritualizers, emphasize exposure paired with response prevention. For example, a patient might be exposed to a dreaded situation, event, or stimulus by various techniques (e.g., imaginal exposure, systematic desensitization, flooding) and then prevented from carrying out the compulsive behavior that usually results. For instance, a compulsive washer may be asked to handle "contaminated" objects (e.g., a dirty tissue) and then be prevented from washing his or her hands. Thought-stopping techniques may be used to interrupt obsessional thoughts (e.g., the therapist may announce in a loud voice "Stop!" to interrupt the cycle of thinking). Proponents of behavior therapies state that 60%–70% of the patients who persevere with the treatment have marked improvement. Unfortunately, many patients refuse to participate in the therapy because they fear the temporary increase in anxiety or drop out. (See Chapter 26 for a more detailed description of behavior therapy.)

Pharmacotherapy has been growing in importance, primarily because of studies showing that clomipramine (a tricyclic antidepressant) and the SRIs—citalopram, fluoxetine, fluvoxamine, paroxetine, and sertraline—have clear antiobsessional properties. The first drug marketed for OCD, clo-

Recommendations for management of obsessive-compulsive disorder (OCD)

1. The patient should be educated about his or her illness.
   - Education will diminish the patient's feelings of isolation, fear, and confusion.
   - The worried patient should be reassured that people with OCD rarely act on their frightening or violent obsessions.
   - The clinician should point out the "up" side of OCD—that people with this disorder are usually conscientious, dependable, and likable.
   - The clinician should recommend lay literature and suggest that the patient join the OC Foundation (New Haven, CT).
2. An empathic relationship should be established.
   - The clinician should not tell patients to stop their rituals. They cannot. That is why they are seeing a clinician.
   - The clinician should explain that talking about the obsessions and compulsions will not make them worse.
3. The clinician should set limited goals with behavior therapy—all rituals should not be tackled at once.
   - The clinician needs to find out what makes the rituals worse and what alleviates them.
   - One ritual at a time should be treated, and treatment should start with simple goals (e.g., reducing the amount of time spent in the shower from 40 to 35 minutes).
   - The patient may need to be referred to an experienced behavior therapist, particularly when compulsive rituals are prominent.
4. Medication should be used in moderate and severe cases.
   - Clomipramine or a serotonin reuptake inhibitor should be administered, and the clinician must be patient. A full trial should last at least 3 months.
   - Higher doses will be needed: clomipramine (150–250 mg/day), citalopram (20–60 mg/day), fluoxetine (20–80 mg/day), fluvoxamine (150–300 mg/day), paroxetine (20–60 mg/day), sertraline (50–200 mg/day).
   - Expectations for the treatment should be realistic. Most patients will still have substantial symptoms after successful treatment.
   - The Yale-Brown Obsessive Compulsive Scale (Y-BOCS), located in the Appendix, may be used to monitor treatment response.
5. Patient support groups, family therapy, and marital counseling each may play a role in patient care.
   - Support groups can provide patients with a supportive atmosphere where they can meet others with the disorder.
   - Family therapy can be useful in educating the family about OCD, as well as in addressing other problems such as anger, guilt, and hostility.
   - Marital therapy can be helpful when OCD has disrupted the spousal relationship.

mipramine, is a relatively specific serotonin reuptake blocker like the SRIs. It is administered in doses ranging from 150 to 250 mg/day, but its many side effects—sedation, orthostatic hypotension, constipation, and urinary hesitancy—limit its usefulness. The SRIs, a relatively new group of antidepressants, are effective in treating OCD. Typically, higher doses of the SRIs are required to treat OCD than depression, and response is often delayed. Thus, patients should have lengthy trials (i.e., 12–16 weeks) at relatively high doses (see box). The SRIs are generally well tolerated, but jitteriness, sedation, insomnia, gastrointestinal disturbance, and sexual dysfunction are problematic for some patients.

The drugs work well at relieving both obsessions and compulsions, although only about three-quarters of patients will respond well. Treatment is long term because patients tend to relapse when the drug is discontinued, often within weeks. Patients who complete a course of behavior therapy are less likely to relapse.

Patients whose symptoms do not respond to the first agent should have serial trials of the other antiobsessional drugs. Augmenting strategies generally are not helpful. An exception is the addition of an antipsychotic drug (e.g., risperidone, 2–6 mg/day) when the patient has a concomitant tic disorder or schizotypal personality disorder.

Psychosurgery has been reported to benefit up to 80% of the patients receiving the surgery, although more recent research shows that 25%–30% of treatment-refractory patients benefit from stereotactic cingulotomy, the most commonly used surgical procedure. Patients should not be referred for psychosurgery unless they fail to respond to proven therapies. Some patients may need to have the surgery repeated, and weeks or months are typically required for optimal improvement.

Supportive psychotherapy is an important adjunct to both behavioral and pharmacological treatments. It is particularly beneficial in helping to restore a patient's low morale and self-esteem, in helping the patient to solve day-to-day problems, and in encouraging treatment compliance. Patients should be encouraged to take risks, such as exposing themselves to feared situations.

Family therapy also has a role in managing OCD. Family members are often ignorant about OCD and get drawn into their relative's rituals in a misguided effort to be helpful. A mother, for example, may be asked to assist in her daughter's cleaning and checking rituals ("Is the stove turned off? Can you check it for me, please?"). In family therapy, the relatives can learn to accept the illness, learn to cope with its manifestations, and learn how not to encourage obsessive-compulsive behavior. Patient support groups are now available in many parts of the United States and are helpful in providing illness education in an atmosphere of mutual support.

Bibliography

Akhtar S, Wig NN, Varma VK, et al: A phenomenological analysis of symptoms in obsessive-compulsive neurosis. Br J Psychiatry 127:342–348, 1975

American Psychiatric Association: Diagnostic and Statistical Manual of Mental Disorders, 4th Edition. Washington, DC, American Psychiatric Association, 1994

American Psychiatric Association: Diagnostic and Statistical Manual of Mental Disorders, 4th Edition Text Revision. Washington, DC, American Psychiatric Association, 2000

Baer L, Jenike MA, Black DW, et al: Effect of Axis II diagnoses on treatment outcome in 55 patients with obsessive-compulsive disorder. Arch Gen Psychiatry 49:862–866, 1992

Baer L, Rauch SL, Ballentine T, et al: Cingulotomy for intractable obsessive-compulsive disorder: prospective long-term follow-up of 18 patients. Arch Gen Psychiatry 52:384–392, 1995

Black DW, Noyes R Jr: Obsessive-compulsive disorder and axis II. Int Rev Psychiatry 9:111–118, 1997

Black DW, Noyes R, Goldstein RB, et al: A family study of obsessive-compulsive disorder. Arch Gen Psychiatry 49:362–368, 1992

Clomipramine Collaborative Study Group: Clomipramine in the treatment of patients with obsessive-compulsive disorder. Arch Gen Psychiatry 48:730–738, 1991

Foa EB, Wilson R: Stop Obsessing! How to Overcome Your Obsessions and Compulsions. New York, Bantam Books, 1991

Greist JH, Jefferson JW, Kobak KA, et al: Efficacy and tolerability of serotonin transport inhibitors in obsessive-compulsive disorder. Arch Gen Psychiatry 52:53–60, 1995

Jenike MA, Buttolph L, Baer L, et al: Open trial of fluoxetine in obsessive-compulsive disorder. Am J Psychiatry 146:909–911, 1989

Jenike MA, Breiter HC, Baer L, et al: Cerebral structural abnormalities in obsessive-compulsive disorder: a quantitative morphometric magnetic resonance imaging study. Arch Gen Psychiatry 53:625–632, 1996

Karno M, Golding JM, Sorenson SB, et al: The epidemiology of obsessive-compulsive disorder in five U.S. communities. Arch Gen Psychiatry 45:1094–1099, 1988

Koran LM, Sallee FR, Pallanti S: Rapid benefit of intravenous pulse loading of clomipramine in obsessive-compulsive disorder. Am J Psychiatry 154:396–401, 1997

Leonard HL, Swedo SE, Lenane MC, et al: A 2-to-7-year follow-up study of 54 obsessive-compulsive children and adolescents. Arch Gen Psychiatry 50:427–439, 1993

Osborn I: Tormenting Thoughts and Secret Rituals. New York, Dell, 1998

Pato MT, Zohar-Kadovich R, Zohar T, et al: Return of symptoms after discontinuation of clomipramine in patients with obsessive-compulsive disorder. Am J Psychiatry 145:1521–1525, 1988

Pauls DL, Alsobrook JP, Goodman W, et al: A family study of obsessive-compulsive disorder. Am J Psychiatry 151:76–84, 1995

Rappoport JL: The Boy Who Couldn't Stop Washing. New York, EP Dutton, 1989

Rasmussen SA, Eisen JL: Epidemiology and clinical features of obsessive-compulsive disorder, in Obsessive-Compulsive Disorders: Theory and Management, 3rd Edition. Edited by Jenike MA, Baer L, Minichiello WE. St. Louis, MO, Mosby, 1998, pp 12–43.

Schwartz JM, Stoessel PW, Baxter LR, et al: Systematic changes in cerebral glucose metabolic rate after successful behavior modification treatment of obsessive-compulsive disorder. Arch Gen Psychiatry 53:109–113, 1996

Skoog G, Skoog I: A 40-year follow-up of patients with obsessive-compulsive disorder. Arch Gen Psychiatry 56:121–127, 1999

Swedo SE, Leonard HL, Garvey M: Pediatric autoimmune neuropsychiatric disorders associated with streptococcal infections: clinical descriptions of the first 50 cases. Am J Psychiatry 155:264–271, 1998

Self-Assessment Questions

1. How is OCD diagnosed?
2. What is the prevalence and gender distribution of OCD?
3. What defense mechanisms are thought to operate in OCD?
4. What evidence supports the neurobiological model?
5. What is the prognosis in OCD? What may change the prognosis of OCD in the future?
6. What is the differential diagnosis of OCD?
7. How are obsessions distinguished from delusions?
8. What are some of the behavioral techniques used to treat OCD?
9. What is the purported mechanism of action of antiobsessional medications?
10. What type of psychosurgery is occasionally performed in patients with OCD?

12 Somatoform and Related Disorders

So it is that a patient can confront his doctor with his symptoms, and put on him the whole onus of their cure.

Mayer-Gross, Slater, and Roth, *Clinical Psychiatry*

Somatoform disorders are characterized by physical complaints that occur in the absence of an identifiable medical explanation. These conditions have been noted throughout recorded time and continue to baffle patients and practitioners alike. These disorders are typically seen by primary care physicians and other specialists, such as neurologists and cardiologists, rather than by psychiatrists. In studies of primary care patients, the proportion with somatic complaints for which no physical cause was detected ranged from 10% to 30%; in specialty clinics, the proportion is even higher.

Seven somatoform disorders are described in DSM-IV-TR (see Table 12–1). They all share the common feature of excessive concern with bodily symptoms unexplained by physical or laboratory evidence.

History

Although we now recognize several discrete somatoform disorders, their history has overlapped. Somatization disorder, formerly known as *hysteria,*

TABLE 12–1.   DSM-IV-TR somatoform disorders

Somatization disorder

Conversion disorder

Hypochondriasis

Body dysmorphic disorder

Pain disorder

    With psychological factors

    With both psychological factors and a general medical condition

Undifferentiated somatoform disorder

Somatoform disorder not otherwise specified

was recognized in ancient Greece, wherein physicians thought it resulted from a displaced uterus. Their treatment was to draw the "wandering uterus" back to its proper place by placing aromatic substances in the region of the vagina. Although Galen rejected this idea, the theory of uterine pathology persisted until Willis suggested that hysteria was caused by a brain disturbance.

Hypochondriasis, meanwhile, is a term derived from the Greek, with the literal meaning of "below the cartilage," which refers to the area under the ribs where various organs are located. The term has been used since the seventeenth century to refer to changes in mental state thought to be due to diseased organs of the hypochondrium, which, it was believed, led to a preoccupation with bodily symptoms. In the seventeenth century, Sydenham suggested a close relation between hysteria and hypochondriasis, and over the next two centuries, clinicians viewed hypochondriasis as the masculine version of hysteria, which occurred mostly in women.

In the nineteenth century, Charcot, a distinguished neurologist working at the Salpêtrière in Paris, became interested in the bizarre and baffling manifestations of hysteria. He believed that intense emotions could produce hysterical symptoms in suggestible people. Hysteria later drew Freud's attention in the early years of psychoanalysis. His interest began while working in Paris with Charcot, who had been treating hysteria with hypnosis. Psychoanalysts focused their theories on hysteria, which they viewed as a manifestation of unconscious conflicts.

In their seminal book on hysteria, Freud and his associate Breuer argued that hysterical patients have emotionally charged memories stored out of reach in the unconscious mind. *Conversion* was believed to be the ego-defense mechanism whereby psychic energy was converted into physical symptoms, and this was thought to give rise to both *primary gain* (i.e., the anxiety arising from a psychological conflict) and *secondary gain* (i.e., support and sympathy from family and friends).

Gradually, the term *hysteria* lost its original meaning, and the adjective *hysterical* was used to label any demanding patient whose symptoms were unexplained. For that reason, a neutral term, *Briquet's syndrome,* was proposed in the 1960s. Paul Briquet, a French physician, had described hysteria as a polysymptomatic disorder in 1859. His concept was used to develop diagnostic criteria (i.e., Briquet's checklist), which were later modified for inclusion in DSM-III, DSM-III-R, DSM-IV, and DSM-IV-TR as *somatization disorder.*

Although hysteria and hypochondriasis were once believed to be similar, the latter term became restricted to more vague, less clearly delineated complaints of pain and discomfort. Hypochondriacal persons were viewed as morbidly preoccupied with bodily sensations and function, unlike hysterical persons, who showed *la belle indifférence* (i.e., a strange lack of concern with the symptoms). Freud furthered the distinction between these disorders by classifying hypochondriasis as a true neurosis, which implied that common everyday disturbances (e.g., sexual frustration) played a role in its etiology, whereas hysteria was conceptualized as a psychoneurosis (e.g., determined by early life experiences).

The acceptance of hypochondriasis as a distinct disorder has continued to wax and wane. In the early twentieth century, it was considered a valid disorder, but this view was later challenged by some who regarded hypochondriacal symptoms as secondary to other disorders, such as depression.

Somatization Disorder

Somatization disorder begins early in life, affects mostly women, and is characterized by multiple somatic symptoms that are medically unexplained. The physical complaints, often dramatically described, involve most organ systems and include pain, anxiety and depression, and pseudoneurological, gastrointestinal, and sexually related symptoms. To receive the diagnosis, patients must have at least eight unexplained symptoms, including four pain, two gastrointestinal, one sexual, and one pseudoneurological symptom (see Table 12–2). For the symptoms to meet the criteria, they cannot be fully explained by a general medical condition, and the complaints or impairment must be greater than would be expected from the history, physical examination, or laboratory findings. In making the diagnosis, it is useful to have old medical charts available and to interview the patient on more than one occasion. Because of their numerous complaints, patients may not recall old symptoms and may not have sufficient time to report new symptoms in one sitting. The frequency of common symptoms in somatization disorder is summarized in Table 12–3, and complaints from a typical patient are presented in Table 12–4.

TABLE 12–2. DSM-IV-TR diagnostic criteria for somatization disorder

A. A history of many physical complaints beginning before age 30 years that occur over a period of several years and result in treatment being sought or significant impairment in social, occupational, or other important areas of functioning.

B. Each of the following criteria must have been met, with individual symptoms occurring at any time during the course of the disturbance:

   (1) *four pain symptoms*:   a history of pain related to at least four different sites or functions (e.g., head, abdomen, back, joints, extremities, chest, rectum, during menstruation, during sexual intercourse, or during urination)

   (2) *two gastrointestinal symptoms:*   a history of at least two gastrointestinal symptoms other than pain (e.g., nausea, bloating, vomiting other than during pregnancy, diarrhea, or intolerance of several different foods)

   (3) *one sexual symptom:*   a history of at least one sexual or reproductive symptom other than pain (e.g., sexual indifference, erectile or ejaculatory dysfunction, irregular menses, excessive menstrual bleeding, vomiting throughout pregnancy)

   (4) *one pseudoneurological symptom*   a history of at least one symptom or deficit suggesting a neurological condition not limited to pain (conversion symptoms such as impaired coordination or balance, paralysis or localized weakness, difficulty swallowing or lump in throat, aphonia, urinary retention, hallucinations, loss of touch or pain sensation, double vision, blindness, deafness, seizures; dissociative symptoms such as amnesia; or loss of consciousness other than fainting)

C. Either (1) or (2):

   (1) after appropriate investigation, each of the symptoms in Criterion B cannot be fully explained by a known general medical condition or the direct effects of a substance (e.g., a drug of abuse, a medication)

   (2) when there is a related general medical condition, the physical complaints or resulting social or occupational impairment are in excess of what would be expected from the history, physical examination, or laboratory findings

D. The symptoms are not intentionally produced or feigned (as in Factitious Disorder or Malingering).

Although a simple count of symptoms appears arbitrary, research has shown that this approach identifies a homogeneous group of patients who have a predictable course and outcome. The diagnosis is reliable and stable

TABLE 12–3. Common symptoms in somatization disorder

Symptom	%	Symptom	%
Nervousness	92	Sexual indifference	44
Back pain	88	Dysuria	44
Weakness	84	Aphonia	44
Joint pain	84	Other bodily pains	36
Dizziness	84	Vomiting	32
Extremity pain	84	Anesthesia	32
Fatigue	84	Thoughts of suicide	28
Abdominal pain	80	Burning pains in rectum,	28
Nausea	80	vagina, mouth	
Headache	80	Lump in throat	28
Dyspnea	72	Felt life was hopeless	28
Trouble doing anything because of	72	Weight loss	28
feeling bad		Anorgasmia	24
Chest pain	72	Diarrhea	20
Abdominal bloating	68	Vomiting all 9 months of	20
Constipation	64	pregnancy	
Anxiety attacks	64	Blindness	20
Depressed feeling	64	Fits or convulsions	20
Visual blurring	64	Fluctuations in weight	16
Anorexia	60	Unconsciousness	16
Palpitations	60	Paralysis	12
Fainting	56	Visual hallucinations	12
Dyspareunia	52	Attempted suicide	12
Menstrual irregularity	48	Amnesia	8
Food intolerance	48	Urinary retention	8
Excessive menstrual bleeding	48	Dysmenorrhea (prepregnancy	8
Dysmenorrhea (other)	48	only)	
Phobias	48	Dysmenorrhea (premarital	4
		only)	
		Deafness	4

Source. Adapted from Perley and Guze 1962.

over time. The following case example illustrates the variety and stability of symptoms found in somatization disorder. The case also illustrates how these patients receive inappropriate diagnoses and unnecessary diagnostic evaluations by physicians unfamiliar with the syndrome.

> Carol, a 26-year-old housewife, first presented for medical evaluation with a chief complaint of weakness and malaise of 1 year's duration. She report-

TABLE 12–4. Complaints from a typical somatization disorder patient

Organ system	Complaint
Neuropsychiatric	"The two hemispheres of my brain aren't working properly." "I couldn't name familiar objects around the house when asked." "I was hospitalized with tingling and numbness all over, and the doctors didn't know why."
Cardiopulmonary	"I had extreme dizziness after climbing stairs." "It hurts to breathe." "My heart was racing and pounding and thumping....I thought I was going to die."
Gastrointestinal	"For 10 years I was treated for nervous stomach, spastic colon, and gall bladder, and nothing the doctor did seemed to help." "I got a violent cramp after eating an apple and felt terrible the next day." "The gas was awful—I thought I was going to explode."
Genitourinary	"I'm not interested in sex, but I pretend to be to satisfy my husband's needs." "I've had red patches on my labia, and I was told to use boric acid." "I had difficulty with bladder control and was examined for a tipped bladder, but nothing was found." "I had nerves cut going into my uterus because of severe cramps."
Musculoskeletal	"I have learned to live with weakness and tiredness all the time." "I thought I pulled a back muscle, but my chiropractor says it's a disc problem."
Sensory	"My vision is blurry. It's like seeing through a fog, but the doctor said that glasses wouldn't help." "I suddenly lost my hearing. It came back, but now I have whistling noises, like an echo."
Metabolic/endocrine	"I began teaching half days because I couldn't tolerate the cold." "I was losing hair faster than my husband."

ed other symptoms as well: burning pain in her eyes, muscular aches and pains in her lower back, headaches, a stiff neck, abdominal pain "on both sides and below the navel," and vomiting "glassy white stuff—as if I were poisoned." Nine months earlier, Carol had been hospitalized for evaluation of the abdominal pain and had a barium enema examination and upper gastrointestinal X-ray series. The test results were normal.

Six months before her clinic visit, Carol had developed blurry vision and a sharp shooting pain in her rectum with walking and had reported passing blood and mucus in her stools. A sigmoidoscopic examination was unremarkable, but she was nevertheless given a diagnosis of mild ulcerative colitis and started on sulfasalazine therapy. Another barium enema examination had negative results. Five months before her clinic visit, she noted "wasting" of her hands and reported needing a larger glove size for the right hand. She also was concerned with a pulsating vessel and whitish nodules on her hand.

Other medical complaints developed, including joint pains, malaise, blotching and red spots on her skin in response to sun exposure, and swelling of her right ankle, both knees, elbows, wrists, and shoulders. Carol noticed multiple bruises that were slow to heal. Three months before her clinic visit, a physician had diagnosed rheumatoid arthritis (despite a normal sedimentation rate) and had administered injections of cortisone and adrenocorticotropic hormone.

At her clinic visit, Carol identified additional symptoms: a burning pain in her pelvis, hands, and feet; heavy vaginal bleeding passing "clots as large as a fist"; abdominal bloating; malodorous stools with "bits of sudsy mucus"; urinary urgency; cough incontinence; tingling in hands and feet; and a belief that her bowel movements "just don't look right." She also disclosed a 10-year history of recurrent tonsillitis and quinsy during her childhood.

Carol was next seen at the same clinic 21 years later after referral by her primary care physician for evaluation of multiple somatic complaints. Her symptoms were remarkably similar to those reported earlier, and it soon became clear that she had never been free of them. Her complaints included a right-sided tremor that caused her to spill food, migratory aches and pains, a feeling of coldness in her extremities, and a heavy menstrual flow ("I used 48 sanitary pads in a single day"). In addition, she reported feeling sick; having abdominal bloating, flatulence, and frequent nausea and vomiting; and being constipated. She was concerned that her skin was becoming darker and that her scalp hair was falling out.

A lengthy medical workup followed and included thyroid function studies, a thyroid uptake scan, a rheumatoid factor, an antinuclear antibody titer, electromyography, and consultations from neurology, ophthalmology, and gynecology. Carol reported to the neurologist a history of convulsions 10 years earlier, which she believed had left her with a residual tremor. She told the consultant of having been concerned with facial sagging, which had prompted a previous neurologist to consider the diagnosis of myasthenia gravis. The ophthalmologist obtained a history of double vision requiring six changes in eyeglass prescription during the past year because of deteriorating vision. She confirmed a history of heavy and painful bleeding to the gynecologist and also a history of five dilation and curettage procedures over the previous 10 years. She also complained of a yellowish discharge during the last 4 days of her cycle that had an "odor of semen."

Six years later, she was admitted to the University of Iowa Psychiatric Hospital. During the intervening years, she had received a total hysterectomy and oophorectomy, but apart from menstrually related symptoms, she continued to have the same unrelenting physical complaints. Again, a protracted medical workup was negative.

Carol's remarkable history of illness spanning 27 years leaves little doubt that she had an unrecognized somatization disorder. Her complaints were consistent over the years and had led to many unnecessary evaluations and procedures. Despite the multiplicity of her complaints, many quite alarming, Carol remained fit and physically healthy.

In the Epidemiologic Catchment Area study, somatization disorder was shown to have a lifetime prevalence of about 0.4% in the general population. The disorder is more common in rural areas and among those with less education. Many women with the disorder report histories of sexual molestation as children. Few patients experience significant improvement or complete remission of symptoms.

Somatization disorder often leads to repeated surgeries, drug abuse, marital instability, major depression, and suicide attempts. Most patients with somatization disorder also have personality disorders; between one-half and two-thirds meet criteria for an unstable or dramatic personality disorder (e.g., histrionic, borderline).

Somatization disorder runs in families, and hereditary factors may be important in the etiology; about 20% of the first-degree female relatives of patients with somatization disorder have the disorder themselves. Family studies also show a link between somatization disorder and antisocial personality. First-degree male relatives of patients with somatization disorder have high rates of both antisocial personality and alcoholism. These findings have led to the hypothesis that depending on the gender of the individual, genetic and/or environmental factors lead to different, but overlapping, clinical syndromes.

The differential diagnosis of somatization disorder includes panic disorder, major depression, and schizophrenia. Patients with panic disorder typically report multiple physical symptoms, but they occur almost exclusively during panic attacks. Patients with major depression often present with physical complaints, but dysphoria and vegetative symptoms of depression (e.g., appetite loss, lack of energy, insomnia) are prominent. Schizophrenic patients sometimes have physical complaints, but they are typically bizarre or delusional (e.g., "my spine is a set of twirling plates"). Although somatic complaints are common in these disorders, the syndromes are sufficiently distinctive that the diagnosis of somatization disorder should not be difficult.

Conversion Disorder

Conversion disorder involves symptoms (or deficits) affecting motor or sensory functions that suggest a neurological or general medical condition; pain is purposely excluded from the definition. (Patients whose major complaint is limited to pain are given pain disorder diagnoses.) In addition, the physician will have determined that the symptom is not under voluntary control and cannot, after appropriate investigation, be explained by a known neurological or medical illness. Psychological factors are associated with the symptoms, as suggested by their initiation or exacerbation after stressful situations. Furthermore, the symptom must not be intentionally produced or feigned and is not a culturally sanctioned behavior. (The criteria are listed in Table 12–5.)

TABLE 12–5.   DSM-IV-TR diagnostic criteria for conversion disorder

A.   One or more symptoms or deficits affecting voluntary motor or sensory function that suggest a neurological or other general medical condition.

B.   Psychological factors are judged to be associated with the symptom or deficit because the initiation or exacerbation of the symptom or deficit is preceded by conflicts or other stressors.

C.   The symptom or deficit is not intentionally produced or feigned (as in Factitious Disorder or Malingering).

D.   The symptom or deficit cannot, after appropriate investigation, be fully explained by a general medical condition, or by the direct effects of a substance, or as a culturally sanctioned behavior or experience.

E.   The symptom or deficit causes clinically significant distress or impairment in social, occupational, or other important areas of functioning or warrants medical evaluation.

F.   The symptom or deficit is not limited to pain or sexual dysfunction, does not occur exclusively during the course of Somatization Disorder, and is not better accounted for by another mental disorder.

Specify type of symptom or deficit:

   With Motor Symptom or Deficit
   With Sensory Symptom or Deficit
   With Seizures or Convulsions
   With Mixed Presentation

Typical conversion symptoms include paralysis, abnormal movements, inability to speak (aphonia), blindness, and deafness. Conversion symptoms usually conform to the patient's concept of disease rather than to recognized physiological patterns. For example, anesthesia may follow a stocking-and-glove pattern, not a dermatomal distribution. Conversion symptoms sometimes occur in patients with mood disorders, somatization disorder, or schizophrenia. In these situations, both diagnoses are made.

Conversion symptoms are surprisingly common. An estimated 20%–25% of the patients admitted to neurology wards have conversion symptoms. In a survey of consecutive psychiatric consultations in a general hospital, 5% of the patients had conversion symptoms. Conversion symptoms are more common in women than in men, in patients from rural areas, and in persons with less education or low socioeconomic status.

Conversion disorder has been explained in psychodynamic, biological, cultural, and behavioral terms. According to the psychodynamic interpretation, patients with certain developmental predispositions respond to particular types of stress with conversion symptoms. The stress causes anxiety by awakening unconscious conflicts, usually over issues involving sexuality, aggression, or dependency. The high frequency of conversion symptoms in patients with earlier brain injury, however, suggests a biological etiology. A study of conversion disorder patients in Australia and Great Britain found that 64% of the patients had coexisting or antecedent brain disorders, such as epilepsy, tumor, or stroke, compared with only 6% of the control patients. Sociologists point out that various ethnic and social (generally non-European) groups are more likely to respond to emotional stress with conversion symptoms than are other groups. Behaviorists see conversion symptoms as a learned excess or deficit that follows a particular event or psychological state and is reinforced by a particular event or set of conditions.

The diagnosis of conversion disorder is established by ruling out medical or neurological illness as a cause of the symptoms and by identifying psychological factors involved in the initiation or exacerbation of the symptom. It is usually not difficult to rule out medical illness when a patient's somatic complaints are inconsistent with physical examination findings and evidence of psychological stress is clear. Yet research shows that up to 30% of patients given diagnoses of conversion disorder are later found to have medical or neurological illnesses that, in retrospect, accounted for their symptoms.

There are many useful clues that the clinician can use to help establish a diagnosis of conversion disorder. Studies of patients with conversion symptoms have found that coexisting mood and anxiety disorders, somatization disorder, schizophrenia, and various personality disorders are frequent. Thus, an unexplained symptom in a patient with a serious psychiatric disorder or a history of conversion symptoms is likely to represent a new conversion symptom. Patients sometimes mimic symptoms based on their experience with an illness or model them on the symptoms of an illness observed in an important person in their life (e.g., a figure from childhood). Contrary to common belief, *la belle indifférence* is not typical of patients with conversion disorder, who are generally quite interested in their symptoms.

A favorable outcome is generally associated with acute onset, a precipitating stressful event, good premorbid adjustment, and the absence of medical or neurological comorbidity. One follow-up study found that 83% of the inpatients and outpatients were well or improved at a 4- to 6-year follow-up; another study found that 100% of the outpatients with conversion symptoms had an immediate favorable response to treatment, with only 20% experiencing a relapse at the end of a 1-year follow-up. Because conversion disorder usually occurs in the context of another psychiatric disorder, it is likely that the outcome reflects the natural history of the primary disorder, such as major depression, somatization disorder, or borderline personality disorder.

Hypochondriasis

Hypochondriasis is defined as a preoccupation with fears of having, or the belief that one has, a serious disease based on the person's misinterpretation of bodily symptoms (Table 12–6). This preoccupation persists after appropriate medical evaluation has ruled out the presence of a medical disorder that could account for the symptoms; furthermore, other mental disorders such as schizophrenia, major depression, or somatization disorder have been ruled out as a cause of the disturbance. Hypochondriasis has a duration of 6 months or more.

TABLE 12–6. DSM-IV-TR diagnostic criteria for hypochondriasis

---

A. Preoccupation with fears of having, or the idea that one has, a serious disease based on the person's misinterpretation of bodily symptoms.

B. The preoccupation persists despite appropriate medical evaluation and reassurance.

C. The belief in Criterion A is not of delusional intensity (as in Delusional Disorder, Somatic Type) and is not restricted to a circumscribed concern about appearance (as in Body Dysmorphic Disorder).

D. The preoccupation causes clinically significant distress or impairment in social, occupational, or other important areas of functioning.

E. The duration of the disturbance is at least 6 months.

F. The preoccupation is not better accounted for by Generalized Anxiety Disorder, Obsessive-Compulsive Disorder, Panic Disorder, a Major Depressive Episode, Separation Anxiety, or another Somatoform Disorder.

Specify if:

> **With Poor Insight:** if, for most of the time during the current episode, the person does not recognize that the concern about having a serious illness is excessive or unreasonable

---

Hypochondriacal patients show an abnormal concern with their health and tend to amplify normal physiological sensations and misinterpret them as signs of disease. These patients often fear a particular disease (e.g., cancer or acquired immunodeficiency syndrome [AIDS]) and cannot be reassured despite careful and repeated examinations. The following vignette illustrates a case of hypochondriasis seen in our hospital:

> Mabel, an 80-year-old retired schoolteacher, was admitted for evaluation of an 8-month preoccupation with having colon cancer. The patient had a history of single vessel coronary artery disease and diabetes mellitus (controlled by oral hypoglycemic agents) but was otherwise well. She had no history of mental illness. On admission, Mabel reported her concern about having colon cancer, which her two brothers had developed. As evidence of a possible tumor, she reported having diffuse abdominal pain and cited an abnormal barium enema examination 1 year earlier. (The examination had revealed diverticulosis.) Because of her concern about having cancer, Mabel had seen 11 physicians, but each in turn had been unable to reassure her that she did not have cancer.
>
> Despite her complaint, Mabel denied depressed mood and displayed a full affect. She reported sleeping less than usual but attributed this to her abdominal discomfort.
>
> Mabel was pleasant and cooperated well with the ward team. She chose not to socialize with other patients, whom she characterized as "crazy." She remained preoccupied with the possibility that she had cancer despite our reassurance. A benzodiazepine was prescribed for her sleep disturbance, but she refused any other type of psychiatric treatment.

Unlike somatization disorder, which starts early in life and mainly affects women, hypochondriasis may begin at any age and appears to be equally common in men and women. The prevalence of hypochondriasis in the general population is unknown, but 2%–7% of the patients seen by primary care physicians have the disorder. Of course, unexplained physical symptoms are relatively common, and from 60% to 80% of healthy persons report such symptoms in any given week; intermittent worry about illness occurs in about 10%–20% of well persons. Most persons can be reassured by physicians that their symptoms are benign, but the hypochondriacal patient is rarely reassured for very long.

Like patients with somatization disorder, hypochondriacal patients may have complaints involving many organ systems, "doctor-shop," and receive multiple workups and unnecessary surgery. Hypochondriacal patients also are at risk for drug addiction as a result of their ongoing physical complaints.

Hypochondriacal symptoms commonly occur in the course of mood or anxiety disorders, which must be ruled out. When hypochondriacal symptoms occur in the course of another illness, such as panic disorder, treatment of the primary disorder often will lead to a reduction in hypochondriacal symptoms. When hypochondriasis is the primary disorder, remission appears unlikely, and a waxing and waning course is typical.

Pain Disorder

Pain in one or more anatomical sites is the major symptom in pain disorder; psychological factors are believed to have an important role in its etiology (see Table 12–7). Two subtypes are specified: pain associated with psychological factors and pain associated with both psychological factors and a general medical condition. The disorder is termed *acute* if the duration is less than 6 months and *chronic* if the duration is 6 months or longer. Some researchers believe that the pain associated with this disorder represents a conversion symptom. Such pain often appears to be related to environmental stressors, such as the loss of a loved one. It generally occurs in the absence of identifiable medical or neurological illness or is grossly out of proportion to that expected from the physical pathology. A patient seen in our clinic illustrated this disorder:

> Nancy, a 34-year-old schoolteacher, developed disabling lower back pain coincidental to a work-related lawsuit in which she alleged unfair treatment by her co-workers. She attributed her back pain to a fall 6 months earlier in which she had twisted her ankle; extensive neurological and orthopedic evaluations had failed to document any physiological abnormality. She became preoccupied with her back pain and stopped working. Her social life became constricted and consisted mainly of attending a support group for persons with chronic pain.

Chronic pain is one of the most common reasons that patients consult physicians. One study found that 13% of the patients in an internal medicine practice had chronic pain; in a health maintenance organization–based sample, 8% of the patients had severe persistent pain, and 2.7% had at least 7 days of pain-related restricted activity within the past 6 months. Low back pain is estimated to affect more than 7 million persons in the United States. Pain disorders are also costly economically because of health care costs and loss of work productivity. Patients with pain disorder are more likely to be seen by internists and general practitioners than by psychiatrists because their complaints are viewed as physical, and psychiatric symptoms (e.g., depressed mood) are often denied.

Chronic pain is one of the most vexing symptoms a patient can develop.

TABLE 12–7. DSM-IV-TR diagnostic criteria for pain disorder

A. Pain in one or more anatomical sites is the predominant focus of the clinical presentation and is of sufficient severity to warrant clinical attention.

B. The pain causes clinically significant distress or impairment in social, occupational, or other important areas of functioning.

C. Psychological factors are judged to have an important role in the onset, severity, exacerbation, or maintenance of the pain.

D. The symptom or deficit is not intentionally produced or feigned (as in Factitious Disorder or Malingering).

E. The pain is not better accounted for by a Mood, Anxiety, or Psychotic Disorder and does not meet criteria for Dyspareunia.

Code as follows:

307.80 **Pain Disorder Associated With Psychological Factors:** psychological factors are judged to have the major role in the onset, severity, exacerbation, or maintenance of the pain. (If a general medical condition is present, it does not have a major role in the onset, severity, exacerbation, or maintenance of the pain.) This type of Pain Disorder is not diagnosed if criteria are also met for Somatization Disorder.

Specify if:

Acute: duration of less than 6 months

Chronic: duration of 6 months or longer

307.89 **Pain Disorder Associated With Both Psychological Factors and a General Medical Condition:** both psychological factors and a general medical condition are judged to have important roles in the onset, severity, exacerbation, or maintenance of the pain. The associated general medical condition or anatomical site of the pain (see below) is coded on Axis III.

Specify if:

Acute: duration of less than 6 months

Chronic: duration of 6 months or longer

Note: The following is not considered to be a mental disorder and is included here to facilitate differential diagnosis.

Pain Disorder Associated With a General Medical Condition: a general medical condition has a major role in the onset, severity, exacerbation, or maintenance of the pain. (If psychological factors are present, they are not judged to have a major role in the onset, severity, exacerbation, or maintenance of the pain.) The diagnostic code for the pain is selected based on the associated general medical condition if one has been established or on the anatomical location of the pain if the underlying general medical condition is not yet clearly established—for example, low back (724.2), sciatic (724.3), pelvic (625.9), headache (784.0), facial (784.0), chest (786.50), joint (719.40), bone (733.90), abdominal (789.0), breast (611.71), renal (788.0), ear (388.70), eye (379.91), throat (784.1), tooth (525.9), and urinary (788.0).

Pain sensitivity and expression depend not only on personality and prior emotional adjustment but also on cultural factors about how pain is experienced and biological factors relating to neural pathways. Following injury, the sensitivity of pain receptors and the excitability of neurons in the spinal cord may change. Pain thresholds may change after neurological injury, and pain-producing substances such as substance P and histamine can alter pain threshold.

Unexplained pain often occurs in the course of other psychiatric disorders, including mood and anxiety disorders and other somatoform disorders. In one study, 60% of depressed patients reported pain. Depression is a frequent consequence of chronic pain, although few pain patients have the marked vegetative symptoms typical of major depression. Thus, the clinician must determine whether a major depression is also present in the patient with a pain disorder. If present, the depression may respond to antidepressant medication, and the distress related to the pain may be alleviated. Suicide always must be kept in mind as a possible consequence of chronic pain.

Other Somatoform Disorders

DSM-IV-TR has three residual categories—body dysmorphic disorder (BDD), undifferentiated somatoform disorder, and somatoform disorder not otherwise specified—for patients who do not show the characteristics of the four major somatoform disorders.

Body Dysmorphic Disorder

A patient with BDD, or dysmorphophobia, usually is preoccupied with an imagined defect in appearance rather than having more diffuse complaints. For this reason, BDD is sometimes referred to as a disease of imagined ugliness. This condition must be differentiated from monohypochondriacal paranoia (delusional disorder, somatic type), in which a patient has a delusional belief that a body part is grossly deformed and distorted. In BDD, the patient is not delusional and is willing to acknowledge that his or her concerns may be exaggerated. Patients with BDD tend to focus on imagined defects involving their face and head, but any body part may become a focus of concern, including the genitals. Mirror checking, comparing oneself with others, camouflaging the affected body part, ritualized grooming, and requesting reassurance are typical. Many patients with BDD, particularly those concerned with their facial appearance, undergo repeated plastic surgery

procedures in their search for a defect-free appearance but are rarely satisfied. The following case example is of a patient with BDD seen in our clinic:

> Arthur first began to think of his face as a problem when he was a senior in
> high school. He noticed that when his face was in repose, his brows would
> droop over his eyes and give him a "devious look." He also noticed that his
> jawline seemed weak and receding. He tried to camouflage these "defects"
> by keeping his lower jaw jutted forward and his eyebrows raised. His at-
> tempts at camouflage became almost habitual, but he consulted a surgeon
> to obtain a jaw augmentation and have his eyebrows raised because he felt
> the camouflaging made him self-conscious and decreased his spontaneity.
>
> Arthur was a good student in high school, participated in a few activ-
> ities, and dated occasionally. He had not had a close relationship with a girl
> and had not had sexual intercourse. He described a brief "bad period" in
> high school during which he rebelled against family standards, stopped
> studying, and smoked marijuana. After several months of this behavior, he
> began to feel depressed, apathetic, guilt-ridden, and paranoid, although he
> did not meet criteria for major depression and did not have any delusions
> or hallucinations. The episode passed when he stopped rebelling and using
> marijuana. He later completed 1 year of college but then dropped out to
> work and thus obtain money for cosmetic surgery. After the surgery, he
> planned to return to college. One day he hoped to attend medical school
> and pursue a career in psychiatry.
>
> Arthur was a rather handsome young man with heavy, dark eyebrows
> but a perfectly normal, perhaps even prominent, jawline. He related his
> motivation for seeking surgery to his general pattern of pursuing perfection
> in all aspects of life. He considered himself well adjusted and normal and,
> in fact, superior to most people. He saw no need for psychiatric treatment
> and refused a recommendation for a trial of serotonin reuptake inhibitors.

BDD may be a variant of obsessive-compulsive disorder, and the treatment is similar. In one study, 70% of the patients receiving a serotonin reuptake inhibitor improved. A positive response leads to decreased distress,
less time spent preoccupied with the "defect," and improved social and occupational functioning. In near delusional forms of BDD, an antipsychotic
added to the serotonin reuptake inhibitor may be helpful. Cognitive-behavioral therapy also can be beneficial. Patients are instructed to stay away from
mirrors, remove their makeup, or take off their hats. Supportive counseling
can help to boost morale, provide hope, and offer insight into the disorder.

Undifferentiated Somatoform Disorder and Somatoform Disorder Not Otherwise Specified

The diagnosis of undifferentiated somatoform disorder is reserved for patients with one or more physical complaints not explained by a known gen-

eral medical condition or pathophysiological mechanism. It lasts at least 6 months, and symptoms do not meet criteria for another somatoform disorder.

The category somatoform disorder not otherwise specified is reserved for patients whose somatoform symptoms do not meet criteria for a more specific disorder.

Clinical Management of the Somatoform Disorders

The development of effective treatments has caused a revolution in contemporary psychiatric practice, particularly for patients with psychotic, mood, or anxiety disorders. The same cannot be said of patients with somatoform disorders. The fundamental management of these disorders has not changed substantially in several decades. Nonetheless, physicians are now more aware of these disorders and recognize that even simple management strategies can have a profound effect on the care and treatment of somatizing patients.

Recommendations for the management of somatization disorder, hypochondriasis, and pain disorder are similar, so they are discussed together. Based on their experience, clinicians generally agree on treatment approaches. First, the physician should follow the Hippocratic oath and "do no harm." Because symptoms are often exaggerated or misidentified (e.g., minor spotting during the menses may be reported as "gushing"), physicians frequently overreact and pursue the diagnostic equivalent of a "wild goose chase." Patients with somatoform disorders often provoke unnecessary evaluations, surgical procedures, or medication that may have little relevance to the underlying condition. Thus, it is essential that physicians who evaluate patients with multiple unexplained symptoms make a proper diagnosis. The nonpsychiatric physician may find a psychiatric consultation helpful in pinpointing the diagnosis and in formulating a treatment plan. A proper diagnosis will help to place the patient's symptoms into proper perspective. A sensible treatment plan will help to ensure that unnecessary interventions and surgeries are avoided.

Second, the physician should see somatizing patients at regular intervals; implicit in this approach is the message that new symptoms are not required to see a physician. In fact, it is advisable initially to set specific appointments at brief intervals. The purpose of these visits is to listen attentively and convey concern without inquiring in detail about the physical symptoms. By avoiding placing the focus on the patient's symptoms, the physician conveys the message that physical complaints are not the most important or interesting feature about the patient.

Third, the physician should minimize the use of psychotropic drugs and prescription analgesics. Somatoform disorder patients often request—or demand—medications, but there is usually little indication for them. Whether medication is ever justified, given that these patients are at risk for substance abuse, is debatable. No data show that medication is beneficial in treating somatization disorder; therefore, drug treatment is not indicated unless another psychiatric syndrome develops that may be amenable to such treatment (e.g., major depression or panic disorder). Antidepressant medications may help relieve major depression, or block panic attacks, yet have little effect on an underlying somatization disorder. As a general rule, benzodiazepines should be avoided because of their abuse potential.

Finally, the physician should realize that the lives of patients with these disorders revolve around their symptoms and that many patients will resist referral for psychiatric treatment. The most important therapeutic approach available to the primary physician, therefore, is an empathic doctor-patient relationship. Ideally, he or she should become the patient's primary and only physician. The physician's goal is not to cure the patient but to help him or her function at as high a level as possible.

These simple measures (see box) have been shown to lower health care costs in patients with somatization disorder. A group of patients receiving a psychiatric consultation with recommendations for conservative care (i.e., essentially these measures) had a 53% decline in health care costs, mostly as a result of fewer hospitalizations. The patients' health status or satisfaction with their health care remained the same. Health care costs of control subjects did not change.

The patient with hypochondriasis may additionally benefit from individual psychotherapy that involves education about illness and selective perception of symptoms. Cognitive-behavioral therapy can help to correct misinterpretations of internal stimuli reported by hypochondriacal persons. Serotonin reuptake inhibitors have been reported to be effective in treating hypochondriasis. One particular form of hypochondriasis, illness phobia, has been reported to respond to imipramine, a tricyclic antidepressant.

The treatment of conversion disorder has not been well established, but reassurance and suggestion usually are appropriate measures, along with efforts to resolve any stressful situation that may have provoked the symptoms. The spontaneous remission rate for acute conversion symptoms is high, so that even without any specific intervention, most patients will improve and probably not have any serious complications. A treatment approach using behavioral modification has been described in which the patient is placed at complete bed rest with the use of a bedpan and is in-

Recommendations for management of somatoform disorders
1. The patient should be scheduled for brief but frequent visits.
• As the patient improves, the time between visits can be extended.
2. An empathic relationship should be established to reduce the patient's tendency to doctor-shop.
• The primary physician should become the patient's only physician.
3. The clinician should focus on psychosocial problems, not the physical symptoms.
• The clinician should not try to talk patients out of their symptoms or tell them it is "all in their head."
• To the patient, the symptom is real and distressing.
4. The use of psychotropic drugs should be minimized.
• No medication has proven value in somatoform disorders. Exceptions may be hypochondriasis and body dysmorphic disorder, in which serotonin reuptake inhibitors appear to be of benefit.
• These patients may become dependent on drugs, particularly sedative-hypnotics.
5. Medical evaluations should be minimized to reduce expense and iatrogenic complications.
• Simple (i.e., conservative) management is proven to reduce costs.

formed that use of ward facilities will parallel his or her improvement. As the patient improves, the time out of bed is gradually increased until full privileges are restored. Nearly all patients (84%) who had conversion symptoms (ranging from blindness to bilateral wrist drop) treated in this manner experienced full remission. By allowing the patient to save face, this method has the advantage of keeping secondary gain (e.g., escaping from noxious activities, obtaining desired attention from family, friends, and others) to a minimum.

In treating conversion disorder, hospital staff should remain supportive and show concern while encouraging self-help. The disorder can be explained to the patient as the body's involuntary response to psychological stress. It is rarely helpful to confront patients about their symptoms or make them feel ashamed or embarrassed ("It's all in your head"). The pain or weakness is quite real to patients; it may be helpful for the physician to communicate his or her awareness of this as he or she explains that the treatment will be conservative and will emphasize rehabilitation rather than medication.

Some experts believe that hypnosis or intravenous amobarbital sodium (e.g., Amytal interview) may help the patient to relive the events that provoked the conversion symptoms and to abreact (or express) accompanying emotions. Other clinicians have recommended psychodynamic psychotherapy, focusing on childhood sexual behavior and other problems that they believe are central to the etiology of conversion. These techniques are probably no more effective than the conservative approach just described.

Related Disorders

Several conditions are related to the somatoform disorders in which physical illnesses are mimicked. Factitious disorders are given their own category in DSM-IV-TR, whereas malingering is grouped with the V-code conditions, which are diagnoses that are not attributable to mental illness but are a focus of clinical attention or treatment.

Factitious Disorders

Factitious disorders involve the intentional production (or feigning) of physical or psychological symptoms. Patients with factitious disorders have no obvious external incentive for the behavior, such as economic gain, better care, or improved physical well-being (see Table 12–8). It is thought that these patients fake physical or emotional illnesses for unconscious reasons.

TABLE 12–8.   DSM-IV-TR diagnostic criteria for factitious disorder

---

A. Intentional production or feigning of physical or psychological signs or symptoms.

B. The motivation for the behavior is to assume the sick role.

C. External incentives for the behavior (such as economic gain, avoiding legal responsibility, or improving physical well-being, as in Malingering) are absent.

Code based on type:

> 300.16 **With Predominantly Psychological Signs and Symptoms:**   if psychological signs and symptoms predominate in the clinical presentation
>
> 300.19 **With Predominantly Physical Signs and Symptoms:**   if physical signs and symptoms predominate in the clinical presentation
>
> 300.19 **With Combined Psychological and Physical Signs and Symptoms:**   if both psychological and physical signs and symptoms are present but neither predominates in the clinical presentation

---

Some persons with the disorder appear to make hospitalization a way of life and have been called "hospital hobos" or "peregrinating problem patients." The term *Munchausen syndrome* also has been used to describe patients who move from hospital to hospital simulating various illnesses. The name Munchausen comes from the fictitious wanderings of the nineteenth-century Baron Von Munchausen, known for his tall tales and fanciful exaggeration. Cases of Munchausen syndrome by proxy have even been noted: a parent induces illness or simulates illness in his or her child so that the child is repeatedly hospitalized.

The frequency of factitious disorder is unknown because many cases go undetected. In one study involving persons with a fever of unknown origin, up to 10% of the fevers were diagnosed as factitious. The variety of maladies induced by patients with such disorders is limited only by their imagination. Patients with factitious disorders typically use one of three strategies: 1) they report symptoms suggesting an illness, without having them; 2) they produce false evidence of an illness (e.g., a factitious fever produced by applying friction to a thermometer to raise the temperature); or 3) they intentionally produce symptoms of illness (e.g., by injecting feces into a knee joint or taking warfarin orally to induce a bleeding disorder). Some of the more common methods for producing symptoms are presented in Table 12–9.

Although most cases of factitious disorder involve the simulation of physical illness, some patients feign mental illness. This form of factitious disorder is probably less common, and the diagnosis can be extremely difficult to make because of the lack of objective physical or laboratory abnormalities associated with psychiatric illness. Patients may report depression, delusions, or auditory hallucinations, or they may behave in a bizarre manner—all in an attempt to simulate mental illness. In a follow-up of nine patients with factitious psychosis, the patients remained emotionally disturbed and had poor social functioning. All had severe personality disorders.

Research suggests that factitious disorders are chronic and begin in early adulthood. They often develop in persons who have had experience with hospitalization or severe illness, involving either themselves or someone close to them, such as a parent. The disorder causes severe impairment of social and occupational functioning and is usually associated with severe character pathology (e.g., borderline, antisocial personality). In one study, most of the factitious disorder patients had worked in health care occupations, including medicine, nursing, and medical technology. Most subjects had abnormal personality traits, but none was given a diagnosis of a major mental disorder (i.e., Axis I disorder). Nearly all were women.

Some experts believe that the patient with factitious disorder conscious-

TABLE 12–9.   Methods used to produce symptoms in patients with a factitious disorder

Method	%
Injection or insertion of contaminated substance	29
Surreptitious use of medications	24
Exacerbation of wounds	17
Thermometer manipulation	10
Urinary tract manipulation	7
Falsification of medical history	7
Self-induced bruises or deformities	2
Phlebotomy	2

Source.   Adapted from Reich and Gottfried 1983.

ly produces the signs or symptoms of physical illness to obtain medical care. Although patients are aware of their role in producing signs and symptoms of illness, they are typically unaware of their motivation for doing so. According to one interpretation, factitious disorder patients experienced emotional deprivation at the hands of absent or inattentive parents but received love and caring from health care givers. By producing illness, these patients re-create the nurturing atmosphere that they had experienced earlier in life from health care givers. Yet, not all patients with factitious disorders have a background of emotional deprivation or nurturance from health care professionals, so this theory applies to only some patients.

The differentiation of factitious disorder from somatoform disorders and malingering, based on presumed psychological mechanisms, is shown in Table 12–10.

The diagnosis of a factitious disorder requires almost as much inventiveness as is shown by the patient in producing symptoms. Clues to the diagnosis include a lengthy and involved medical history that does not correspond to the patient's apparent health and vigor, a clinical presentation that too closely resembles textbook descriptions, a sophisticated medical vocabulary, demands for specific medications or treatments, and a history of excessive surgeries. Previous hospital charts should be gathered and prior clinicians contacted when a factitious disorder is suspected. In one intriguing case reported in the literature, the authors were able to document at least 15 different hospitalizations in a 2-year period and found that the medical evaluations had included repeated cardiac catheterizations and angiograms and had resulted in the loss of a limb. In this particular patient, clues to the diagnosis included the manner in which the patient presented his story, the absence of family or friends at the hospital, the presence of multiple surgical scars, and an absence of distress despite complaints of crushing retrosternal pain.

TABLE 12–10. Differentiating among the somatoform disorders, factitious disorders, and malingering

Disorder	Mechanism of illness production	Motivation for illness production
Somatoform disorders[a]	Unconscious	Unconscious
Factitious disorder	Conscious	Unconscious
Malingering	Conscious	Conscious

[a]Includes somatization disorder, conversion disorder, hypochondriasis, and pain disorder.
Source. Adapted from Eisendrath 1984.

The treatment of factitious disorder is difficult and frustrating. The first task is to make the diagnosis so that additional and potentially harmful procedures are avoided. Because many of these patients are hospitalized on medical and surgical wards, a psychiatric consultation should be obtained. The psychiatrist can help make the diagnosis and educate the treatment team about the nature of factitious disorders. Once sufficient evidence has been gathered to support the diagnosis, the patient should be confronted in a nonthreatening manner by the attending physician and the consulting psychiatrist. In a follow-up of 42 patients with factitious disorder, 33 were confronted. None signed out of the hospital or became suicidal, but only 13 acknowledged causing their disorders; most improved after the confrontation, and 4 became asymptomatic. The authors reported that their lawyers had advised that room searches could be justified legally and ethically in their pursuit of a diagnosis. Like the suicidal patient whose belongings are searched for dangerous objects, the factitious disorder patient also has a potentially life-threatening condition.

Malingering

Malingering is defined as the intentional production of false or grossly exaggerated physical or psychological symptoms motivated by external incentives, such as avoiding military conscription or duty, avoiding work, obtaining financial compensation, evading criminal prosecution, obtaining drugs, or securing better living conditions.

Unlike factitious disorder, in which symptoms are produced for presumably unconscious reasons, malingering is produced intentionally for reasons that are apparent to the malingerer. Most malingerers are male, and most have obvious reasons to feign illness. They are often prisoners, factory workers, or persons living in unpleasant settings where an illness may provide a temporary escape from harsh responsibilities and hospitalization a temporary sanctuary.

Malingering should be suspected when any of the following clues are present: medicolegal context of presentation (e.g., the person is being referred by his or her attorney for examination); marked discrepancy between the person's claimed disability and objective findings; lack of cooperation during the diagnostic evaluation and noncompliance with the treatment regimen; and the presence of an antisocial personality disorder. Symptoms that malingering patients report are often vague, subjective, and unverifiable.

There is some debate about the correct approach to take with the malingerer. Some experts believe that malingering patients should be confronted once sufficient evidence has been collected to confirm the diagnosis. Others feel that confrontations will simply disrupt the doctor-patient relationship and make the patient even more alert to possible detection in the future. Clinicians who take the second position feel that the best approach is to treat the patient as though the symptoms were real. The symptoms can then be given up in response to treatment without the patient losing face.

Bibliography

American Psychiatric Association: Diagnostic and Statistical Manual of Mental Disorders, 3rd Edition Revised. Washington, DC, American Psychiatric Association, 1987

American Psychiatric Association: Diagnostic and Statistical Manual of Mental Disorders, 4th Edition. Washington, DC, American Psychiatric Association, 1994

American Psychiatric Association: Diagnostic and Statistical Manual of Mental Disorders, 4th Edition Text Revision. Washington, DC, American Psychiatric Association, 2000

Andreasen NC, Bardach J: Dysmorphophobia: symptom or disease? Am J Psychiatry 134:673–676, 1977

Barsky AJ, Fama JM, Bailey ED, et al: A prospective 4- to 5-year study of DSM-III-R hypochondriasis. Arch Gen Psychiatry 55:737–744, 1998

Bash IY, Alpert M: The determination of malingering. Ann N Y Acad Sci 347:86–99, 1980

Blumer D, Heilbronn M: Antidepressant treatment for chronic pain: treatment outcome of 1,000 patients with the pain prone disorders. Psychiatric Annals 14:796–800, 1984

Eisendrath SJ: Factitious illness: a clarification. Psychosomatics 25:110–117, 1984

Fallon BA, Klein BW, Liebowitz MR: Hypochondriasis: treatment strategies. Psychiatric Annals 23:374–381, 1993

Gureje O, Simon GE, Ustun TB, et al: Somatization in cross-cultural perspective: a World Health Organization study in primary care. Am J Psychiatry 154:989–995, 1997

Kellner R: Hypochondriasis and somatization. JAMA 258:2718–2722, 1987

Lilienfeld SO, VanValkenberg C, Larntz K, et al: The relationship of histrionic personality disorder to antisocial personality and somatization disorders. Am J Psychiatry 143:718–722, 1986

Morrison J: Childhood sexual histories of women with somatization disorder. Am J Psychiatry 146:239–241, 1989

Noyes R, Reich J, Clancy J, et al: Reduction in hypochondriasis with treatment of panic disorder. Br J Psychiatry 149:631–635, 1986

Noyes R, Kathol RG, Fisher MM, et al: The validity of DSM-III-R hypochondriasis. Arch Gen Psychiatry 50:961–970, 1993

Noyes R, Holt CS, Kathol RG: Somatization: diagnosis and management. Arch Gen Psychiatry 4:790–795, 1995

Noyes R, Holt CS, Happel RL, et al: A family study of hypochondriasis. J Nerv Ment Dis 185:223–232, 1997

Perley MJ, Guze SB: Hysteria: the stability and usefulness of clinical criteria. N Engl J Med 266:421–426, 1962

Phillips KA: The Broken Mirror: Understanding and Treating Body Dysmorphic Disorder. New York, Oxford University Press, 1996

Pope HG, Jonas JM, Jones B: Factitious psychosis: phenomenology, family history, and long-term outcome of nine patients. Am J Psychiatry 139:1480–1483, 1982

Reich P, Gottfried LA: Factitious disorders in a teaching hospital. Ann Intern Med 99:240–247, 1983

Shah KA, Forman MB, Freedman HS: Munchausen's syndrome and cardiac catheterization: a case of a pernicious interaction. JAMA 248:3008–3009, 1982

Simon GE, Von Korff M: Somatization and psychiatric disorder in the NIMH Epidemiologic Catchment Area study. Am J Psychiatry 148:1494–1500, 1991

Slater ETO, Glithero E: A follow-up of patients diagnosed as suffering from "hysteria." J Psychosom Res 9:9–13, 1965

Smith GR, Monson RA, Ray DC: Psychiatric consultation in somatization disorder. N Engl J Med 314:1407–1413, 1986

Turner M: Malingering. Br J Psychiatry 171:409–411, 1997

Warwick HMC, Clark DM, Cobb AM, et al: A controlled trial of cognitive behavioral therapy of hypochondriasis. Br J Psychiatry 169:189–195, 1996

Wesner RB, Noyes R: Imipramine, an effective treatment for illness phobia. J Affect Disord 22:43–48, 1991

Self-Assessment Questions

1. What is the origin of the terms *hysteria* and *hypochondriasis?*
2. How is somatization disorder diagnosed?
3. What do family studies of somatization disorder show?
4. Explain conversion as an ego-defense mechanism.
5. What are the risk factors for conversion disorder?
6. What is the natural history of the different somatoform disorders?
7. How does somatization disorder differ from hypochondriasis?
8. How are the somatoform disorders managed?
9. How do the somatoform disorders, factitious disorders, and malingering differ?

13 Dissociative Disorders

> In a bright, unfamiliar voice that sparkled, the woman said "Hi, there, Doc!"
>
> Corbett Thigpen and Hervey Cleckley,
> *The Three Faces of Eve*, 1957

The hallmark of dissociative disorders is a disturbance of or alteration in the normally well-integrated functions of identity, memory, and consciousness. They include the amnestic states (dissociative amnesia and dissociative fugue), dissociative identity disorder (formerly multiple personality disorder), and depersonalization disorder. A residual category exists for dissociative disorders that do not meet the criteria for a more specific disorder (see Table 13–1).

From their initial description in the nineteenth century, dissociative symptoms—dramatic personality changes and strange memory disturbances—have baffled physicians and patients alike. Early observers generally viewed these phenomena as being part of a hysterical syndrome. Charcot, the great neurologist at the Salpêtrière in Paris, proposed that specific mental functions could be separated from conscious awareness and function independently. His extensive description of *la grande hysterie* mainly focused on the sensorimotor symptoms observed in his patients: paralyses, convulsions, and contractures. It was his disciple Janet who attributed disorders of memory and consciousness to hysteria. He thought that psychological stress or

TABLE 13–1.   Dissociative disorders

Amnestic states

   Dissociative amnesia

   Dissociative fugue

Dissociative identity disorder (formerly multiple personality disorder)

Depersonalization disorder

Dissociative disorder not otherwise specified

hereditary factors could cause a split—or dissociation—of memories and their associations from other mental elements, leading to amnesia, fugues, or multiple personality. Freud, also a pupil of Charcot, hypothesized that hysterical phenomena—both physical and mental—resulted when memories of childhood sexual abuse (real or imagined) were reactivated later in life. Repression is considered a mental mechanism in which unacceptable memories are pushed out of conscious awareness.

Despite the intense interest of physicians in these disorders at the turn of the century, dissociative syndromes—especially multiple personality—fell into disrepute. Many psychiatrists came to believe that these symptoms were caused by hypnosis and that they were being manipulated by patients. Yet, as professional interest waned, cases of multiple personality continued to accumulate in the literature, and experience with soldiers in both world wars showed that complaints of amnesia were relatively common. In the last few decades, interest has grown as new generations of psychiatrists have begun to study these disorders, and surveys show that up to 10% of the general population experience dissociative symptoms at some point during their lives.

Amnestic States

Psychologically motivated memory loss is called *dissociative amnesia* (see Table 13–2). The disorder is defined as one or more episodes of inability to recall important personal information, usually of a traumatic or stressful nature, considered too extensive to be explained by ordinary forgetfulness. With dissociative amnesia, the person is typically confused and perplexed. The individual may not recall significant personal information or even his or her own identity. The amnesia typically develops suddenly and can last from minutes to days, or even longer. In one case series, 79% of the amnestic episodes lasted less than a week.

TABLE 13–2. DSM-IV-TR diagnostic criteria for dissociative amnesia

A. The predominant disturbance is one or more episodes of inability to recall important personal information, usually of a traumatic or stressful nature, that is too extensive to be explained by ordinary forgetfulness.
B. The disturbance does not occur exclusively during the course of Dissociative Identity Disorder, Dissociative Fugue, Posttraumatic Stress Disorder, Acute Stress Disorder, or Somatization Disorder and is not due to the direct physiological effects of a substance (e.g., a drug of abuse, a medication) or a neurological or other general medical condition (e.g., Amnestic Disorder Due to Head Trauma).
C. The symptoms cause clinically significant distress or impairment in social, occupational, or other important areas of functioning.

The prevalence of dissociative amnesia is unknown, but it has been reported to occur after severe physical or psychosocial stressors (e.g., natural disasters, war). In a study of combat veterans, between 5% and 20% were amnesic for their combat experiences. It has been estimated that from 5% to 14% of all military psychiatric casualties experience amnesia to some extent.

Dissociative fugue is characterized by amnesia with inability to recall one's past and the assumption of a new identity, which may be partial or complete (see Table 13–3). The fugue usually involves sudden, unexpected travel away from home or one's workplace, is not due to a dissociative identity disorder, and is not induced by a substance or a general medical condition (e.g., temporal lobe epilepsy). Like dissociative amnesia, fugue states are reported to occur in psychologically stressful situations, such as natural disasters or war. Personal rejections, losses, or financial pressures are reported to have preceded the fugue in some cases. Fugues can last for months and lead to a complicated pattern of travel and identity formation.

TABLE 13–3. DSM-IV-TR diagnostic criteria for dissociative fugue

A. The predominant disturbance is sudden, unexpected travel away from home or one's customary place of work, with inability to recall one's past.
B. Confusion about personal identity or assumption of a new identity (partial or complete).
C. The disturbance does not occur exclusively during the course of Dissociative Identity Disorder and is not due to the direct physiological effects of a substance (e.g., a drug of abuse, a medication) or a general medical condition (e.g., temporal lobe epilepsy).
D. The symptoms cause clinically significant distress or impairment in social, occupational, or other important areas of functioning.

A case example of a woman who had a fugue follows:

Carrie, a 31-year-old attorney from a small midwestern town, was reported as missing for 4 days under mysterious circumstances. Carrie was known to have finished her day at work and to have exercised at a health spa but had failed to return home. Her car was found abandoned. A search was mounted, and it was assumed that she had been abducted or murdered, especially after a headless corpse was found. Candlelight vigils were held, psychics were consulted, and friends blanketed the community with posters offering rewards for help in locating her.

One month after her disappearance, Carrie called her father from Las Vegas, where she had been the entire time. She was at a local hospital and claimed to have had amnesia. Carrie reported that she was physically assaulted while jogging on the night of her disappearance. During the struggle, she had been knocked unconscious: "When I came to, I was dazed, confused, and disoriented." She felt that the assault had prompted the amnesia, leading her to forget her past. She later hitchhiked to Las Vegas, where she was found wandering aimlessly. The police took her to a nearby hospital, where she claimed a new identity.

With the help of a psychologist who used hypnosis, Carrie quickly recovered her memory and her identity. She returned home and resumed her legal practice. Her family and friends had described her as a "creature of habit," but otherwise normal, and were as baffled as Carrie about her amnesia. She had no prior mental illness.

The differential diagnosis of dissociative amnesia or fugue includes many medical and neurological conditions that can cause memory impairment (e.g., a brain tumor, closed head trauma, dementia), as well as the effects of a substance (e.g., alcohol-induced blackouts). Before assuming that the amnesia or fugue is psychologically motivated, medical and neurological conditions and substance abuse must be ruled out. A workup should include a thorough physical examination, mental status examination, toxicological studies, an electroencephalogram, and other tests when indicated. (See Table 6–5 in Chapter 6 for a complete medical workup.) The chief distinction will be among the various dissociative disorders, medical or neurological conditions, the direct effects of a substance, and malingering.

As a general rule, the onset and termination of amnestic and fugue states due to medical illness or to the effect of a substance are unlikely to be associated with psychological stress. Memory impairment is more likely to be severe for recent than for remote events and to resolve slowly if at all; in these cases, memory only rarely recovers fully. Disturbances in attention, disorientation, and labile affect are characteristic of many brain disorders (e.g., brain tumors, strokes, Alzheimer's disease) but are unlikely in dissociative amnesia. Memory loss from alcohol intoxication (blackouts) is characterized by impaired short-term recall and evidence of heavy substance abuse. Malingering involves claiming amnesia for behaviors that are alleged to be out of character when obvious reasons exist for secondary gain (e.g., claiming amnesia for a crime). Careful observation in a hospital setting can help to clarify the diagnosis.

Recovery from dissociative amnesia or fugue tends to occur spontaneously. In fugue states, recovery of past memories and the resumption of the former identity may occur abruptly over several hours but can take much longer. Both conditions can reoccur, particularly when the precipitating stressors remain or return. Hypnosis and interviews conducted under the influence of intravenous sodium amobarbital (Amytal) have been reported to help patients recover missing memories. (See Chapter 27 for a discussion of the "Amytal interview.") When memories return, patients should be helped to understand their motivation behind the memory loss and to resolve any issues that may have led to the disturbance.

Dissociative Identity Disorder

Dissociative identity disorder (DID) is characterized by the presence of two or more distinct identities or personality states, each with its own relatively enduring pattern of perceiving, relating to, and thinking about the environment and self (see Table 13–4). A personality state is not as well developed or as well integrated in both thinking and behavior as an identity. In some cases, there may be at least two fully developed identities, whereas in others there may be only one distinct identity and one or more personality states. According to DSM-IV-TR, at least two of these identities or personality states recurrently take full control of the person's behavior. Although DID has been described for centuries, most lay conceptions are based on media presentations. The most famous portrayals are found in *The Three Faces of Eve* and *Sybil,* both of which provide detailed accounts of women with many strikingly different personalities.

The prevalence of DID is unknown, but it is reportedly rare. In the past few decades, the number of reported cases has grown, and some experts believe that the disorder is common in both inpatient and outpatient settings. This reported increase in the frequency of DID has led some to question whether cases of the disorder are the creation of well-meaning therapists who unwittingly induce the phenomenon. They point out that through attention, suggestion, and the process of hypnosis itself, additional personalities can be created in suggestible patients. These same experts observe that

TABLE 13–4. DSM-IV-TR diagnostic criteria for dissociative identity disorder

A. The presence of two or more distinct identities or personality states (each with its own relatively enduring pattern of perceiving, relating to, and thinking about the environment and self).

B. At least two of these identities or personality states recurrently take control of the person's behavior.

C. Inability to recall important personal information that is too extensive to be explained by ordinary forgetfulness.

D. The disturbance is not due to the direct physiological effects of a substance (e.g., blackouts or chaotic behavior during Alcohol Intoxication) or a general medical condition (e.g., complex partial seizures). **Note:** In children, the symptoms are not attributable to imaginary playmates or other fantasy play.

when ignored, the different personalities subside because they no longer gain the therapist's attention.

From 75% to 90% of the patients with DID are women. The disorder is thought to have a childhood onset, usually before age 9 years, and is chronic. DID may be familial because it has been described as occurring in multiple generations and in siblings within families.

The cause of DID is unknown. Some experts believe that the disorder is causally related to the effects of severe physical and sexual abuse during early childhood. They hold that DID results from self-induced hypnosis, which the person uses as a means of coping with the psychological effects of abuse, emotional maltreatment, or neglect. Some experts compare DID with posttraumatic stress disorder, a condition caused by the psychological effects of a life-threatening situation.

According to one large case series, the mean number of personalities in DID patients is 7, although approximately one-half had more than 10 personalities. During the course of the disorder, different personalities vary in the percentage of the time they control an individual's behavior. The transition from one personality to another may be sudden or gradual. The switches are thought to be brought on by stressful situations, disputes among the personalities, or deep-seated psychological conflicts. The personalities may or may not be aware of the other *alters.*

Some of the more common symptoms reported by patients with DID, as well as characteristics of their alternate personalities, are presented in Table 13–5.

A case example of a relatively typical patient with DID seen at our hospital follows:

TABLE 13–5. Common symptoms in patients with dissociative identity disorder and characteristics of alternate personalities ("alters") in 50 patients

Symptoms	%	Alternate personality characteristics	%
Markedly different moods	94	Amnestic personalities	100
Exhibiting an alter	84	Personalities with proper names	98
Different accents	68	(e.g., Nick, Sally)	
Inability to remember angry outbursts	58	Angry alternate personality	80
Inner conversations	58	Depressed alternate personality	74
Different handwriting	34	Personalities of different ages	66
Different dress or makeup	32	Suicidal alternate personality	62
Unfamiliar people know them well	18	Protector alternate personality	30
Amnesia for a previously learned subject	14	Self-abusive alternate personality	30
Discovery of unfamiliar possessions	14	Opposite-sexed alternate personality	26
Different handedness	14	Personality with nonproper names (e.g., "observer," "teacher")	24
		Unnamed alternate personality	18

Source. Adapted from Coons et al. 1988.

Cindy, a 24-year-old, was transferred to our hospital to facilitate community placement. Cindy had received a diagnosis of multiple personality disorder, although in the past she had received diagnoses of chronic schizophrenia, borderline personality disorder, schizoaffective disorder, and bipolar disorder.

Cindy had been well until 3 years before admission. At that time, she developed depression, "voices," multiple somatic complaints, periods of amnesia, and repeated wrist cutting. Her family and friends became concerned with her abrupt changes in mood and thought that Cindy had become a pathological liar because she would do or say things that she would later deny. Her chronic depression and recurrent suicidal behavior led to frequent hospitalization. Cindy received trials of antipsychotics, antidepressants, mood stabilizers, and anxiolytics, all with little or no benefit. Cindy's condition continued to worsen.

Cindy was friendly, neatly groomed, and diminutive. She reported that she had heard voices from nine separate personalities but had no formal thought disorder. She had learned about her many personalities with the help of a therapist during one of her earlier hospitalizations. The alters ranged in age from 2 to 48 years, and two were masculine. Cindy's main concern was her inability to control the switches among the personalities, which made her feel out of control. Cindy reported that she had been sexually abused by her father as a child. She described visual hallucinations consisting of visions of her father coming at her with a knife. We were unable to confirm the history of sexual abuse but thought that it was likely based on what we learned of her early chaotic home life.

Cindy was cooperative with the treatment team. Nursing staff observed several episodes when the patient switched to one of her troublesome alters. Cindy's voice would change in inflection and tone, and she became childlike. (Cindy told us that at these times, Joy, an 8-year-old alter, took control.) Arrangements were made for individual psychotherapy, and Cindy was discharged to the community.

At a follow-up 3 years later, Cindy still had many personalities but was functioning better, had fewer switches, and lived independently. She continued to see a therapist weekly and hoped to one day integrate her many alters.

Patients with DID often meet criteria for other psychiatric disorders. Like Cindy, many have unexplained physical complaints and may fulfill criteria for somatization disorder; headaches and amnesia ("losing time") are particularly common. Borderline personality disorder is found in up to 70% of DID patients and is diagnosed on the basis of mood instability, identity disturbance, deliberate self-harm, and other symptoms characteristic of the disorder. Many DID patients report psychotic symptoms such as auditory hallucinations (voices) and may have a prior diagnosis of schizophrenia, schizoaffective disorder, or psychotic mood disorder, all of which must be ruled out. Both their symptoms and their ability to function may fluctuate, and multiple prior diagnoses are the rule.

Observant clinicians note that patients with DID tend to report that voices originate within their heads, are not experienced with the ears (or as a percept), and are not associated with mood changes; insight generally is preserved. Patients with psychotic disorders usually report that auditory hallucinations "come from the outside," have the quality of a percept (as opposed to one's own thoughts), and often produce corresponding changes in mood or affect (delusional mood); insight is minimal. The hallucinations reported with DID are best considered *pseudohallucinations,* that is, hallucinations brought about by the exercise of one's imagination and accompanied by the realization that the experience is due to illness and is not real.

Many experts believe that long-term psychotherapy is of value in helping patients to integrate their personalities, and at least one study has shown that motivated patients treated by experienced therapists achieved integration of their personalities and remission of symptoms. Other aspects of treatment remain controversial. Some experts use hypnosis or intravenous amobarbital sodium, or both, to help access the different personalities in the course of psychotherapy. Some therapists now use cognitive-behavioral therapy to help patients achieve reintegration. All experts agree that therapy is lengthy and difficult.

Although the core features of DID do not respond to medication, typical patients have many mood and anxiety symptoms that do respond to drug therapy. For example, antidepressants may relieve coexisting major depression and block panic attacks. Some experts claim that different personalities require different medications. Although this claim may have some theoretical value, it runs counter to known pathophysiological mechanisms of the major disorders.

Depersonalization Disorder

Depersonalization disorder is characterized by periods in which a person feels detached from his or her own mental processes (or body) and feels that he or she is an outside observer. A person may describe experiencing a dream-like state (see Table 13–6). Depersonalization makes the person feel mechanical and separated from his or her thoughts, emotions, or identity. Some individuals describe themselves as feeling like robots or automatons. Depersonalization may be accompanied by *derealization,* a sense of detachment, unreality, and altered relation to the outside world.

The prevalence of depersonalization disorder is unknown, but it is more common in women. Many people who are otherwise normal have transiently experienced mild forms of depersonalization. For example, transient depersonalization can occur when a person is sleep deprived, travels to unfamiliar places, or is intoxicated with hallucinogens, marijuana, or alcohol. In a study of college students, between one-third and one-half of the respondents reported having experienced depersonalization. A similarly high frequency has been reported in persons exposed to life-threatening situations, such as traumatic accidents. For these reasons, depersonalization disorder is diagnosed only when it is severe and persistent and causes marked distress.

The disorder typically starts in adolescence or early adulthood but rarely after age 40 years. Many persons vividly recall their first episode of depersonalization, which is often abrupt and without a precipitating stressor. Some report a precipitating event, such as smoking marijuana. The duration of depersonalization episodes is highly variable. Episodes can last hours, days, or weeks. The symptoms of depersonalization disorder tend to wax and wane; although it is typically chronic and continuous, some persons ex-

---

TABLE 13–6. DSM-IV-TR diagnostic criteria for depersonalization disorder

A. Persistent or recurrent experiences of feeling detached from, and as if one is an outside observer of, one's mental processes or body (e.g., feeling like one is in a dream).

B. During the depersonalization experience, reality testing remains intact.

C. The depersonalization causes clinically significant distress or impairment in social, occupational, or other important areas of functioning.

D. The depersonalization experience does not occur exclusively during the course of another mental disorder, such as Schizophrenia, Panic Disorder, Acute Stress Disorder, or another Dissociative Disorder, and is not due to the direct physiological effects of a substance (e.g., a drug of abuse, a medication) or a general medical condition (e.g., temporal lobe epilepsy).

---

perience periods of remission. Exacerbations may follow psychologically stressful situations, such as the loss of an important relationship.

The cause of depersonalization disorder is unknown. Freud postulated that depersonalization allowed a person to deny painful or unacceptable feelings by denying one's experience of self. Depersonalization also could represent an adaptive response to overwhelming stress, perhaps explaining why some cases begin after serious traumatic accidents. The fact that depersonalization frequently accompanies several central nervous system disturbances (e.g., temporal lobe epilepsy, tumors, stroke, encephalitis, migraine) suggests a biological basis. One recent theory of depersonalization holds that the state of increased alertness seen in patients with depersonalization disorder results from an activation of prefrontal attentional systems combined with a reciprocal inhibition of the anterior cingulate, which causes "mind emptiness."

Some have linked depersonalization with obsessive-compulsive disorder; these investigators point out that patients may be preoccupied with their depersonalization symptoms and repetitively scrutinize themselves to check out feelings of unreality. Conditions in which depersonalization symptoms can occur, including schizophrenia, major depression, phobias, panic disorder, obsessive-compulsive disorder, drug abuse, and sleep deprivation, must be ruled out. Medical illness (e.g., partial complex seizures or migraine) and drug-induced states need to be ruled out as well.

There are no proven treatments for this disorder, but benzodiazepines may be of help in managing the accompanying anxiety (e.g., diazepam, 5 mg three times daily). Serotonin reuptake inhibitors (e.g., fluoxetine, 20 mg/day) and clomipramine (150–250 mg/day) have been reported to relieve symptoms of depersonalization. Patients also have been reported to benefit from hypno-therapy or cognitive-behavioral therapy to help control their episodes of dep-ersonalization. With cognitive-behavioral therapy, patients learn to confront their distorted thoughts and challenge their feelings of unreality.

Management of Dissociative Disorders

Recommendations for the clinical management of dissociative disorders are summarized in the box.

Recommendations for management of dissociative disorders

1. Medical causes of dissociation must be ruled out.

2. The therapist should be patient and supportive. In most cases of amnesia, return of memory is rapid and complete.

3. The sodium amobarbital (Amytal) interview may be helpful both diagnos-tically and therapeutically in patients with amnesia (see Chapter 27).

   • The interview will help many patients to recover missing memories.

   • The interview can be helpful diagnostically in separating psychological from medical causes of amnesia. The patient with psychologically moti-vated amnesia may experience a return of memory, and the patient with medically induced amnesia will become more confused.

4. Patients with dissociative identity disorder are especially problematic, and therapy may be long term. The clinician may want to refer the patient to a therapist experienced in treating dissociative identity disorder.

   • It may be best to help the patient gradually learn about the number and nature of their personalities.

   • A goal with these patients should be to help them learn how to control their switches and accept responsibility for their actions.

5. Medications have no proven value in treating dissociative disorders; an ex-ception is that depersonalization disorder may respond to serotonin reuptake inhibitors (e.g., fluoxetine, paroxetine, sertraline) or clomipramine.

   • Benzodiazepines may be of help in reducing the anxiety that often ac-companies depersonalization (e.g., diazepam, 5 mg three times daily).

Bibliography

American Psychiatric Association: Diagnostic and Statistical Manual of Mental Disorders, 4th Edition. Washington, DC, American Psychiatric Association, 1994

American Psychiatric Association: Diagnostic and Statistical Manual of Mental Disorders, 4th Edition Revised. Washington, DC, American Psychiatric Association, 2000

Andreasen PJ, Seidel JA: Behavioral techniques in the treatment of patients with multiple personality disorder. Ann Clin Psychiatry 4:29–32, 1992

Coons PM, Bohman ES, Milstein V: Multiple personality disorder: a clinical investigation of 50 cases. J Nerv Ment Dis 176:519–527, 1988

Ellason JW, Ross CA: Two year follow-up of inpatients with dissociative identity disorder. Am J Psychiatry 154:832–839, 1997

Fahy TA: The diagnosis of multiple personality disorder: a critical review. Br J Psychiatry 153:597–600, 1988

Guralnik O, Schmeidler J, Simeon D: Feeling unreal: cognitive processes in depersonalization. Am J Psychiatry 157:103–109, 2000

Lauer J, Black DW, Keen P: Multiple personality disorder and borderline personality disorder: distinct entities or variations on a common theme? Ann Clin Psychiatry 5:129–134, 1993

Mersky H: The manufacture of personalities—the production of multiple personality disorder. Br J Psychiatry 160:327–340, 1992

Piper A: Multiple personality disorder. Br J Psychiatry 164:600–612, 1994

Rifkin A, Ghisalbert D, Dimatov S, et al: Dissociative identity disorder in psychiatric inpatients. Am J Psychiatry 155:844–845, 1998

Ross CA, Miller SD, Reagor P, et al: Structured interview data on 102 cases of multiple personality disorder from four centers. Am J Psychiatry 147:596–601, 1990

Saxe GN, Vander Kolk BA, Berkowitz R, et al: Dissociative disorders in psychiatric inpatients. Am J Psychiatry 150:1037–1042, 1993

Schenk L, Bear D: Multiple personality and related dissociative phenomena in patients with temporal lobe epilepsy. Am J Psychiatry 138:1311–1315, 1981

Schreiber FR: Sybil. Chicago, IL, Henry Regnery, 1973

Sierra M, Berrios GE: Depersonalization: neurobiologic perspectives. Biol Psychiatry 44:898–908, 1998

Simeon D, Gross S, Guralnik O, et al: Feeling unreal: 30 cases of DSM-III-R depersonalization disorder. Am J Psychiatry 154:1107–1113, 1997

Simeon D, Stein DJ, Hollander E: Treatment of depersonalization disorder with clomipramine. Biol Psychiatry 44:302–303, 1998

Thigpen CH, Cleckley HM: The Three Faces of Eve. New York, McGraw-Hill, 1957

Tutkun H, Sar V, Yarte I, et al: Frequency of dissociative disorder among psychiatric inpatients in a Turkish insanity clinic. Am J Psychiatry 155:800–805, 1998

Self-Assessment Questions

1. What is dissociation?
2. How does dissociative amnesia differ from dissociative fugue?
3. What is the differential diagnosis of the dissociative disorders?
4. What is the current popular etiological theory of DID?
5. What is depersonalization, and how common is it?
6. Why has depersonalization disorder been compared with obsessive-compulsive disorder?

14 Alcohol-Related Disorders

At such gruesome moments, I would solace myself with thoughts of the wondrous gifts of alcohol, the manna that mankind so seldom appreciates.

W.C. Fields

Persons in virtually all cultures have consumed alcoholic beverages for medicinal purposes, for religious ceremony, and for recreation. It is likely that since the days when cave dwellers first drank beverages made from fermented juices and grains, alcohol has also led to trouble. Drunkenness was condemned in the Old Testament as early as the story of Noah and in later years was thought to represent Satan's influence. Nonetheless, production of all types of liquors, wine, and beer flourished over the centuries, and attempts at controlling alcohol production and distribution, such as during the Prohibition era in the United States, largely failed. Only Islamic countries have successfully proscribed the use of alcohol.

The disease concept of alcoholism took root in the nineteenth century, starting with the work of the American physician Benjamin Rush and the British physician Thomas Trotter. By the turn of the century, institutions had opened for the treatment of alcoholism, and societies and journals devoted to the study of the disorder were established. The disease concept lost popularity during Prohibition but was revived after World War II, due in part to the influence of Jellinek's *Disease Concept of Alcoholism,* published in 1960, and in part to the great number of returning veterans with alcohol-related problems. Whether alcoholism is a disease is still being debated, yet both the American Medical Association and the American Psychiatric Association have endorsed the disease model. Its value has been to encourage problem drinkers to seek help in a humane and nonjudgmental way.

Definition

The concept of a general drug-dependent syndrome is embedded in DSM-IV-TR and has been endorsed by the World Health Organization. As a result, all substance use disorders, including alcohol abuse and dependence, follow the same set of criteria (Tables 14–1 and 14–2). The definition of substance abuse requires a maladaptive pattern of substance use leading to significant impairment or distress, as manifested by at least one of four problem areas (e.g., job, physical hazard, legal, interpersonal) occurring during a 12-month period. Furthermore, the person has never met criteria for substance dependence.

TABLE 14–1. DSM-IV-TR criteria for substance abuse

A. A maladaptive pattern of substance use leading to clinically significant impairment or distress, as manifested by one (or more) of the following, occurring within a 12-month period:

    (1) recurrent substance use resulting in a failure to fulfill major role obligations at work, school, or home (e.g., repeated absences or poor work performance related to substance use; substance-related absences, suspensions, or expulsions from school; neglect of children or household)

    (2) recurrent substance use in situations in which it is physically hazardous (e.g., driving an automobile or operating a machine when impaired by substance use)

    (3) recurrent substance-related legal problems (e.g., arrests for substance-related disorderly conduct)

    (4) continued substance use despite having persistent or recurrent social or interpersonal problems caused or exacerbated by the effects of the substance (e.g., arguments with spouse about consequences of intoxication, physical fights)

B. The symptoms have never met the criteria for Substance Dependence for this class of substance.

TABLE 14–2. DSM-IV-TR criteria for substance dependence

A maladaptive pattern of substance use, leading to clinically significant impairment or distress, as manifested by three (or more) of the following, occurring at any time in the same 12-month period:

(1) tolerance, as defined by either of the following:

    (a) a need for markedly increased amounts of the substance to achieve intoxication or desired effect

    (b) markedly diminished effect with continued use of the same amount of the substance

(2) withdrawal, as manifested by either of the following:

    (a) the characteristic withdrawal syndrome for the substance (refer to Criteria A and B of the criteria sets for Withdrawal from the specific substances)

    (b) the same (or a closely related) substance is taken to relieve or avoid withdrawal symptoms

(3) the substance is often taken in larger amounts or over a longer period than was intended

(4) there is a persistent desire or unsuccessful efforts to cut down or control substance use

(5) a great deal of time is spent in activities necessary to obtain the substance (e.g., visiting multiple doctors or driving long distances), use the substance (e.g., chain-smoking), or recover from its effects

(6) important social, occupational, or recreational activities are given up or reduced because of substance use

(7) the substance use is continued despite knowledge of having a persistent or recurrent physical or psychological problem that is likely to have been caused or exacerbated by the substance (e.g., current cocaine use despite recognition of cocaine-induced depression, or continued drinking despite recognition that an ulcer was made worse by alcohol consumption)

Specify if:

    With Physiological Dependence: evidence of tolerance or withdrawal (i.e., either Item 1 or 2 is present)

    Without Physiological Dependence: no evidence of tolerance or withdrawal (i.e., neither Item 1 nor 2 is present)

Course specifiers (see text for definitions):

Early Full Remission

Early Partial Remission

Sustained Full Remission

Sustained Partial Remission

On Agonist Therapy

In a Controlled Environment

The definition of dependence requires that the person have at least three of seven behaviors at any time during a 12-month period. The criteria focus on drinking behavior, impairment caused by drinking, and the development of tolerance or withdrawal symptoms. Substance dependence is subtyped as occurring with or without physiological dependence (i.e., evidence of either withdrawal or tolerance).

Epidemiology

Nearly two-thirds of American adults occasionally drink alcoholic beverages, whereas 12% are heavy drinkers—that is, they drink almost every day and become intoxicated several times a month. Drinkers tend to be young, relatively prosperous, well educated, and urban. According to the Epidemiologic Catchment Area study, the lifetime prevalence for alcohol dependence is almost 14%; in any given 6-month period, 5% of persons will meet criteria for alcohol dependence. In hospitals, the prevalence is far greater; from 25% to 50% of medical-surgical patients in general hospitals have alcoholism, and an estimated 50%–60% of psychiatric inpatients in some settings have coexisting alcoholism or another substance use disorder.

There are about four alcoholic men to each alcoholic woman, and the usual age at onset is between 16 and 30 years. Onset in men occurs earlier than in women, although the medical complications of alcoholism progress more rapidly in women. Alcoholism is the third leading cause of death in the United States.

Rates of alcoholism are high in certain countries, including Russia, France, Ireland, and Korea, and low in other countries. China and several Islamic nations (e.g., Saudi Arabia, Syria) have among the lowest rates of alcoholism in the world. People in certain occupations are prone to alcoholism, including waitpersons, bartenders, longshoremen, and writers. Other groups prone to alcoholism include patients with antisocial personality, anxiety, and mood disorders and homosexual persons.

A simple classification for alcoholism has been developed based on demographic and clinical distinctions. Type I alcoholic persons are characterized by an adult onset; gradually increasing consumption; personality characteristics of guilt, worry, dependency, and introversion; little or no family history of alcoholism; equal prevalence in men and women; and a better response to treatment than Type II alcoholism. Nearly 75% of all alcoholic persons fit this description.

Type II alcoholic persons are characterized by early onset; personality characteristics of impulsivity, distractibility, and recklessness; presence of antisocial personality disorder; a strong family history of alcoholism; male gender; and poor treatment response. About 25% of alcoholic persons fit this description.

Clinical Findings

No general clinical picture applies to the alcoholic person because both drinking patterns and symptoms vary widely. In its earliest stages, alcoholism is difficult to identify because symptoms are minimal, and the alcoholic person may deny excessive drinking. Family members and co-workers are often in the best position to identify early symptoms in alcoholic persons, which may include a subtle change in work habits or productivity, lateness or unexplained absences, or minor personality changes such as irritability or moodiness.

As alcoholism progresses, minor physical changes begin to occur, including acne rosacea (i.e., an enlarged red nose); palmar erythema (i.e., reddened palms associated with higher estrogen levels circulating in the blood of alcoholic persons); or painless enlargement of the liver consistent with fatty infiltration, the earliest form of alcoholic liver disease. Other manifestations of early alcoholism include cigarette-burned fingers, unexplained respiratory or other infections, unexplained bruises, periods of amnesia (blackouts), minor traumatic accidents, complaints by others about the drinker's driving skills, and in some cases an arrest or accident from driving while intoxicated. Advancing signs of liver disease can develop, including jaundice or ascites. Testicular atrophy, gynecomastia, and Dupuytren's contractures also may occur. By this point, alcoholism is likely to disrupt the person's life and to lead to job loss, marital discord, and family problems.

The following case example illustrates many of the clinical symptoms and findings of alcoholism and is an example of a person with Type I alcoholism:

> John, a 66-year-old attorney, was brought to an alcohol rehabilitation unit by his wife and son. On arrival, he smelled of alcohol and was mildly disheveled. In a belligerent manner, and slurring his words, John said that he would not stay. His wife intervened and told him firmly that she would file for divorce if he refused to stay and get help. He stayed.
>
> John had a 20-year history of excessive drinking. He had started drinking while in the army and had enjoyed drinking with his friends, mostly on social occasions. He had grown up in a household where alcohol was prohibited for religious reasons. Following his military service, he married, obtained his law degree, and established a successful career as a

trial attorney. Although he sometimes enjoyed a single beer or cocktail after work, the drinking never progressed. Then, in his mid-40s, his alcohol consumption began to escalate. John would drink several beers or cocktails during the evening and then fall asleep. He and his wife began to fight, mainly about his drinking, which he denied was a problem. He paid little attention to his four children because he preferred to drink in solitude.

A series of personal crises followed. John had an affair with a divorcee, separated from his wife, and eventually sought a divorce. He had a falling out with his law partners and withdrew from his longtime friends. His drinking took a more serious turn. Although he was still able to practice law, his case load decreased as lawyers in his small town became increasingly aware of his impairment. He began to drink in the morning (to calm his nerves, he said), had several cocktails at lunch, and continued his drinking in the evening, finally passing out on the davenport. He continued to deny his alcoholism, even when confronted by his new wife and all his children. He pointed out that he was still able to work and was not a skid row bum.

His doctor also was concerned. John was overweight and hypertensive and had developed the stigmata of alcoholism: spider angiomata, acne rosacea, palmar erythema, and testicular atrophy. The progression of his alcoholism was so gradual that by the time of hospital admission, no one could remember what John's personality had once been like. All that people could recall were his drunken appearance, his occasional belligerence, and his social withdrawal.

The inpatient program consisted of individual, group, and family therapy sessions following an uneventful period of alcohol withdrawal. By the end of his 30-day stay, he was noticeably happier, was more optimistic, and seemed motivated once more. He had new ideas for improving his law practice and looked forward to the future. Three years later, he was still abstinent, had developed a satisfying relationship with his wife and children, and had a growing law practice.

Complications

Alcoholism can affect a person's medical and emotional health and lead to a broad array of social problems (summarized in Table 14–3). Medical problems range from benign fatty infiltration of the liver to fulminant liver failure. Almost all organ systems, especially the gastrointestinal tract, are affected by the heavy use of alcohol. Minor problems include gastritis and diarrhea. Peptic ulcers may develop or be aggravated by the direct toxic effect that alcohol has on the mucosa. Fatty infiltration of the liver occurs in almost all alcoholic persons, but cirrhosis occurs in only about 10% of heavy drinkers. Pancreatitis may develop and lead to impaired digestion and diabetes mellitus. Cardiomyopathy, thrombocytopenia, anemia, and myopathy all have been reported to occur.

TABLE 14–3. Medical and psychosocial hazards associated with alcoholism

Drug interactions	**Alcohol withdrawal syndromes**
Gastrointestinal	Uncomplicated alcohol withdrawal
Esophageal bleeding	(the "shakes")
Mallory-Weiss tear	Withdrawal seizures
Gastritis	Alcoholic hallucinosis
Intestinal malabsorption	Alcohol withdrawal delirium
Pancreatitis	(delirium tremens)
Liver disease	**Infectious disease**
Fatty infiltration	Pneumonia
Alcoholic hepatitis	Tuberculosis
Cirrhosis	**Cardiovascular**
Nutritional deficiency	Cardiomyopathy
Malnutrition	Hypertension
Vitamin B deficiency	**Cancer**
Neuropsychiatric	Oral cavity
Wernicke-Korsakoff syndrome	Esophagus
Cortical atrophy/ventricular dilation	Large intestine/rectum
Alcohol-induced dementia	Liver
Peripheral neuropathy	Pancreas
Myopathy	**Birth defects**
Depression	Fetal alcohol syndrome
Suicide	**Psychosocial**
Endocrine system	Accidents
Testicular atrophy	Crime
Increased estrogen levels	Spouse and child abuse
	Job loss
	Divorce, separation
	Legal entanglements

The central and peripheral nervous systems may be damaged by the direct and indirect effects of alcohol. Peripheral neuropathy commonly occurs in a stocking-and-glove distribution, probably from alcohol-induced vitamin B deficiency. Cerebellar damage can cause dysarthria and ataxia. Wernicke's encephalopathy can result from thiamine deficiency and consists of nystagmus, ataxia, and mental confusion (which usually reverses with an injection of thiamine). The Wernicke-Korsakoff syndrome occurs when cognitive and memory impairment endures, although it may be reversible in up to one-third of patients. It involves an anterograde amnesia characterized by the presence of *confabulation*, in which patients invent stories to fill in memory gaps. The syndrome is associated with necrotic lesions of the mamillary bodies, thalamus, and other brain stem regions.

Severely alcoholic persons can develop a frank dementia as a result of either vitamin deficiency or the direct effects of alcohol, although the exact cause is unknown. Chronic alcoholism also has been associated with enlarged cerebral ventricles and widened cortical sulci, effects that may be partially reversible when the individual stops drinking. Careful neuropsychological testing of alcoholic persons generally reveals mild to moderate cognitive deficits which, like the structural abnormalities, partially reverse with sobriety.

A *fetal alcohol syndrome* (FAS) has been described in children whose mothers have alcoholism. This syndrome is induced by excessive maternal consumption of alcohol during pregnancy, especially when binge drinking produces a surge in blood alcohol levels. Abnormalities associated with this disorder include facial anomalies (i.e., small head circumference, epicanthic folds, indistinct philtrum, small midface), low IQ, and behavior problems. FAS affects about one to two infants per 100,000 live births. Women should be warned that FAS can result from alcohol consumption during pregnancy.

Alcohol consumption is a frequent cause of traumatic injuries; alcohol contributes to more than one-half of all motor vehicle deaths each year. Household injuries also are common, which is not surprising because alcoholic persons are often unsteady on their feet. This can lead to falls, with resulting bruises, fractures, and lacerations. The highly publicized deaths of actor William Holden and actress Natalie Wood testify to the lethal nature of these accidents. Subdural hematomas occur in many elderly alcoholic persons who fall and sustain head injuries; the impact tears the bridging veins within the skull.

Cancer rates of the mouth, tongue, larynx, esophagus, stomach, liver, and pancreas are increased. The precise role that alcohol plays in these cancers is uncertain because its effects are confounded by those of smoking and tobacco use. Alcohol interferes with male sexual function and can cause impotency and affect fertility by lowering serum testosterone levels. Increased circulating levels of female hormones (e.g., estrogen) can cause breast enlargement (gynecomastia) and a female escutcheon (pubic hair pattern) in men.

The direct psychiatric complications of alcoholism include acute intoxication, alcohol withdrawal disorders, amnestic syndromes such as Wernicke-Korsakoff syndrome, and dementia. Depression occurs in up to 60% of alcoholic patients; alcohol itself can induce depression through its direct effects on the brain. Depression can contribute to an increased risk of suicide, which occurs in 2%–3% of alcoholic persons. Alcoholic persons at greatest risk for suicide include those with a history of interpersonal loss within the past year (best defined as the loss of an intimate relationship).

Other problems associated with alcoholism are largely social and occupational. Marital and family problems can lead to domestic abuse, separation, and divorce; work-related problems such as absenteeism and job loss; and legal entanglements stemming from arrests for public intoxication, drunk driving, or bar fights. Alcoholism also increases the risk that individuals have for abuse or dependence of other substances.

Etiology

Although the cause of alcoholism is unknown, strong evidence has supported a role for genetics. Family studies have consistently shown high rates of the disorder among first-degree relatives of alcoholic persons. In fact, nearly 25% of the fathers and brothers of alcoholic persons themselves have alcoholism. The relatives of alcoholic persons also have high rates of depression, criminal behavior, and antisocial personality disorder. Typically, depression occurs in the female relatives of alcoholic persons, and alcoholism or antisocial personality disorder occurs in the male relatives.

Identical twins have a higher concordance rate for alcoholism than do nonidentical twins. Adoption studies have shown that the biological relatives of alcoholic adoptees are more likely to have alcoholism than are the relatives of control adoptees. Genetic transmission may be gender specific: in men, alcoholism tends to run in families, but in women, alcoholism tends to occur sporadically. Molecular genetic techniques have been used to search for an alcoholism gene. An association between the dopamine D_2 receptor gene and alcoholism was reported, but the evidence is inconclusive.

Social and environmental factors are also important elements in the development of alcoholism. In one study, alcoholism was related not only to the biological background of adult adoptees but also to the environment in which they were reared.

Research suggests that environmental stressors lead to alcoholism in persons with an inherited predisposition. One hypothesis is that alcohol leads to increased activity of endorphins (or morphine-like substances), which contributes to an individual's preference for alcohol. Another hypothesis is that alcohol might, at least initially, increase relaxation in susceptible persons (e.g., sons of alcoholic persons), as evidenced by slow-wave alpha activity on the electroencephalogram, or that these persons have a particularly high tolerance to alcohol and require more than others to produce the desired effect. Along these lines, some persons may be protected from developing alcoholism. For example, it has been suggested that the *oriental flush*, an unpleasant physiological response to alcohol, might protect persons of Chinese descent from developing alcoholism.

Behaviorists have suggested that learning plays an important role in the genesis of alcoholism and point to the fact that children tend to imitate their parents' drinking patterns. Boys are encouraged to drink more than girls, reinforcing the gender difference in alcoholism. Learning processes also may contribute to the development of the disorder through the repeated experience with alcohol withdrawal; relieving the symptoms with alcohol only reinforces further drinking.

Course and Outcome

In a major review of 10 large studies, the authors concluded that 2%–3% of alcoholic persons become abstinent each year and about 1% return to asymptomatic or controlled drinking. These findings were true for both treated and untreated samples of alcoholic persons, supporting the hypothesis that alcoholism is self-limiting for some persons. In the 10 studies, 46%–87% of the subjects had alcoholism at follow-up; 8%–39% achieved abstinence; and 0%–33% were asymptomatic drinkers.

Diagnosis

Alcoholism usually can be diagnosed on the basis of a careful history and mental status examination. Because many alcoholic persons deny their illness or underestimate the extent of their drinking, it is helpful to gather information from family members or other informants when alcoholism is suspected. The four-question CAGE test is a simple screen for the presence of alcohol abuse or dependence (see Table 14–4). Any positive or overly defensive answer suggests that a problem exists.

TABLE 14–4.   CAGE: Screening test for alcohol abuse or dependence

C	Have you felt the need to CUT DOWN on your drinking?
A	Have you felt ANNOYED BY CRITICISM of your drinking?
G	Have you felt GUILTY (or had regrets) about your drinking?
E	Have you felt the need for an EYE-OPENER in the morning?

Blood alcohol levels can be useful in detecting alcohol abuse or dependence. For example, a level of 150 mg/dL in a nonintoxicated person is strong evidence for alcoholism. Blood alcohol levels can be roughly correlated to level of intoxication:

0–100 mg/dL   A sense of well-being, sedation, tranquillity
100–150 mg/dL   Incoordination, irritability
150–250 mg/dL   Slurred speech, ataxia
>250 mg/dL   Passing out, unconsciousness

Other laboratory measures are useful but not diagnostic. Alcoholic persons may develop increased high-density lipoprotein (HDL) cholesterol, increased lactate dehydroxygenase, decreased low-density lipoprotein (LDL) cholesterol, decreased blood urea nitrogen, decreased red blood cell volume, and increased uric acid level. Mean corpuscular volume is increased in up to 95% of alcoholic persons. Thirty percent of alcoholic persons have evidence of an old rib or vertebral fracture on chest X ray (compared with 1% of control subjects). Liver enzymes are frequently abnormal. γ-Glutamyltransferase (GGT) is increased in about 75% of alcoholic persons and may be the earliest laboratory sign of alcoholism. Transaminase (aspartate aminotransferase and alanine aminotransferase) levels also are increased. One study showed that a combination of elevated serum GGT and elevated erythrocyte mean corpuscular volume identified 90% of alcoholic patients.

Clinical Management

Alcohol-induced disorders often require medical intervention. Intoxication is the most common disorder and rarely requires more than simple supportive measures, such as decreasing external stimuli and removing the source of alcohol (see Table 14–5 for the DSM-IV-TR criteria). When respiration is compromised by excessive alcohol intake, intensive care may be required.

Treatment of alcohol withdrawal depends on the syndrome exhibited (see Table 14–3). These syndromes usually are precipitated by the abrupt withdrawal from alcohol but can be seen in alcoholic persons who simply reduce their usual high intake. *Uncomplicated alcohol withdrawal* (the "shakes") begins 12–18 hours after the cessation of drinking and peaks at 24–48 hours (Table 14–6). Uncomplicated alcohol withdrawal subsides within 5–7 days but may linger. Minor symptoms include anxiety, tremors, and nausea and vomiting; heart rate and blood pressure may be increased.

Alcoholic withdrawal seizures ("rum fits") occur 7–38 hours after the

TABLE 14–5.   DSM-IV-TR diagnostic criteria for alcohol intoxication

A. Recent ingestion of alcohol.

B. Clinically significant maladaptive behavioral or psychological changes (e.g., inappropriate sexual or aggressive behavior, mood lability, impaired judgment, impaired social or occupational functioning) that developed during, or shortly after, alcohol ingestion.

C. One (or more) of the following signs, developing during, or shortly after, alcohol use:

    (1) slurred speech

    (2) incoordination

    (3) unsteady gait

    (4) nystagmus

    (5) impairment in attention or memory

    (6) stupor or coma

D. The symptoms are not due to a general medical condition and are not better accounted for by another mental disorder.

TABLE 14–6.   DSM-IV-TR diagnostic criteria for alcohol withdrawal

A. Cessation of (or reduction in) alcohol use that has been heavy and prolonged.

B. Two (or more) of the following, developing within several hours to a few days after Criterion A:

    (1) autonomic hyperactivity (e.g., sweating or pulse rate greater than 100)

    (2) increased hand tremor

    (3) insomnia

    (4) nausea or vomiting

    (5) transient visual, tactile, or auditory hallucinations or illusions

    (6) psychomotor agitation

    (7) anxiety

    (8) grand mal seizures

C. The symptoms in Criterion B cause clinically significant distress or impairment in social, occupational, or other important areas of functioning.

D. The symptoms are not due to a general medical condition and are not better accounted for by another mental disorder.

Specify if:

With Perceptual Disturbances

cessation of drinking and peak between 24 and 48 hours. The patient may have a single burst of one to six generalized seizures; status epilepticus is rare. Withdrawal seizures occur primarily in chronic, long-term alcoholic patients and precede delirium tremens in about 30% of cases.

Alcoholic hallucinosis—vivid and unpleasant auditory hallucinations—begins within 48 hours of cessation of drinking and occurs in the presence of a clear sensorium. The hallucinations typically last about 1 week but have been reported to become chronic. Like withdrawal seizures, they are a sign of severe alcoholism.

The most dramatic withdrawal syndrome is *alcohol withdrawal delirium* (delirium tremens). Delirium tremens occurs in about 5% of hospitalized alcoholic patients but in about one-third of those who have had withdrawal seizures. Manifestations include delirium (confusion and disorientation, perceptual disturbances, sleep cycle disturbance, agitation), mild fever, and autonomic hyperarousal. The delirium may begin 2–3 days after the drinking stops or after a significant reduction of intake. Symptoms peak 4 or 5 days later. The syndrome typically lasts about 3 days but can persist for weeks. With good supportive care, death is rare, although mortality rates of up to 15% were reported in the past.

The following case illustrates the diagnosis and management of alcohol withdrawal delirium:

> Dave, a 34-year-old unemployed veteran, requested admission for alcohol withdrawal treatment. He had a 10-year history of alcoholism and had experienced delirium tremens, alcoholic blackouts, and withdrawal seizures. He had been admitted many times for alcohol withdrawal and rehabilitation services and was well known at the hospital for his unpleasant and critical attitude.
>
> Dave had been drinking heavily—about 1 quart of liquor daily—since his last inpatient stay 3 months earlier, particularly during the week before seeking help. He was tremulous, hypertensive, and diaphoretic. The "Librium protocol" (i.e., chlordiazepoxide taper, see below) was instituted. To the chagrin of the treatment team, Dave insisted on leaving the hospital against medical advice the next day. He claimed that he had "more important things" to do. The night before, nursing staff noted that he was mildly intrusive and had wandered into other patients' rooms.
>
> Dave was brought back to the hospital the next day by the police. He had been found wandering aimlessly around town. He was noticeably paranoid and thought that unnamed persons were plotting against him. He was also disoriented; he knew where he was but was unable to give the date or the year. By the next morning, Dave was globally confused. He also was febrile, had very high diastolic blood pressure, and was diaphoretic. Because of his belligerence and physical restlessness, he was placed in seclusion,

and restraints were used for his protection. Over the next 2 days, he received nearly 1,200 mg of chlordiazepoxide, but he remained loud and agitated. Intravenous hydration was required because of his poor oral intake. The nurses observed him to play an imaginary game of chess with unseen playmates.

On the third day of hospitalization, Dave awakened and was fully oriented. He remained suspicious but was no longer hallucinating. He gradually returned to his baseline over the next week and was discharged.

The management of alcohol withdrawal consists of general support (i.e., adequate food and hydration, careful medical monitoring), nutritional supplementation, and the use of benzodiazepines. Persons who have a history of uncomplicated withdrawal and a physician who is familiar with them probably can be managed as outpatients. Treatment may include 25–50 mg of chlordiazepoxide four times daily, tapered slowly over the next 4–5 days, combined with daily visits to the physician to assess symptoms.

Alcoholic patients with comorbid medical or psychiatric illness, impaired ability to follow instructions, inadequate or absent social support, or a history of severe withdrawal symptoms require careful monitoring and may need to be hospitalized. Patients should receive an adequate diet plus oral thiamine (100 mg), folic acid (1 mg), and multivitamins. Thiamine (100–200 mg intramuscularly) can be administered if oral intake is not possible and should be given before any situation in which glucose loading is required because glucose can deplete thiamine stores. Chlordiazepoxide should be administered in doses ranging from 25 to 100 mg orally four times daily on the first day with a 20% per day decrease in dose over 4–5 days. (A specific protocol is recommended in Table 14–7.) Additional doses may be given for breakthrough signs or symptoms (e.g., tremors or diaphoresis). Chlordiazepoxide and the other benzodiazepines are the preferred drugs for withdrawal because of their safety and cross-tolerance with alcohol. Chlordiazepoxide is most often recommended because of its long half-life and low cost, but other benzodiazepines work just as well. Intermediate- or short-acting benzodiazepines (e.g., lorazepam, oxazepam) are generally preferred in patients with liver damage or in elderly patients because these benzodiazepines lack metabolites and are renally excreted. Diazepam can be given to interrupt seizures should status epilepticus occur. Other drugs, including carbamazepine, clonidine, propranolol, and valproate, have been used to treat alcohol withdrawal, but their role in treating the disorder is not yet clear.

Delirious patients require additional care, which may include seclusion and restraints. To facilitate patient care, 10 mg of intravenous diazepam (or

---

TABLE 14–7.   Management of alcohol withdrawal syndromes

---

1.   Chlordiazepoxide protocol

- 50 mg every 4 hours × 24 hours, then
- 50 mg every 6 hours × 24 hours, then
- 25 mg every 4 hours × 24 hours, then
- 25 mg every 6 hours × 24 hours

The protocol should be started when three of seven parameters are met: systolic blood pressure >160 mm Hg, diastolic blood pressure >100 mm Hg, pulse >110 beats/min, temperature >38.3°C, nausea, vomiting, or tremors. The dose should be held if any of the following signs are present: nystagmus, sedation, ataxia, slurred speech, or the patient is asleep.

2.   Thiamine: 50–100 mg orally or intramuscularly × 1; folic acid: 1 mg/day orally

3.   Haloperidol: 2–5 mg/day; or risperidone: 2–6 mg/day for patients with alcoholic hallucinosis

4.   For delirium tremens:

- 10 mg of intravenous diazepam (or 2–4 mg of lorazepam), followed by 5-mg doses every 5 minutes until calm; once stabilized, the dose may be tapered slowly over 4 or 5 days
- Seclusion and restraints as necessary
- Adequate hydration and nutrition

2–4 mg of lorazepam) may be given, followed by 5-mg doses every 5 minutes (or 1–2 mg of lorazepam) thereafter until the patient is calm. Once the patient has stabilized, the benzodiazepine dose should be tapered slowly over the next 4 or 5 days. Intravenous hydration may also be necessary, although most alcoholic patients are overhydrated, not dehydrated, as is commonly believed. Any electrolyte disturbance should be corrected, and the patient should be examined for injuries or evidence of a physical illness (e.g., pneumonia).

A small dose of haloperidol (2–5 mg/day) or risperidone (2–6 mg/day) may help relieve the frightening auditory hallucinations of the patient with alcoholic hallucinosis. The medication usually is discontinued when the hallucinations stop.

Rehabilitation

Once alcohol detoxification has been accomplished, efforts at rehabilitation can begin. Rehabilitation has two goals: 1) that the patient remain sober and

2) that coexisting disorders be identified and treated. Perhaps two-thirds of alcoholic patients have additional psychiatric diagnoses (including mood or anxiety disorders) that may require treatment. Because alcoholism itself can cause depression and most alcohol-induced depressions lift with sobriety, antidepressants are probably needed only for patients who remain depressed after 2–4 weeks of sobriety.

The first step toward rehabilitation occurs when the physician diagnoses alcohol abuse or dependence. Patients should be told that their disorder is significant and potentially life-threatening and that treatment is recommended. Receiving a diagnosis may be the single most important step in leading the alcoholic person to change.

Patients should be encouraged to attend Alcoholics Anonymous (AA), a worldwide self-help group for recovering alcoholic persons founded in 1935. AA uses a program of 12 steps; new members are asked to admit their problems, to give up a sense of personal control over the disease, to make personal amends, and to help others to achieve sobriety. The meetings provide a blend of acceptance, belonging, forgiveness, and understanding.

A team approach is used for the hospitalized alcoholic patient. Group therapy enables patients to see their own problems mirrored in others and to learn better coping skills. With individual therapy, alcoholic persons can learn to identify triggers that prompt drinking and more effective coping strategies. Family therapy is often important because the family system that has been altered to accommodate the patient's drinking may end up reinforcing it. These issues can be addressed in family therapy. Inpatient programs also provide education about the harmful effects of alcohol on the mind and body.

The U.S. Food and Drug Administration has approved the use of two drugs—disulfiram and naltrexone—for the treatment of alcohol dependence. Disulfiram may help some patients maintain their sobriety. Disulfiram inhibits aldehyde dehydrogenase, an enzyme necessary for the metabolism of alcohol. Inhibiting this enzyme leads to the accumulation of acetaldehyde when alcohol is consumed. Acetaldehyde is toxic and induces noxious symptoms, such as nausea, vomiting, palpitations, and hypotension. Because the effects may be fatal in rare cases, disulfiram should be prescribed only after careful consideration and with the full cooperation of the patient. The usual dose is 250 mg once daily. Although evidence supporting its effectiveness is inconclusive, many physicians and patients believe disulfiram is an effective psychological deterrent to drinking.

Naltrexone, a μ-opioid antagonist, can help lower the alcoholic person's risk of relapse. One theory holds that naltrexone reduces drinking and in-

---

Recommendations for management of alcoholism

1. The alcoholic person needs acceptance, not blame.

2. Although it is tempting to refuse treatment to the chronic alcoholic person based on his or her history of failure, it is always possible that the next rehabilitation may work. The therapist must not give up!

3. Treatment of alcohol withdrawal syndromes should take place in an inpatient setting if the patient has a history of severe "shakes," hallucinations, seizures, or delirium tremens. Other patients (the majority) can be handled as outpatients.

   - Chlordiazepoxide is standard treatment, but other benzodiazepines (e.g., lorazepam) work just as well.

4. The clinician should manage the patient's other emotional problems (e.g., panic disorder, depression) because if untreated, they may lead to a resumption of drinking.

5. The patient should be referred to Alcoholics Anonymous to provide ongoing social support and encouragement from persons similarly affected.

6. The family should be included in the treatment process.

   - Alcoholism affects every member of the family, and unresolved issues may lead to relapse.

   - Family members should be encouraged to attend Al-Anon, a support group for relatives of alcoholic persons.

---

creases abstinence by decreasing the psychologically reinforcing pleasurable effects of alcohol and by reducing the person's craving for alcohol. The recommended daily dose is 50 mg. The drug is generally well tolerated but can produce nausea, headache, anxiety, or sedation. Acamprosate, a drug used in several European countries, is being tested in the United States and also appears to be effective. Other drugs being investigated for their use in treating alcohol dependence include tiapride, bromocriptine, and ondansetron.

Aversive conditioning was once used in the treatment of alcoholism. Drugs that induced either vomiting (e.g., emetine, apomorphine) or apnea (e.g., succinylcholine) or electrical stimulation used to produce pain were paired with the act of drinking. Although aversive conditioning techniques often were effective, both the risk of medical complications and their general unpleasantness contributed to their loss in popularity.

Rehabilitation programs for alcoholic patients have shifted from traditional inpatient to residential and outpatient settings. Outcome studies have shown that these programs are effective, but not all patients do well. In general, patients likely to benefit have a stable marriage and home life, are employed, have fewer comorbid psychiatric disorders (especially antisocial personality disorder), and have no family history of alcoholism. Unfortunately, nearly one-half of treated alcoholic persons relapse, most commonly during the first 6 months after treatment. Even though relapse is common, treatment should be viewed as beneficial and cost-effective. Treatment has the potential to reduce the medical and social complications and the excessive mortality associated with alcoholism. Repeated efforts at treatment may lead to long-term sobriety.

Recommendations for the clinical management of alcoholism are summarized in the box on page 419.

Bibliography

American Psychiatric Association: Diagnostic and Statistical Manual of Mental Disorders, 4th Edition. Washington, DC, American Psychiatric Association, 1994

American Psychiatric Association: Diagnostic and Statistical Manual of Mental Disorders, 4th Edition Revised. Washington, DC, American Psychiatric Association, 2000

Cadoret RJ, O'Gorman TW, Troughton E, et al: Alcoholism and antisocial personality: interrelationships, genetic and environmental factors. Arch Gen Psychiatry 42:162–167, 1985

Cloninger CR: Neurogenic adaptive mechanisms in alcoholism. Science 236:410–416, 1987

DeWit DJ, Adlaf EM, Offord DR, et al: Age at first alcohol use: a risk factor for the development of alcohol disorders. Am J Psychiatry 157:745–750, 2000

Eckardt MJ, Harford TC, Kaelber CT, et al: Health hazards associated with alcohol consumption. JAMA 246:648–666, 1981

Frances RJ, Bucke S, Alexopoulous GS: Outcome study of familial and non-familial alcoholism. Am J Psychiatry 141:1469–1471, 1984

Fuller RK, Branchey L, Brightwell DR, et al: Disulfiram treatment of alcoholism: a Veterans Administration cooperative study. JAMA 256:1449–1455, 1986

Garbutt JC, West SL, Carey TS, et al: Pharmacologic treatment of alcohol dependence: a review of the evidence. JAMA 281:1318–1325, 1999

Gelernter J, Goldman D, Risch N: The A1 allele at the D2 dopamine receptor gene and alcoholism: a reappraisal. JAMA 269:1673–1677, 1993

Goodwin DW: Alcoholism and genetics. Arch Gen Psychiatry 42:171–174, 1985

Grant I, Adams KM, Reed R: Aging, abstinence, and medical risk factors in the prediction of neuropsychologic deficit among long-term alcoholics. Arch Gen Psychiatry 41:710–718, 1984

Helzer JE, Pryzbeck TR: The co-occurrence of alcoholism with other psychiatric disorders in the general population and its impact on treatment. J Stud Alcohol 49:219–224, 1988

Helzer JE, Robins LN, Taylor JR, et al: The extent of long-term moderate drinking among alcoholics discharged from medical and psychiatric treatment facilities. N Engl J Med 312:1678–1682, 1985

Holden C: Is alcoholism treatment effective? Science 236:20–22, 1987

Irwin M, Schuckit M, Smith TL: Clinical importance of age at onset in type I and type II primary alcoholics. Arch Gen Psychiatry 47:320–324, 1990

Jellinek EM: The Disease Concept of Alcoholism. New Haven, CT, College and University Press, 1960

Malcolm R, Ballenger JC, Sturgis ET, et al: Double-blind controlled trial comparing carbamazepine to oxazepam treatment of alcohol withdrawal. Am J Psychiatry 146:617–621, 1989

Nutt D: Alcohol and the brain: pharmacologic insights for psychiatrists. Br J Psychiatry 175:114–119, 1999

Schuckit MA, Smith TL, Anthenelli R, et al: Clinical course of alcoholism in 646 male inpatients. Am J Psychiatry 150:786–792, 1993

Stein LI, Newton JR, Bowman RS: Duration of hospitalization for alcoholism. Arch Gen Psychiatry 32:247–252, 1975

Streissguth AP, Clarren SK, Jones KL: Natural history of the fetal alcohol syndrome: a 10 year follow up of 11 patients. Lancet 2:85–91, 1985

Swift RM: Drug therapy for alcohol dependence. N Engl J Med 340:1482–1489, 1999

Vaillant GE: The Natural History of Alcoholism: Causes, Patterns, and Paths to Recovery. Cambridge, MA, Harvard University Press, 1983

Volpicelli JR, Alterman AI, Hayashida M, et al: Naltrexone in the treatment of alcohol dependence. Arch Gen Psychiatry 49:876–880, 1992

Self-Assessment Questions

1. Who originated the disease concept of alcoholism?
2. How is alcohol dependence diagnosed?
3. How do Type I and Type II alcoholic patients differ?
4. What are the clinical findings in the earliest stage of alcoholism? Middle stage? Late stage?
5. List the medical complications of alcoholism.
6. What laboratory abnormalities are associated with alcoholism?

7. What are the major withdrawal syndromes, and how are they treated?
8. Discuss the role of disulfiram and naltrexone in the treatment of alcoholism.
9. What are the predictors of good outcome for alcohol rehabilitation efforts?

15 Other Substance-Related Disorders

O true apothecary! Thy drugs are quick.

William Shakespeare, *Romeo and Juliet*

Psychoactive substances are compounds that can alter a person's state of mind. Alcohol, the most important psychoactive substance, is discussed in Chapter 14. Other substances also have been around since antiquity, although some new ones are the product of modern organic chemistry techniques. A literal cornucopia of psychoactive substances is readily available in the United States, and many have been subject to both appropriate and inappropriate use.

The problems resulting from substance abuse appear more extensive today than in the past, probably because of the increased availability of a growing number of drugs that are subject to experimentation and use. Drug-related problems cut across all social and economic boundaries. All age groups, but particularly adolescents and young adults, are affected. Because of the near epidemic nature of illicit drug use and growing public concern, the government has acted to increase funding for research on drug abuse. Tough federal and state laws mandating heavy penalties for both drug possession and drug distribution have been enacted. Presidential commissions have been appointed, and, since 1989, a drug "czar" has been in place to coordinate drug containment efforts. Despite these measures, the problem continues to grow.

In this chapter, we review the major categories of substance use disorders, as well as related syndromes that result from their use: sedative, hypnotic, and anxiolytic use disorders; opioid use disorders; central nervous system (CNS) stimulants and their associated disorders; hallucinogen and arylcyclohexylamine use disorders; cannabis (e.g., marijuana) use disorders; and inhalant use disorders.

Other substance use disorders, involving nicotine, caffeine, anabolic steroids, nitrate inhalants, and nitrous oxide—also are discussed in this chapter. (See Table 15–1 for a list of the categories and substances of abuse.)

TABLE 15–1.　Categories of drug use disorders

Sedatives, hypnotics, and anxiolytics	Hallucinogens
Barbiturates	Arylcyclohexylamines
Nonbarbiturates (e.g., meprobamate)	Phencyclidine
Benzodiazepines	Cannabis
Opiates	Inhalants
Heroin	Other substances
Meperidine	Nicotine
Codeine	Caffeine
Hydromorphone	Anabolic steroids
Stimulants	Nitrate inhalants
Amphetamines	Nitrous oxide
Methylphenidate	
Cocaine	

As pointed out in Chapter 14, DSM-IV-TR uses generic criteria for substance dependence and abuse, a concept endorsed by the World Health Organization. *Substance dependence* involves a maladaptive pattern of substance use, as manifested by at least three of seven significant signs or symptoms, occurring at any time in the same 12-month period. These signs and symptoms include evidence of physiological tolerance or withdrawal and psychosocial problems that indicate a serious degree of involvement with the drug. (The DSM-IV-TR criteria for substance dependence appear in Table 14–2.)

Substance abuse is a category for persons who continue to abuse substances despite problems caused by their use but who fail to meet criteria for dependence. (The DSM-IV-TR criteria for substance abuse appear in Table

14–1.) These criteria are geared toward separating individuals whose use of a substance is hazardous (dependence) from those whose use is harmful (abuse), although the distinction is not always clear, and considerable overlap exists between dependence and abuse. These disorders are probably better thought of as lying along a continuum of severity.

Epidemiology

Substance use and abuse are widespread in the United States. It is probably impossible to know their true extent because drug abusers may not cooperate with surveys and because much use is recreational and not necessarily accompanied by signs or symptoms of abuse or dependence. The Epidemiologic Catchment Area survey found that lifetime prevalence of the combined category of drug abuse and dependence ranged from 5.5% to 5.8%. In the more recent National Comorbidity Survey, lifetime prevalence for drug abuse or dependence was 14.6% in men and 9.5% in women. In these surveys, drug abuse and dependence were more common in men, young persons, and those with low incomes.

These data do not show the true extent of illicit drug use. Surveys show, for example, that marijuana has been used by more than one-quarter of Americans and is regularly smoked by about 20 million persons. Cocaine achieved great popularity in the 1980s, particularly among young urban professionals, and nearly one-quarter of young Americans have used it, including nearly 7% of high school seniors. A 1990 household survey found that more than 6 million Americans admitted to using cocaine in the year before the survey. Patterns of use change, however, reflecting the fluctuating popularity of drugs, their availability, and their cost. Opiates and barbiturates peaked in popularity long ago, but the estimated number of persons addicted to heroin has remained stable at about 500,000. Cocaine is more widely available and less expensive than in the past. Crack, a freebased derivative of cocaine, is even cheaper, and its use has become epidemic in inner cities and elsewhere. Another factor in drug use is the introduction of new substances to the black market. Many drugs are easily synthesized in basement laboratories and are widely available at low prices. Methcathinone (cat) is a recent example. A stimulant that is inhaled or injected, methcathinone can be synthesized from battery acid, drain cleaner, paint thinner, and ephedrine, an over-the-counter cold remedy.

Among the more worrisome trends is the use of multiple drugs of abuse. As a general rule, the use of one substance greatly increases the chance that a person will use another. Some drugs are deliberately combined to produce a desired effect (e.g., a speedball, consisting of a combination of cocaine and heroin). The extent of combined drug use is only now becoming apparent. In DSM-IV-TR, this pattern of use is classified as *polysubstance dependence*, that is, three or more drugs have been repeatedly used, but no single agent has predominated.

Etiology

Understanding substance use involves knowledge of the user, his or her environment, and the drug itself. None of these variables works in isolation, and it is the confluence of all three that leads to drug use disorders.

Some users appear to have an inherited vulnerability to drug abuse. Research shows that dependence on certain substances (e.g., tobacco, narcotics, alcohol) is familial; adoptees born to substance-abusing parents and placed in drug-free homes show an increased likelihood of drug use. This work shows that the tendency to use drugs is not only familial but also genetic to some extent.

Although no single personality pattern is associated with drug abuse, the frequency of personality disorders among drug abusers is very high. Antisocial and borderline personality disorders appear to predispose to drug use. Narcissistic traits have been identified as a possible risk factor in cocaine abusers. Other psychological characteristics seen in drug abusers include hostility, low frustration tolerance, inflexibility, and low self-esteem. Several longitudinal studies have shown that many of these traits (e.g., aggressiveness and rebelliousness manifested in childhood) precede and predict the use of psychoactive substances.

Other medical and psychiatric disorders have been linked with drug abuse, including chronic pain, anxiety disorders, and depression. Many patients experiencing physical or emotional pain often seek relief through drugs or alcohol and are at high risk for abuse or dependence.

An individual's neurobiology may predispose to abuse. The presence of opiate receptors in several brain regions may predispose to opiate abuse. Benzodiazepine receptors have been identified in the CNS and may play a role in anxiolytic abuse. Knowledge of these neurotransmitter systems helps us to understand why drug abusers can become increasingly reliant on drugs while progressively ignoring other means to enjoy life (e.g., food, work, sex, family, friends).

The pharmacological properties of the drug itself may contribute to abuse. Some compounds (e.g., opiates, sedatives, hypnotics, anxiolytics) can produce rapid relief of anxiety. Stimulants generally relieve boredom and fatigue and provide a sensation of energy and increased mental alertness. Hallucinogens provide a temporary escape from reality. These properties all contribute to their abuse. Substances that do not give pleasure to the user (e.g., phenothiazines) are rarely abused. In general, drugs with rapid onset and briefer action (e.g., heroin, cocaine) are preferred. Methods of administration that enhance the rapidity of onset—for example, sniffing, smoking, or intravenous use—are often exploited to provide an added kick. Tolerance and withdrawal symptoms also contribute to abuse. Users quickly learn that higher doses of some substances are needed to get the same effect and that the drug itself can be used to prevent unpleasant withdrawal symptoms.

Societal and family values influence the use of illicit drugs. When parents smoke, drink alcoholic beverages, or use psychoactive substances, their offspring are more prone to use illicit drugs, perhaps from learning the implicit lesson that their use is socially acceptable. Persons whose friends use drugs are more likely to use them, too, which suggests that people are prone to peer influence. Susceptibility to peer influence has been associated with the lack of a close bond with one's parents, a large amount of time spent away from home, and increased reliance on peers as opposed to parents.

Laws also can affect illicit drug use. Antidrug laws have been tried with mixed success for millennia (e.g., alcohol, tobacco, opium). Such laws are generally more successful in authoritarian countries (e.g., Singapore) than in more open and pluralistic ones (e.g., Western European countries, United States). In some countries (e.g., Saudi Arabia), drug use is proscribed for religious reasons and has severe consequences. Drug abuse in these countries is rare.

Diagnosis

The diagnosis of a substance use disorder requires a careful history, a thorough physical examination, and a detailed mental status examination. The assessment of drug-addicted persons is rarely easy because few will report their substance use. More commonly, these patients will present for evaluation of medical complaints or symptoms of psychological distress. A careful interview may help to uncover social, marital, occupational, or legal problems that may have contributed to the substance use. The clinician should remember that substance use can induce major psychiatric syndromes, including depression, mania, and psychosis. Likewise, many drug-addicted persons will have co-occurring psychiatric disorders, including major depression, bipolar disorder, or an anxiety disorder, that should be diagnosed and treated. Personality disorders—particularly antisocial and borderline personality disorder—are very frequent in these individuals and may be important factors in promoting continued drug use.

Additional history obtained from relatives or friends, or from other physicians, will help fill in the gaps. Even patients who are straightforward about their abuse may minimize its extent. Once the physician's suspicion has been raised about drug use, he or she should inquire specifically about each class of commonly abused substances and record the patient's pattern of use.

A physical examination will offer signs of intoxication and withdrawal, depending on when the individual presents at a hospital or clinic (see Table 15–2). The clinician should be forthright and nonjudgmental with these patients and help them to get needed treatment.

The following case example from our hospital illustrates many of the symptoms that beset substance abusers, as well as some of the factors that lead to the abuse. Laura's story also points out the dilemma that caregivers face with uncooperative patients and the lack of satisfactory solutions.

Laura was referred to the hospital for evaluation of polydrug abuse. The 21-year-old Native American worked as a nursing assistant in a residential care center.

Laura was adopted at an early age into a middle-class family. Her adoptive parents took care to ensure that she was adequately clothed and fed but provided little emotional nurturing. As a child, Laura was sexually molested for several years by one of her adoptive brothers. At age 12, she became pregnant by him, carried the baby to term, and gave it up for adoption.

Laura had an extensive history of drug abuse. She started smoking marijuana and drinking alcoholic beverages at age 12, was using amphetamines by age 14, and later used cocaine and crack. She also admitted to having tried an assortment of other drugs, including phencyclidine (PCP), lysergic diethylamide (LSD), and heroin. To pay for her drug use, Laura sold drugs and later engaged in prostitution.

In the 6 months before her hospitalization, she had begun to inject cocaine intravenously, sometimes in combination with heroin. She reported that she enjoyed the sexual feelings she received from the injections and had actually lost interest in sexual activity with her boyfriend. She admitted that she used unclean needles despite knowing that they could transmit the human immunodeficiency virus (HIV). Her boyfriend was a drug dealer with an extensive prison record and worked as her pimp.

Laura had received prior psychiatric treatment for depression and had had several prior admissions for drug detoxification, one following a suicide attempt. She had never stayed in the hospital very long and usually left against medical advice.

Laura was referred to our hospital under a court order and told us she had no plans to stop using drugs. She was eventually transferred to a drug

TABLE 15–2. Signs of drug intoxication

Signs	Sedatives, hypnotics, or anxiolytics	Stimulants	Opioids	Cannabis
Eyes	Nystagmus; miosis when severe	Mydriasis, which may require protective sunglasses	Miosis prominent	Injected conjunctivae
Vital signs	Stage dependent; chronic user yields increased blood pressure	Increased—or sometimes decreased—heart rate and blood pressure, varied arrhythmias	Bradycardia, risk of respiratory depression and pulmonary edema	Tachycardia
Neurological	Incoordination to unsteady gait, slurred speech	Dyskinesia, dystonia, muscle weakness, seizures	Slurred speech	Impaired coordination
Psychomotor	Agitation, combativeness	Agitation (sometimes retardation) and stereotyped behaviors	Activity usually outside normal range; may be increased or decreased	Passive
Sensorium	Impaired concentration and memory; stupor to coma	Confusion to coma	Impaired attention and memory; drowsiness to coma	Impaired attention, memory, and sense of time
Autonomic	Diaphoresis, flushed face and skin	Diaphoresis, chills		Dry mouth
Gastrointestinal	Poor nutrition	Nausea, vomiting, marked weight loss, poor nutrition	Constipation, poor nutrition	Increased appetite
Skin and mucosa	Dental neglect	Needle marks and tracks, ulcerated nasal septum, dental neglect	Needle marks and tracks, dental neglect	

Source. Adapted from Barber and O'Brien 1995.

rehabilitation center under court order. The referral was based on our hope that at some point the treatment would "take." Our alternative was to do nothing.

Sedative, Hypnotic, and Anxiolytic Use Disorders

Sedatives, hypnotics and anxiolytics have been used to provide sedation, induce sleep, relieve anxiety, prevent seizures, relax muscles, and induce general anesthesia. All sedatives, hypnotics, and anxiolytics are cross-tolerant with one another and with alcohol. They are also capable of producing physical and psychological dependence and symptoms of withdrawal. Classes of these compounds include the barbiturates, the nonbarbiturate sedative-hypnotics (e.g., meprobamate), and the benzodiazepines.

The history of sedative-hypnotics dates to 1903, when barbital, the first barbiturate, was introduced. Later, other sedative-hypnotics (e.g., meprobamate) were synthesized; benzodiazepines first became available in the 1960s. Because of their wide margin of safety, the benzodiazepines have largely displaced barbiturates and the earlier nonbarbiturate sedative-hypnotics from the market. An overdose of barbiturates is potentially fatal, but the benzodiazepines produce almost no respiratory depression, and the ratio of lethal to effective dosage is extraordinarily high. Although the barbiturate and nonbarbiturate sedative-hypnotics are effective in providing both sedation and hypnosis (e.g., sleep induction), they are rarely used today. The main indication for phenobarbital now is as an anticonvulsant. Methaqualone, a nonbarbiturate sedative-hypnotic, no longer has any accepted medical use and is not manufactured in the United States, although it is readily available on the black market. The benzodiazepines are among the most widely prescribed medications in the United States, and about 15% of the general population is prescribed a benzodiazepine in any given year. Research has shown that most prescriptions for benzodiazepines are appropriate, and only a small percentage of patients abuse the drugs. Nonetheless, prescribing practices contribute to the problem of sedative-hypnotic abuse, and physicians have an obligation to monitor and, if necessary, limit the use of these drugs (see Table 15–3). Further information about the rational use of sedative-hypnotics is found in Chapter 27.

Sedative-hypnotic abuse involves a maladaptive pattern of use leading to clinically significant impairment, as indicated by one or more independent indications of inappropriate use or problems directly attributable to the substance at any time during a 12-month period. Dependence requires the presence of three or more problem behaviors (out of seven) at any time in

---

TABLE 15–3. Rational prescribing of sedative-hypnotic agents

---

1. Avoid or limit prescriptions to patients if risk for substance abuse is suggested by

   • A history of alcohol abuse or dependence

   • A history of drug abuse or dependence

   • A presence of borderline or antisocial personality disorder

   • A strong family history of substance abuse or dependence

2. Learn to recognize "red flag" presentations by patients seeking prescription drugs, as suggested by

   • Dramatic claims of need for a scheduled drug

   • Reports of lost prescriptions

   • Frequent requests for early refills

   • Requests for a specific scheduled drug, reports of allergies to other drugs, or use of nonscheduled drugs for pain relief or anxiety

   • Obtaining prescriptions from many physicians

Source. Courtesy of William R. Yates, M.D.

the same 12-month period, including manifestations of tolerance and withdrawal. (Please refer to Tables 14–1 and 14–2 for the definitions of abuse and dependence, respectively.)

There may be two distinct groups of sedative, hypnotic, and anxiolytic abusers. The first group includes persons in their teens or 20s who obtain the drugs illegally and use them for recreational purposes. Similar to persons with Type II alcoholism, this group likely has coexisting psychopathology, such as an antisocial personality disorder. The second group consists of middle-aged women who obtain the drug from their physician for complaints of nervousness and become physically dependent. There is no special "addictive personality" that is more prone to abusing these agents.

Sedative, hypnotic, and anxiolytic dependence may eventually lead to both medical and social complications, occupational difficulties (e.g., job loss), and problems with relationships. Drug-dependent persons sometimes turn to crime to obtain their drug of choice. Not much is known about the natural history of sedative, hypnotic, and anxiolytic dependence, but like alcoholism, the course probably is chronic and relapsing.

Sedative, hypnotic, and anxiolytic misuse can lead to intoxication, withdrawal, and withdrawal delirium. These syndromes vary little from drug to drug, although the withdrawal phenomena may be more intense with the shorter-acting drugs (e.g., alprazolam) and more prolonged with the longer-acting ones (e.g., phenobarbital). The syndromes are similar to those seen with alcoholism, which is not surprising because these agents are cross-tolerant. As in alcohol withdrawal, symptoms may occur when the substance is abruptly withdrawn or the dose is reduced.

The symptoms of sedative, hypnotic, and anxiolytic intoxication are dose related. Lethargy, impaired mental functioning, poor memory, irritability, self-neglect, and emotional disinhibition all may occur in intoxicated persons. As intoxication progresses, slurred speech, ataxia, and impaired coordination can develop. With higher doses, death may occur as a result of respiratory depression, a complication that rarely occurs with the benzodiazepines. (The DSM-IV-TR criteria for sedative, hypnotic, or anxiolytic intoxication are found in Table 15–4.)

TABLE 15–4.   DSM-IV-TR diagnostic criteria for sedative, hypnotic, or anxiolytic intoxication

A. Recent use of a sedative, hypnotic, or anxiolytic.

B. Clinically significant maladaptive behavioral or psychological changes (e.g., inappropriate sexual or aggressive behavior, mood lability, impaired judgment, impaired social or occupational functioning) that developed during, or shortly after, sedative, hypnotic, or anxiolytic use.

C. One (or more) of the following signs, developing during, or shortly after, sedative, hypnotic, or anxiolytic use:

(1) slurred speech

(2) incoordination

(3) unsteady gait

(4) nystagmus

(5) impairment in attention or memory

(6) stupor or coma

D. The symptoms are not due to a general medical condition and are not better accounted for by another mental disorder.

Withdrawal from sedatives, hypnotics, and anxiolytics can be hazardous and should be carefully monitored (Table 15–5). During the first 24 hours of withdrawal, the patient is typically anxious, restless, and apprehensive. Coarse tremors develop, and deep tendon reflexes become hyperactive. Weakness, nausea and vomiting, orthostatic hypotension, sweating, and other signs of autonomic hyperarousal occur. On the second or third day of withdrawal, grand mal seizures can occur. The seizures generally consist of a single convulsion or burst of several convulsions; status epilepticus rarely develops. A withdrawal delirium, associated with confusion, disorientation, and visual and somatic hallucinations, sometimes develops at this stage. Barbiturate withdrawal can be especially serious, and its symptoms are presented in Table 15–6.

TABLE 15–5. DSM-IV-TR diagnostic criteria for sedative, hypnotic, or anxiolytic withdrawal

A. Cessation of (or reduction in) sedative, hypnotic, or anxiolytic use that has been heavy and prolonged.

B. Two (or more) of the following, developing within several hours to a few days after Criterion A:

    (1) autonomic hyperactivity (e.g., sweating or pulse rate greater than 100)

    (2) increased hand tremor

    (3) insomnia

    (4) nausea or vomiting

    (5) transient visual, tactile, or auditory hallucinations or illusions

    (6) psychomotor agitation

    (7) anxiety

    (8) grand mal seizures

C. The symptoms in Criterion B cause clinically significant distress or impairment in social, occupational, or other important areas of functioning.

D. The symptoms are not due to a general medical condition and are not better accounted for by another mental disorder.

Specify if:

    With Perceptual Disturbances

Patients addicted to sedatives, hypnotics, or anxiolytics should undergo withdrawal from the drug under medical supervision and in some cases in the hospital. Before a tapering withdrawal schedule is initiated, a tolerance test should be given with either pentobarbital or diazepam when the patient's total daily dosage is either unknown or unusually high (Table 15–7). The test should be administered to a patient who is not currently intoxicated.

Once the level of tolerance has been established, the patient is withdrawn by using phenobarbital or diazepam. (Other long-acting benzodiazepines will work just as well.) The initial dose is determined by substituting 30 mg of phenobarbital for every 100 mg of pentobarbital administered during the tolerance test. During withdrawal, the daily dosage of phenobarbital is decreased by 30 mg. When diazepam is used, the daily dosage is decreased by 10 mg from an initial level equal to the intoxicating dose. On this schedule, the patient will be somewhat uncomfortable. If signs of withdrawal

TABLE 15–6.   Barbiturate withdrawal syndrome

Severity	Symptoms	Onset	Duration
Minor	Postural hypotension; nausea, vomiting, anorexia; tremors; sleeplessness; agitation/anxiety	12–24 hours	Up to 14 days
Moderate	Status epilepticus; seizures; myoclonic jerking	2–3 days	Up to 8 days
Dangerous	Death; hyperpyrexia; delirium tremens; hallucinosis	3–4 days	Up to 14 days

worsen or if the patient becomes somnolent or intoxicated, the schedule can be adjusted. Some patients will present at the hospital already experiencing withdrawal symptoms, in which case pentobarbital or diazepam should be administered in sufficient dosages to make them comfortable before the withdrawal procedure is initiated.

Certain general rules apply to all patients who are given these drugs. The drugs should be targeted at specific symptoms or syndromes (e.g., generalized anxiety disorder), and their use should be limited to weeks or months whenever possible; the drugs should be prescribed at the minimum dosage necessary to control the patient's symptoms. Because of the proven safety and efficacy of benzodiazepines, there is no reason to prescribe the more dangerous barbiturates (except for their use as anticonvulsants) or the other nonbarbiturate sedative-hypnotics.

Opioid Use Disorders

The opiates include morphine, heroin, hydromorphine, codeine, and meperidine. (Meperidine is a synthetic opiate pharmacologically similar to morphine.) The opiates are commonly used for pain control, and heroin is the only one of these substances not available in the United States for medicinal use.

Opiate abuse is more common in urban settings, among men, and among African Americans. It is also more common among physicians and other health care professionals than among other occupations, probably because of the availability of these drugs in medical settings. Many persons who are addicted to opiates have other psychiatric disorders as well, including other substance use disorders, mood disorders, and anxiety disorders. Up to 50% of opiate-addicted persons have antisocial personality disorder.

TABLE 15–7. Pentobarbital-diazepam tolerance test

1. Pentobarbital 200 mg (or diazepam 20 mg) is administered orally. Evaluate in 2 hours:

   - No tolerance—the patient is asleep but arousable

   - Tolerance to 400–500 mg of pentobarbital (or 40–50 mg of diazepam)—the patient is grossly ataxic and has a coarse tremor or lateral nystagmus

   - Tolerance to 600 mg of pentobarbital (or 60 mg of diazepam)—the patient is mildly ataxic

   - Tolerance to 800 mg of pentobarbital (or 80 mg of diazepam)—the patient has slight nystagmus

   - Tolerance to 1,000 mg of pentobarbital (or 100 mg of diazepam)—the patient is asymptomatic

2. If the patient remains asymptomatic, an additional oral dose of pentobarbital 200 mg (or diazepam 20 mg) is given.

   - Failure to become symptomatic at this dose suggests a daily tolerance of >1,600 mg of pentobarbital (or 160 mg of diazepam)

Many users turn to crime because of the relatively high cost of opiates.

The natural history of opiate addiction is variable and depends on both availability and exposure to its use. In a 12-year follow-up of opiate-addicted patients treated in a federal treatment center, 98% returned to using opiates within 12 months of release. A follow-up study in London found a relapse rate of 53% within 6 months. A 24-year follow-up of persons addicted to narcotics in California confirmed that substance use and criminal involvement continued over the years and that cessation of drug use was uncommon. However, a study of military veterans who had used opiates in Vietnam found that fewer than 2% continued their use after returning home. These discrepant findings suggest that there may be more than one type of user.

Opiate addiction is associated with high mortality rates because of inadvertent fatal overdoses, accidental deaths, and suicide. Although it is unlikely that addicted persons will outgrow their habit over the years, the death rate is so high that there are relatively few older abusers.

Opiate users need to be carefully evaluated because they are likely to have comorbid medical illness. Opiate-addicted persons also are at high risk for developing medical conditions stemming from their poor nutritional status and use of dirty needles. Serum hepatitis, HIV infection, pneumonia, skin ulcers (at injection sites), and cellulitis are all too common among those addicted to opiates.

Most persons who are addicted to heroin or morphine inject opiates intravenously, producing both euphoria and a sense of well-being; drowsiness, inactivity, psychomotor retardation, and impaired concentration follow. Physical signs that occur after a heroin-addicted person "shoots up" (which may occur three or more times a day) include flushing, pupillary constriction, slurred speech, respiratory depression, hypotension, hypothermia, and bradycardia. Constipation, nausea, and vomiting are also frequent. (The criteria for opioid intoxication are presented in Table 15–8.)

TABLE 15–8.   DSM-IV-TR diagnostic criteria for opioid intoxication

A. Recent use of an opioid.

B. Clinically significant maladaptive behavioral or psychological changes (e.g., initial euphoria followed by apathy, dysphoria, psychomotor agitation or retardation, impaired judgment, or impaired social or occupational functioning) that developed during, or shortly after, opioid use.

C. Pupillary constriction (or pupillary dilation due to anoxia from severe overdose) and one (or more) of the following signs, developing during, or shortly after, opioid use:

  (1) drowsiness or coma

  (2) slurred speech

  (3) impairment in attention or memory

D. The symptoms are not due to a general medical condition and are not better accounted for by another mental disorder.

Specify if:

  With Perceptual Disturbances

Tolerance eventually develops to most of these drug effects, including the euphoria. Sexual interest diminishes, and in women, menstruation may cease. In the chronic user, depending on dose and drug potency, withdrawal symptoms begin approximately 10 hours after the last dose with short-acting opioids (e.g., morphine, heroin) or after a longer period with longer-acting substances (e.g., meperidine). Minor withdrawal symptoms include lacrimation, rhinorrhea, sweating, yawning, piloerection, hypertension, and tachycardia. Symptoms that indicate more severe withdrawal include hot and cold flashes, muscle and joint pain, nausea, vomiting, and abdominal cramps. Seizures sometimes occur during meperidine withdrawal. Psychological symptoms of withdrawal include severe anxiety and restlessness, irritability, insomnia, and decreased appetite. (The criteria for opioid withdrawal are found in Table 15–9.)

Patients addicted to opiates should be gradually withdrawn by using methadone, a long-acting opiate. The initial methadone dose is determined by the presenting signs and symptoms of withdrawal (see Table 15–10). The

TABLE 15–9. DSM-IV-TR diagnostic criteria for opioid withdrawal

A. Either of the following:

  (1) cessation of (or reduction in) opioid use that has been heavy and prolonged (several weeks or longer)

  (2) administration of an opioid antagonist after a period of opioid use

B. Three (or more) of the following, developing within minutes to several days after Criterion A:

  (1) dysphoric mood

  (2) nausea or vomiting

  (3) muscle aches

  (4) lacrimation or rhinorrhea

  (5) pupillary dilation, piloerection, or sweating

  (6) diarrhea

  (7) yawning

  (8) fever

  (9) insomnia

C. The symptoms in Criterion B cause clinically significant distress or impairment in social, occupational, or other important areas of functioning.

D. The symptoms are not due to a general medical condition and are not better accounted for by another mental disorder.

dose is then repeated in 12 hours, and supplemental doses are given when necessary. Once the 24-hour dose is determined, the dose is tapered at the rate of 20% per day for short-acting opiates or 20% every other day for long-acting opiates. Once the patient has stabilized, methadone should be given two to three times daily, and the patient's vital signs should be recorded before each dose. Withdrawal from short-acting substances (e.g., heroin, morphine) typically takes 7–10 days. Withdrawal from longer-acting substances (e.g., methadone) proceeds more slowly (e.g., 2–3 weeks).

Another drug used to withdraw patients from opiates is clonidine, which provides good suppression of the autonomic signs of withdrawal. Patients do better with an abrupt switch to clonidine when the methadone dose is first stabilized at 20 mg or less daily. At the first sign of withdrawal, the patient is given 0.3–0.5 mg (0.006 mg/kg) of clonidine, which is repeated at bedtime. For the next 4 days, the patient receives 0.9–1.5 mg/day in three to four divided doses. The dose should be withheld if the diastolic blood pressure falls below 60 mm Hg or marked sedation occurs. On days 6–8, the dose can be decreased by 50%, and on day 9, clonidine can be discontinued altogether. For long-acting opiates, clonidine reduction should occur on days 11–14, with discontinuation on day 15.

TABLE 15–10.   Methadone withdrawal dosing schedule

Signs and symptoms	Initial methadone dose (mg)
Lacrimation, rhinorrhea, diaphoresis, yawning, restlessness, insomnia	5
Dilated pupils, piloerection, muscle twitching, myalgias, arthralgias, abdominal pain	10
Tachycardia, hypertension, tachypnea, fever, anorexia, extreme restlessness, nausea	15
Diarrhea, vomiting, dehydration, hyperglycemia, hypotension	20

Source. Adapted from Perry et al. 1997.

Naltrexone, a long-acting opioid antagonist, is also used for opiate withdrawal. The drug blocks opioid receptors, thereby preventing the behaviorally reinforcing euphoric effects of opiates. Naltrexone is usually given over 5–10 days after the last opiate use at doses of 25–50 mg/day. The dosage is gradually increased to 100–150 mg three times weekly. Although approved for opioid withdrawal by the U.S. Food and Drug Administration, the effectiveness of naltrexone varies greatly with the population studied. In some groups that have been studied, the drug was poorly accepted and was associated with high dropout rates.

The combination of clonidine and naltrexone also has been used. Naltrexone may act to "reset" or desensitize opiate receptors, thereby facilitating withdrawal. With this approach, withdrawal can be shortened to as little as 3–4 days. Buprenorphine, a mixed opiate agonist-antagonist, also is being studied for use in both opiate withdrawal and maintenance treatment. Low doses (2–4 mg) are agonistic, whereas doses greater than 8 mg are generally antagonistic. Patients can be switched directly from their opiate drug to buprenorphine and are then detoxified.

Other adjunctive therapies are often helpful in opiate withdrawal. Benzodiazepines can treat very mild cases of withdrawal and can help relieve anxiety and promote needed sleep. Mild analgesics, such as the nonsteroidal anti-inflammatory drugs (NSAIDs), can relieve muscle aches and pain. Gastrointestinal distress can be treated with dicyclomine.

It is not uncommon to find patients tolerant to different substances (e.g., both a sedative-hypnotic and an opiate). When this situation occurs, it is safest to stabilize the patient on a dose of methadone and withdraw the sedative-hypnotic first because sedative-hypnotic withdrawal is potentially the more dangerous syndrome.

Participation in a federally approved methadone maintenance program continues to be the major alternative to complete cessation of use. With this approach, methadone is administered orally (e.g., 60–100 mg/day). Because of its long half-life (22–56 hours) and its wide distribution in the body, the drug has few subjective effects and produces almost no withdrawal symptoms. The rationale for methadone maintenance is that by switching addicted patients to methadone, their drug hunger is alleviated so that they are less preoccupied with drug-seeking behavior. For the most part, this approach has been successful, and most patients in these programs show significant decreases in opiate and nonopiate drug use, criminal activity, and depressive symptoms. They also show increases in gainful employment and stability in social relationships. Many programs espouse the view that methadone is a transitional treatment that will eventually lead to total abstinence, yet at least one well-designed study has shown that methadone maintenance programs produce better results than detoxification. Methadone programs also emphasize ongoing individual and group psychotherapy to help keep addicted persons in the program and to assist them in coping with day-to-day problems without resorting to drugs.

An alternative to methadone is levomethadyl acetate, a long-acting μ-opioid agonist that produces opioid blockade. It offers a more subtle and prolonged clinical effect than methadone, and its main advantage is that it can be administered three times weekly instead of daily. It also appears to have less abuse potential than methadone. Like methadone maintenance, its use is confined to specially sanctioned programs.

Central Nervous System Stimulant Use Disorders

CNS stimulants include dextroamphetamine, methylphenidate, methamphetamine, phenmetrazine, and cocaine. The action of these agents is to elevate mood, increase energy and alertness, decrease appetite, and improve task performance. These drugs also cause autonomic hyperarousal, which leads to tachycardia, elevated blood pressure, and pupillary dilation. Amphetamines were first used in the 1930s and have been prescribed for depression, obesity, sleep disorders, and attention-deficit/hyperactivity disorder. (Their rational use in the treatment of attention-deficit/hyperactivity disorder is discussed in Chapter 27.)

The abuse potential of stimulants was recognized relatively early, and illicit use of these drugs is widespread. Because of their overuse in the 1970s as diet pills, changes in the regulation of their legitimate distribution were made to stem the tide of abuse. Even though their legal use has declined, many of these compounds are easy to synthesize, and their illegal use continues to grow. One of the newest drugs to hit the black market, "ice," is a crystallized form of the easily synthesized drug methamphetamine.

Cocaine differs structurally from the amphetamines but has similar stimulant effects. Derived from the coca plant, which is indigenous to certain countries in South America, cocaine has legitimate medical use as a local anesthetic. Cocaine has always had a following in the United States because of its pleasurable effects. In fact, it was used in the late nineteenth century in a variety of elixirs and tonics, including the original Coca-Cola formulation. Freud, the founding father of psychoanalysis, was one of its earliest advocates. However, cocaine became increasingly associated with sudden death, emotional and domestic problems, and addiction. It was finally declared an illegal narcotic in the Harrison Act of 1914. Cocaine has continued to be a popular recreational drug, although its use has generally been restricted to affluent groups because of its high cost. A low-cost derivative, crack, became available in the 1980s.

The clinical syndromes produced by the CNS stimulants include those of abuse and dependence, intoxication, delirium, psychosis, mood disorders, and withdrawal. Amphetamine intoxication (Table 15–11) and cocaine intoxication are quite similar and are diagnosed on the basis of their recent use, maladaptive behavior, and evidence of autonomic hyperarousal.

Unlike intoxication with the other stimulants, cocaine intoxication can cause tactile hallucinations (e.g., "coke bugs"). Psychological symptoms of intoxication include a sense of euphoria, disinhibition, sexual arousal, enhanced feelings of mastery, and improved self-esteem. Depending on how the drug is administered (e.g., intranasally, intravenously), users may experience a rapid onset of euphoria, or rush. By smoking a purified cocaine base that has been freed from its salts and cutting agents by a chemical process (i.e., freebasing), users report an even more rapid but short-lived high. Table 15–12 presents a list of common psychological and physical symptoms seen in freebase cocaine abusers.

Stimulant intoxication can induce aggression, agitation, and impaired judgment. Transient psychosis may occur, involving persecutory delusions similar to those seen in patients with paranoid schizophrenia; the psychosis usually subsides 1–2 weeks after the drug use stops. If a stimulant-induced psychosis persists, a diagnosis of schizophrenia should be considered as long as it is clear that there is no continuing source of the drug. Delirium is a rare complication that gradually resolves once the drug has been discontinued. Cocaine also has been associated with serious medical complications such as acute myocardial infarction due to coronary artery constriction and anox-

---

TABLE 15–11. DSM-IV-TR diagnostic criteria for amphetamine intoxication

A. Recent use of amphetamine or a related substance (e.g., methylphenidate).
B. Clinically significant maladaptive behavioral or psychological changes (e.g., euphoria or affective blunting; changes in sociability; hypervigilance; interpersonal sensitivity; anxiety, tension, or anger; stereotyped behaviors; impaired judgment; or impaired social or occupational functioning) that developed during, or shortly after, use of amphetamine or a related substance.
C. Two (or more) of the following, developing during, or shortly after, use of amphetamine or a related substance:
  (1) tachycardia or bradycardia
  (2) pupillary dilation
  (3) elevated or lowered blood pressure
  (4) perspiration or chills
  (5) nausea or vomiting
  (6) evidence of weight loss
  (7) psychomotor agitation or retardation
  (8) muscular weakness, respiratory depression, chest pain, or cardiac arrhythmias
  (9) confusion, seizures, dyskinesias, dystonias, or coma
D. The symptoms are not due to a general medical condition and are not better accounted for by another mental disorder.
Specify if:
  With Perceptual Disturbances

---

ic brain damage due to cocaine-induced seizures.

Cessation or reduction of amphetamine (or cocaine) use may lead to a withdrawal syndrome often referred to as a crash (Table 15–13). Symptoms include fatigue and depression, nightmares, headache, profuse sweating, muscle cramps, and hunger. Withdrawal symptoms usually peak in 2–4 days. Intense dysphoria can occur, peaking between 48 and 72 hours after the last dose of the stimulant.

Because amphetamine intoxication and amphetamine psychotic disorder are generally self-limiting, no specific treatment is necessary. Benzodiazepines (e.g., diazepam, lorazepam) can be used to treat agitation or anxiety. Antipsychotics have been used to treat the symptoms of stimulant-induced psychosis but may be unnecessary because the psychosis is generally short lived once the offending drugs have been stopped. Elimination of the drug can be accelerated by acidifying the urine with ammonium chloride, but this step is rarely necessary. A withdrawal depression that persists longer than 2 weeks can be treated with antidepressants, although their use in these cases

TABLE 15–12. Common psychological and physical symptoms in 32 freebase cocaine abusers

Psychological symptoms	%	Physical symptoms	%
Paranoia	63	Blurred vision	34
Visual hallucinations	50	Coughing	34
Craving	47	Muscle aches	34
Asocial behavior	41	Dry skin	28
Impaired concentration	38	Tremors	28
Irritability	31	Weight loss	25
Bad dreams	31	Chest pains	22
Hyperexcitability	28	Episodic unconsciousness	16
Violence	28	Difficult urination	16
Auditory hallucinations	25	Respiratory problems	9
Lethargy	25	Edema	9
Depression	25	Seizures	3

Source. Adapted from Vereby and Gold 1988.

TABLE 15–13. DSM-IV-TR diagnostic criteria for amphetamine withdrawal

A. Cessation of (or reduction in) amphetamine (or a related substance) use that has been heavy and prolonged.

B. Dysphoric mood and two (or more) of the following physiological changes, developing within a few hours to several days after Criterion A:

   (1) fatigue

   (2) vivid, unpleasant dreams

   (3) insomnia or hypersomnia

   (4) increased appetite

   (5) psychomotor retardation or agitation

C. The symptoms in Criterion B cause clinically significant distress or impairment in social, occupational, or other important areas of functioning.

D. The symptoms are not due to a general medical condition and are not better accounted for by another mental disorder.

has not been systematically evaluated. Desipramine and other antidepressants have been used to treat cocaine withdrawal, as have the dopamine agonists bromocriptine and amantadine, but their success in reducing cocaine craving has been mixed. Flupenthixol, an antipsychotic not available in the United States, also has been used to facilitate cocaine withdrawal. None of these drugs is routinely used in clinical practice, however.

Hallucinogen and Arylcyclohexylamine Use Disorders

Hallucinogens are a diverse group of compounds; most are synthetic, but two (peyote, mescaline) are of botanical origin. These drugs can induce psychotic-like experiences, including hallucinations, perceptual disturbances, and feelings of unreality. Some persons believe that hallucinogens bring them closer to God or can expand their minds. The drugs achieved popularity in the late 1960s and early 1970s when psychedelic substances were romanticized, and self-styled drug gurus like the late Timothy Leary advocated their use. Their use continues, although they are probably not as popular now.

As sympathomimetics, hallucinogens can cause tachycardia, hypertension, sweating, blurry vision, pupillary dilation, and tremors. They affect the neurotransmitters dopamine, serotonin, acetylcholine, and γ-aminobutyric acid (GABA). Tolerance can develop to some (e.g., LSD) but not others (e.g., PCP). Hallucinogens are probably not physically addicting, but many persons have become psychologically dependent on them.

The hallucinogens differ in quality and duration of their subjective effects. As the prototype, LSD is short acting and rapidly absorbed. Onset of action occurs within an hour of ingestion, and its effects last between 8 and 12 hours. In addition to autonomic hyperarousal, the drug causes varied psychological effects, including profound alterations in perception (e.g., colors may be experienced as brighter and more intense), and senses appear heightened. Emotions seem to intensify, and many users report becoming more introspective. Many users claim that their use leads to spiritual and philosophical insight. DSM-IV and DSM-IV-TR have termed this reaction *hallucinogen intoxication* (see Table 15–14). In fact, these properties led psychiatrists to experiment with LSD and other hallucinogens in the early 1960s for therapeutic purposes, such as to facilitate communication, improve insight, and increase self-esteem.

"Bad trips" occasionally occur, in which patients become markedly anxious or paranoid. Another undesirable outcome is the flashback, a brief reexperiencing of the drug's effects that occurs in situations unrelated to

TABLE 15–14.   DSM-IV-TR diagnostic criteria for hallucinogen intoxication

A. Recent use of a hallucinogen.

B. Clinically significant maladaptive behavioral or psychological changes (e.g., marked anxiety or depression, ideas of reference, fear of losing one's mind, paranoid ideation, impaired judgment, or impaired social or occupational functioning) that developed during, or shortly after, hallucinogen use.

C. Perceptual changes occurring in a state of full wakefulness and alertness (e.g., subjective intensification of perceptions, depersonalization, derealization, illusions, hallucinations, synesthesias) that developed during, or shortly after, hallucinogen use.

D. Two (or more) of the following signs, developing during, or shortly after, hallucinogen use:

   (1) pupillary dilation

   (2) tachycardia

   (3) sweating

   (4) palpitations

   (5) blurring of vision

   (6) tremors

   (7) incoordination

E. The symptoms are not due to a general medical condition and are not better accounted for by another mental disorder.

taking the drug. Flashbacks consist of visual distortions, geometric hallucinations, and misperceptions. In DSM-IV-TR, flashbacks that cause marked distress are diagnosed as *hallucinogen persisting perception disorder* (see Table 15–15). The disorder is usually self-limiting, but it may become chronic in rare cases.

Chronic psychosis has been reported in some hallucinogen users, and it was once thought that these drugs could induce schizophrenia. Although these drugs may cause psychotic episodes in some individuals, users who develop schizophrenia probably would have developed the illness regardless of their hallucinogen use.

PCP, the prototypical arylcyclohexylamine, has become a significant drug of abuse since the late 1960s. Common street terms for the drug include *angel dust* and *crystal*. PCP originally was developed as an anesthetic agent for animals, and although it affects several neurotransmitter systems, its mechanism of action is still unknown. The drug may produce intoxication, delirium, psychosis, or mood disorders and has been known to cause flashbacks. Because PCP is easy to manufacture and is relatively cheap, it is often used to adulterate other illicit compounds.

TABLE 15–15.   DSM-IV-TR diagnostic criteria for hallucinogen persisting perception disorder (flashbacks)

A. The reexperiencing, following cessation of use of a hallucinogen, of one or more of the perceptual symptoms that were experienced while intoxicated with the hallucinogen (e.g., geometric hallucinations, false perceptions of movement in the peripheral visual fields, flashes of color, intensified colors, trails of images of moving objects, positive afterimages, halos around objects, macropsia, and micropsia).

B. The symptoms in Criterion A cause clinically significant distress or impairment in social, occupational, or other important areas of functioning.

C. The symptoms are not due to a general medical condition (e.g., anatomical lesions and infections of the brain, visual epilepsies) and are not better accounted for by another mental disorder (e.g., delirium, dementia, Schizophrenia) or hypnopompic hallucinations.

PCP can be taken in a variety of ways (e.g., orally, intravenously, intranasally). Onset of action occurs in as short as 5 minutes and peaks in about 30 minutes. Users report feelings of euphoria, derealization, tingling, and warmth. With moderate doses, bizarre behavior may occur, along with myoclonic jerks, confusion, and disorientation. Higher doses can produce coma and seizures. Death can result from respiratory depression. Unlike hallucinogen users, who tend to have dilated pupils, PCP users have normal or small pupils. Chronic psychotic episodes can follow its use, and unlike other hallucinogens, PCP may cause long-term neuropsychological damage. (The criteria for phencyclidine intoxication are found in Table 15–16.)

Treatment may be required for adverse reactions. Diazepam can be used to treat agitation, but severe behavioral disturbances may require short-term antipsychotic use, preferably one with a relative lack of anticholinergic side effects (e.g., haloperidol). Phentolamine or other antihypertensive drugs can be used to reduce elevated blood pressure. Ammonium chloride can be used to acidify the urine to promote the drug's elimination, although its use is generally unnecessary.

Cannabis Use Disorders

The active ingredient in marijuana is thought to be delta-9-tetrahydrocannabinol (THC). Marijuana is a hemp plant (*Cannabis sativa*) that has been used for centuries for medicinal and recreational purposes. The plant contains varying amounts of THC; plants used today tend to have much higher THC concentrations than in the past. Marijuana achieved popularity among the drug subculture in the 1960s and 1970s and is still widely used.

TABLE 15–16.   DSM-IV-TR diagnostic criteria for phencyclidine intoxication

---

A.   Recent use of phencyclidine (or a related substance).

B.   Clinically significant maladaptive behavioral changes (e.g., belligerence, assaultiveness, impulsiveness, unpredictability, psychomotor agitation, impaired judgment, or impaired social or occupational functioning) that developed during, or shortly after, phencyclidine use.

C.   Within an hour (less when smoked, "snorted," or used intravenously), two (or more) of the following signs:

   (1) vertical or horizontal nystagmus

   (2) hypertension or tachycardia

   (3) numbness or diminished responsiveness to pain

   (4) ataxia

   (5) dysarthria

   (6) muscle rigidity

   (7) seizures or coma

   (8) hyperacusis

D.   The symptoms are not due to a general medical condition and are not better accounted for by another mental disorder.

Specify if:

   With Perceptual Disturbances

Marijuana is generally smoked as a cigarette (often called a joint), causing intoxication within 10–30 minutes. THC and its metabolites are highly lipid soluble and accumulate in fat cells; the half-life is approximately 50 hours. Intoxication can last 2–4 hours depending on the dose, although behavioral changes may continue for many hours. Oral ingestion (e.g., from adding marijuana to baked goods) produces a slower onset of action but leads to more powerful intoxicant effects.

Psychological effects of marijuana intoxication include feelings of euphoria and serenity and drowsiness. Users also report feeling that time has slowed. Users develop increased appetite and thirst, feel that their senses are heightened, and report improved self-confidence. Physical symptoms include conjunctivitis (red eyes), tachycardia, dry mouth (cotton mouth), and coughing fits (Table 15–17). Many effects reported by marijuana users are similar to those reported by LSD users, such as the development of perceptual distortions, sensitivity to sound, and a feeling of oneness with the environment. Unwanted effects include feelings of anxiety and paranoia (e.g., hyperalertness, suspiciousness), impaired attention, and decreased motor coordination. Marijuana rarely causes severe psychological or physical reactions.

TABLE 15–17. DSM-IV-TR diagnostic criteria for cannabis intoxication

A. Recent use of cannabis.
B. Clinically significant maladaptive behavioral or psychological changes (e.g., impaired motor coordination, euphoria, anxiety, sensation of slowed time, impaired judgment, social withdrawal) that developed during, or shortly after, cannabis use.
C. Two (or more) of the following signs, developing within 2 hours of cannabis use:
    (1) conjunctival injection
    (2) increased appetite
    (3) dry mouth
    (4) tachycardia
D. The symptoms are not due to a general medical condition and are not better accounted for by another mental disorder.
Specify if:
    With Perceptual Disturbances

Marijuana has been shown to impair the transfer of material from immediate to long-term memory. Electroencephalographic studies show a suppression of rapid eye movement (REM) sleep and diffuse slowing of background activity. Chronic use has been associated with an *amotivational syndrome* characterized by impersistence at schoolwork or any task that requires a prolonged attention period. Patients may seem apathetic or inert. It is often difficult to isolate the effects of marijuana because many of its regular users also take other drugs.

Professional help usually is not needed to treat the adverse effects of marijuana. Anxiolytics (e.g., diazepam) may help to calm highly anxious users. Because no characteristic withdrawal syndrome occurs, detoxification is unnecessary.

Inhalant Use Disorders

The inhalants are a group of compounds that produce psychoactive vapors, including airplane glue, paint thinner, nail polish remover, gasoline, and many other substances found in aerosol cans (e.g., hair spray, room deodorizers). The active substances in the inhalants include toluene, acetone, benzene, and other organic hydrocarbons. Methods of inhalation may vary, but usually a substance is sprayed into a plastic bag and inhaled. (The criteria for inhalant intoxication are presented in Table 15–18.)

The use of volatile solvents is widespread, and it is estimated that 1 in 10 persons younger than 17 years has experimented with them. Because they are widely available and cheap, inhalants are mostly used by young per-

TABLE 15–18.   DSM-IV-TR diagnostic criteria for inhalant intoxication

A. Recent intentional use or short-term, high-dose exposure to volatile inhalants (excluding anesthetic gases and short-acting vasodilators).

B. Clinically significant maladaptive behavioral or psychological changes (e.g., belligerence, assaultiveness, apathy, impaired judgment, impaired social or occupational functioning) that developed during, or shortly after, use of or exposure to volatile inhalants.

C. Two (or more) of the following signs, developing during, or shortly after, inhalant use or exposure:

  (1) dizziness
  (2) nystagmus
  (3) incoordination
  (4) slurred speech
  (5) unsteady gait
  (6) lethargy
  (7) depressed reflexes
  (8) psychomotor retardation
  (9) tremor
  (10) generalized muscle weakness
  (11) blurred vision or diplopia
  (12) stupor or coma
  (13) euphoria

D. The symptoms are not due to a general medical condition and are not better accounted for by another mental disorder.

sons who have trouble gaining access to other psychoactive substances.

Most users of inhalants are male. Latinos and Native Americans are overrepresented among inhalant users. Although experimentation with inhalants is extremely common, regular use is found primarily among the lower socioeconomic classes, children of alcoholic parents, and children from abusive or disruptive homes.

Inhalants act as CNS depressants and produce an intoxication similar to that of alcohol but of shorter duration. Effects can last 5–45 minutes and include feelings of excitation, disinhibition, and euphoria. Adverse effects include dizziness, slurred speech, and ataxia. Inhalants also may induce an acute delirium characterized by impaired concentration and disorientation. Hallucinations and delusions have been reported with their use. Other effects include loss of appetite, lateral nystagmus, hypoactive reflexes, and double vision. At higher doses, patients may become stuporous or comatose.

Inhalants do not cause a specific withdrawal syndrome. Because inhalants often contain high concentrations of heavy metals, permanent neuro-muscular and brain damage can occur, along with serious risk of damage to the kidneys, liver, and other organs from benzene and other hydrocarbons.

Other Substance Use Disorders

Nicotine

Nicotine is a highly addictive compound found in cigarettes, chewing tobac-co and snuff, and other tobacco products. Currently, about 25% of adult Americans smoke, although smoking is even more frequent in certain groups (e.g., minority groups, persons of low socioeconomic status, less-educated persons). Rates among psychiatric patients are also very high; for example, up to 90% of patients with schizophrenia smoke.

Smoking has been implicated as a cause of lung cancer, emphysema, and cardiovascular disease. Snuff and chewing tobacco have been associated with oropharyngeal cancers. Secondary smoke has been associated with res-piratory and cardiovascular diseases.

Dependence on nicotine develops quickly and is often reinforced by peer pressure. Society has clearly changed its views on smoking, and in re-cent years, smokers' rights have been increasingly limited.

Nicotine withdrawal usually begins within 1 hour after the last cigarette is smoked and peaks within 24 hours. Withdrawal may last weeks or months and consists of nicotine craving, irritability, anxiety, restlessness, and de-creased heart rate. Weight gain and depression often follow smoking cessa-tion.

Relapse is common among former smokers, especially during the first year. Nicotine transdermal patches and nicotine-containing gum help moti-vated persons to quit, but even with these aids, relapse remains distressingly high. Bupropion, an antidepressant, also is marketed as an aid for smoking cessation under the trade name of Zyban. Controlled studies show that it is more effective than placebo in helping people to quit smoking. Because the consequences of tobacco use are so potentially harmful, all physicians have a responsibility to urge their patients, particularly young patients, not to smoke or to use tobacco products and to assist patients who do use them to quit.

Caffeine

Caffeine is found in coffee, tea, chocolate, cola drinks, and many over-the-counter pain and cold remedies. Except for certain religious groups that proscribe its use (e.g., Mormons), use of caffeine is nearly universal.

The mild stimulant effects of caffeine occur at doses of 50–150 mg (i.e., one cup of coffee). These effects include increased alertness and improved verbal and motor performance. At higher doses, unless tolerance has been achieved, signs of intoxication occur, including restlessness, irritability, and insomnia. Doses higher than 1 g/day can lead to seizures and coma. Withdrawal from caffeine can induce headaches, lethargy, irritability, and depression. Higher daily doses are more likely to lead to withdrawal.

Chronic use of caffeine can contribute to excess gastric acidity and aggravate esophageal and gastric disorders, can exacerbate fibrocystic breast disease in women, and can worsen anxiety disorders such as panic disorder or generalized anxiety disorder. Chronic use can itself cause excessive anxiety; in DSM-IV-TR, this condition is called *caffeine-induced anxiety disorder*. Once the disorder is identified, treatment consists of reducing or eliminating caffeine from the diet. Decaffeinated cola drinks, tea, and coffee are now widely available.

Anabolic Steroids

Anabolic steroids are widely abused by athletes who believe that their performance and muscle mass will be enhanced by their use. Although these drugs may initially produce a sense of well-being, this feeling is later replaced by anergy, dysphoria, and irritability. Frank psychosis can develop, as can serious medical problems, such as liver disease.

Nitrate Inhalants

Nitrate inhalants ("poppers") produce an intoxicated state characterized by a feeling of fullness in the head, mild euphoria, a change in time perception, relaxation of the smooth muscles, and possibly an increase in sexual feelings. These drugs carry the possible risk of immune system impairment, respiratory system irritation, and a toxic reaction that may lead to vomiting, severe headaches, and hypotension. They are commonly abused by the gay community and at least initially were thought to be a risk factor for the acquired immunodeficiency syndrome (AIDS).

Nitrous Oxide

Nitrous oxide ("laughing gas") can cause intoxication characterized by light-headedness and a floating sensation that quickly clear once the administration of gas stops. Temporary confusion or paranoia can occur when this substance is used regularly.

Clinical Management of Psychoactive Substance Use

Specific treatment approaches differ depending on the primary agent of abuse, the pattern of abuse, and the characteristics of the abuser. Nonetheless, general guidelines apply to all psychoactive substance abusers. These guidelines are similar to those applied to the alcoholic patient, which are summarized in Chapter 14.

Treatment can be thought of as having two phases—an acute phase and a continuation phase. In the acute phase, detoxification is the major goal. This goal may be difficult to achieve in some patients, such as those with potentially serious withdrawal syndromes (e.g., barbiturate or opiate abusers). Detoxification may be easier in others (e.g., marijuana abusers) who have no specific withdrawal syndrome. Hospitalization is necessary for safe detoxification in some patients so that tolerance can be determined and a slow drug taper can be monitored under medical supervision. The circumstances of detoxification should be determined by the patient and physician working together.

Many persons addicted to drugs have serious medical conditions that the physician also must address during this phase of treatment. For example, a heroin-addicted person may have an antecubital cellulitis and be seropositive for HIV; a cocaine-addicted person may have an eroded nasal septum (from sniffing the drug) that has become secondarily infected.

Psychiatric comorbidity is also important to assess during the acute phase of treatment. Many, if not most, substance abusers have additional psychiatric diagnoses that can have a profound effect on their treatment outcome. Abuse of other substances is the most common comorbidity, followed by mood disorders, anxiety disorders, and personality disorders. Comorbidity always complicates treatment efforts and reduces the likelihood of success. Examples include the amphetamine abuser who develops a suicidal depression during withdrawal and the heroin-addicted person with an antisocial personality disorder whose use seems, in part, motivated by his membership in a street gang that celebrates drug use.

The continuation phase of treatment consists of efforts to rehabilitate the patient and to prevent future use of psychoactive substances. The success of this phase is almost completely dependent on the motivation of the patient because there is no way to truly assess or enforce compliance (except, of course, by frequent and random drug screening tests and threats of punishment for noncompliance). Such strict enforcement is neither possible nor desirable, except in the military, in certain professions (e.g., pilots), and in authoritarian societies.

Multimodel approaches are necessary for rehabilitation. Individual psychotherapy is important to help patients learn about their motivation for using drugs and to learn alternative methods for handling stressful situations. Group therapy, especially in the hospital, is useful in confronting patients with the seriousness of their problem and how the drug significantly affects their lives. Peer groups are unequaled in their ability to achieve confrontation. At least among cocaine-dependent persons, the combination of individual and group psychotherapy works best at preventing relapse, as one recent study showed.

Among other approaches, cognitive-behavioral therapy may help the patient reverse habits that lead to or promote drug use or may correct cognitive distortions (e.g., "If I don't use drugs, I won't be popular with my friends"). Social skills training may help some patients break a cycle of getting in with the wrong crowd and learn to meet and be accepted by more appropriate peers. Family therapy and marital counseling are necessary adjuncts in other patients. Examples include the teenager whose inhalant use has led to considerable disruption of his family life and the young man whose marriage is falling apart because of his cocaine addiction.

Medical approaches for the continuation phase of treatment can be important. Methadone maintenance for those persons addicted to opiates has been popular for years and seems to have an established role in the treatment of at least some opiate addiction. The user is given a carefully monitored substitute addiction that allows him or her to function in society. Patients with comorbid psychiatric disorders may, of course, benefit from ongoing treatment of anxiety, depression, or psychosis.

Self-help groups have become an integral part of a comprehensive treatment approach to substance use disorders. Alcoholics Anonymous (AA) has led the way for the creation of sister groups, such as Cocaine Anonymous (CA), Narcotics Anonymous (NA), and Drugs Anonymous (DA). These groups, now available in many parts of the United States, are organized along the same lines as AA and follow a 12-step model. They provide an atmosphere of mutual support in which recovering addicted persons can share their experiences.

Recommendations for the clinical management of substance use disorders are provided in the box.

Recommendations for management of substance use disorders

1. The clinician should not allow his or her personal beliefs and attitudes about drug abuse to interfere with the care of the addicted patient.

   - Patients need consistent yet firm handling.
   - The clinician should neither condemn addicted persons nor condone their behavior.

2. The clinician should consider both medical and psychiatric comorbidity. Many addicted persons have potentially serious medical problems that require treatment, significant addictions to other substances, mood disorders, or personality disorders.

3. The clinician should be prepared for relapses during the continuation phase of treatment. Relapse is almost inevitable, but it does not represent failure of the treatment program. The clinician must be there to help the patient get back on the wagon.

4. Support groups can be very helpful to the patient, and referral to community-based organizations is essential.

Bibliography

American Psychiatric Association: Diagnostic and Statistical Manual of Mental Disorders, 4th Edition. Washington, DC, American Psychiatric Association, 1994

American Psychiatric Association: Diagnostic and Statistical Manual of Mental Disorders, 4th Edition Revised. Washington, DC, American Psychiatric Association, 2000

American Psychiatric Association: Practice guidelines for the treatment of patients with substance use disorders: alcohol, cocaine, opioids. Am J Psychiatry 152 (suppl 11):1–80, 1995

American Psychiatric Association: Practice guidelines for the treatment of patients with nicotine dependence. Am J Psychiatry 153 (suppl 10):1–31, 1996

Barber WS, O'Brien CP: Early identification and intervention in an office setting. Primary Psychiatry 2:49–55, 1995

Breslau N, Kilbey M, Andreski P: Nicotine withdrawal symptoms and psychiatric disorders: findings from an epidemiologic study of young adults. Am J Psychiatry 149:464–469, 1992

Busto U, Sellers EM, Naranjo CA, et al: Withdrawal reaction after long-term therapeutic use of benzodiazepines. N Engl J Med 315:854–859, 1986

Cadoret RJ, Troughton E, O'Gorman TW, et al: An adoption study of genetic and environmental factors in drug abuse. Arch Gen Psychiatry 43:1131–1136, 1986

Cadoret RJ, Yates WR, Troughton E, et al: An adoption study of drug abuse/dependency in females. Compr Psychiatry 37:88–94, 1996

Cregler LL, Mark H: Medical complications of cocaine abuse. N Engl J Med 315:1495–1500, 1986

Crits-Christoph P, Siqueland L, Blaine J, et al: Psychosocial treatments for cocaine dependence. Arch Gen Psychiatry 56:493–502, 1999

Dinwiddie SH, Zorumski CF, Rubin EH: Psychiatric correlates of chronic solvent abuse. J Clin Psychiatry 48:334–337, 1987

Fishbain DA, Rosomoff HL, Cutler R, et al: Opiate detoxification protocols: a clinical manual. Ann Clin Psychiatry 5:53–65, 1993

Gawin FH, Kleber HD, Byck R, et al: Desipramine facilitation of initial cocaine abstinence. Arch Gen Psychiatry 46:117–121, 1989

Gossop M, Green L, Phillips G, et al: What happens to opiate addicts immediately after treatment: a prospective follow-up study. BMJ 294:1377–1380, 1987

Halikas JA, Weller RA, Morse CL, et al: Regular marijuana use and its effect on psychosocial variables: a longitudinal study. Compr Psychiatry 24:229–235, 1983

Hser YI, Anglin MD, Powers K: A 24-year follow-up of California narcotic addicts. Arch Gen Psychiatry 50:577–584, 1993

Hughes JR, Goldstein MG, Hurt RD, et al: Recent advances in the pharmacotherapy of smoking. JAMA 281:72–76, 1999

Jones HE, Strain EL, Bigelow GE, et al: Induction with levomethadyl acetate: safety and efficacy. Arch Gen Psychiatry 55:729–736, 1998

Jorenby DE, Leischow SJ, Nides MA, et al: A controlled trial of sustained release bupropion, a nicotine patch, or both for smoking cessation. N Engl J Med 340:685–691, 1999

Little KY, Zhang L, Desmond T, et al: Striatal dopamine abnormalities in human cocaine users. Am J Psychiatry 156:238–245, 1999

McNagney SE, Parker RM: High prevalence of recent cocaine use and the unreliability of patient self-report in an inner city walk-in clinic. JAMA 267:1106–1108, 1992

Merikangas KR, Stolar M, Stevens DE, et al: Familial transmission of substance use disorders. Arch Gen Psychiatry 55:973–979, 1998

National Consensus Development Panel on Effective Medical Treatment of Opiate Addiction: Effective medical treatment of opiate addiction. JAMA 280:1936–1943, 1998

Perry P, Anderson K, Yates W: Illicit anabolic steroid use in athletes: a case series analysis. Am J Sports Med 184:422–428, 1990

Perry PJ, Alexander B, Liskow BI: Psychotropic Drug Handbook, 7th Edition. Washington, DC, American Psychiatric Press, 1997, p 566

Pope HG, Yurgelun-Todd D: The residual cognitive effects of heavy marijuana use in college students. JAMA 275:521–527, 1996

Pope HG, Kouri EM, Powell KF, et al: Anabolic-androgenic steroid use among 133 prisoners. Compr Psychiatry 37:322–327, 1996

Schlaepfer TE, Strain EC, Greenberg BD, et al: Site of opioid action in the human brain: mu and kappa agonists' subjective and cerebrospinal blood flow effects. Am J Psychiatry 155:470–473, 1998

Sees KL, Delucchi KL, Masson C, et al: Methadone maintenance vs 180-day psychosocially enriched detoxification for treatment of opioid dependence: a randomized controlled trial. JAMA 283:1303–1310, 2000

Vaillant GE: A 12-year follow-up of New York narcotic addicts. Arch Gen Psychiatry 15:599–609, 1966

Vardy M, Kay S: LSD psychosis or LSD induced schizophrenia? Arch Gen Psychiatry 40:877–883, 1983

Vereby K, Gold MS: From coca leaves to crack: the effects of dose and routes of administration in abuse liability. Psychiatr Ann 18:513–520, 1988

Warner EA: Cocaine abuse. Ann Intern Med 119:226–235, 1993

Yates WR, Fulton AI, Gabel J, et al: Personality risk factors for cocaine abuse. Am J Public Health 79:891–892, 1989

Young CR: Sertraline treatment of hallucinogen persisting perception disorder (letter). J Clin Psychiatry 58:85, 1997

Self-Assessment Questions

1. How widespread are substance abuse and dependence, and what are their risk factors?
2. What appear to be the two types of sedative-hypnotic abusers?
3. Describe the withdrawal syndrome from sedatives, hypnotics, and anxiolytics.
4. Why are barbiturates especially dangerous?
5. Describe the pentobarbital-diazepam tolerance test.
6. Describe the opiate withdrawal syndrome and how it differs from sedative-hypnotic withdrawal.
7. What are the pharmacokinetics of cocaine?
8. Does the use of LSD lead to schizophrenia?
9. What are the symptoms of PCP intoxication?
10. What is the amotivational syndrome associated with marijuana use?
11. Why are the inhalants potentially dangerous?
12. Why do athletes abuse anabolic steroids?

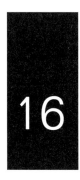

16 Personality Disorders

> All is caprice, they love without measure those whom
> they will soon hate without reason.
>
> Thomas Sydenham, 1682

Maladaptive character traits have been recognized since Cain killed his brother Abel. In ancient Greece, Hippocrates observed and classified many of the mental illnesses that are recognized today. Although he had no category for personality disorders, he described four temperaments believed to embody the elements of earth, air, fire, and water: the optimistic sanguine, the irritable choleric, the sad melancholic, and the apathetic phlegmatic. Variations of this simple classification of temperament were used right up to the twentieth century; the German psychiatrist Kraepelin, in fact, described the personalities he found in manic-depressive patients and their relatives as depressive, hypomanic, or irritable, terms that roughly correspond to the melancholic, sanguine, and choleric temperaments.

Formal efforts to describe abnormal personality traits began in the early nineteenth century, as European psychiatrists Pinel, Esquirol, and Prichard and the American psychiatrist Rush described persons whose behavior violated social norms. Patients receiving these diagnoses now would probably be regarded as having antisocial personality disorder. At the turn of the twentieth century, more specific personality types were described. Janet and Freud wrote about the psychological traits associated with hysteria, the fore-runner of today's histrionic personality disorder. Soon after, early psychoanalysts were setting forth the view that an arrest at one of the three stages of psychosexual development could lead to abnormal personality formation, as described later in the chapter. Object relations theorists later proposed that the early parent-child relationship was instrumental in shaping personality development, and an abnormal or disturbed relationship could result in specific defects in how a person views himself or herself and related to others. These defects could contribute to personality traits such as dependency, obsessionality, or narcissism.

Attempts to list the variety of personality types took root with the publication of DSM-I in 1952, in which seven different types of personality disturbances were described. With the arrival of DSM-III in 1980, personality disorders were accorded new status on a separate axis in the multiaxial evaluation system; criteria for 11 different personality disorders were enumerated, including several new disorders created in response to clinical and research observations. The list of personality disorders was pared to 10 in DSM-IV, which was published in 1994 (see Table 16–1), and did not change with the recent text revision, DSM-IV-TR, published in 2000.

TABLE 16–1.   DSM-IV-TR personality disorders

Cluster A (the eccentric disorders)

    Paranoid

    Schizoid

    Schizotypal

Cluster B (the dramatic disorders)

    Antisocial

    Borderline

    Histrionic

    Narcissistic

Cluster C (the anxious disorders)

    Avoidant

    Dependent

    Obsessive-compulsive

The 10 personality disorders are divided among three clusters. Each cluster is characterized by phenomenologically similar disorders, or personality disorders whose criteria overlap. Cluster A consists of the eccentric disorders—paranoid, schizoid, and schizotypal personality disorders. They are characterized by a pervasive pattern of abnormal cognition (e.g., suspiciousness), self-expression (e.g., odd speech), or relating to others (e.g., seclusiveness). Cluster B consists of the dramatic disorders—antisocial, borderline, histrionic, and narcissistic personality disorders. They are characterized by a pervasive pattern of violating social norms (e.g., criminal behavior), impulsivity, excessive emotionality, grandiosity, or "acting out" (e.g., tantrums, self-abusive behavior, angry outbursts). Cluster C consists of the anxious disorders—avoidant, dependent, and obsessive-compulsive personality disorders. They are characterized by a pervasive pattern of abnormal fears involving social relationships, separation, and need for control. In addition to the 10 distinct personality disorders listed in DSM-IV-TR, a residual category exists for individuals with mixed or atypical traits that do not fit into the better-defined categories (personality disorder not otherwise specified).

Personality disorders are defined in DSM-IV-TR as an enduring pattern of inner experience and behavior that deviates markedly from the expectations of the individual's culture, is pervasive and inflexible, has an onset in adulthood, is stable over time, and leads to distress or impairment. As a general rule, personality disorders are representative of long-term functioning and are not limited to episodes of illness. A personality disorder is not diagnosed, for instance, in a person who develops transient personality changes during an episode of major depression.

These disorders are coded on Axis II in order to separate them from the major mental disorders, which are coded on Axis I. A person can—and often does—have both Axis I and Axis II disorders, with some exceptions. For example, personality disorders are not diagnosed in persons with chronic psychotic disorders (e.g., schizophrenia) that are so devastating to the personality that the concept of personality disorder becomes meaningless. The most frequently diagnosed Axis I disorder in persons with personality disorders is major depression.

Although the DSM approach offers more rigorously defined subtypes than were available before, many psychiatrists and psychologists feel that they are artificial constructs that have little relevance to clinical reality and are not helpful in treating patients. These clinicians generally prefer a dimensional approach to the diagnosis of personality disorder, in which scales are used to measure different qualities, such as obsessionality or narcissism.

Another criticism of the DSM system is that normal personality variations, and the way these shade into more dysfunctional types, are left out. Few persons with personality disorders show exclusively the traits of the diagnosed personality disorder, and they usually manifest traits belonging to several of the defined types.

Some mental health professionals refuse to treat people with personality disorders, devalue their suffering, or view treatment as long term, complicated, and ineffective. This situation is particularly unfortunate because it is based on misinformation and prejudice, which have no place in medical practice. In fact, most patients with personality disorders are not difficult or unpleasant, their treatment is not always long term, and their treatment results are often successful and rewarding. The different personality disorders themselves are so varied that it is rarely useful to make generalizations about all patients with personality disorders based on one's experience with a particular type (e.g., borderline personality disorder).

Epidemiology

Surveys show that from 10% to 20% of the general population have a personality disorder. The prevalence is far greater in psychiatric samples (see Table 16–2, which is based on data collected at our hospital). In this table, the prevalence of personality disorders diagnosed with the Personality Diagnostic Questionnaire, a self-report instrument, is compared in four groups: control subjects who had been screened to exclude those with Axis I disorders, persons with major depression, persons with obsessive-compulsive disorder, and persons with panic disorder. Although the prevalence of specific personality disorders differed among the four groups, and no particular personality disorder was specific to Axis I pathology, the prevalence of personality disorder was high in all three patient groups. More than 50% of the hospitalized patients with major depression had a diagnosable personality disorder. The table also indicates the great overlap among the personality disorders because most patients with a personality disorder meet criteria for more than one disorder.

Abnormal personality traits are even more frequent than specific personality disorders. Data from Iowa showed that nearly 30% of the general population, 20% of the subjects screened to exclude those with Axis I disorders, and nearly two-thirds of psychiatric outpatients have maladaptive personality traits (see Table 16–3).

These disorders tend to have an onset in adolescence and are established by young adulthood. Late-onset personality changes suggest the presence of

TABLE 16–2. Prevalence of the DSM-III personality disorders among psychiatric patients and screened control subjects

Disorder	Screened control subjects (*n*=35)	Major depression (*n*=78)	Obsessive-compulsive disorder (*n*=37)	Panic disorder (*n*=83)
Cluster A				
Paranoid	0	1	19	6
Schizoid	0	1	0	0
Schizotypal	3	9	19	0
Cluster B				
Histrionic	3	18	11	10
Narcissistic	3	0	5	0
Antisocial	0	1	0	1
Borderline	0	23	19	7
Cluster C				
Avoidant	0	15	27	20
Dependent	0	17	46	18
Obsessive-compulsive	3	6	30	8
Passive-aggressive	9	4	49	2

Source. Adapted from Pfohl et al. 1991.

a major mental illness (e.g., the prodrome of schizophrenia), a brain disorder, or a disorder caused by medical illness or the effects of a substance. Antisocial personality disorder is the only personality disorder in which an age requirement is specified (18 years). Gender distribution differs among the 10 personality disorders, and some (e.g., antisocial, schizoid, obsessive-compulsive) have a male preponderance, whereas others (e.g., borderline, histrionic, avoidant, dependent) have a female preponderance. Others have a more equal distribution (e.g., schizotypal).

Personality disorders can cause enormous problems for individuals and society. These disorders are frequently associated with impaired social, interpersonal, and occupational adjustment. Family life, marriages, and academic and work performance suffer. Rates of unemployment, homelessness, divorce and separation, and domestic violence are high. These disorders also

TABLE 16–3. Prevalence (in percentages) of the DSM-III personality traits in a community sample, psychiatric outpatients, and screened subjects

Traits	Community sample (*n*=235)	Outpatient sample (*n*=82)	Screened subjects (*n*=40)
Any	29	67	20
Cluster A	13	32	7
Paranoid	1	1	5
Schizoid	1	4	3
Schizotypal	13	30	8
Cluster B	6	42	5
Narcissistic	0	0	0
Histrionic	4	28	5
Borderline	0	0.5	0
Antisocial	1	30	3
Cluster C	26	53	18
Avoidant	0	16	8
Dependent	15	43	10
Obsessive-compulsive	15	26	5
Passive-aggressive	0	4	0

Note. The numbers are not additive because many patients have traits of several different disorders.

Source. Adapted from Reich et al. 1989.

are associated with increased rates of health care utilization and excessive rates of traumatic accidents, emergency room visits, and hospitalization. As a group, individuals with personality disorders are at risk for early death, mainly from suicide or accidents.

Personality disorders tend to be stable and enduring. Relatively few long-term follow-up studies of the various personality disorders have been done. Research shows that schizotypal, borderline, and antisocial personality disorders are all stable on follow-up but tend to improve as the patient ages. Some evidence indicates that certain Axis II disorders are variable over time and are influenced by significant life events.

Attention has recently focused on the importance of the interrelation (comorbidity) between personality disorders and Axis I disorders because many differences exist between patients who have personality disorders and those who do not. For example, depressed patients with personality disorders are younger, are more likely to be female, are more likely to have a history of marital instability, are more likely to report precipitating stressors for the depression, and are more likely to have a history of nonserious suicide attempts. Depressed patients with personality disorders also are less likely to have a positive dexamethasone suppression test result and are more likely to have a family history of alcoholism and antisocial personality disorder. (The dexamethasone suppression test, which measures serum cortisol 12 hours after taking a 1-mg dose of dexamethasone, has a positive result in about 50% of the persons with major depression and is viewed as an indicator of a more biological or genetic form of the disorder.) These findings suggest that depressed patients with personality disorders may form an important subgroup that differs genetically and biochemically from depressed patients with primary depressive illness. The presence of a personality disorder also is associated with a poorer response to treatment, particularly antidepressant medication and electroconvulsive therapy. These interesting findings also seem to be true for some patients with obsessive-compulsive disorder, panic disorder, and probably other diagnoses as well.

Etiology

Early psychoanalysts theorized that personality disorders occurred when a person failed to progress through appropriate stages of psychosexual development. Several of the DSM-IV-TR disorders derive from the oral, anal, and phallic character types that were described. Fixation at the oral stage was thought to result in a personality characterized by demanding and dependent behavior (i.e., dependent personality disorder). Fixation at the anal stage was thought to lead to a personality characterized by obsessionality, rigidity, and emotional aloofness (i.e., obsessive-compulsive personality disorder). Fixation at the phallic stage was believed to cause shallowness and an inability to engage in intimate relationships (i.e., histrionic personality). These broad character types have, in fact, been supported by factor analytic studies, but little evidence shows that they are related to developmental fixations early in life.

A growing body of evidence suggests that childhood abuse or maltreatment is associated with risk for personality disorder in general and perhaps borderline and antisocial personality disorders specifically. The resulting trauma is thought to cause difficulty in developing trust and intimacy. An early home environment in which domestic abuse, divorce, separation, or parental absence is found also can contribute to the risk of developing a personality disorder.

Genetic factors help to explain some of the personality disorders. Family, twin, and adoption studies suggest that schizotypal personality is genetically related to schizophrenia. Family and adoption studies also have confirmed a strong genetic factor in the etiology of antisocial and borderline personality disorders. Antisocial personality disorder, for instance, has been found more frequently in identical than in nonidentical twins, and offspring of antisocial parents adopted in childhood are more likely to develop antisocial behavior than are adoptees without an antisocial parent. Less evidence is available for the heritability of the other DSM-IV-TR personality disorders. Some evidence suggests that basic dimensions of personality (e.g., callousness, intimacy problems) are inherited along a continuum with normality.

Some effort has been made to explore the neurobiology of personality disorders. Schizotypal personality has been associated with low platelet monoamine oxidase activity and impaired smooth pursuit eye movement. Low levels of cerebrospinal fluid 5-hydroxyindoleacetic acid (5-HIAA)—a metabolite of serotonin—have been linked with impulsive and aggressive behaviors typical of both borderline and antisocial personality disorders. Chronic nervous system underarousal is thought by some researchers to underlie antisocial personality disorder. Research shows that antisocial patients as a group have low resting pulse rates, low skin conductance, and an increased amplitude on event-related potentials. One theory is that individuals with chronically low arousal seek out potentially dangerous or risky situations to raise their arousal to more optimal levels to satisfy their craving for excitement.

Subtle forms of brain injury have been hypothesized to cause some personality disorders. Electroencephalographic abnormalities—mostly slow-wave activity—have been reported in persons with antisocial personality disorder for many years, and at least one study of patients with borderline personality disorder reported similar findings. Recent brain imaging studies have linked antisocial behavior to abnormal function in the prefrontal cortex.

Diagnosis

Personality disorders are often ingrained such that individuals have little awareness of the difficulties their maladaptive traits create for themselves and others. For that reason, only rarely does the personality disorder itself lead the individual to seek help. When these patients seek help, it is generally for marital or work-related problems, depression, anxiety, or substance abuse. The clinician's task is to help the patients understand how their personality traits contribute to their ongoing troubles and to help them modify their maladaptive traits whenever possible.

The diagnosis of a personality disorder requires a thorough personal and social history and a careful mental status examination. Several structured interviews and self-report instruments are available to help with diagnosis but are mainly used in research. (Several of these interviews and questionnaires are described in Chapter 4.) When a personality disorder is suspected—as is often the case when the patients' immediate problem and social history intertwine—the clinician should inquire about the kinds of symptoms found in these patients. One of our colleagues developed a series of six questions to screen for the presence of a personality disorder. A "yes" answer on two or more items suggests a better than 80% chance of a personality disorder being present. These questions appear in Table 16–4.

Collateral information also is important when a personality disorder is suspected but the patient denies or seems unaware of his or her maladaptive traits. A person with antisocial personality disorder may deny criminal activity or minimize its significance. Information from relatives, the police, or a parole officer can be helpful in confirming its severity and extent. An informant also can be helpful in determining whether a personality disorder is present when a patient seems unconcerned with the trait or behavior. A person suspected of having a schizoid personality disorder, for instance, may be comfortable with his or her social isolation and not view it as a problem.

A frequent concern with a personality disorder diagnosis is that it may be made prematurely. Patients with major depression are often socially anxious and dependent on others, traits that tend to recede or disappear when the depression is successfully treated. Therefore, caution needs to be exercised in making the diagnosis, particularly when the patient has an Axis I disorder such as major depression.

Long-term observation is often necessary to confirm the diagnosis of personality disorder. Sometimes the clinician will defer diagnosis of a personality disorder—even when it is suspected—until he or she has seen the patient several times and has had the opportunity to gather additional information. In this case, the word "defer" should be coded on Axis II. This word alerts other clinicians that a personality disorder is suspected but that information to confirm the diagnosis is insufficient.

TABLE 16–4. Screening questions for the presence of a DSM-IV personality disorder

I'd like to ask you a few questions about some of your thoughts and feelings. Your answers will help me better understand what you are usually like. If the way you have been in recent weeks or months is different from the way you usually are, please look back to when you were your usual self when you answer these questions.

1. **Experiences marked shifts in mood: throughout the course of a typical day, experiences sudden spells of depression, irritability, anxiety, or anger**

   Y   N

   How often do you have days when your mood is constantly changing—days when you shift back and forth from feeling as you usually do to feeling angry or depressed or anxious? (**IF PRESENT**): How long has this been going on?

2. **Feels inadequate and uncomfortable in situations where he or she is not the center of attention**

   Y   N

   Some people prefer to be the center of attention, while others are content to remain on the edge of things. How would you describe yourself? (**IF CENTER**): How do you feel when you're not the center of attention?

3. **Actions usually directed toward obtaining immediate satisfaction; difficulty persisting with long-term goals**

   Y   N

   Do you frequently insist on having what you want right now, even when waiting a little longer would get you something much better? Do you get excited by a new project or job but then lose interest before it's done?

4. **Is reluctant to confide in others because of unwarranted fear that the information will be used against him or her**

   Y   N

   Do you think it's best if other people don't get to know you too well? (**IF YES**): What are the reasons for this?

   Are you concerned that certain friends or co-workers are not really loyal or trust-worthy? (**IF YES**): What has caused you concern?

5. **Excessive social anxiety, e.g., extreme discomfort in social situations involving unfamiliar people**

   Y   N

   Are you concerned about saying the wrong things in front of other people? (**IF YES**): Does this keep you from speaking up?

TABLE 16–4. Screening questions for the presence of a DSM-IV personality disorder *(continued)*

How would you feel at a gathering where you didn't know many people? (**IF UNCOMFORTABLE**): Even if you're uncomfortable at first, do you relax after a while and enjoy yourself? How often would you make the first move in starting a conversation with someone?

6. **Unwilling to get involved with people unless certain of being liked, such that the number of friends has been limited**

    Y   N

    How often do you avoid getting to know someone because you are worried they may not like you? (**IF OFTEN**): How has this affected the number of friends you have?

Source. Used with permission of Bruce Pfohl, M.D.

The DSM-IV-TR Personality Disorders

Cluster A Disorders

Paranoid Personality Disorder

Paranoid personality was first described by Adolph Meyer in the early twentieth century. Early formulations of the disorder came from a psychoanalytic perspective, which emphasized the defense mechanisms of reaction formation and projection. Some researchers have hypothesized that paranoid personality disorder lies within the schizophrenic spectrum and is the product of a common genetic predisposition. A behavioral model has been suggested in which suspiciousness and mistrust are learned, leading to social withdrawal, testing of others, and ruminative suspiciousness. These patients are chronically suspicious, distrust others, and fulfill their suspicious prophecies by leading others to be overly cautious and deceptive (see Table 16–5).

Patients with paranoid personality disorder rarely seek treatment, probably because of their general suspiciousness of others, including psychiatrists and therapists. The disorder is often recognized when the patient seeks treatment for a mood or anxiety disorder. Apart from diagnosing and managing the patients' main complaint, the clinician should take care to be supportive and to listen patiently to their accusations and complaints, while being open, honest, and respectful. Once rapport has been established, alternative explanations for the patients' misperceptions can be suggested. Group therapy should be avoided because patients with paranoid personality disor-

TABLE 16–5.   DSM-IV-TR diagnostic criteria for paranoid personality disorder

A. A pervasive distrust and suspiciousness of others such that their motives are interpreted as malevolent, beginning by early adulthood and present in a variety of contexts, as indicated by four (or more) of the following:

(1) suspects, without sufficient basis, that others are exploiting, harming, or deceiving him or her

(2) is preoccupied with unjustified doubts about the loyalty or trustworthiness of friends or associates

(3) is reluctant to confide in others because of unwarranted fear that the information will be used maliciously against him or her

(4) reads hidden demeaning or threatening meanings into benign remarks or events

(5) persistently bears grudges, i.e., is unforgiving of insults, injuries, or slights

(6) perceives attacks on his or her character or reputation that are not apparent to others and is quick to react angrily or to counterattack

(7) has recurrent suspicions, without justification, regarding fidelity of spouse or sexual partner

B. Does not occur exclusively during the course of Schizophrenia, a Mood Disorder With Psychotic Features, or another Psychotic Disorder and is not due to the direct physiological effects of a general medical condition.

Note: If criteria are met prior to the onset of Schizophrenia, add "Premorbid," e.g., "Paranoid Personality Disorder (Premorbid)."

der tend to misinterpret statements and situations that arise in the course of the therapy. Antipsychotics may help to reduce their suspiciousness, although these drugs have not been specifically studied in these patients.

Schizoid Personality Disorder

The term *schizoid* was originally used to characterize the premorbid seclusiveness of schizophrenic patients and their eccentric relatives. Gradually, it came to be used to describe almost all persons who had difficulty achieving intimacy. The concept of schizoid personality disorder was narrowed in 1980 in DSM-III. At that time, odd, eccentric people were relegated to a new category, schizotypal personality disorder. Persons who were isolated because of an unwillingness to confront rejection were placed in another new category, avoidant personality disorder. Schizoid personality disorder became restricted to persons with a profound defect in the ability to form personal relationships and to respond to others in a meaningful way (see Table 16–6). The following case example from our hospital illustrates the disorder:

TABLE 16–6. DSM-IV-TR diagnostic criteria for schizoid personality disorder

A. A pervasive pattern of detachment from social relationships and a restricted range of expression of emotions in interpersonal settings, beginning by early adulthood and present in a variety of contexts, as indicated by four (or more) of the following:

   (1) neither desires nor enjoys close relationships, including being part of a family
   (2) almost always chooses solitary activities
   (3) has little, if any, interest in having sexual experiences with another person
   (4) takes pleasure in few, if any, activities
   (5) lacks close friends or confidants other than first-degree relatives
   (6) appears indifferent to the praise or criticism of others
   (7) shows emotional coldness, detachment, or flattened affectivity

B. Does not occur exclusively during the course of Schizophrenia, a Mood Disorder With Psychotic Features, another Psychotic Disorder, or a Pervasive Developmental Disorder and is not due to the direct physiological effects of a general medical condition.

Note: If criteria are met prior to the onset of Schizophrenia, add "Premorbid," e.g., "Schizoid Personality Disorder (Premorbid)."

Michael, a 24-year-old white male, was transferred to the psychiatric inpatient unit after receiving treatment for a self-inflicted gunshot wound to the head. The bullet grazed his scalp but did not cause a brain injury. Michael had had prior depressive spells. According to his family, he had been depressed for several weeks before shooting himself. After transfer, Michael denied feeling depressed and believed that there was no reason for him to be in the hospital.

Michael had always been considered shy by his relatives, was socially isolated, and had no friends that his family was aware of. He had done poorly in school and had dropped out before graduating from high school. Michael had never dated and had no interest in sexual activity, apart from masturbation. Michael admitted that he was not emotionally close to any of his family members, and although he lived with his elderly father, he showed little interest or affection in describing their relationship. Despite average intelligence, Michael had never persisted with a job and was currently unemployed. He preferred to stay home and watch television or play computer games. He never bothered to obtain a driver's license.

Michael believed that his only problem was his episodic depression. He neither complained about his social isolation and emotional aloofness nor accepted the fact that these symptoms could reflect an underlying disorder. He had no interest in changing his ways and refused referral for psychotherapy.

Like Michael, patients with schizoid personality disorder have no close relationships and choose solitary activities. They rarely experience strong emotions, express little desire for sexual experience with another person, are indifferent to praise or criticism, and have a constricted affect. The disorder is not diagnosed in persons with schizophrenia or other psychotic disorders because these conditions are typically accompanied by a schizoid adjustment.

Schizoid personality disorder is uncommon in clinical settings because persons with this disturbance rarely seek psychiatric help except for a co-occurring disorder such as depression, anxiety, or substance abuse. Persons with schizoid personality disorder lack the insight and motivation necessary for individual psychotherapy and would likely find the intimacy of group therapy threatening. When the patient is motivated to change, simple behavioral techniques may be helpful, such as graded exposure to a variety of social tasks. For example, the clinician might encourage the patient to attend a concert, then join a bridge club, and eventually enter a dance class.

Schizotypal Personality Disorder

Schizotypal personality disorder was created during the development of DSM-III. Researchers had observed that relatives of schizophrenic patients often had a cluster of schizophrenic-like traits, a fact noted earlier by Krae-pelin and Bleuler around the turn of the twentieth century. Forerunners of this disorder included Bleuler's categories of simple and latent schizophrenia, which were diagnosed in nonpsychotic persons who showed mild symptoms of schizophrenia such as avolition or apathy. Schizotypal personality disorder now is considered part of the schizophrenia spectrum, along with schizophreniform disorder, schizoaffective disorder, and perhaps psychotic mood disorders.

Schizotypal personality disorder is characterized by a pattern of peculiar behavior, odd speech and thinking, and unusual perceptual experiences. Schizotypal patients are frequently socially isolated and have "magical" beliefs, mild paranoia, inappropriate or constricted affect, and social anxiety (see Table 16–7).

Community surveys show that schizotypal personality disorder has a prevalence of around 3%–5%, making it one of the more common personality disorders. As noted in Table 16–3, up to 30% of psychiatric outpatients have one or more schizotypal traits. Comorbidity with mood, substance use, and anxiety disorders is common; men and women are equally likely to have the disorder.

The treatment of schizotypal personality disorder often centers on issues that led the person to seek treatment, such as feelings of alienation or

---

TABLE 16–7. DSM-IV-TR diagnostic criteria for schizotypal personality disorder

---

A. A pervasive pattern of social and interpersonal deficits marked by acute discomfort with, and reduced capacity for, close relationships as well as by cognitive or perceptual distortions and eccentricities of behavior, beginning by early adulthood and present in a variety of contexts, as indicated by five (or more) of the following:

   (1) ideas of reference (excluding delusions of reference)

   (2) odd beliefs or magical thinking that influences behavior and is inconsistent with subcultural norms (e.g., superstitiousness, belief in clairvoyance, telepathy, or "sixth sense"; in children and adolescents, bizarre fantasies or preoccupations)

   (3) unusual perceptual experiences, including bodily illusions

   (4) odd thinking and speech (e.g., vague, circumstantial, metaphorical, overelaborate, or stereotyped)

   (5) suspiciousness or paranoid ideation

   (6) inappropriate or constricted affect

   (7) behavior or appearance that is odd, eccentric, or peculiar

   (8) lack of close friends or confidants other than first-degree relatives

   (9) excessive social anxiety that does not diminish with familiarity and tends to be associated with paranoid fears rather than negative judgments about self

B. Does not occur exclusively during the course of Schizophrenia, a Mood Disorder With Psychotic Features, another Psychotic Disorder, or a Pervasive Developmental Disorder.

Note: If criteria are met prior to the onset of Schizophrenia, add "Premorbid," e.g., "Schizotypal Personality Disorder (Premorbid)."

---

isolation, paranoia, or suspiciousness. Exploratory and group psychotherapies are overly threatening to these patients, but social skills training can be helpful. The goal is to make eccentric, odd persons feel more comfortable with themselves and others.

Antipsychotics are sometimes prescribed to patients with schizotypal personality disorder. Atypical antipsychotics (e.g., risperidone, 1–6 mg/day; olanzapine, 5–20 mg/day) are well tolerated and may help to reduce the intense anxiety, paranoia, and unusual perceptual experiences these individuals experience.

Cluster B Disorders

Antisocial Personality Disorder

Antisocial personality disorder was first recognized in the early nineteenth century as *manie sans délire* ("mania without delirium") or *moral insanity,* phrases used to describe immoral or guiltless behavior in the absence of impaired reasoning. By the turn of the twentieth century, the disorder was known as *psychopathic personality.* In DSM-I, the disorder was called *sociopathic personality* and was renamed antisocial personality disorder in DSM-III in 1980; the definition emphasized the continuity between childhood conduct disorder and adult antisocial behavior.

Antisocial patients typically report a history of childhood behavior problems such as fighting with peers, conflicts with adults, lying, cheating, and stealing. Fire setting and cruelty to animals and other children are particularly worrisome symptoms. As the antisocial youth reaches adulthood, other problems develop reflecting age-appropriate responsibilities such as uneven job performance or domestic abuse. Unreliability, reckless behavior, and inappropriate aggression are frequent problems. Criminal behavior, pathological lying, and the use of the aliases are also characteristic of the disorder (Table 16–8). Marriages are often marked by instability or emotional and physical abuse of the spouse; separation and divorce are common. One of the best descriptions of this disorder appears in Cleckley's *The Mask of Sanity*, originally published in 1941. Cleckley, who is better known as the coauthor of *The Three Faces of Eve,* enumerated 16 traits he considered descriptive of the disorder, thus creating the first operational, criteria-based definition in psychiatry.

The following case example is of a patient treated at our hospital in the 1950s and followed up 30 years later. The case illustrates the personal and interpersonal difficulties that arise from the disorder and that affect individuals for a lifetime.

Douglas, aged 18 years, was admitted for evaluation of antisocial behavior. His early childhood was chaotic and abusive. His alcoholic father had married five times and abandoned his family when Douglas was 6. Because his mother had a history of incarceration and was unable to care for him, Douglas was placed in foster care until he was adopted at age 8. His adoptive father was a university professor; his adoptive mother was described as compulsive and strict.

Since early childhood, Douglas had a criminal streak. He lied, cheated at games, shoplifted, and stole money from his mother's purse. He once burglarized a church and, when older, stole an automobile. Despite an above-average IQ, Douglas's school performance was poor, and he was frequently in detention for breaking rules. Because of continued lawbreaking, he was sent to a juvenile reformatory at age 16 for 2 years. While in the reformatory, he slashed another boy with a razor blade in a fight. Douglas had his first sexual experience before his peers and since leaving the reformatory had had several different sexual partners. He chain-smoked and admitted to regular alcohol abuse.

TABLE 16–8. DSM-IV-TR diagnostic criteria for antisocial personality disorder

A. There is a pervasive pattern of disregard for and violation of the rights of others occurring since age 15 years, as indicated by three (or more) of the following:

  (1) failure to conform to social norms with respect to lawful behaviors as indicated by repeatedly performing acts that are grounds for arrest

  (2) deceitfulness, as indicated by repeated lying, use of aliases, or conning others for personal profit or pleasure

  (3) impulsivity or failure to plan ahead

  (4) irritability and aggressiveness, as indicated by repeated physical fights or assaults

  (5) reckless disregard for safety of self or others

  (6) consistent irresponsibility, as indicated by repeated failure to sustain consistent work behavior or honor financial obligations

  (7) lack of remorse, as indicated by being indifferent to or rationalizing having hurt, mistreated, or stolen from another

B. The individual is at least age 18 years.

C. There is evidence of Conduct Disorder with onset before age 15 years.

D. The occurrence of antisocial behavior is not exclusively during the course of Schizophrenia or a Manic Episode.

An electroencephalogram was normal, and his IQ was measured at 112. He was discharged after a 16-day stay and was thought to be unimproved. He had poorly cooperated with attempts at both individual and group therapy.

Douglas used an alias, which complicated efforts to locate him for follow-up. He was finally discovered living in an impoverished area of a small midwestern community. A poorly groomed man, Douglas, now 48, appeared nervous and tremulous. His dilapidated home was dark and cold because the furnace did not work.

Douglas acknowledged more than 20 arrests and more than 5 felony convictions for charges ranging from attempted murder and armed robbery to driving while intoxicated. He had spent more than 17 years in prison. While in prison, Douglas had escaped with the help of his biological mother, with whom he then had a sexual relationship. He was returned to prison 2 months later. His most recent arrest occurred within the past year and was for public intoxication and simple assault.

Douglas reported at least nine hospitalizations for alcohol detoxification, the latest occurring earlier that year. He admitted to having used marijuana, amphetamines, tranquilizers, cocaine, and heroin in the past.

He had never held a full-time job in his life; the longest job he had held lasted 60 days. He was currently doing body work on cars in his own garage to earn a living but had not done any work for several months. He estimated that he had held about 150 jobs in the past 10 years. His family received public assistance.

Douglas reported that nine persons lived in his home, including his four children. He had met his common-law wife in a psychiatric hospital. He told us that she required tranquilizers for emotional problems and that the marriage was unsatisfactory.

He had lived in six different states and in the last 10 years had moved more than 20 times. He reported occasionally attending Alcoholics Anonymous at a local church but otherwise did not socialize outside his family.

He reported being afraid of closed places, which he related to graphic memories of prison life. He claimed to have witnessed several murders of "snitches" and to have committed murder himself during a prison riot. He admitted that he had not yet settled down and told us that he still spent money foolishly, was frequently reckless, and got into frequent fights and arguments. He said that he got a "charge out of doing dangerous things."

Research shows that from 2% to 4% of men and 0.5% to 1% of women meet criteria for antisocial personality disorder. The percentages are much higher in psychiatric hospitals and clinics, prisons, the homeless, and alcohol- and drug-addicted persons. The disorder is chronic but tends to be worse early in its course, and patients tend to improve with advancing age. In a 30-year follow-up survey of 82 subjects, 12% were in remission, and another 20% had improved; the remaining subjects were considered as disturbed as or more disturbed than at the study onset. The median age for improvement in this study was 35 years. Although the most dangerous and destructive behaviors associated with antisocial personality disorder may improve or remit, other troubling symptoms continue, including domestic abuse, alcoholism or drug abuse, and general irresponsibility toward others.

Nearly two-thirds of antisocial persons have an alcohol or drug use disorder. Mood disorder and anxiety disorder, sexual dysfunction, paraphilias, other personality disorders (e.g., borderline personality), and pathological gambling are also common. Antisocial persons frequently attempt suicide, and mortality studies show high rates of death from natural causes as well as accidents, suicides, and homicides.

Several drugs have been shown to reduce aggression, the chief problem of many antisocial patients. Lithium carbonate and phenytoin, specifically, have been shown to reduce anger, threatening behavior, and assaultiveness among prisoners. Other drugs, including carbamazepine, valproate, propranolol, buspirone, trazodone, and the antipsychotics, have been used with varying degrees of success to treat aggression in brain-injured or mentally retarded patients. Tranquilizers from the benzodiazepine class should not be used to treat antisocial personality disorder because they are potentially addictive and may lead to behavioral dyscontrol. Medication targeted at co-morbid mood or anxiety disorders or attention-deficit/hyperactivity disorder may help to reduce antisocial behavior.

Cognitive-behavioral therapy recently has been used to treat antisocial personality disorder and involves evaluating situations in which the patient's distorted beliefs and attitudes (e.g., "My actions have no consequences") interfere with his or her functioning. The major goal of therapy is to help patients understand how they create their own problems and how their distorted perceptions prevent them from seeing themselves as others see them. Working with antisocial patients can be very difficult; they tend to blame others, have a low tolerance for frustration, are impulsive, and rarely form trusting relationships.

Antisocial patients with spouses (or partners) and families may benefit from marriage or family counseling. Clinicians who specialize in family therapy may be helpful by addressing the antisocial person's trouble maintaining an enduring attachment to his or her spouse or partner, inability to be an effective parent, problems with honesty and responsibility, and anger and hostility that can lead to domestic violence.

Borderline Personality Disorder

Borderline personality disorder was introduced in DSM-III, although the concept has a much longer history. As currently conceptualized, the disorder represents a pervasive pattern of mood instability, unstable and intense interpersonal relationships, impulsivity, inappropriate or intense anger, lack of control of anger, recurrent suicidal threats and gestures, self-mutilating behavior, marked and persistent identity disturbance, chronic feelings of emptiness or boredom, and frantic efforts to avoid real or imagined abandonment (see Table 16–9). Patients also may experience transient paranoid ideation or dissociative symptoms. Thomas Sydenham, an English physician best known for describing Saint Vitis' dance, captures the essence of borderline personality in his quotation at the beginning of this chapter. In DSM-I, these features would have been recognized as *emotionally unstable personality*. Early theorists considered borderline personality to be a variant of schizophrenia, and the term *borderline schizophrenia* was coined to describe persons who experienced transient episodes of psychosis during periods of regression or during psychotherapy.

The disorder is of great interest to psychoanalysts. Kernberg, for example, used the term *borderline personality organization* to describe a broad diagnostic concept and diagnosed borderline personality on the basis of

---

TABLE 16–9.   DSM-IV-TR diagnostic criteria for borderline personality disorder

---

A pervasive pattern of instability of interpersonal relationships, self-image, and affects, and marked impulsivity beginning by early adulthood and present in a variety of contexts, as indicated by five (or more) of the following:

(1) frantic efforts to avoid real or imagined abandonment.   Note: Do not include suicidal or self-mutilating behavior covered in Criterion 5.

(2) a pattern of unstable and intense interpersonal relationships characterized by alternating between extremes of idealization and devaluation

(3) identity disturbance: markedly and persistently unstable self-image or sense of self

(4) impulsivity in at least two areas that are potentially self-damaging (e.g., spending, sex, substance abuse, reckless driving, binge eating).   Note: Do not include suicidal or self-mutilating behavior covered in Criterion 5.

(5) recurrent suicidal behavior, gestures, or threats, or self-mutilating behavior

(6) affective instability due to a marked reactivity of mood (e.g., intense episodic dysphoria, irritability, or anxiety usually lasting a few hours and only rarely more than a few days)

(7) chronic feelings of emptiness

(8) inappropriate, intense anger or difficulty controlling anger (e.g., frequent displays of temper, constant anger, recurrent physical fights)

(9) transient, stress-related paranoid ideation or severe dissociative symptoms

---

presence of identity diffusion, primitive defense mechanisms such as splitting (e.g., exaggerated dichotomies of good and evil, black and white), and the maintenance of reality testing except in the perception of self and others.

The diagnosis of borderline personality disorder identifies a large group of patients and overlaps with many other personality disorders, especially the schizotypal, histrionic, and antisocial types. One of the more common personality disorders among psychiatric patients, as indicated in Table 16–2, its frequency in the general population has been estimated at 1%–2%. Borderline personality disorder is relatively stable in long-term follow-up studies. The disorder is associated with poor treatment response and has a suicide rate exceeding 5%. Better long-term outcome is associated with higher intelligence, self-discipline, and social support from friends and relatives. Anger, antisocial behavior, suspiciousness, and vanity are traits associated with poor outcome. Patients frequently have comorbid major depression, dysthymia, anxiety disorders, and substance use disorders.

Some researchers have argued that borderline personality disorder is a form of depression, as evidenced by its association with depression in family studies, follow-up studies showing that most patients with borderline personality develop major depression, and positive response to antidepressant medication. In their view, the chronic mood instability creates the personality disturbance, not vice versa. On the other hand, it can be argued that patients with borderline personality disorder develop depression because of either a psychosocial predisposition (e.g., history of verbal and sexual abuse during childhood) or a biological vulnerability.

There is little agreement on the appropriate treatment for borderline personality disorder. Treatment recommendations range from Kernberg's intensive, interpretive, and confrontational psychotherapy focusing on the transference relationship to psychotherapy emphasizing practical support and problem solving. Borderline patients can form an intense transference; countertransference can be a problem because these patients often stimulate intense feelings of frustration, guilt, or anger in their therapists. Family or group psychotherapy may help dilute the transference. Cognitive-behavioral therapy may be effective in correcting dysfunctional attitudes and ambivalent perceptions of others and oneself. At least one specific form of cognitive-behavioral therapy—dialectical behavior therapy—administered in both individual and group therapy formats appears to be effective in reducing deliberate self-harm behaviors, hospitalization rates, and anger dyscontrol.

Pharmacotherapy for borderline personality disorder tends to focus on the patients' target symptoms. Antipsychotics can be helpful in treating perceptual distortions; lithium carbonate, valproate, or other mood stabilizers can be useful in treating mood swings; and monoamine oxidase inhibitors can be useful in treating dysphoria secondary to interpersonal rejection. In one study, four treatments were compared, including an antipsychotic (trifluoperazine), a mood stabilizer (carbamazepine), a tranquilizer (alprazolam), and a monoamine oxidase inhibitor (phenelzine). All drugs were somewhat effective, except for alprazolam, which caused behavioral disinhibition and anger dyscontrol.

Serotonin reuptake inhibitors, such as fluoxetine, also may be helpful in reducing depressive symptoms and suicidal ideations and behavior. The fact that these drugs are not fatal in overdose is an important consideration in patients known for impulsive suicide attempts. Because suicide attempts are a frequent complication in these patients, physicians should be cautious about prescribing any medication that could be fatal in overdose.

Histrionic Personality Disorder

Histrionic personality takes its name from *hysteria,* a disorder first described in the nineteenth century and associated with conversion, somatization, and dissociation. Self-dramatizing and attention-seeking behaviors were observed to be associated with hysteria. *Hysterical personality* was included in DSM-II and was renamed *histrionic personality* in DSM-III, so as not to be confused with hysteria (renamed *somatization disorder*). Many persons with somatization disorder have histrionic personality disorder, but there is no one-to-one relationship.

Persons with histrionic personality show a pattern of excessive emotionality and attention-seeking behavior. Typical symptoms include excessive concern with appearance and wanting to be the center of attention (see Table 16–10). Histrionic persons are often gregarious and superficially charming but can be manipulative, vain, and demanding.

TABLE 16–10.   DSM-IV-TR diagnostic criteria for histrionic personality disorder

---

A pervasive pattern of excessive emotionality and attention seeking, beginning by early adulthood and present in a variety of contexts, as indicated by five (or more) of the following:
(1) is uncomfortable in situations in which he or she is not the center of attention
(2) interaction with others is often characterized by inappropriate sexually seductive or provocative behavior
(3) displays rapidly shifting and shallow expression of emotions
(4) consistently uses physical appearance to draw attention to self
(5) has a style of speech that is excessively impressionistic and lacking in detail
(6) shows self-dramatization, theatricality, and exaggerated expression of emotion
(7) is suggestible, i.e., easily influenced by others or circumstances
(8) considers relationships to be more intimate than they actually are

---

The disorder has a prevalence of nearly 2% in the general population but is more common in women. Persons with this disorder tend to seek out medical attention and to make frequent use of available health services.

The cause of histrionic personality is unknown, although the disorder has been linked through family studies to somatization disorder and antisocial personality disorder. It also has been suggested that histrionic personality is a gender-biased diagnosis that merely describes a caricature of stereotypic femininity because it is frequently diagnosed among females in clinical samples.

The treatment of histrionic personality disorder has traditionally involved psychodynamic psychotherapy and for that reason is considered by some the treatment of choice. Other experts recommend a more supportive, problem-solving approach or cognitive-behavioral therapy to help patients counter their distorted thinking, such as the inflated self-image that many histrionic patients have. With interpersonal psychotherapy, the patient can focus on conscious (or unconscious) motivations for seeking out disappointing lovers and being unable to commit oneself to a stable, meaningful relationship. Group therapy may be useful in addressing provocative and attention-seeking behavior. Patients may not be aware of their annoying behaviors, and it may be helpful to have others point them out. A condition that may be related, *hysteroid dysphoria,* described in depressed women who have a history of sensitivity to rejection in relationships, is reported to preferentially respond to monoamine oxidase inhibitors.

Narcissistic Personality Disorder

Narcissistic personality disorder was introduced in DSM-III and is named after Narcissus from Greek mythology, who fell in love with his own reflection. Freud used the term to describe persons who were self-absorbed; the term was later expanded to describe the more general concept of excessive self-love and grandiosity. Pathological narcissism became of great interest to psychoanalysts and the concept was heavily influenced by the contributions of Kohut. In his view, narcissism develops as a response to parental failures in conveying empathy to a child's need for idealization and admiration; the child becomes self-centered and views others only in their role of satisfying his or her narcissistic needs.

The disorder is characterized by grandiosity, lack of empathy, and hypersensitivity to evaluation by others (see Table 16–11). Narcissistic persons are egotistical, inflate their accomplishments, and often manipulate or exploit those around them to achieve their own aims. They have an exaggerated sense of entitlement and believe that they deserve special treatment. They expect to receive love and admiration but have little empathy for others. Narcissistic individuals are often irritating, haughty, or difficult; although they appear outwardly charming, relationships tend to be superficial and cold. They often have little insight into their own narcissism.

The following case vignette illustrates many of the symptoms of narcissistic personality disorder:

> Dr. Smith, a 53-year-old psychiatrist, formerly on the faculty at an Ivy League medical school, was known for having an expansive and grandiose attitude and for belittling the accomplishments of his colleagues. He made others constantly aware of his own scholarly productivity and the later success of his private practice.
>
> While seeking the admiration and adulation of others, he rarely reciprocated, displaying superficial charm without a genuine capacity for empa-

TABLE 16–11. DSM-IV-TR diagnostic criteria for narcissistic personality disorder

A pervasive pattern of grandiosity (in fantasy or behavior), need for admiration, and lack of empathy, beginning by early adulthood and present in a variety of contexts, as indicated by five (or more) of the following:

(1) has a grandiose sense of self-importance (e.g., exaggerates achievements and talents, expects to be recognized as superior without commensurate achievements)

(2) is preoccupied with fantasies of unlimited success, power, brilliance, beauty, or ideal love

(3) believes that he or she is "special" and unique and can only be understood by, or should associate with, other special or high-status people (or institutions)

(4) requires excessive admiration

(5) has a sense of entitlement, i.e., unreasonable expectations of especially favorable treatment or automatic compliance with his or her expectations

(6) is interpersonally exploitative, i.e., takes advantage of others to achieve his or her own ends

(7) lacks empathy: is unwilling to recognize or identify with the feelings and needs of others

(8) is often envious of others or believes that others are envious of him or her

(9) shows arrogant, haughty behaviors or attitudes

thy. His nurse remarked to a colleague, "When you talk to him, it's like you're not even really there as a person. It's like he can't connect."

Dr. Smith's sense of entitlement led him to bill Medicare and other insurance carriers for services that he had never rendered or that were inflated on the bills. He believed that changes in the reimbursement system penalized him and that he was entitled to a higher level of payment because of his training, experience, and keen intelligence.

At the urging of his colleagues in practice, and after being repeatedly caught and confronted about his billing fraud, Dr. Smith entered therapy with a well-known psychoanalyst and psychiatrist, Dr. Brown. Dr. Smith told a colleague, months into therapy: "I think Dr. Brown envies me; he knows how much money I make. I can tell the size of my practice, and my success, bothers him."

Dr. Smith eventually was investigated, indicted on 37 criminal fraud counts, and tried in federal court. Many of his colleagues testified against him in federal court. "I can't believe they would *do* this to me," he was heard to say. Convicted on 35 counts, Dr. Smith was sentenced to 5 years in a federal penitentiary.

Narcissistic personality disorder is relatively uncommon; in one community survey, no cases were found among a sample of nearly 800 persons. Some experts argue that the disorder is not a distinctive syndrome because narcissistic traits are common to some extent in most individuals who have a personality disorder. The criteria also overlap with those of other disorders, such as borderline personality disorder, leading some to question its distinctiveness. Some clinicians believe that the diagnosis can be made only on the basis of the emerging transferential relationship in psychoanalytic psychotherapy. Narcissistic personality disorder, like other Axis II disorders, is generally viewed as stable over time, although recent research suggests that it may vary under the influence of significant life events, such as achievement and new relationships.

There is no consensus on the treatment of narcissistic personality, and recommendations range from intensive psychodynamic psychotherapy to interpersonal or cognitive-behavioral psychotherapy. Narcissistic patients can be very difficult to work with. They develop unrealistic expectations, may devalue the therapist, and sometimes abruptly terminate therapy.

Cluster C Disorders

Avoidant Personality Disorder

Avoidant personality disorder was introduced in DSM-III and represents a variant of what had previously been called *schizoid personality*. Another predecessor was *inadequate personality*, a term used to describe individuals who had experienced failure in several spheres of life (e.g., interpersonal relationships, occupation).

Avoidant behavior is described as inhibited, introverted, and anxious. Persons with avoidant personality disorder tend to have low self-esteem, hypersensitivity to rejection, apprehension and mistrust, social awkwardness, timidity, social discomfort, and self-conscious fears of being embarrassed or acting foolish (see Table 16–12).

A current issue is whether avoidant personality disorder represents a dimension along a spectrum of anxiety disorders, similar to the way borderline personality disorder has been linked to the mood disorders and schizotypal personality disorder to schizophrenia. Clearly, many features of avoidant personality disorder are indistinguishable from those of social phobia, and the two disorders frequently overlap. Avoidant personality disorder may involve a genetic predisposition to chronic anxiety.

Several psychotherapeutic strategies have evolved for the treatment of avoidant personality disorder. Group therapy may help the person to overcome social anxiety and to develop interpersonal trust. Assertiveness and social skills training may be helpful, as might systematic desensitization to treat anxiety symptoms, shyness, and introversion. Cognitive-behavioral therapy has been recommended to help correct dysfunctional attitudes (e.g.,

TABLE 16–12.   DSM-IV-TR diagnostic criteria for avoidant personality disorder

A pervasive pattern of social inhibition, feelings of inadequacy, and hypersensitivity to negative evaluation, beginning by early adulthood and present in a variety of contexts, as indicated by four (or more) of the following:

(1) avoids occupational activities that involve significant interpersonal contact, because of fears of criticism, disapproval, or rejection
(2) is unwilling to get involved with people unless certain of being liked
(3) shows restraint within intimate relationships because of the fear of being shamed or ridiculed
(4) is preoccupied with being criticized or rejected in social situations
(5) is inhibited in new interpersonal situations because of feelings of inadequacy
(6) views self as socially inept, personally unappealing, or inferior to others
(7) is unusually reluctant to take personal risks or to engage in any new activities because they may prove embarrassing

"I had better not open my mouth because I'll probably say something stupid"). Benzodiazepines can be useful while the patient is attempting to reverse previously avoided behavior. It is best to limit the use of these drugs to short periods (i.e., weeks or months), although some patients will benefit from long-term use. Serotonin reuptake inhibitors (e.g., fluoxetine, paroxetine) also may be helpful because they have been effective in treating social phobia.

Dependent Personality Disorder

Dependent personality disorder was listed as a subtype of the DSM-I passive-aggressive personality, was not included in DSM-II, but was reintroduced in DSM-III. The disorder is characterized by a pattern of relying excessively on others for emotional support (see Table 16–13). Psychoanalysts have linked dependency to fixation at the oral stage of development, which focuses on the biological gratification that arises from feeding. Other theorists have tied dependent personality to the disruption of attachments early in life. Others view dependency as stemming from overprotectiveness and parental authoritarianism experienced early in life. The following patient, in whom dependency issues were important, was seen at our hospital:

Bob, a 45-year-old farm laborer, presented for evaluation of major depression, which had been chronic for several years. He also reported a long-standing eating disorder, which had resulted in significant weight loss. For 10 years, Bob had feared becoming fat like his father, who had died unexpectedly of a myocardial infarction.

TABLE 16–13. DSM-IV-TR diagnostic criteria for dependent personality disorder

A pervasive and excessive need to be taken care of that leads to submissive and clinging behavior and fears of separation, beginning by early adulthood and present in a variety of contexts, as indicated by five (or more) of the following:

(1) has difficulty making everyday decisions without an excessive amount of advice and reassurance from others
(2) needs others to assume responsibility for most major areas of his or her life
(3) has difficulty expressing disagreement with others because of fear of loss of support or approval.   Note: Do not include realistic fears of retribution.
(4) has difficulty initiating projects or doing things on his or her own (because of a lack of self-confidence in judgment or abilities rather than a lack of motivation or energy)
(5) goes to excessive lengths to obtain nurturance and support from others, to the point of volunteering to do things that are unpleasant
(6) feels uncomfortable or helpless when alone because of exaggerated fears of being unable to care for himself or herself
(7) urgently seeks another relationship as a source of care and support when a close relationship ends
(8) is unrealistically preoccupied with fears of being left to take care of himself or herself

In addition to these problems, Bob described a dull and passive lifestyle. The third of eight children, Bob left school after eighth grade to work on the family farm, as had his siblings. The family remained close because there were few opportunities for outside friendships. Bob reported that he had rarely dated, although he had once been "sweet on a girl." He denied any current interest in developing a relationship.

Bob lived with his mother until she insisted he move out at age 44, which he did reluctantly. Although he lived alone, he remained in close contact with his mother, eating meals with her twice daily and phoning her 10–20 times a day. He relied on her to make decisions for him, even minor ones about day-to-day activities.

Bob had no interests or hobbies apart from his farm chores. He admitted that he was uncomfortable being alone in his mobile home, which prompted him to telephone his mother. He cried when he was asked how he would handle his mother's eventual death. (She was then older than 80 years.)

Although Bob gained weight steadily on a refeeding protocol, it became clear that he would need supervision outside the hospital. Because his mother was too old to help (and her supervision would only worsen his dependency on her), a decision was made by his family to place Bob in a residential care facility.

Although there has been considerable research on the psychology of dependency, there have been few studies of dependent personality disorder. One criticism of the disorder is that it is not sufficiently distinctive to stand alone and that dependency on others is common in other personality disorders; it is also found in persons with chronic medical or psychiatric disorders. One recent study showed that persons with dependent personality are older than patients with other types of personality disorders and are more likely to be women. Comorbid psychiatric disorders are common, particularly mood and anxiety disorders. Persons with dependent personality have poor social and family life, in part because their dependency on others accentuates and promotes interpersonal conflicts.

There is little consensus on the treatment of dependent personality disorder. Cognitive-behavioral psychotherapy is recommended as a way to promote emotional growth, assertiveness, effective decision making, and independence. To encourage this process, a therapist might have the patient set goals for each session and challenge his or her assumptions related to dependency ("I won't be able to make up my mind without mother's input"). Some patients benefit from more focused assertiveness training, or social skills training. Marital counseling is indicated when the patient's dependence on his or her spouse is adversely affecting their relationship.

Obsessive-Compulsive Personality Disorder

Obsessive-compulsive personality disorder is thought by psychoanalysts to represent a fixation at the anal stage of development, characterized by obstinacy, parsimony, and orderliness. Originally termed *compulsive personality* in DSM-I, this disorder was long thought to lead to the development of obsessive-compulsive disorder (OCD). Although early studies showed that some patients with OCD were likely to have a premorbid obsessional personality, it became clear that obsessive-compulsive personality and OCD do not have a one-to-one relation. (The relation between obsessive-compulsive personality disorder and OCD is more fully explored in Chapter 11.)

Obsessive-compulsive personality disorder represents a lifelong pattern of perfectionism and inflexibility typically associated with overconscientiousness and constricted emotions (see Table 16–14). Patients with obsessive-compulsive personality are prone to develop major depression, particularly as they get older. Comorbidity with various anxiety disorders also is common.

Obsessive-compulsive personality disorder is relatively difficult to treat. Some experts recommend psychodynamic psychotherapy; however, these

TABLE 16–14. DSM-IV-TR diagnostic criteria for obsessive-compulsive personality disorder

A pervasive pattern of preoccupation with orderliness, perfectionism, and mental and interpersonal control, at the expense of flexibility, openness, and efficiency, beginning by early adulthood and present in a variety of contexts, as indicated by four (or more) of the following:

(1) is preoccupied with details, rules, lists, order, organization, or schedules to the extent that the major point of the activity is lost

(2) shows perfectionism that interferes with task completion (e.g., is unable to complete a project because his or her own overly strict standards are not met)

(3) is excessively devoted to work and productivity to the exclusion of leisure activities and friendships (not accounted for by obvious economic necessity)

(4) is overconscientious, scrupulous, and inflexible about matters of morality, ethics, or values (not accounted for by cultural or religious identification)

(5) is unable to discard worn-out or worthless objects even when they have no sentimental value

(6) is reluctant to delegate tasks or to work with others unless they submit to exactly his or her way of doing things

(7) adopts a miserly spending style toward both self and others; money is viewed as something to be hoarded for future catastrophes

(8) shows rigidity and stubbornness

patients tend to intellectualize and may be insightful, but they develop little feeling or emotion. Cognitive-behavioral therapy may help these individuals develop a greater tolerance to the notion that the world is mostly made up of gray and not clearly defined black and white lines of rigidly held beliefs. Serotonin reuptake inhibitors (e.g., fluoxetine, paroxetine) may be helpful in reducing the need for perfectionism and the unnecessary ritualizing that sometimes develop.

Management of Personality Disorders

Recommendations for the clinical management of personality disorders are summarized in the box.

Recommendations for management of personality disorders

1. Some patients with personality disorders are difficult, unpleasant, and manipulative. The therapist should not let this fact interfere with or color his or her understanding of *all* patients with personality disorders.

2. Patients have enduring, long-term problems, and therapy may be long term as well. Decades of maladaptive behavior cannot be easily understood or reversed.

3. The therapist should maintain a professional distance from the patient. The therapist is not a friend or collaborator.

   • Therapists must avoid becoming overinvolved with patients, doing favors (e.g., giving out home telephone number), or relating their problems. These "boundary" issues can create enormous problems if not dealt with from the outset.

4. Ground rules for therapy must be established (e.g., that the therapist is willing to see the person regularly, at a specified time).

   • The therapist should spell out what the patient should do or whom the patient should call in a crisis.

   • The therapist should spell out the consequences of self-damaging acts (e.g., hospitalization, referral to another therapist).

5. The therapist should avoid fantasies of becoming a "savior" to the patient. If the personality disorder is chronic, the patient has undoubtedly seen other therapists without success.

6. The therapist should seek support for himself or herself from peers or supervisors. Patients with personality disorders can be a handful, and the therapist will probably need advice or consultation now and then.

7. Support groups can be very helpful to the patient, and referral to community-based organizations is essential.

Bibliography

Akhtar S, Thompson JA: Full review: narcissistic personality disorder. Am J Psychiatry 139:12–20, 1982

American Psychiatric Association: Diagnostic and Statistical Manual of Mental Disorders. Washington, DC, American Psychiatric Association, 1952

American Psychiatric Association: Diagnostic and Statistical Manual of Mental Disorders, 3rd Edition. Washington, DC, American Psychiatric Association, 1980

American Psychiatric Association: Diagnostic and Statistical Manual of Mental Disorders, 4th Edition. Washington, DC, American Psychiatric Association, 1994

American Psychiatric Association: Diagnostic and Statistical Manual of Mental Disorders, 4th Edition Revised. Washington, DC, American Psychiatric Association, 2000

Barrett MS, Stanford MS, Felthaus A, et al: The effects of phenytoin on impulsive and premeditated aggression: a controlled study. J Clin Psychopharmacol 17:341–349, 1997

Beck A: Cognitive Therapy of Personality Disorders. New York, Guilford, 1990

Benedetti F, Sforzini C, Columbo C, et al: Low dose clozapine in acute and continuation treatment with severe borderline personality disorder. J Clin Psychiatry 59:103–107, 1998

Black DW: Bad Boys, Bad Men: Confronting Antisocial Personality Disorder. New York, Oxford University Press, 1999

Black DW, Bell S, Hulbert J, et al: The importance of Axis II in patients with major depression: a controlled study. J Affect Disord 14:115–122, 1988

Cacciola JS, Alterman AI, Rutherford M, et al: Treatment response of antisocial substance abusers. J Nerv Ment Dis 183:166–171, 1995

Cadoret RJ, Yates WR, Troughton E, et al: Genetic-environment interaction in the genesis of aggressivity and conduct disorders. Arch Gen Psychiatry 52:916–924, 1995

Cardasis W, Hochman JA, Silk KR: Transitional objects and borderline personality disorder. Am J Psychiatry 154:250–255, 1997

Cleckley H: The Mask of Sanity. St. Louis, MO, Mosby, 1941

Coid JW: Aetiological risk factors for personality disorders. Br J Psychiatry 174:530–538, 1999

Cornelius JR, Soloff PH, Perel JM, et al: A preliminary trial of fluoxetine in refractory borderline patients. J Clin Psychopharmacol 11:116–120, 1991

Cornelius JR, Soloff PH, Perel JM, et al: Continuum pharmacotherapy of borderline personality disorder with haloperidol and phenelzine. Am J Psychiatry 150:1843–1848, 1993

Cowdry RW, Gardner D: Pharmacotherapy of borderline personality disorder. Arch Gen Psychiatry 45:111–119, 1988

Ferco T, Klein DN, Schwartz JE, et al: 30 month stability of personality disorder diagnoses in depressed outpatients. Am J Psychiatry 155:653–659, 1998

Fulton M, Winokur G: A comparative study of paranoid and schizoid personality disorders. Am J Psychiatry 150:1363–1367, 1993

Gabbard GO: Psychotherapy of personality disorders. Journal of Practical Psychiatry and Behavioral Health 3:327–333, 1997

Goldman SJ, D'Angelo EJ, De Maso DR: Psychopathology in the families of children and adolescents with borderline personality disorder. Am J Psychiatry 150:1832–1835, 1993

Johnson JG, Cohen P, Brown J, et al: Childhood maltreatment increases risk for personality disorders during young adulthood. Arch Gen Psychiatry 56:600–606, 1999

Kavoussi RJ, Cocaro EF: Divalproex sodium for impulsive aggressive behavior in patients with personality disorders. J Clin Psychiatry 59:676–680, 1998

Kernberg O: Severe Personality Disorders. New Haven, CT, Yale University Press, 1984

Langbehn DR, Pfohl BM, Reynolds S, et al: The Iowa Personality Disorders Screen: development and preliminary validation of a brief screening interview. J Personal Disord 13:75–89, 1999

Lewis G, Appleby L: Personality disorders: the patients psychiatrists dislike. Br J Psychiatry 153:44–49, 1988

Livesley WJ, Jang LL, Jackson DN, et al: Genetic and environmental contributions to dimensions of personality disorder. Am J Psychiatry 150:1826–1831, 1993

McGlashan TH: Schizotypal personality disorder. Arch Gen Psychiatry 43:329–334, 1986

Nestadt G, Romanoski AJ, Chahal R, et al: An epidemiological study of histrionic personality disorder. Psychol Med 20:413–422, 1990

Paris J: Social Factors in the Personality Disorders. New York, Cambridge University Press, 1996

Pfohl B, Blum N: Obsessive-compulsive personality disorder: a review of available data and recommendations for DSM-IV. J Personal Disord 5:363–375, 1991

Pfohl B, Black DW, Noyes R, et al: Axis I and Axis II comorbidity findings: implications for validity, in Personality Disorders: New Perspective on Diagnostic Validity. Edited by Oldham J. Washington, DC, American Psychiatric Press, 1991, pp 145–161

Pollack J: Obsessive-compulsive personality. J Personal Disord 1:248–262, 1987

Reich J: Sex distribution of DSM-III personality disorders in psychiatric outpatients. Am J Psychiatry 144:485–488, 1987

Reich J: The morbidity of DSM-III-R dependent personality disorder. J Nerv Ment Dis 84:22–26, 1996

Reich J, Green AI: Effect of personality disorders on outcome of treatment. J Nerv Ment Dis 179:74–82, 1991

Reich J, Yates W, Nguaguba M: Prevalence of DSM-III personality disorders in the community. Soc Psychiatry Psychiatr Epidemiol 24:12–16, 1989

Ronningstam E, Gundersen J, Lyons M: Changes in pathological narcissism. Am J Psychiatry 152:253–257, 1995

Siever L: A psychobiological perspective on the personality disorders. Am J Psychiatry 148:1647–1658, 1991

Skodol AE: Classification, assessment, and differential diagnosis of personality disorders. Journal of Practical Psychiatry and Behavioral Health 3:261–274, 1997

Stone MH: Long-term outcome in personality disorders. Br J Psychiatry 162:299–313, 1993

Tarnepolsky A, Berelowitz M: Borderline personality: a review of recent research. Br J Psychiatry 151:724–734, 1987

Zanarini MC, Frankenburg FR, Dubo ED, et al: Axis I comorbidity of borderline personality disorder. Am J Psychiatry 155:1733–1739, 1998

Zimmerman M, Coryell W: DSM-III personality disorder diagnosis in a non-patient sample. Arch Gen Psychiatry 46:682–689, 1989

Self-Assessment Questions

1. What are the Greek temperaments, and why are they still useful descriptively?

2. How are the personality disorders defined? What is the difference between trait and disorder?

3. Why is the term *personality disorder* considered pejorative?

4. How common are personality disorders? Which ones are more common in men? Which ones are more common in women? Are the disorders stable?

5. What are Freud's character types? How well do they correspond to present-day categories?

6. What evidence is there for genetic or biological origin for the personality disorders? Which personality disorders?

7. Describe the three personality disorder clusters.

8. How do schizoid and schizotypal personality disorders differ? How do these two categories differ from avoidant personality disorder?

9. Are medications useful in treating Cluster A disorders? Which medications?

10. For which disorders might social skills training or assertiveness training be useful?

11. What is the childhood precursor of antisocial personality disorder? What biological abnormalities have been found in these patients? Why is transference a problem with treatment of patients with antisocial personality disorder? Are medications of any value?

12. What features characterize the Cluster C disorders? What are the general treatment recommendations for these disorders? How does obsessive-compulsive personality disorder differ from OCD?

17 Sexual and Gender Identity Disorders

Lolita, light of my life, fire of my loins. My sin, my soul. Lo-lee-ta.

Vladimir Nabakov, *Lolita*

The three categories of sexual disorders are 1) *sexual dysfunctions,* which involve either a disturbance of sexual arousal or a disturbance of psychophysiological performance; 2) *paraphilias,* which involve culturally inappropriate or dangerous patterns of sexual arousal, such as exhibitionism; and 3) *gender identity disorders* (e.g., transsexualism), which involve dissatisfaction with one's biological gender and a desire to become a member of the opposite gender. Sexual dysfunctions are very common, and, in fact, a recent survey of adult Americans showed that 43% of women and 31% of men acknowledged having one or more forms of sexual dysfunction. Paraphilias are less common but are more problematic because they may lead to behavior that endangers, or at a minimum annoys, unsuspecting persons. Gender identity disorders are relatively rare yet remain of interest to psychiatrists and other mental health professionals because of the distress and unhappiness they create. The sexual disorders are listed in Table 17–1.

Sexual Dysfunctions

DSM-IV-TR identifies four major categories of sexual dysfunction: sexual desire disorders, sexual arousal disorders, orgasmic disorders, and sexual

TABLE 17-1.   Sexual and gender identity disorders

Sexual disorders	Sexual dysfunction not otherwise specified
Sexual dysfunctions	Paraphilias
Sexual desire disorders	Exhibitionism
Hypoactive sexual desire	Fetishism
disorder	Frotteurism
Sexual aversion disorder	Pedophilia
Sexual arousal disorders	Sexual masochism
Female sexual arousal	Sexual sadism
disorder	Transvestic fetishism
Male erectile disorder	Voyeurism
Orgasmic disorders	Paraphilia not otherwise specified
Female orgasmic disorder	Other sexual disorders
Male orgasmic disorder	Sexual disorder not otherwise specified
Premature ejaculation	Gender identity disorder not otherwise
Sexual pain disorders	specified
Dyspareunia	Gender identity disorders
Vaginismus	Gender identity disorder

pain disorders. Each category tends to correspond with the different phases of the sexual response cycle. Two residual categories, sexual dysfunction not otherwise specified and sexual disorder not otherwise specified, may be used to diagnose sexual disorders that do not meet the criteria for a more specific disorder. All of the sexual dysfunctions can be classified as due to either psychological factors or a combination of psychological factors and a general medical condition.

Human Sexual Response Cycle

According to DSM-IV-TR, the normal human sexual response cycle consists of four stages:

1. The *appetitive stage* lasts minutes to hours. In this stage, sexual fantasies and the desire for sexual intimacy occur.
2. The *excitement stage* ("foreplay") consists of a) an early phase lasting minutes to hours characterized by penile erection in males and vaginal lubrication, nipple erection, and vasocongestion of the external genitalia in females and b) a late phase lasting seconds to minutes characterized by the appearance of drops of fluid at the head of the penis in males

and a tightening of the outer one-third of the vagina and breast engorgement in females.

3. The *orgasmic stage* typically lasts 5–15 seconds and is accompanied in males by ejaculation and involuntary muscular contractions of the pelvis and in females by contractions of the outer one-third of the vagina and involuntary pelvic thrusting. Females are capable of having multiple orgasms, but the male has an obligatory refractory period before another orgasm is possible.

4. The *resolution stage* consists of detumescence and feelings of both relaxation and well-being.

Sexual Desire Disorders

Hypoactive sexual desire disorder and sexual aversion disorder correspond to the appetitive stage of the sexual response cycle.

Persons with *hypoactive sexual desire disorder* have a persistent or recurrent deficiency in or absence of sexual fantasies and desire for sexual activity that does not result from major depression or another Axis I disorder, such as schizophrenia. (These disorders are often associated with low sex drive.) The direct effects of a substance or a general medical condition (e.g., diabetes mellitus) also must be ruled out as causing the disturbance. Many persons with this disorder have significant trouble with social uneasiness, lack self-confidence, and avoid social situations. The disorder is common among married couples, and more women are affected than men. In one study, 35% of the women and 16% of the men reported having little or no desire for sexual activity for at least some temporary period. (See Table 17–2 for additional findings from this study.) In a community survey of women, 17% of the respondents reported having little sexual interest. Among women treated for sexual disorders, the frequency of hypoactive sexual desire disorder may exceed 75%.

For many persons, low sexual interest temporarily results from stressful situations such as overwork, lack of privacy, or lack of opportunity for sexual relationships. Many persons with this disorder are poorly educated about sexual matters or are unduly inhibited for reasons of religion. Before making a diagnosis of hypoactive sexual desire disorder, a clinician must take into account factors that affect sexual functioning, including age, gender, and the context of a person's life (e.g., it may be culturally appropriate for a celibate priest to report a lack of sexual desire).

Sexual aversion disorder represents a persistent and recurrent aversion to and avoidance of genital contact with a sexual partner. The disorder is not

TABLE 17–2. Frequency of self-reported sexual problems in "normal couples"

Sexual dysfunction	%
Women	
Difficulty getting excited	48
Difficulty in reaching orgasm	46
Difficulty maintaining excitement	33
Inability to have an orgasm	15
Reaching orgasm too quickly	11
Men	
Ejaculating too quickly	36
Difficulty maintaining an erection	9
Difficulty getting an erection	7
Difficulty in ejaculating	4
Inability to ejaculate	0

Source. Adapted from Frank et al. 1978.

due to obsessive-compulsive disorder, major depression, or another serious Axis I condition. Many experts believe that persons with this disorder have been sexually victimized in the past and harbor unpleasant memories or beliefs about sexual intimacy.

Sexual Arousal Disorders

The sexual arousal disorders include male erectile disorder (impotence) and female sexual arousal disorder.

Primary impotence occurs when a man has never been able to achieve an erection sufficient for vaginal insertion. With *secondary impotence*, the man has successfully achieved an erection sufficient for vaginal penetration at some time during the past but is currently unable to do so. Primary impotence is rare, but secondary impotence is reported to occur in up to one-quarter of all men. Among men treated for sexual disorders, more than 50% report this problem.

Female sexual arousal disorder occurs in up to one-third of all married women and is defined as the partial or complete failure to attain or maintain the lubrication-swelling response characteristic of the excitement stage or the complete lack of sexual excitement and pleasure. The disorder can be due to physical factors (e.g., dyspareunia) and is usually associated with anorgasmia.

Orgasmic Disorders

The orgasmic disorders include female orgasmic disorder (anorgasmia), male orgasmic disorder, and premature ejaculation. *Female orgasmic disorder* is manifested by the delay in or absence of orgasm following a normal sexual excitement stage; the clinician judges the woman's orgasmic capability to be less than expected for her age, sexual experience, and amount of sexual stimulation received. *Male orgasmic disorder* occurs when a man achieves ejaculation during intercourse only with great difficulty, if at all. Again, the clinician must take into account the man's age, sexual experience, and amount of sexual stimulation received.

Premature ejaculation is a common disorder reported by more than one-quarter of married men and is the second most frequent complaint among men seeking help for a sexual disorder. The disorder is diagnosed when the man has persistent or recurrent ejaculation with minimal sexual stimulation before, on, or shortly after vaginal penetration and before the man wants to ejaculate. There is no corresponding disorder in women.

Sexual Pain Disorders

The sexual pain disorders include dyspareunia—painful intercourse in males or females—and vaginismus, in which involuntary muscle contractions sufficient to prevent penile insertion occur in the outer one-third of the vagina.

Dyspareunia should not be diagnosed when it is better accounted for by an Axis I disorder, such as somatization disorder, or when it is thought to be due to the direct effects of a substance or a general medical condition. Furthermore, it is not diagnosed when caused exclusively by vaginismus or lack of lubrication. Dyspareunia is a frequent complaint of women evaluated for sexual therapy and is common, at least temporarily, among women who have undergone pelvic surgery or recent childbirth; it is rare in men.

Other Sexual Dysfunctions

Less common sexual dysfunctions include *postcoital headaches* (i.e., headaches that occur immediately after intercourse); *orgasmic anhedonia*, a condition in which there is no physical sensation of orgasm even though ejaculation may have occurred; and *masturbatory pain*, in which pain is experienced with masturbation in the absence of a physical abnormality. The latter disorder is usually caused by a small vaginal tear, Peyronie's disease (which causes an abnormal curvature of the penis), or some other physical disorder.

Etiology of Sexual Dysfunctions

Sexual dysfunction may be caused by psychological or physical factors or sometimes a combination of the two. For example, lack of sexual desire can result from chronic stress, anxiety, or depression or can result from medications that either depress the central nervous system or decrease testosterone production. Prolonged sexual abstinence itself may suppress desire. Major physical stresses, such as illness or surgery, especially when they alter body image (e.g., mastectomy, ileostomy), also may depress sexual desire.

Impotence may be caused by both physical and psychological conditions (Table 17–3). Research shows that up to 75% of the men evaluated for impotency have a physical cause for the disorder, including cardiovascular disease (e.g., atherosclerotic disease), renal disorders (e.g., chronic renal failure), liver disease (e.g., cirrhosis), malnutrition, diabetes mellitus, multiple sclerosis, traumatic spinal cord injury, abuse of alcohol and other psychoactive drugs, psychotropic medication, prostate surgery, and pelvic irradiation.

TABLE 17–3. Causes of male erectile disorder (impotence)

Medical illness	Psychiatric illness
Acromegaly	Anxiety disorders
Addison's disease	Dementia
Diabetes	Major depression
Hyperthyroidism	Schizophrenia
Hypothyroidism	Drugs
Klinefelter's syndrome	Alcohol
Multiple sclerosis	Antiandrogens
Parkinson's disease	Anticholinergics
Pelvic surgery or irradiation	Antidepressants
Peripheral vascular disease	Antihypertensives (especially centrally acting ones)
Pituitary adenoma	Antipsychotics
Spinal cord injury	Barbiturates
Syphilis	Marijuana
Temporal lobe epilepsy	Opiates
	Stimulants

In assessing the cause of impotence, it is important to determine whether spontaneous erections occur at times when the man does not plan to have intercourse (e.g., morning erections or erections with masturbation). A psychological cause is likely if erections occur at these times. The workup for a medical cause may include 1) measuring nocturnal penile tumescence, 2) measuring blood pressure in the penis with a penile plethysmograph or Doppler flow meter, or 3) measuring pudendal nerve latency time. A glucose tolerance test, thyroid and liver function tests, serum prolactin, luteinizing hormone, and follicle stimulating hormone can help to rule out metabolic or endocrinological causes of impotence, such as diabetes mellitus. Invasive tests (e.g., penile arteriography, infusion cavernosography, or radioactive xenon penography) are used in evaluating the rare patient who is a candidate for vascular reconstructive surgery.

Anorgasmia also may result from physical factors, such as the effects of medication or surgery, or psychological factors, such as fears of impregnation, rejection by the sexual partner, or clinical depression. Cultural factors also may contribute. In Victorian times, for instance, girls were commonly told by their mothers that sexual intercourse was a duty and not for pleasure.

Male orgasmic disorder is relatively uncommon and must be differentiated from retrograde ejaculation, in which ejaculation occurs, but the seminal fluid passes backward into the bladder. Both male orgasmic disorder and retrograde ejaculation most likely have a physiological cause, such as the effects of medication, genitourinary surgery (e.g., prostatectomy), or neurological disorders involving the lumbosacral section of the spinal cord. Centrally acting antihypertensives (e.g., guanethidine, α-methyldopa), tricyclic antidepressants (e.g., amitriptyline), or antipsychotics, particularly the phenothiazines (e.g., chlorpromazine, thioridazine), may be responsible for the disorder. Serotonin reuptake inhibitor (SRI) antidepressants (e.g., citalopram, fluoxetine, paroxetine) frequently cause ejaculatory delay or failure. Age itself is an important factor; older men may not ejaculate at every sexual encounter, but perhaps only every second or third time.

Clinical Management of Sexual Dysfunctions

The most widely used approach for the treatment of sexual dysfunction disorders was pioneered by Masters and Johnson in the 1970s. Their "dual" sex therapy involves both partners because the sexual problem affects both persons in a relationship; the principles apply equally to heterosexual and homosexual couples. In this approach, therapy begins with a review of the psychological and physiological aspects of sexual functioning and an evaluation of the couple's attitudes about sexual behavior and of their ability to communicate. After the sexual disturbance has been diagnosed (e.g., male erectile disorder), assignments are given for specific sexual activities that the couple is expected to carry out in private. Sexual relations are emphasized as natural and healthy behaviors that should enhance the couple's relationship. The relatively brief sex therapy (e.g., 8–12 sessions) focuses on correcting dysfunctional behavior, not interpreting presumed underlying psychodynamics. These methods can be used for a variety of sexual disorders and are modified depending on whether the problem represents a disorder of the appetitive, excitement, or orgasmic stage of the sexual response cycle.

As an example of sex therapy for male erectile disorder, the couple is prohibited from engaging in sexual activity other than that prescribed by the therapist. Exercises focus on increasing sensory awareness of erogenous zones, so that couples can learn to give and receive bodily pleasure (i.e., "sensate focus"). Sensate focus exercises are a technique in which the patient engages initially in nongenital, nondemanding caressing with his or her partner with the focus on the patient's own pleasure and feelings. At this point, intercourse is prohibited. Couples are encouraged to separate sexual pleasure from intercourse.

Genital stimulation is gradually included in the exercises; couples are instructed to try various positions for sexual intercourse but not to concern themselves with completing the act. In time, the couple gains confidence and learns to communicate better. They also learn to give and receive pleasure without the pressure of sexual intercourse. Without that pressure, the man is eventually able to have erections and to successfully complete vaginal intercourse.

Specific instructions are altered depending on the presenting complaint. For example, in cases of male orgasmic disorder, the woman may be instructed to insert her partner's penis herself. With anorgasmia, therapy may first involve training the woman to have an orgasm by masturbation before treating the couple. Vaginismus may require individual therapy, relaxation techniques (e.g., progressive muscle relaxation), or the use of Hegar's dilators, which are inserted into the vagina. The size of the dilators is slowly increased over 3–5 days to gradually enlarge the vaginal opening. The "squeeze method" is used to treat premature ejaculation. When the man feels he is about to ejaculate, the woman is instructed to squeeze her partner's penis (for up to 5 seconds) by placing her thumb on the frenulum and her first and second fingers on the opposite side. This action effectively aborts ejaculation so that the couple may prolong foreplay. SRIs are now commonly prescribed for this disorder because a common side effect is delayed ejaculation. Alternatively, men may benefit from 1% dibucaine (Nupercaine) ointment applied to the coronal ridge and frenulum of the penis to reduce stimulation. A case example of male orgasmic disorder and its treatment follows:

> Robert, a 34-year-old bank officer, had been happily married for 6 months but reported that he was now having trouble achieving orgasm. Although he had no sexual experience before marriage, he and his more experienced wife quickly developed a satisfying sexual relationship. They both had versatile sexual interests and were both able to achieve orgasm with adequate stimulation.
>
> Robert reported that for the past month he had been having difficulty achieving orgasm, even with adequate foreplay. Although he was able to reach orgasm through masturbation, he was unable to achieve orgasm with vaginal intercourse, despite trying a variety of positions.
>
> An evaluation showed no evidence of an anxiety disorder or major depression or a physical disorder. Robert had denied any recent change in his marital relationship but had disclosed to the therapist a deep-seated fear that he was unworthy of his new mate and felt that he could not satisfy her sexually. The therapist met with the couple, recommended that Robert abstain from masturbation, prescribed sensate focus exercises to be tried initially without intercourse, and suggested that, as intercourse was attempted, the wife take a dominant role. Learning that he could give and receive pleasure without the pressure of sexual intercourse apparently allowed Robert and his wife to experience intercourse and each to achieve a satisfactory orgasm.

Two oral medications have been approved by the U.S. Food and Drug Administration for the treatment of impotence, or erectile dysfunction. Sildenafil increases blood flow to the penis; although it is well tolerated, it may cause headache, nausea, and sinus congestion. The dose ranges from 25 to 100 mg. Apomorphine acts centrally to increase levels of dopamine, which facilitates erection. Nausea and dizziness are common side effects. The typical dose is 4 mg. Both drugs are taken about 1 hour before anticipated sexual activity. Alprostadil is another drug approved for the treatment of impotence. The drug is placed directly into the urethra with a special syringe and works to increase penile blood flow within 5–10 minutes. The main drawback to this drug is the inconvenience and discomfort involved with the applicator.

Surgical treatments for impotence are also available. The most common technique involves the insertion of a penile prosthesis. These devices are generally either semi-rigid or inflatable; each has its advantages and disadvantages. Most penile implant recipients report satisfaction with the results. As an alternative, vacuum pump devices can be used to produce an erection by increasing blood flow to the penis. Once an erection is achieved, a metal ring is placed around the base of the penis to maintain the erection for about 30 minutes.

Recommendations for the clinical management of sexual dysfunctions are summarized in the box.

Recommendations for management of sexual dysfunction disorders

1. The clinician must learn to take a sexual history without shame or embarrassment. Patients will detect the clinician's anxiety, which will only serve to increase their own.

2. The clinician should not apologize for asking intimate questions. How couples behave sexually is important to assess.

   - Most couples will be surprisingly forthcoming in describing their sex life.

3. Both members of the couple need to participate in the therapy, which may be used with equal success in heterosexual and homosexual couples.

4. The principles of dual sex therapy are relatively simple to learn and emphasize education about sexual functioning, helping couples to communicate better, and correcting dysfunctional attitudes about sex that one or both partners may hold.

5. Therapy involves homework assignments, which assist the couple in learning to increase sensory awareness. Techniques may include self-masturbation, sensate focus experiences, special coital techniques, and learning to separate pleasure from physiological response (e.g., erection).

6. Male erectile disorders now can be treated pharmacologically, whether the disorder is primarily psychologically motivated or medically based. Medications include two oral drugs: sildenafil and apomorphine. Another drug, alprostadil, is placed directly into the urethra with a special applicator.

   - Surgical techniques are available and involve the placement of a semi-rigid or an inflatable device.

   - Vacuum pump devices that draw blood into the penis also are available; a metal ring is then placed around the base of the penis to maintain the erection.

Paraphilias (Sexual Deviations)

The paraphilias are characterized by a disturbance in the object, or expression, of sexual gratification (Table 17–4). To be considered paraphilic, sexual activity must be characterized by a preference for the use of nonhuman objects in achieving sexual arousal, by imposing sexual humiliation or suffering, or by the involvement of nonconsenting sexual partners, such as children. Common paraphilias include *exhibitionism,* in which an individual exposes his or her genitals to unprepared strangers for the purpose of achieving sexual gratification; *fetishism,* in which inanimate objects are the preferred or only means of achieving sexual excitement; *pedophilia,* in which repeated sexual activity with prepubertal children is the preferred or exclusive method of obtaining sexual release (e.g., the character Humbert Humbert in Nabakov's *Lolita*); *transvestic fetishism,* in which a person experiences sexual excitement from dressing in the clothes of the opposite sex; and *voyeurism,* in which observing the sexual activity of others is the preferred means of sexual arousal. Other much less common paraphilias include sexual sadism, sexual masochism, frotteurism, and necrophilia.

DSM-IV-TR provides specific criteria for eight paraphilias and includes a residual category, paraphilia not otherwise specified, for other disorders that fail to meet criteria for any of the specific paraphilias. One of the more unusual paraphilias is *infantilism,* in which the person obtains sexual gratification by behaving like an infant. In one such case seen at our hospital, a 30-year-old former fighter pilot reported that he could function sexually only while wearing a diaper and sucking on a pacifier. He enjoyed having his partner change the diaper, apply baby powder, and bottle-feed him. Although the role-play initially was used for sexual gratification, he later found it comforting and generally wore a diaper under his clothing at all times.

Sexual deviations are seen as having three aspects. First, the behavior does not conform to the generally accepted views of what constitutes normal sexual activity. (The accepted view of normal sexual behavior varies from society to society and has changed over time.) Second, the behavior may cause harm to another person involved in the sexual behavior, such as intercourse with young children or extreme forms of sexual sadism. Third, the behavior may result in subjective distress. The distress may result from societal attitudes that cause persons to see their sexual urges at odds with their moral standards or to be aware of the distress caused to another person from their sexual practices. A patient with a paraphilia treated in our hospital follows:

> Frank, a 38-year-old mechanic, presented to the emergency room requesting help. He had left his wife 3 days earlier, fearing that another arrest for

TABLE 17–4.   Paraphilias (sexual deviations)

Preferential sex act	Behaviors/objects of gratification
Exhibitionism	Exposing self to others
Fetishism	Using inanimate object (e.g., shoe)
Frotteurism	Rubbing against nonconsenting persons
Pedophilia	Preferring prepubertal children
Sexual masochism	Enjoying pain and humiliation
Sexual sadism	Inflicting pain on others
Transvestic fetishism	Cross-dressing
Voyeurism	Window peeping
Paraphilia not otherwise specified	
Coprophilia	Feces
Hypoxophilia	Desire to achieve altered state of consciousness secondary to hypoxia
Infantilism	Acting as though one is an infant
Klismania	Enemas
Oralism	Focusing on oral-genital contact to the exclusion of intercourse
Necrophilia	Dead persons
Partialism	Focusing on one part of the body (e.g., feet) to the exclusion of all else
Telephone scatologia	Obscene telephone calls
Urophilia	Urine
Zoophilia (bestiality)	Animal contacts

indecent exposure would humiliate his family and friends. His story soon unfolded.

At age 10, Frank had lost a testicle in an accident—a fact that was known to his classmates. He was teased endlessly, leading to feelings of insecurity and inadequacy. He began to masturbate at age 12 and was soon masturbating up to five times daily. Although he could not remember when it first occurred, he began to masturbate in public settings—not out in the open, but in areas where he might be discovered. He found the challenge of avoiding detection sexually exciting. He would often masturbate where he could observe women, such as in shopping centers, in libraries, or even from his parked car where he could watch women walk by. Although he denied genital exposure, he admitted that occasionally women would "accidentally" observe him masturbating, adding to his excitement. His masturbation had a compulsive quality, and he felt powerless to stop.

The behavior continued over a 25-year period, leading to several arrests for indecent exposure. Feeling guilty and wanting to make amends, Frank sought psychotherapy after each arrest, but he would soon drop out. One psychiatrist prescribed thioridazine to dampen his sex drive, but it only caused retrograde ejaculation. Another physician recommended that he read pornography and masturbate in private.

Frank denied other paraphilic behaviors and thought that pedophilia was "disgusting." He admitted to two episodes of exhibitionism, first at age 18 to a girl sitting next to him in class and once during his honeymoon. Although he was socially awkward with women and did not date until age 21, Frank had married at age 23. He described the marriage as stable and viewed his sexual relationship with his wife as satisfying. He admitted that he preferred masturbation to sexual intercourse.

Frank was admitted to the hospital for further evaluation. Physical examination confirmed the absence of the right testicle, but results of the examination were otherwise normal. Serum testosterone level was 288 ng/dL (normal serum level=200–800 ng/dL). Treatment was begun with medroxyprogesterone. At a follow-up visit 1 month later, his serum testosterone had fallen to 41 ng/dL. He had been able to resist masturbating in public and no longer had spontaneous erections. He felt that he could control his behavior. Six months later, he chose to discontinue the medication and within 1 month had returned to his old ways.

Frank presented for follow-up 10 years later after an arrest for soliciting a prostitute. He described himself as a "sex addict" and acknowledged that he continued to compulsively masturbate and to expose himself to unsuspecting women. He had received no treatment in the interim. He was given paroxetine, 40 mg/day, and over the following year reported that the drug helped him to control his sexual urges and behaviors. He also became involved in a support group.

Epidemiology of Paraphilias

The paraphilias are relatively uncommon in psychiatric practice. Most cases are noted only if treatment is sought or if there are legal entanglements. Many paraphilias would scarcely be reported at all because the activity takes place between consenting adults or by a lone individual (e.g., fetishism). Individuals who are comfortable with their paraphilias are completely underrepresented in all samples. The best statistics regarding prevalence are legal and medical. In 1998, more than 90,000 persons were arrested on sexually related charges in the United States, excluding forcible rape and prostitution, and a similar number were incarcerated in state and federal prisons; perpetrators are overwhelmingly male. These figures are biased toward impulsive individuals and persons with paraphilias that are considered dangerous or a public nuisance. Among the legally identified cases, pedophilia is the most common paraphilia, probably because of its unsavory nature and the great effort made in apprehending pedophiles. Exhibitionism is commonly reported, possibly because it involves repeated public displays to young girls. Sexual masochism and sexual sadism are underrepresented in crime statistics because it is unlikely that these disorders would come to public attention unless a tragedy occurred (e.g., autoerotic suffocation).

Etiology of Paraphilias

For centuries, variations of the sexual act were regarded as offenses against nature, God, or the law rather than as disorders that physicians should study and treat. The systematic study of the paraphilias began in the 1870s with the work of Krafft-Ebing, Hirschfeld, Ellis, and others. In 1886, Krafft-Ebing, a Viennese psychiatrist, compiled the first systematic account of sexual deviations in his book *Psychopathia Sexualis*. He considered the sexual deviations to be hereditary and believed that they could be modified by social and psychological factors. Freud, also active at this time, explained sexual deviations as resulting from failures of the developmental processes during childhood.

Much of the recent work on paraphilias has focused on learning theory. In this model, persons with inappropriate fantasies and urges attempt to suppress these desires. They inadvertently pair paraphilic fantasies with masturbation, which intensifies their interest and links the fantasy with the positive experience of orgasm. Paraphilic arousal strengthens, control breaks down, and the fantasy is acted on. Once this process becomes established, it is likely to reoccur because orgasm is such a powerful reinforcement.

Paraphilic acts also may result from poor impulse control that occurs in the context of schizophrenia, a dementing illness, or a brain injury. Patients with antisocial personality disorder occasionally commit deviant sexual acts to gratify their immediate urges, although a true paraphilia may not exist.

A small body of research has suggested that sexually deviant behavior has a biological basis. Evidence that supports this view includes the finding of an increased frequency of abnormal results on neuropsychological tests and electroencephalograms (EEGs) in sex offenders. Abnormal brain computed tomography scans have been reported in pedophiles and other sexually aggressive men; dilation of the temporal horns, especially the right horn, is the major finding. Familial transmission and hypothalmic-pituitary-gonadal axis dysfunction have been reported in pedophilia.

Clinical Findings, Course, and Outcome of Specific Paraphilias

Paraphilias are generally established in adolescence and occur almost exclusively among men, although cases are described in women. Most paraphilic patients are heterosexual, not homosexual, contrary to widely held views. These demographic features appear to be true for fetishists, pedophiles, exhibitionists, and voyeurs. People with paraphilias often meet criteria for several paraphilias simultaneously. Co-occurring psychiatric disorders are common and include substance abuse, mood disorders, and personality disorders.

The person with fetishism often uses rubber garments, women's underclothing, and high-heeled shoes as objects of gratification. Contact with the object produces sexual arousal, which is followed by masturbation. Fetishists may spend considerable time seeking their desired objects. No reliable follow-up data are available, but the disorder typically begins in adolescence or young adulthood and may diminish when satisfying heterosexual relationships are established. A case example of fetishism seen in our clinic follows:

> A 41-year-old attorney had his law license suspended after admitting to breaking into and entering more than 100 homes to obtain women's underwear for sexual gratification. He entered the houses through unlocked doors or would sometimes jimmy a lock with a credit card or knife. Once inside the house, he would seek undergarments to use later in solitary acts of masturbation. He was finally caught after he had entered a neighbor's home, where he was found searching for the woman's underwear. He was apprehended and charged with criminal trespass, convicted, and placed on probation. He denied subsequent episodes of pilfering undergarments at a follow-up 5 years later, but he admitted that the interest remained. A renewed interest in religion was responsible for his self-control, he claimed.

Transvestic fetishism often begins at puberty. Persons may start by putting on only a few garments of the opposite sex. In time, the individual may dress entirely in the clothes of the opposite sex. Early on, the person experiences the cross-dressing as sexually stimulating. As the person gains confidence, the clothes may be worn in public. Although data are limited, the disorder continues for years, although the urge to cross-dress may decline as the sexual drive diminishes.

Persons with pedophilia choose a child of the same or opposite sex as a sexual partner. Although the condition may begin at any age, most pedophiles seen by physicians are middle-aged. Prognosis has not been reliably

studied but probably depends on the length of the history of pedophilic behavior, the frequency of the behavior, the absence of other social and sexual
relationships, and the underlying personality.

Exhibitionists make up about one-third of the sexual offenders referred
for treatment and generally involve two groups of men—those with an inhibited temperament who struggle with their urges and expose a flaccid
penis and those with aggressive traits who expose an erect penis and masturbate. When exhibitionism begins in the middle or older years, the behavior may indicate the presence of a dementia. Exhibitionists who repeat are
likely to persist for years, according to evidence from the courts. In keeping
with clinical impression, the evidence suggests that the reconviction rate for
indecent exposure is low after the first conviction but high after a second
conviction.

Voyeurism is often an expression of sexual curiosity in adolescents. The
behavior is gradually replaced by direct sexual experience, although voyeurism may persist. The following case of voyeurism was reported in a local
paper:

> A 27-year-old law student pleaded guilty to five counts of criminal trespass
> after admitting that he had repeatedly spied on women in dormitory show-
> ers. He was arrested near the dormitory one morning after students had
> caught him lying on the floor outside the women's shower and looking
> through the ventilation grate. He was chased out of the dormitory by the
> women who had found him there.
>
> Residents of the dorm had banded together and would watch for him
> daily from 5:00 A.M. to 9:00 A.M., believing that he would repeat his act. The
> "peeper" was well known at the dorm for his voyeurism and for making a
> nuisance of himself.

Although homosexuality has traditionally been included with the sexual deviations, most psychiatrists now believe it to be an alternative form of
sexual behavior that should be of little concern to physicians, other than as
a risk factor for various conditions such as genital herpes or HIV-related diseases. In fact, members of the American Psychiatric Association voted in
1973 to delete homosexuality from its list of mental disorders. Currently, homosexuality is not considered a mental disorder, unless the patient is chronically distressed by it (i.e., ego-dystonic homosexuality), although most
homosexual persons will experience a transient phase during which they are
disturbed or distressed by their sexual orientation. Ego-dystonic homosexuality is classified in DSM-IV-TR as a sexual disorder not otherwise
specified.

Clinical Management of the Paraphilias

In the last two decades, behavioral interventions have become the mainstay of treatment of the paraphilias. Methods have been developed to reduce deviant arousal patterns through masturbatory satiation (i.e., satiating or boring the patient with his own deviant fantasies) or covert sensitization (i.e., replacing fantasies with unpleasant images) and to generate arousal in response to nondeviant themes through masturbatory conditioning. Social skills training is used to help the patient learn to communicate more effectively with appropriate adult partners. Cognitive-behavioral techniques are used to help the paraphiliac patient restructure faulty cognitions used to justify behavior (e.g., erroneously interpreting a child's docility as an expression of desire). Relaxation training may help reduce the anxiety and stress that frequently precede paraphilic behavior. A follow-up study of 194 child molesters treated with behavior modification techniques showed an 82% success rate (defined as no recidivism) at 12 months posttreatment. Although these results are encouraging, it is not known whether they can be generalized to the other paraphilias and to persons not motivated by threats of arrest or incarceration.

Reports on the use of antiandrogen medications, such as medroxyprogesterone or cyproterone (not available in the United States), indicate promising results for the treatment of repeat offenders, such as our patient Frank, whose case is presented earlier in the chapter. These medications act peripherally to reduce serum testosterone levels and centrally to reduce sexual drive. The goal is to decrease paraphilic fantasies and their associated behaviors, while avoiding erectile dysfunction. Medroxyprogesterone is given orally starting with doses of 100–200 mg/day; some patients will need up to 400 mg/day. A long-acting preparation (Depo-Provera) may be given intramuscularly at doses of 200–400 mg every 7–10 days. Sustained use is necessary because relapse generally follows drug discontinuation. The long-term risk of these medications has not been adequately studied, and because there may be a risk of liver disease or cancer, they should be used with caution, and the patient's health should be carefully monitored. The gonadotropin-releasing hormone analogue triptorelin also has been used to reduce serum testosterone levels in men with paraphilias. This drug has fewer side effects than medroxyprogesterone (or cyproterone) and can be administered by monthly injections. At least one well-designed study showed that it was effective when compared with placebo. However, triptorelin is not presently available in the United States.

SRIs recently have been used to reduce both paraphilic fantasies and behavioral impulsivity. An open-label study with sertraline showed that individuals with widely varying paraphilias experienced substantial benefit. No direct comparisons of SRIs and medroxyprogesterone have been done, but because SRIs are well tolerated and may be effective, they should be used initially. Antiandrogens should be reserved for patients whose symptoms do not respond to SRIs and whose hypersexuality is uncontrolled or dangerous. Other drug therapy, including antipsychotic or antidepressant medication, is indicated when the paraphilia is associated with schizophrenia or major depression.

Recommendations for the clinical management of paraphilias are summarized in the box.

Recommendations for management of paraphilias

1. The history is of utmost importance in treating paraphilias. The therapist must learn where and when the behavior occurs, who or what the desired object is, and what occurs in the presence of the object.

   • Most patients with paraphilias have a variety of abnormal behaviors, and the therapist is safe in assuming that more are present than are initially disclosed by the patient.

2. Paraphilias are difficult to treat, but behavior therapy techniques may offer the best hope for success. The purpose of these techniques is to reduce deviant arousal patterns and to generate new arousal in response to nondeviant themes.

   • Methods may include masturbatory satiation and conditioning, social skills training, and cognitive restructuring.

3. Medications may help reduce paraphilic fantasies and inappropriate behavior.

   • Serotonin reuptake inhibitors have been used with some success.

   • Antiandrogens are generally reserved for repeat offenders whose actions are uncontrolled or potentially dangerous.

4. Difficult cases should be referred to clinicians who have experience in treating these disorders.

Gender Identity Disorders

Gender identity disorders are relatively rare and usually have their onset in childhood and adolescence. Their essential feature is the desire to become a member of the opposite sex. Individuals with this disorder, also referred to as *transsexualism*, typically manifest a strong and persistent cross-gender identification and a sense of inappropriateness about their assigned gender. In adults, this often leads to a persistent preoccupation with getting rid of their primary and secondary sex characteristics and acquiring the sex characteristics of the opposite gender. In children, this may be manifested in a boy by an assertion that his penis or testes are disgusting. The diagnostic criteria for gender identity disorder are listed in Table 17–5. A residual category, gender identity disorder not otherwise specified, exists for disorders that do not meet the full syndromal criteria (e.g., a person preoccupied with castration but with no desire to acquire the sex characteristics of the opposite gender). The case of a patient with transsexualism evaluated in our clinic follows:

> William, a 25-year-old felon, was referred for evaluation of gender dysphoria. He had recently filed a lawsuit requesting that the state pay for his gender reassignment surgery, as well as allow him to wear women's clothing. He asked for transfer to a women's prison and to have hormone injections. Corrections officials had refused all of these requests.
>
> William reported that he had never felt comfortable with his gender. He was effeminate as a child and enjoyed playing house, in which he would assume feminine roles such as playing the mother or sister. He also liked games associated with girls, such as hopscotch and jump rope, and was not very good at team sports. He began to cross-dress at age 9 and said that he felt more comfortable and natural when dressed as a girl. He wished that he had been born a girl and was unhappy with his male genitals: "I can't stand them. I don't consider them mine."
>
> William began to cross-dress full-time in his early 20s and for a 5-month period lived as a woman, calling himself Julie. Although he never had a desire for heterosexual relationships, he was able to perform sexually with a woman and achieve orgasm, but he "didn't like it." During sexual intercourse, William would fantasize about being made love to as a woman. He had had homosexual experiences with more than 100 partners and had developed several relationships of 5 or 6 months' duration. He would generally assume a passive role, for example, performing oral sex on others or being the receptive partner of anal sex. He refused to allow any of his male partners to touch his genitals and refused mutual masturbation.
>
> William had read about transsexualism and had written to many different medical centers for information. Imprisonment had been difficult for him because he claimed that other inmates would make fun of his personal habits, including shaving his chest, arms, legs, and axilla. He had attempted to mutilate his genitals on three occasions and several months before his evaluation had managed to lacerate his penis with a shard of glass.
>
> In addition to his gender dysphoria, William had a lifelong history of disciplinary and behavior problems and as a young boy had been temporarily placed in detention. He had a history of abusing both alcohol and marijuana and had many run-ins with the law for shoplifting, theft, and

TABLE 17–5. DSM-IV-TR diagnostic criteria for gender identity disorder

A. A strong and persistent cross-gender identification (not merely a desire for any perceived cultural advantages of being the other sex).

    In children, the disturbance is manifested by four (or more) of the following:

   (1) repeatedly stated desire to be, or insistence that he or she is, the other sex

   (2) in boys, preference for cross-dressing or simulating female attire; in girls, insistence on wearing only stereotypical masculine clothing

   (3) strong and persistent preferences for cross-sex roles in make-believe play or persistent fantasies of being the other sex

   (4) intense desire to participate in the stereotypical games and pastimes of the other sex

   (5) strong preference for playmates of the other sex

    In adolescents and adults, the disturbance is manifested by symptoms such as a stated desire to be the other sex, frequent passing as the other sex, desire to live or be treated as the other sex, or the conviction that he or she has the typical feelings and reactions of the other sex.

B. Persistent discomfort with his or her sex or sense of inappropriateness in the gender role of that sex.

    In children, the disturbance is manifested by any of the following: in boys, assertion that his penis or testes are disgusting or will disappear or assertion that it would be better not to have a penis, or aversion toward rough-and-tumble play and rejection of male stereotypical toys, games, and activities; in girls, rejection of urinating in a sitting position, assertion that she has or will grow a penis, or assertion that she does not want to grow breasts or menstruate, or marked aversion toward normative feminine clothing.

    In adolescents and adults, the disturbance is manifested by symptoms such as preoccupation with getting rid of primary and secondary sex characteristics (e.g., request for hormones, surgery, or other procedures to physically alter sexual characteristics to simulate the other sex) or belief that he or she was born the wrong sex.

C. The disturbance is not concurrent with a physical intersex condition.

D. The disturbance causes clinically significant distress or impairment in social, occupational, or other important areas of functioning.

Code based on current age:

   302.6   Gender Identity Disorder in Children

   302.85   Gender Identity Disorder in Adolescents or Adults

Specify if (for sexually mature individuals):

   Sexually Attracted to Males

   Sexually Attracted to Females

   Sexually Attracted to Both

   Sexually Attracted to Neither

writing bad checks. He also had several psychiatric hospitalizations, mostly for depression or suicidal behavior. None of his suicide attempts had been medically serious.

William crossed his legs in an effeminate manner, was limp-wristed, and had long, greasy hair parted down the middle, covering half of his face. There was no evidence of a mood disorder, formal thought disorder, hallucinations, or delusions. Although somewhat guarded during the interview, he summarized everything with the comment, "It's all a confused mess."

Although he clearly met criteria for gender identity disorder, his lawsuit ultimately failed, and he remained in the men's prison.

The diagnosis of transsexualism is easily made, but it is important to rule out schizophrenia, transvestic fetishism, and effeminate homosexuality. In schizophrenia, a desire to change one's anatomical gender is generally part of a complex delusion (e.g., the belief that the FBI is conspiring to change the patient's sex). Transvestites who cross-dress occasionally may come to feel that sex change surgery is a natural extension of their cross-dressing. Effeminate homosexual persons, on the other hand, might request a sex change to make themselves more appealing to potential sex partners.

Transsexualism almost always begins in childhood, when gender identity is established. In boys, early features of transsexualism include overidentification with the mother, overtly feminine behavior (e.g., playing with dolls), little interest in typical male pursuits (e.g., disliking sports), and peer relationships primarily with girls. Tomboyishness is found in young transsexual girls, but the behavior is more acceptable in our society than is feminine behavior in boys and tends to draw less attention. The prevalence of the disorder is estimated at 1 in 30,000 men and 1 in 100,000 women.

DSM-IV-TR subtypes transsexuals according to their attraction to males or females. Those not attracted to either gender generally have a history of either no sexual activity or little pleasure derived from the genitals. The homosexual transsexual person reports sexual arousal from same-sex partners. The heterosexual transsexual person reports arousal from opposite-sex partners. Male and female transsexuals generally deny any interest in homosexuality because they believe themselves to be members of the opposite sex.

Depression, substance abuse, and personality disorders are frequent complications among persons with gender identity disorders. Narcissistic, histrionic, and borderline traits are relatively frequent because many transsexuals are viewed as being self-absorbed and demanding, being interpersonally shallow, having persistent identity problems, engaging in self-mutilation, and having angry outbursts. The self-mutilation may include damage to their genitals; autocastration occurs in extreme cases. These acts are generally not suicide attempts because they are designed to force the physician to deal with the patient's transsexualism.

Many transsexual persons seek hormonal therapy and request sex reassignment surgery. Clinics in the United States and elsewhere offering sex reassignment surgery often require that the patient live as a member of the opposite sex for more than 1 year before considering him or her for surgery. A new birth certificate designating the new sexual status is typically sought after surgery.

In the transition from male to female, the individual is prescribed hormones (e.g., estradiol, progesterone) to promote breast development; laser treatment and electrolysis are used to remove hair. Finally, surgery is performed to remove the testes and penis and to create an artificial vagina (vaginoplasty). The female-to-male transsexual patient undergoes mastectomy, hysterectomy, and oophorectomy; is prescribed testosterone to help develop muscle mass and deepen the voice; and may have an artificial penis constructed. Male-to-female sex reassignment surgery is relatively successful; many of these individuals have excellent cosmetic results and are able to function sexually and to achieve orgasm.

Transsexual patients who adjust well after surgery tend to have had a lifelong cross-gender identification, were able to "pass" convincingly as a member of the opposite sex before surgery, have good social support, have a college education, and have a steady job. Patients without these characteristics tend to do less well. The overwhelming majority are satisfied with the outcome of surgery and their new anatomical contours. Many patients will continue to benefit from psychotherapy following surgery to assist them in handling day-to-day problems, as well as adjusting to their new gender role.

Psychotherapeutic strategies for patients who do not seek surgery include individual and group sessions aimed at helping them to accept their anatomical sex, helping them to develop an ability to experience pleasure from their genitals, and helping them to make a successful adjustment in other important domains of life.

Bibliography

Abel GG, Osborn C: Stopping sexual violence. Psychiatric Annals 22:301–306, 1992

American Psychiatric Association: Diagnostic and Statistical Manual of Mental Disorders, 4th Edition. Washington, DC, American Psychiatric Association, 1994

American Psychiatric Association: Diagnostic and Statistical Manual of Mental Disorders, 4th Edition Text Revision. Washington, DC, American Psychiatric Association, 2000

Black DW: Compulsive sexual behavior: a review. Journal of Practical Psychiatry and Behavioral Health 4:219–229, 1998

Black DW, Goldstein RB, Blum N, et al: Personality characteristics in 60 subjects with psychosexual dysfunction: a non-patient sample. J Personal Disord 9:275–285, 1995

Brown GR: A review of clinical approaches to gender dysphoria. J Clin Psychiatry 51:57–64, 1990

Brown GR, Wise TN, Costa PT, et al: Personality characteristics and sexual functioning of 188 cross dressing men. J Nerv Ment Dis 184:265–273, 1996

Frank E, Anderson C, Rubinstein D: Frequency of sexual dysfunction in "normal couples." N Engl J Med 229:111–115, 1978

Fuller AK: Child molestation and pedophilia: an overview for the physician. JAMA 261:602–606, 1989

Gaffney GR, Berlin FS: Is there a gonadal dysfunction in pedophilia? A pilot study. Br J Psychiatry 145:657–660, 1984

Gaffney GR, Lurie SF, Berlin FS: Is there familial transmission of pedophilia? J Nerv Ment Dis 172:546–548, 1984

Green R: Gender identity in childhood and later sexual orientation: follow-up of 78 males. Am J Psychiatry 142:339–341, 1985

Heiman J, LoPiccolo J: Clinical outcome of sex therapy. Arch Gen Psychiatry 40:443–449, 1983

Kafka MP: Sertraline pharmacotherapy for paraphilias and paraphilia-related disorders—an open trial. Ann Clin Psychiatry 6:189–196, 1994

Kafka M: Psychopharmacologic treatments for nonparaphilic compulsive behaviors. CNS Spectrums 5:49–59, 2000

Langevin R: Biological factors contributing to paraphilic behavior. Psychiatric Annals 22:307–314, 1992

Laumann EO, Paik A, Rosen RC: Sexual dysfunction in the United States: prevalence and predictors. JAMA 281:537–544, 1999

Meyer JK, Reter DJ: Sex reassignment follow-up. Arch Gen Psychiatry 36:1010–1015, 1979

Osborn M, Hawton K, Gath D: Sexual dysfunction among middle-aged women in the community. BMJ 296:959–962, 1988

Reissig ED, Binik YM, Khalifé S: Does vaginismus exist? A critical review of the literature. J Nerv Ment Dis 187:261–273, 1999

Rendell MS, Raifer J, Wicker PA, et al: Sildenafil for treatment of erectile dysfunction in men with diabetes: a randomized controlled trial. JAMA 281:421–426, 1999

Schiavi RC, Schreiner-Engel P, Mandeli J, et al: Healthy aging and male sexual function. Am J Psychiatry 147:766–771, 1990

Segraves RJ: Effects of psychotropic drugs on human erection and ejaculation. Arch Gen Psychiatry 46:275–284, 1989

Seidman SN, Rieder RO: A review of sexual behavior in the United States. Am J Psychiatry 151:330–341, 1994

Smith RS: Voyeurism, a review of the literature. Arch Sex Behav 5:585–609, 1975

Spector KR, Boyle M: The prevalence and perceived aetiology of male sexual problems in a non-clinical sample. Br J Med Psychol 59:351–358, 1986

Sternbach H: Age-associated testosterone decline in men: clinical issues for psychiatry. Am J Psychiatry 155:1310–1318, 1998

Wise TN: Fetishism, etiology and treatment: a review from multiple perspectives. Compr Psychiatry 26:249–256, 1985

Self-Assessment Questions

1. What are the three major types of sexual disorders?
2. What are the stages of the sexual response cycle?
3. What are the disorders of the appetitive stage?
4. What are the causes of male erectile disorder (impotence)?
5. How is impotence treated?
6. How common are paraphilias?
7. How can learning experiences lead to paraphilic behavior?
8. Is homosexuality a sexual deviation?
9. What are the antecedent behavioral characteristics of transsexuals?
10. What are the treatments for gender identity disorder?

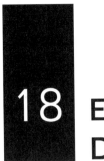
18 Eating Disorders

O! that this too too solid flesh would melt.

William Shakespeare, *Hamlet*

Anorexia nervosa and bulimia nervosa, the two major eating disorders, are each characterized by the presence of disturbed eating behaviors combined with an intense preoccupation with body weight and shape. Many persons believe that these syndromes have developed relatively recently, perhaps reflecting contemporary society's obsession with youth, beauty, and slimness. In fact, the disorders have been recognized for centuries. Richard Morton, an English physician, is generally credited with describing the syndrome of anorexia nervosa in 1694, although it was Sir William Gull who coined the term in 1873. Gull's patients were mostly young women who showed emaciation, amenorrhea, constipation, slow pulse, and remarkable overactivity. His account of anorexia nervosa as a disorder of starvation motivated by the pursuit of thinness is still noteworthy for its attention to detail.

Definition

Anorexia nervosa is diagnosed when a person induces weight loss leading to a body weight of less than 85% of a healthy norm or refuses to gain appropriate weight while growing taller; has an intense fear of gaining weight or becoming fat even though underweight; has a disturbance in the perception of his or her body shape; and (in women) has missed three consecutive menstrual cycles (see Table 18–1). The patient's body mass index (weight in kilograms/height in meters^2) is generally less than 17.5. The requirement that the person with anorexia be 15% underweight for body height emphasizes severity, and the requirement for amenorrhea adds to the specificity of the diagnosis. (In men, there is no comparable requirement for reproductive hormone abnormality.) The clinician should further specify whether the disorder is the restricting type (i.e., no bingeing or purging) or the binge-eating/purging type.

TABLE 18–1.   DSM-IV-TR diagnostic criteria for anorexia nervosa

A. Refusal to maintain body weight at or above a minimally normal weight for age and height (e.g., weight loss leading to maintenance of body weight less than 85% of that expected; or failure to make expected weight gain during period of growth, leading to body weight less than 85% of that expected).

B. Intense fear of gaining weight or becoming fat, even though underweight.

C. Disturbance in the way in which one's body weight or shape is experienced, undue influence of body weight or shape on self-evaluation, or denial of the seriousness of the current low body weight.

D. In postmenarcheal females, amenorrhea, i.e., the absence of at least three consecutive menstrual cycles. (A woman is considered to have amenorrhea if her periods occur only following hormone, e.g., estrogen, administration.)

Specify type:

Restricting Type: during the current episode of Anorexia Nervosa, the person has not regularly engaged in binge-eating or purging behavior (i.e., self-induced vomiting or the misuse of laxatives, diuretics, or enemas)

Binge-Eating/Purging Type: during the current episode of Anorexia Nervosa, the person has regularly engaged in binge-eating or purging behavior (i.e., self-induced vomiting or the misuse of laxatives, diuretics, or enemas)

Bulimia nervosa consists of recurrent episodes of binge eating; a feeling of lack of control over eating during the binges; recurrent use of inappropriate compensatory behaviors to prevent weight gain, such as vomiting, use of laxatives or diuretics, strict dieting or fasting, or vigorous exercise; an average of two binge episodes weekly for 3 months; and persistent overconcern with body shape and weight. Furthermore, the disturbance does not occur exclusively in the course of anorexia nervosa (see Table 18–2). The clinician should specify whether the disorder is the purging type (e.g., self-induced vomiting) or the nonpurging type.

TABLE 18–2.   DSM-IV-TR diagnostic criteria for bulimia nervosa

A. Recurrent episodes of binge eating. An episode of binge eating is characterized by both of the following:
   (1) eating, in a discrete period of time (e.g., within any 2-hour period), an amount of food that is definitely larger than most people would eat during a similar period of time and under similar circumstances
   (2) a sense of lack of control over eating during the episode (e.g., a feeling that one cannot stop eating or control what or how much one is eating)
B. Recurrent inappropriate compensatory behavior in order to prevent weight gain, such as self-induced vomiting; misuse of laxatives, diuretics, enemas, or other medications; fasting; or excessive exercise.
C. The binge eating and inappropriate compensatory behaviors both occur, on average, at least twice a week for 3 months.
D. Self-evaluation is unduly influenced by body shape and weight.
E. The disturbance does not occur exclusively during episodes of Anorexia Nervosa.
Specify type:
   Purging Type: during the current episode of Bulimia Nervosa, the person has regularly engaged in self-induced vomiting or the misuse of laxatives, diuretics, or enemas
   Nonpurging Type: during the current episode of Bulimia Nervosa, the person has used other inappropriate compensatory behaviors, such as fasting or excessive exercise, but has not regularly engaged in self-induced vomiting or the misuse of laxatives, diuretics, or enemas

Although anorexia nervosa and bulimia nervosa differ, there is considerable diagnostic overlap between the two disorders, and their natural histories frequently intertwine.

The discrepancy between weight and perceived body image is key to the diagnosis of anorexia nervosa. Most underweight persons are concerned about their weight. They recognize when it is too low and express a desire to gain weight. Patients with anorexia, on the other hand, take delight in their weight loss and express a fear of gaining weight. Bulimic patients often successfully hide their binge-eating and purging behaviors and often have normal weight.

Another category, *eating disorder not otherwise specified,* is used for symptoms that do not meet the criteria for a more specific eating disorder. A woman who has features of anorexia nervosa but who still menstruates would fit this category. Another example is the person with eating binges but no compensatory purging behavior, who would receive a diagnosis of *binge-eating disorder,* which tends to occur in older persons and is found in about one-quarter of morbidly obese individuals.

Epidemiology

There has been some concern that eating disorders are increasing in prevalence, and several investigators have suggested that anorexia nervosa is more common than it was decades ago. It seems more likely that increasing public awareness has simply led to increased recognition of the disorder. Also, because treatments have become available, patients may be more likely to seek help. Estimates from high school and college-age populations yield a prevalence among women of approximately 1% for anorexia nervosa and up to 4% for bulimia nervosa. For either disorder, the frequency in men is about one-tenth that for women. Isolated symptoms, such as bingeing, purging, or fasting, are far more common than the disorders themselves. The gender difference is probably not artifactual because population surveys confirm what clinicians have noted.

Eating disorders have an onset during adolescence or young adulthood. Studies comparing anorexia and bulimia generally find an earlier age at onset for anorexia (early teens) than for bulimia (late teens, early 20s). These disorders are found in all social strata, although in the past they were thought to be more common in the higher socioeconomic groups. Anorexia nervosa, however, is uncommon in nonindustrialized countries and is less frequent among African Americans in the United States. Eating disorders are overrepresented in occupations that require rigorous control of body shape (e.g., modeling, ballet). Male athletes—particularly wrestlers and jockeys— often develop eating disorders because they must meet strict weight criteria.

The following case example illustrates a patient who developed anorexia nervosa first and later achieved normal weight complicated by bulimia nervosa.

> Mary, a 36-year-old registered nurse, had a 16-year history of abnormal eating behaviors. Although she now maintained a normal weight and had regular periods, she had frequent binge-purge episodes.
>
> Mary grew up in a competitive, upper-middle-class family. The middle of five children, Mary always felt unloved and ignored by her parents, whom she felt favored the other children. Apart from occasional temper outbursts during her childhood and teen years, Mary was well adjusted, performed well in school, was active in clubs, and had many friends. Yet Mary felt insecure and unattractive; she rarely dated.
>
> At age 20, she and a friend toured Europe together and would skip meals to save money. Both felt that they could afford to lose some weight, although Mary then weighed about 120 pounds (height 5 feet, 3 inches). On her return, she weighed less than 85 pounds; her family became concerned with her scarecrowlike appearance, but Mary was happy with her

weight loss and felt more attractive. In fact, she expressed a desire to lose more weight.

Over the next 5 years, her weight fluctuated, but she remained underweight. Family members remained concerned about her eating habits. She refused to eat meals with her family, adopted a vegetarian diet, and was often seen in the kitchen preparing high-caloric snacks. Her mother noted that cakes, cookies, and other desserts prepared for the family would mysteriously disappear, or a cake might be found with all of the frosting removed. Mary eventually moved into her own apartment. Her brother remembers running into her at a grocery store and finding only diet soda, a single head of lettuce, and several bags of candy in the shopping cart.

Her family also had found evidence of purging behavior. Early on, Mary had learned to induce vomiting, which later occurred spontaneously. She would keep empty jars in her room to hold her emesis. After she had moved out of the family home, several filled jars were found under her bed.

Always active, Mary became obsessed with exercise. She jogged 10 miles each day and placed highly in several marathons. She finally cut back on her jogging when bone spurs and an old back injury flared up. She developed a new routine involving less running but added a 10-mile bicycle ride, followed by a 45-minute swim. Mary was so busy with her exercise routine that she had little time for friends and lost interest in dating. Nonetheless, she lived independently, maintained a full-time job, and attended school part time, eventually obtaining a bachelor's degree in nursing.

When Mary was 25, her mother talked her into seeing a physician for evaluation of her thinness, but the physician was not familiar with eating disorders and explained that Mary's thinness and abnormal eating behaviors were a harmless idiosyncrasy. Mary later sought help from a counselor for relationship problems but never sought help for her eating disorder.

Nine years later, Mary continued to engage in occasional bingeing and purging but maintained a normal weight. She continued to work full time, had married, and had two healthy children.

Etiology and Pathophysiology

The cause of eating disorders is unknown but, like other psychiatric illnesses, probably involves a combination of biological vulnerability, psychological predisposition, and societal influences. Genetic factors seem important in anorexia nervosa, which has a concordance rate of nearly 70% for identical twins and only about 20% for nonidentical twins. Several studies have shown an increased frequency of bulimia nervosa among the relatives of bulimic persons.

Another important biological factor may be a disturbance in the central nervous serotonergic system. In the hypothalamus, the neurotransmitter serotonin helps to modulate feeding behavior by producing feelings of fullness and satiety. Patients with anorexia frequently complain of being very full after eating. Another effect of the central nervous serotonin pathways involves regulation of mood, impulses, and obsessionality. Patients with anorexia nervosa are often rigid, inhibited, and perfectionistic. One study showing high levels of central nervous system 5-hydroxyindoleacetic acid (5-HIAA)—a metabolite of serotonin—in recovered anorectic patients suggested that an overactive serotonin system could contribute to behavioral restraint, obsessionality, and an inhibited appetite.

Once dieting begins, psychological and physiological changes occur that perpetuate abnormal eating behavior. Anorexia nervosa often serves a positive function in the person's life by providing a refuge from upsetting life events or developmental issues involving relationships and sexuality. Some clinicians believe that anorexia nervosa represents an attempt to prolong childhood and escape the responsibilities of adulthood. Patients cling to their disorder and take comfort in their success with dieting. The tension relief gained from the avoidance of food or purging behavior is strongly reinforcing.

Physiological changes that occur in anorexia nervosa also reinforce the disorder. Corticotropin-releasing hormone (CRH) secretion is enhanced in anorexia nervosa and may act to maintain abnormal eating behavior. Levels of vasopressin are high and oxytocin levels are low in the cerebrospinal fluid of underweight persons with anorexia. One hypothesis is that both hormones work together to promote distorted thinking patterns and obsessional concerns about food.

Clinical Findings

The patient with anorexia quickly develops a repertoire of behaviors in the pursuit of weight loss. Examples include extreme dieting, adoption of special diets (or vegetarianism), and refusal to eat meals with family members or in restaurants. Persons with anorexia often show an unusual interest in food that belies their fear of gaining weight. The individual may clip and collect recipes or prepare elaborate meals for friends and relatives; some persons develop an interest in nutrition. At mealtime, some patients play with the food on their plate or cut meat into tiny pieces. Despite the concern of friends and family, persons with anorexia will insist that their weight is normal and, in fact, that they are overweight. Many anorectic persons develop an intense, obsessive interest in physical exercise and develop elaborate workout routines. Abuse of laxatives, diuretics, or stimulants in an effort to enhance weight loss is relatively frequent.

Anorectic persons with bulimic behavior and persons with bulimia carry out their binge eating and purging in private. Enormous amounts of food can be consumed during a binge (e.g., an entire cake, a quart of ice cream, and a package of cookies). Although families may be unaware of the bingeing, they may observe that the family food bill is increasing or that certain foods, particularly those high in calories or carbohydrates, seem to disappear. Binge eating may initially provide tension relief for the patient, but this relief is short-lived and generally leads to feelings of guilt and disgust. The patient then induces vomiting, typically by placing her or his fingers in the throat; later, she or he may be able to vomit at will. Ipecac or other emetics are sometimes abused to facilitate vomiting. Many bulimic persons, perhaps more than 10%, steal food by shoplifting or other means.

Patients with anorexia develop profound weight loss that makes many of them appear emaciated. Along with severe weight loss, hypothermia, dependent edema, bradycardia, and hypotension may occur. Anorexic persons may complain of sensitivity to cold weather and experience near-chronic constipation. They may have hormonal abnormalities, including elevated growth hormone levels, increased plasma cortisol, and reduced gonadotropin levels. Thyroxin and thyroid-stimulating hormone may be normal, even though triiodothyronine (T_3) may be reduced. Men with anorexia nervosa generally have low levels of circulating testosterone and may show signs of clinical hypogonadism. For these reasons, many persons with anorexia tend to have delayed sexual development and show a diminished interest in sex. Amenorrhea precedes the onset of obvious weight loss in one-fifth of female patients.

Bulimic persons may develop calluses on the dorsal surface of the hands (resulting from the irritation caused by placing fingers down the throat), dental erosion, and caries. Rarely, esophageal erosion or tears occur. All are complications of frequent vomiting.

Medical complications caused by bulimic behavior include hypocalcemia or hypokalemic alkalosis (in those who engage in self-induced vomiting or who abuse laxatives and diuretics); electrolyte disturbances, resulting in weakness, lethargy, or electrocardiographic changes, such as depressed T waves; elevated serum transaminases, reflecting fatty degeneration of the liver; elevated serum cholesterol and carotenemia, reflecting malnutrition; and parotid gland enlargement and elevated serum amylase. The medical complications of the eating disorders are summarized in Table 18–3.

TABLE 18–3. Medical complications of the eating disorders

Physical manifestations	Laboratory abnormalities
Amenorrhea	Dehydration[a]
Sensitivity to cold	Hypokalemia[a]
Constipation	Hypochloremia[a]
Low blood pressure	Alkalosis
Bradycardia	Leukopenia
Hypothermia	Elevated transaminases
Lanugo hair	Elevated serum cholesterol
Hair loss	Carotenemia
Petechia	Elevated BUN[a]
Carotenemic skin	Elevated amylase levels[a]
Parotid gland enlargement[a]	
Dental erosion, caries[a]	
Pedal edema	
Dry skin	

Endocrine abnormalities
  Increased growth hormone levels
  Increased plasma cortisol and loss of
    diurnal variation
  Reduced gonadotropin levels (LH, FSH,
    impaired response to LHRH)
  Low T_3, high T_3RU impaired TRH
    responsiveness[a]
  Abnormal glucose tolerance test results
  Abnormal dexamethasone suppression
    test results[a]

Note. BUN = blood urea nitrogen; FSH = follicle-stimulating hormone; LH = luteinizing hormone; LHRH = luteinizing hormone–releasing hormone; T_3RU = triiodothyronine reuptake; TRH = thyrotropin-releasing hormone.
[a]Seen in patients who binge and purge.

Course and Outcome

The long-term course of the eating disorders ranges from full recovery to malignant weight loss and rapid death. One study of patients with anorexia showed a death rate of 11% during a 12-year follow-up, a rate significantly higher than expected. From 25% to 40% of eating disorder patients have a good outcome, meaning that they eat normally, do not binge or purge, and are emotionally well adjusted. In the remaining patients, characteristic symptoms of the illness, such as having a distorted body image or abnormal eating behaviors, persist. Poor outcome is generally associated with longer duration of illness, older age at onset, prior psychiatric hospitalizations, poor premorbid adjustment, and the presence of a comorbid personality disorder.

Diagnosis and Assessment

The diagnosis of an eating disorder is based on the patient's history and a careful mental status examination. In addition, a thorough physical examination should be part of the workup. Particular attention should be given to vital signs, weight, skin, and the cardiovascular system. The patient's weight and height should be measured, and the appropriateness of weight for height, age, and gender should be determined according to his or her expected body weight or the body mass index (see Figure 18–1). This information can help guide decisions with respect to medical and nutritional management.

Laboratory studies should be individualized based on the patient's condition to rule out alternative diagnoses. These tests should include a complete blood count, urinalysis, blood urea nitrogen, and serum electrolytes. For malnourished and severely symptomatic patients, other tests are indicated, including serum cholesterol and lipids; serum calcium, magnesium, phosphorus, and amylase; liver enzymes; and an electrocardiogram. Brain imaging with magnetic resonance or computed tomography is indicated in some patients to rule out a mass lesion. Thyroid function tests are indicated when hyperthyroidism is suspected as a cause of weight loss. Bone mineral densitometry is helpful in assessing and monitoring osteoporosis; bone-density measurements are more than two standard deviations below normal in about 50% of the females with anorexia nervosa.

Other major psychiatric illnesses must be excluded before a diagnosis of anorexia or bulimia nervosa is made. Schizophrenia is sometimes accompanied by bizarre eating habits, but they are usually related to the patient's psychosis. Major depressive disorder is frequently accompanied by poor appetite and significant weight loss, but this weight loss is not associated with a distorted body image and is unwanted. Ritualistic eating behaviors resulting in weight loss sometimes occur in patients with obsessive-compulsive disorder, but the weight loss is not accompanied by a distorted body image or fears of gaining weight.

Psychiatric comorbidity is common, and many patients with anorexia nervosa or bulimia nervosa will fulfill criteria for another psychiatric disor-

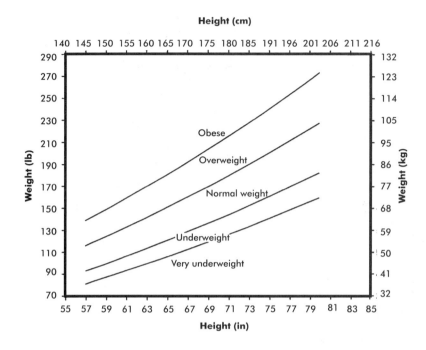

FIGURE 18–1.   Weight ranges for adults according to the body mass index (BMI). Anorexia nervosa is characterized by a BMI of 17.5 or lower.
Source.   Reprinted from Becker et al. 1999. Used with permission of the Massachusetts Medical Society.

der. Examples include major depressive disorder, anxiety disorders, or a personality disorder, such as borderline personality. Obsessive-compulsive disorder, specific phobias, and agoraphobia are the most frequent anxiety disorders diagnosed in patients with anorexia nervosa. Bulimic persons are at high risk for substance use disorders.

Medical illnesses also need to be ruled out as a cause of the eating disorder and weight loss. Conditions associated with severe weight loss include gastrointestinal disorders (e.g., a malabsorption syndrome) and endocrine disorders (e.g., hyperthyroidism). Midline tumors in the brain can be associated with anorexia and weight loss in the absence of localizing neurological abnormalities. Nevertheless, when the core features of an eating disorder are present—morbid fear of fatness and self-induced starvation, for example—a medical cause is highly unlikely.

Clinical Management

The treatment of eating disorders has three fundamental goals. The first and most important goal is to restore the patient's nutritional state. In patients with anorexia, this goal means restoring weight to within a normal range. In bulimic patients, it means ensuring that metabolic balance is achieved. The second goal is to modify the patients' distorted eating behaviors. This will help patients maintain their weight within a normal range and reverse (or lessen) binge eating, purging, and other abnormal eating behaviors. The third goal is to help change the patient's distorted and erroneous beliefs about the benefits of weight loss.

Treatment usually occurs on an outpatient basis, but many patients will need to be hospitalized. Severe starvation and weight loss, hypotension or hypothermia, and electrolyte imbalance are the main indications for hospitalization. Depressed patients with eating disorders who have suicidal ideations or psychosis also require hospitalization. Failure of outpatient treatment, as indicated by failure to gain weight, or failure to reverse severe binge-purge cycles are other reasons to hospitalize the patient. Partial hospital (or day treatment) programs are helpful to patients who need more supervision and support than can be obtained in an outpatient clinic but who do not require inpatient care. In these programs, patients attend the hospital during the day but live at home.

The psychological treatment of anorexia nervosa or bulimia nervosa generally involves behavioral modification combined with individual and group psychotherapy. The purpose of behavior therapy is to restore normal eating behavior. In the hospital, this goal is accomplished by setting goals for both eating and weight gain and by targeting certain abnormal behaviors for correction (e.g., reducing the number of vomiting episodes for bulimic patients). Positive reinforcement is used to help patients achieve the goals outlined in a treatment contract that is agreed to by the patient. For example, patients who are able to achieve their weight goals are rewarded with special privileges, such as a pass with a family member.

The patient should be weighed regularly, early in the morning after emptying the bladder and while wearing only a hospital gown. Daily fluid intake and output should be recorded. Patients should be observed for at least 2 hours after meals to prevent vomiting, even if attendants must accompany them to the bathroom. Patients are typically started on a diet providing about 500 calories more than the amount required to maintain their present weight; the caloric intake is slowly increased. At first, to prevent discomfort, it may be advisable to spread meals out over six feedings throughout the day.

Patients who are significantly underweight or are having trouble gaining weight may need tube feedings.

An electrocardiogram is essential for determining the presence of hypokalemia or palpitations. Prolongation of the Q-T interval contraindicates the use of tricyclic antidepressants and should lead to immediate medical intervention because it may increase the risk of ventricular tachycardia and sudden death. Gastric motility agents rarely relieve bloating sensations associated with refeeding, but use of stool softeners or bulk laxatives may be needed to alleviate the severe constipation associated with long-term use of stimulant laxatives or their withdrawal. The use of estrogen supplementation usually is not necessary, but patients should receive vitamins, including calcium, at a dose of 1,000–1,500 mg/day and a multivitamin to ensure that vitamin D intake is adequate (400 IU/day).

Psychotropic medication can be helpful in selected patients, particularly those with bulimic behaviors. Several classes of antidepressant medications have been shown to decrease both bingeing and purging but have no specific role in treating anorexia nervosa. The best-studied and most easily tolerated drugs are fluoxetine (60 mg/day), the only drug approved by the U.S. Food and Drug Administration for the treatment of bulimia nervosa; desipramine (up to 300 mg/day); and imipramine (up to 300 mg/day). Trazodone and phenelzine are effective but are not considered first-line agents. Bupropion is contraindicated because it can lower seizure threshold in eating disorder patients with electrolyte disturbances. Other serotonin reuptake inhibitors are routinely used but have not been studied in controlled trials. Fluoxetine and clomipramine may be useful in preventing relapse in patients with anorexia whose weight has been restored to within 80% of normal. Antidepressants often have a minimal effect in relieving depression in emaciated patients with anorexia nervosa; weight gain itself may have an antidepressant effect.

Other medications have been used to reduce the anxiety that often accompanies early refeeding effects, including the phenothiazines (e.g., chlorpromazine) and the benzodiazepines (e.g., diazepam, lorazepam). An example of how these medications can be helpful follows:

> Allan, a 25-year-old man weighing 85 pounds, presented for treatment of anorexia nervosa. A program was instituted with a primary emphasis on refeeding.
>
> Allan made slow but steady progress. When his weight exceeded 100 pounds, he began to regularly vomit. The frequency of vomiting, which occurred immediately after eating, gradually increased. Allan told us that he hated the foods given him and that they made him "gag."

Because the vomiting had no medical explanation and because it interfered with refeeding efforts, chlorpromazine (25 mg) was given before meals. Within a day, Allan stopped vomiting and appeared more relaxed at mealtime. Although he still did not enjoy his meals, he was able to keep the food down and gain needed weight.

Many patients with eating disorders will not seek treatment on their own and will deny their illness. They are sometimes brought unwillingly to a physician by their family or friends and may resist treatment; if hospitalized, they may leave against medical advice. For these reasons, the physician must use tact and skill to enlist the patient's cooperation. Once in treatment, the physician and patient should agree on a behavioral contract. The contract often becomes a focus of criticism, and the patient may make repeated requests of the physician to change it. The best approach is to refuse any modifications once the contract has been set to avoid repeated battles with patients over additional requests that are sure to follow.

Individual psychotherapy should be practical and goal oriented at first. The therapy should focus on educating the patient about the illness, helping the patient to understand his or her symptoms, and explaining the need for treatment. Later, psychodynamic approaches that aim to promote insight can be used to help the patient resolve problems and conflicts that may have contributed to (or reinforced) their abnormal eating behavior. Family therapy is often helpful, especially when the patient is living at home and the disturbed eating behavior has been prompted by family interactions or when the disturbed eating behavior has created problems within the family. Intensive programs that emphasize a behavioral approach, such as nutritional education, cognitive restructuring techniques, and psychosocial support, seem to be the most effective.

Cognitive-behavioral therapy and interpersonal psychotherapy have both been shown to be effective in patients with bulimia nervosa. Cognitive-behavioral therapy has as its goal correcting inappropriate thoughts and beliefs that bulimic patients have about themselves and their disorder. With interpersonal psychotherapy, interpersonal sources of stress thought to precede or contribute to the person's eating disorder are addressed. Both therapies help to normalize the patient's eating behavior by reducing the number of binge-purge episodes. These therapies also are effective in patients with binge-eating disorder.

Recommendations for the clinical management of eating disorders are summarized in the box.

Recommendations for management of eating disorders

1. An empathic relationship should be encouraged. This goal may be difficult to achieve because patients with anorexia can be manipulative and unmotivated. Many will lack insight and refuse treatment.

2. Reasonable targets for behavioral modification should be developed.

   - Antidepressants should be used in the patient with bingeing and purging who does not respond to behavioral measures alone.

3. Therapists should set a firm but nonpunitive behavioral contract with patients and have them sign it.

   - The goals should be set and not changed. Minor changes in the protocol will open a Pandora's box.

4. The therapist should examine the patient carefully for psychiatric comorbidity. Eating disorder patients are highly likely to have comorbid major depression, anxiety disorders, substance abuse, or a personality disorder.

   - Remember, the presence of a personality disorder complicates treatment of almost all psychiatric disorders, including eating disorders.

5. Medication is of limited value in treating anorexia nervosa.

   - Fluoxetine and clomipramine may help the patient to maintain weight once initial refeeding goals have been achieved.

6. Medication is an important treatment adjunct in patients with bulimia nervosa.

   - Serotonin reuptake inhibitors are the drugs of first choice; fluoxetine has received the most study.

   - Tricyclic antidepressants, monoamine oxidase inhibitors, and trazodone are effective but considered second-line choices because of their potential side effects.

   - Bupropion is contraindicated because of its tendency to lower seizure threshold.

7. Family therapy is especially helpful with patients who still live at home or whose behavior has created problems within the family.

Bibliography

American Psychiatric Association: Diagnostic and Statistical Manual of Mental Disorders, 4th Edition Text Revision. Washington, DC, American Psychiatric Association, 2000

American Psychiatric Association: Practice guidelines for eating disorders (revision). Am J Psychiatry 157:1–39, 2000

Becker AE, Grinspoon SK, Klibanski A, et al: Eating disorders. N Engl J Med 340:1092–1098, 1999

Crisp AH, Hsu LKG, Harding B, et al: Clinical features of anorexia nervosa: a study of 102 cases. J Psychosom Res 24:179–191, 1980

Deter HC, Herzog W: Anorexia nervosa in a long-term perspective: results of the Heidelberg-Mannheim Study. Psychosom Med 56:20–27, 1994

Dorian BT, Garfinkel PE: The contributions of epidemiologic studies to the etiology and treatment of the eating disorders. Psychiatric Annals 29:187–191, 1999

Drewnowski A, Hopkins SA, Kessler RC: Prevalence of bulimia nervosa in the U.S. college student population. Am J Public Health 78:1322–1325, 1988

Fairburn CG, Jones R, Peveler RC, et al: Psychotherapy and bulimia nervosa: long-term effects of interpersonal psychotherapy, behavior therapy, and cognitive behavior therapy. Arch Gen Psychiatry 50:419–428, 1993

Fairburn CG, Norman PA, Welch SL, et al: A prospective study of outcome in bulimia nervosa and the long-term effects of three psychological treatments. Arch Gen Psychiatry 52:304–312, 1995

Fava M, Copeland PM, Schweiger U, et al: Neurochemical abnormalities of anorexia nervosa and bulimia nervosa. Am J Psychiatry 146:963–971, 1989

Fluoxetine Bulimia Nervosa Collaborative Study Group: Fluoxetine in the treatment of bulimia nervosa: a multicenter, placebo controlled, double blind trial. Arch Gen Psychiatry 49:139–147, 1992

Holland AJ, Hall A, Murray R, et al: Anorexia nervosa study of 34 twin pairs and one set of triplets. Br J Psychiatry 145:414–419, 1984

Howard WT, Evans KK, Quintero-Howard CV, et al: Predictors of success or failure of transition to day hospital treatment for inpatients with anorexia nervosa. Am J Psychiatry 156:1697–1702, 1999

Kaye W, Strober M, Stein M, et al: New directions in treatment research of anorexia and bulimia nervosa. Biol Psychiatry 45:1285–1292, 1999

Keel PK, Mitchell JE: Outcome in bulimia nervosa. Am J Psychiatry 154:313–321, 1997

Lilienfeld LR, Kaye WH, Greeno CG, et al: A controlled family study of anorexia nervosa and bulimia nervosa: psychiatric disorders in first-degree relatives and effects of proband comorbidity. Arch Gen Psychiatry 55:603–610, 1998

Logue CM, Crowe RR, Bean JA: A family study of anorexia nervosa and bulimia. Compr Psychiatry 30:179–188, 1989

Mehler PS, Andersen AE: Eating Disorders: A Guide to Medical Care and Complication. Baltimore, MD, Johns Hopkins Press, 1999

Mitchell JE, Pyle RL, Eckert ED, et al: A comparison study of antidepressants and structured intensive group psychotherapy in the treatment of bulimia nervosa. Arch Gen Psychiatry 47:149–157, 1990

Pope HG, Keck PE, McElroy S, et al: A placebo controlled study of trazodone in bulimia nervosa. J Clin Psychopharmacol 9:254–259, 1989

Sharp CW, Freeman CPL: The medical complications of anorexia nervosa. Br J Psychiatry 162:452–463, 1993

Yates WR, Sieleni B, Reich J, et al: Comorbidity of bulimia nervosa and personality disorder. J Clin Psychiatry 50:57–59, 1989

Self-Assessment Questions

1. How do bulimia nervosa and anorexia nervosa differ? How do they overlap?
2. What are the sociodemographic characteristics of eating disorder patients?
3. What are some of the theories about the cause of anorexia nervosa?
4. What are typical clinical findings in anorexia and bulimia?
5. What potential medical complications may result form anorexia nervosa? From bulimia nervosa?
6. What are the major goals in the treatment of eating disorders?

 # Adjustment Disorders

> Whether 'tis nobler in the mind to suffer the slings and arrows of outrageous fortune or to take arms against a sea of troubles, and, by opposing, end them.
>
> William Shakespeare, *Hamlet*

Whether one is a homemaker caring for small children or a bank president, stressful situations arise nearly daily for all of us. The homemaker may need to calm a colicky child and clean up the spilled ice cream cone her other child has accidentally dropped on the new living room carpet. The bank president may have to reprimand an errant employee or handle the consequences of learning about her husband's love affair with his secretary. In these examples, both the people involved and the circumstances differ tremendously, but they illustrate the universality of stressful situations.

Most of us learn to handle everyday stressful events. Some people, however, feel overwhelmed by these situations and develop symptoms of emotional distress, such as depression, anxiety, or impaired work ability. These symptoms may be sufficiently severe to require brief periods of psychiatric care, usually on an outpatient basis. People with these problems often represent the "walking wounded"—the wife of an abusive alcoholic person, the person rejected by a lover or spouse, or the teenager failing in school.

Definition

The term *adjustment disorder* was introduced in DSM-III in 1980 to describe conditions in which a person develops psychological symptoms in response

531

to stressful events. The concept of adjustment disorders was categorized in DSM-I as *transient situational personality disorders* and in DSM-II as *transient situational disturbances.* These categories were used to diagnose disorders in persons who adjusted poorly to difficult situations or to newly experienced environmental factors in the absence of serious underlying personality defects. These disorders could be of any severity, including reactions of psychotic proportions.

Specific criteria for adjustment disorders were first enumerated in DSM-III. The maladaptive reaction had to occur within 3 months of the stressor. The diagnosis could be made in addition to another mental disorder but could not be part of a characterological pattern or an exacerbation of an existing mental disorder, such as major depression. DSM-III excluded psychotic disturbances from being categorized as adjustment disorders. In DSM-IV and DSM-IV-TR, the definition specifies that a maladaptive reaction cannot persist for more than 6 months after the termination of the stressor or its consequences (see Table 19–1).

Five subtypes of adjustment disorder are listed, so that the specific diagnosis depends on the predominant symptoms that develop in response to the stressor, such as depressed mood, anxiety, disturbance of conduct, mixed disturbance of emotions and conduct, or mixed anxiety and depressed mood. An unspecified subtype exists for reactions that do not fit into any specific categories, such as a patient responding to a new diagnosis of acquired immunodeficiency syndrome (AIDS) with denial and noncompliance with his or her treatment regimen.

Epidemiology

Adjustment disorders are undoubtedly common, but no good prevalence estimates are available. The frequency in psychiatric clinics and hospitals probably ranges from 5% to 10%. Adjustment disorders are commonly diagnosed on psychiatric consultation-liaison services at general hospitals. On these services, the frequency of the diagnosis may exceed 50% among certain groups of patients. One study of cardiac surgery patients reported a rate of 51%, whereas a study of newly hospitalized cancer patients reported a rate of 32%. Among adolescents who recently received a diagnosis of diabetes mellitus, the rate of adjustment disorders was 36%.

The diagnosis appears to be more common in women, unmarried persons, and young persons. Among adolescents, common symptoms include behavioral changes or acting out, whereas adults typically manifest mood or anxiety symptoms. Although adjustment disorders may occur at any age, the

---

TABLE 19–1. DSM-IV-TR diagnostic criteria for adjustment disorders

A. The development of emotional or behavioral symptoms in response to an identifiable stressor(s) occurring within 3 months of the onset of the stressor(s).

B. These symptoms or behaviors are clinically significant as evidenced by either of the following:

(1) marked distress that is in excess of what would be expected from exposure to the stressor

(2) significant impairment in social or occupational (academic) functioning

C. The stress-related disturbance does not meet the criteria for another specific Axis I disorder and is not merely an exacerbation of a preexisting Axis I or Axis II disorder.

D. The symptoms do not represent Bereavement.

E. Once the stressor (or its consequences) has terminated, the symptoms do not persist for more than an additional 6 months.

Specify if:

Acute: if the disturbance lasts less than 6 months

Chronic: if the disturbance lasts for 6 months or longer

Adjustment Disorders are coded based on the subtype, which is selected according to the predominant symptoms. The specific stressor(s) can be specified on Axis IV.

309.0	**With Depressed Mood**
309.24	**With Anxiety**
309.28	**With Mixed Anxiety and Depressed Mood**
309.3	**With Disturbance of Conduct**
309.4	**With Mixed Disturbance of Emotions and Conduct**
309.9	**Unspecified**

---

average age for patients is in the mid-20s.

In one study of patients with adjustment disorders who were seen on a consultation service, medical illness was the identified stressor in more than two-thirds of the patients. These patients were largely free of preexisting psychiatric illness and had endured prolonged hospitalizations for serious physical illnesses, such as cancer or diabetes. The one-third of patients in whom medical illness was not the stressor were more likely to have established psychiatric histories and recurrent problems with relationships or finances.

Etiology

According to DSM-IV-TR, adjustment disorders must occur in reaction to identifiable psychosocial stressors within 3 months of their onset. As a result of this definition, adjustment disorder is one of the few psychiatric diagnoses in which a cause-and-effect relationship is presumed. Posttraumatic stress disorder is another example. Most people are remarkably resilient and do not develop psychiatric symptoms in response to stressful situations, which suggests that individuals who develop an adjustment disorder have an underlying psychological vulnerability.

Psychodynamic explanations are sometimes used to infer why stressful situations produce illness in some persons and not others; for example, unpleasant childhood experiences could lead to fixation at certain stages of development, which later triggers a regression when sufficient stress is applied. Thus, each person has his or her own "breaking point," depending on the amount of stress applied, underlying constitution, personality structure, and temperament. To draw an analogy, if enough pressure is applied to a bone, it will fracture; however, the amount of pressure applied will differ from person to person, depending on age, gender, and physical well-being. To carry the analogy a bit further, adjustment disorders can occur in psychiatrically "normal" people, just as healthy bones will break if subjected to sufficient stress. At the other end of the continuum, people with fragile personalities, like bones with osteoporosis, will "break" more readily.

Clinical Findings

Different subtypes of adjustment disorder reflect the varied symptoms that can occur. These include depressed mood, manifested by dysphoria, tearfulness, and hopelessness; anxiety, manifested by psychic anxiety, palpitations, jitteriness, or hyperventilation; disturbance of conduct, in which the rights of others are violated or age-appropriate societal norms and rules are disregarded, such as vandalism, reckless driving, or fighting; and mixed disturbance of emotions and conduct, manifested by emotional symptoms such as depression or anxiety, in addition to a disturbance of conduct such as truancy or vandalism. Other examples not listed in DSM-IV-TR include work disturbance (or academic inhibition), manifested by difficulty functioning at work (or in school), and withdrawal, manifested by socially withdrawn behavior that is not typical for the person.

Table 19–2 presents the frequency of psychosocial stressors thought to have provoked adjustment disorders in a study of adults and adolescents. Few of the listed stressors can be considered overwhelming, and, in many cases, the stressors were multiple, recurrent, or continuous. Among adolescents, school problems were the most common stressor. Parental rejection, alcohol and/or drug problems, and parental separation or divorce also were quite common. Among adults, the most common stressors were marital problems, separation or divorce, moving, and financial problems. Many of the stressors were chronic. For example, among the adolescents, nearly 60% of the stressors had been present for a year or more, and only 9% had been present for 3 months or less. Among adults, stressors showed more variation, but 36% had been present for a year or more, and nearly 40% had been present for 3 months or less.

TABLE 19–2. Precipitants occurring in adolescents and adults with adjustment disorders

Adolescents		Adults	
Stressor	%	Stressor	%
School problems	60	Marital problems	25
Parental rejection	27	Separation or divorce	23
Alcohol and/or drug problems	26	Move	17
Parental separation or divorce	25	Financial problems	14
Girlfriend or boyfriend problems	20	School problems	14
Marital problems in parents	18	Work problems	9
Move	16	Alcohol and/or drug problems	8
Legal problems	12	Illness	6
Work problems	8	Legal problems	6
Other	60	Other	81

Source. Adapted from Andreasen and Wasek 1980.

A relatively typical patient seen at our hospital who developed an adjustment disorder with depressed mood is described below:

> Carol, a 34-year-old housewife, was admitted to the hospital after a tricyclic antidepressant overdose. Carol had felt well until earlier that day, when she learned that she had lost custody of her 13-year-old daughter to her ex-husband. She became upset, anxious, sad, and tearful. That evening, feeling desperate, Carol gulped a handful of nortriptyline tablets that she had in her medicine chest (prescribed months earlier for migraine) because she felt life was no longer worth living. When her husband returned home from work, Carol told him what she had done. He called for an ambulance, and Carol was taken to the hospital emergency room, where she underwent charcoal lavage. Carol had had no prior psychiatric treatment.
>   When Carol's condition had stabilized, and she had calmed sufficiently, she explained that her current husband had been accused of sexually molesting her daughter, an allegation that had been reported to local social service agencies. This led to her daughter's placement in foster care. Al-

though the patient denied that her husband had ever touched her daughter inappropriately, she conceded that such an allegation was serious and would be taken into account by a judge in determining custody. After thinking through her situation, Carol reported that she was no longer depressed or suicidal and that she was now in an appropriate frame of mind to work with her lawyer in an attempt to regain custody of her child.

Course and Outcome

Adjustment disorders are generally transient, lasting days or weeks, although some are more chronic (e.g., a woman with an alcoholic husband). By definition, however, adjustment disorders can persist no longer than 6 months after termination of the stressor (or its consequences). When a disturbance lasts longer, it will presumably meet criteria for another disorder, such as generalized anxiety disorder, major depression, or dysthymia.

Research suggests that the diagnosis of adjustment disorder in adults has a relatively good outcome. In a 5-year follow-up of 100 adults with this diagnosis, 79% were well at follow-up, with 8% having an intervening problem. In a more recent study, adults with adjustment disorder had shorter hospital stays and fewer readmissions during a 2-year follow-up than comparison subjects with other psychiatric diagnoses. These data suggest that, at least in adults, the diagnosis identifies persons with acute-onset disorders who recover quickly and do not have underlying psychopathology that causes chronic maladjustment.

The data are somewhat mixed for adolescents who receive the diagnosis. In the 5-year follow-up referred to in the previous paragraph, 57% of the adolescents with an adjustment disorder were well at follow-up, but 43% had a current mental disorder, including schizophrenia, major depression, alcohol or drug abuse, and antisocial personality disorder. In the more recent study also cited above, adolescents were likely to be suicidal at admission but had readmission rates similar to those of comparison subjects. These findings suggest that the diagnosis may be less useful in adolescents because they tend to have more varied outcomes. Some clinicians consider the diagnosis of adjustment disorder particularly useful for younger patients because it is relatively nonpejorative. They believe the diagnosis avoids stereotyping patients with a harsher, more severe diagnosis that may lead to self-fulfilling prophecies.

Diagnosis and Differential Diagnosis

In making the diagnosis of adjustment disorder, the crucial question is "What is the patient having trouble adjusting to?" Without a stressor to cause maladjustment, no adjustment disorder is present. Yet, even when a stressor exists, other major mental disorders must be ruled out as causing the symptoms, and the stressor cannot represent bereavement. Thus, a person who experiences an important stressor (e.g., recent marital separation) and develops depression is given a diagnosis of adjustment disorder when their symptoms fail to meet criteria for major depression. Other Axis I disorders take precedence over a diagnosis of adjustment disorder.

The differential diagnosis reflects the broad range of symptoms seen in adjustment disorders. The differential diagnosis includes mood disorders (such as major depression), anxiety disorders (such as panic disorder or generalized anxiety disorder), or conduct disorders in the child or adolescent. Personality disorders should be considered because they are frequently associated with mood instability and behavior problems. Patients with personality disorders typically react to stressful situations in maladaptive ways, so an additional diagnosis of adjustment disorder usually is unnecessary, unless the new reaction differs from their usual maladaptive pattern. Psychotic disorders are often preceded by the development of social withdrawal, work or academic inhibition, or dysphoria and need to be differentiated from adjustment disorders. Other psychiatric disorders that are believed to occur in reaction to a stressor also must be considered, including brief psychotic disorder, in which a person develops psychotic symptoms in response to a stressor, and posttraumatic stress disorder, which develops after a traumatic event that involves actual or threatened death or serious injury (e.g., wartime experiences).

As with the assessment of any mental disorder, the patient being evaluated for an adjustment disorder should undergo a thorough physical examination and mental status examination to rule out alternative diagnoses.

Clinical Management

The management of adjustment disorders has not been systematically evaluated, but psychotherapy is probably the most widely used intervention. Individual psychotherapy may give the patient an opportunity to review the meaning and significance of the psychosocial stressor that led to the disturbance. The therapist can help the patient to adapt to the stressor when it is ongoing or to better understand the stressor once it has passed. Group psychotherapy can provide a supportive atmosphere for persons who have experienced similar stressors, such as patients who have received a diagnosis of AIDS.

Medications also may be beneficial and should be prescribed based on the patient's predominant symptoms. For example, a patient with depressed mood who has initial insomnia may benefit from a hypnotic (e.g., zolpidem, 5–10 mg) at bedtime for a few days. A patient experiencing anxiety may benefit from a brief course (e.g., days to weeks) of a benzodiazepine tranquilizer (e.g., lorazepam, 0.5–2.0 mg twice daily). If the disorder persists, it may be worthwhile to reconsider the diagnosis. At some point, an adjustment disorder with depressed mood, for example, may develop into a major depressive disorder, which would respond best to antidepressant medication.

Recommendations for the clinical management of adjustment disorders are summarized in the box.

Recommendations for management of adjustment disorders

1. The key question is "What is the patient having trouble adjusting to?" When there is no stressor, there is no adjustment disorder.

2. Adjustment disorders frequently evolve into other, better-defined disorders, such as major depression.
   - Be alert to changes in mental status and to symptoms.

3. Most adjustment disorders are transient. Tincture of time and supportive psychotherapy are usually all that is necessary.

4. Patients with common psychosocial stressors (e.g., diagnosis of cancer or AIDS, chronic back pain, breakup of a relationship) often benefit from attending support groups with others who have experienced the same stressor.

5. Psychotropic medication should be targeted to the predominant symptoms:
   - Hypnotics (e.g., zolpidem, 5–10 mg at bedtime) for those with insomnia.
   - Benzodiazepines (e.g., lorazepam, 0.5–2.0 mg twice daily) for those with anxiety.

6. If long-term therapy is needed, the patient may have another disorder (e.g., major depression, generalized anxiety disorder), which will need to be diagnosed and treated.

Bibliography

American Psychiatric Association: Diagnostic and Statistical Manual of Mental Disorders. Washington, DC, American Psychiatric Association, 1952

American Psychiatric Association: Diagnostic and Statistical Manual of Mental Disorders, 2nd Edition. Washington, DC, American Psychiatric Association, 1968

American Psychiatric Association: Diagnostic and Statistical Manual of Mental Disorders, 3rd Edition. Washington, DC, American Psychiatric Association, 1980

American Psychiatric Association: Diagnostic and Statistical Manual of Mental Disorders, 4th Edition. Washington, DC, American Psychiatric Association, 1994

American Psychiatric Association: Diagnostic and Statistical Manual of Mental Disorders, 4th Edition Revised. Washington, DC, American Psychiatric Association, 2000

Andreasen NC, Hoenk PR: The predictive value of adjustment disorders: a follow-up study. Am J Psychiatry 139:584–590, 1982

Andreasen NC, Wasek P: Adjustment disorders in adolescents and adults. Arch Gen Psychiatry 37:1166–1170, 1980

Derogatis LR, Morrow GR, Fetting J, et al: The prevalence of psychiatric disorders among cancer patients. JAMA 249:751–757, 1983

Despland JN, Monod L, Ferrero F: Clinical relevance of adjustment disorder in DSM-III-R and DSM-IV. Compr Psychiatry 36:454–460, 1995

Fabrega H, Mezzich JE, Mezzich AC: Adjustment disorder as a marginal or transitional illness category in DSM-III. Arch Gen Psychiatry 44:567–572, 1987

Greenberg WM, Rosenfeld DN, Ortega EA: Adjustment disorder as an admission diagnosis. Am J Psychiatry 152:459–461, 1995

Kovacs M, Ho V, Pollock MH: Criterion and predictive validity of the diagnosis of adjustment disorder: a prospective study of youths with new-onset insulin dependent diabetes mellitus. Am J Psychiatry 152:523–528, 1995

Looney JG, Gunderson EKE: Transient situational disturbances: course and outcome. Am J Psychiatry 135:660–663, 1978

Oxman TE, Barrett JE, Freeman DH, et al: Frequency and correlates of adjustment disorder related to cardiac surgery in older patients. Psychosomatics 35:557–568, 1994

Popkin MK, Callies AL, Colon EA, et al: Adjustment disorders in medically ill inpatients referred for consultations in a university hospital. Psychosomatics 31:410–414, 1990

Strain JJ, Smith GC, Hammer JS, et al: Adjustment disorder: a multisite study of its utilization and intervention in the consult-action-liaison psychiatry setting. Gen Hosp Psychiatry 20:139–149, 1998

Self-Assessment Questions

1. What is the evolution of the adjustment disorder diagnosis from DSM-I to DSM-IV and DSM-IV-TR?

2. How common are adjustment disorders, and what are their typical precipitants and manifestations?

3. What is the differential diagnosis for adjustment disorders?

4. How do the precipitants differ between adolescents and adults?

5. How are adjustment disorders managed clinically?

 # Impulse-Control Disorders

The king, sir, hath laid, that in a dozen passes between you and him, he shall not exceed you three hits; he laid on twelve for nine.

William Shakespeare, *Hamlet*

F ive types of impulse-control disorders are listed in DSM-IV-TR: intermittent explosive disorder, kleptomania, pyromania, pathological gambling, and trichotillomania. Another category exists for impulse-control disorders that do not meet criteria for a more specific disorder, such as compulsive spending or buying (see Table 20–1 for a list of these disorders).

Disorders of impulse control are frequently underdiagnosed and underappreciated. In fact, some are quite common, such as pathological gambling, and all can lead to considerable emotional distress and to social or occupational impairment. All are characterized by the presence of irresistible urges or impulses to carry out potentially harmful or self-destructive behaviors.

Intermittent Explosive Disorder

Intermittent explosive disorder is diagnosed when a person has several discrete episodes of losing control over his or her aggressive impulses that are out of proportion to any stressor; these episodes may involve assaultive acts or destruction of property. The diagnosis is used in persons in whom the loss

TABLE 20–1.   Impulse-control disorders

Disorder	Uncontrolled behavior
Intermittent explosive disorder	Aggression
Kleptomania	Stealing
Pyromania	Fire setting
Pathological gambling	Gambling
Trichotillomania	Hairpulling
Impulse-control disorder not otherwise specified	
Compulsive buying	Shopping

of control is out of character and not merely part of a pattern of overreacting to life's problems. Therefore, psychiatric conditions in which assaultive behaviors occur as a matter of course need to be ruled out, such as antisocial or borderline personality disorders, psychotic disorders, mania, or alcohol or drug intoxication. A sudden behavioral change accompanied by outbursts in an otherwise healthy person suggests a brain disorder, which needs to be ruled out; these conditions are discussed in Chapter 6.

Intermittent explosive disorder was first recognized in DSM-III in 1980 but has received little study. Patients who receive the diagnosis are largely young men with relatively low frustration tolerance. "Pure" cases of intermittent explosive disorder—which occur in the absence of any indication of a brain disorder, such as abnormal electroencephalogram findings, neurological soft signs, or the presence of abnormal personality traits—are rare.

There is little consensus on the proper management of intermittent explosive disorder because treatments have not been well studied. Individual psychotherapy may be helpful in teaching patients how to recognize when they are becoming angry and in identifying typical stressors that lead to aggressive outbursts. At that point, patients can be taught alternative ways to grapple with the stimuli that would otherwise trigger rages, which can then be defused.

Medication to reduce or eliminate aggressive impulses may be helpful in selected cases. Lithium carbonate, valproate, carbamazepine, and propranolol all have been tried with some success. Benzodiazepines may be helpful in treating the unbearable tension that some patients describe as leading to outbursts, although they may cause behavioral disinhibition as well.

Kleptomania

Kleptomania involves the recurrent failure to resist impulses to steal objects not needed for personal use or for their monetary value; an increasing sense of tension immediately before committing the theft; and pleasure, gratification, or relief at the time of the theft. The stealing is not committed to express anger or vengeance, is not in response to hallucinations or delusions, and is not better accounted for by antisocial personality disorder, conduct disorder, or a manic episode.

The prevalence of kleptomania has been estimated at 6 per 1,000, which may be an underestimate because most persons with this disorder are ashamed of their behavior and probably do not report it to physicians. The disorder probably begins in adolescence or early adulthood and tends to be chronic; nearly three-quarters of the individuals with kleptomania are women. One of us (D.W.B.) is currently following up with an 82-year-old woman with a history of impulsive stealing since age 16. Only the humiliation of an arrest at age 78, and the resultant publicity, has kept her from stealing again, despite her nearly continuous urges and temptations.

Mood disorders frequently co-occur with kleptomania. Stealing impulses and behaviors often change in frequency or intensity consistent with the patient's mood alteration. Anxiety disorders, including obsessive-compulsive disorder, panic disorder, and social phobia, also are common, as are substance use and eating disorders.

Antidepressant medication has been used to reduce stealing behavior. In a case series of 20 patients with kleptomania, 10 of the 18 patients receiving various antidepressants and/or mood stabilizers improved after several weeks of treatment with dosages typical of those used to treat mood disorders. In 2 of the patients, stealing behavior resumed when the medication was discontinued. Serotonin reuptake inhibitors are probably the most commonly used antidepressants in this disorder.

Various forms of behavioral treatment for kleptomania, including aversive therapy and covert sensitization, have been used. In covert sensitization, patients are instructed to pair images of nausea and vomiting with the urge to steal. Psychodynamic psychotherapy also has been used, in which kleptomania is conceptualized as a symptom of an underlying emotional conflict.

Many persons with kleptomania are arrested for shoplifting and are handled through the courts, and the embarrassment and shame they experience may keep some from acting on their urges, such as the 82-year-old woman described earlier. Furthermore, probation may help by providing a regular reminder of what might occur if the person is caught stealing. Perhaps the most common treatment method is the self-imposed banning of all shopping in an attempt to head off potential thefts.

Pyromania

Pyromania as defined in DSM-IV-TR is relatively uncommon. The disorder is characterized by deliberate and purposeful fire setting on more than one occasion; tension or affective arousal before the act; fascination with, interest in, curiosity about, or attraction to fire and its contents and characteristics; and pleasure, gratification, or relief when setting fires or when witnessing or participating in their aftermath. Based on this definition, the arsonist who sets fires for monetary gain or for political or criminal purposes does not qualify for the diagnosis. Persons with antisocial personality disorder, conduct disorder, or mania sometimes set fires but generally do not have the sense of fascination with fire or experience the associated tension and relief with fire setting. Deliberate fire setting is probably motivated most frequently by anger or revenge.

Fire setting is more common among psychiatrically ill boys from large families of low socioeconomic status. These patients usually have a history of serious delinquent behavior. Fire setting is considered a poor prognostic sign for children with conduct disorders and is highly correlated with adult aggression.

Treatment of pyromania begins with the identification of other psychiatric disorders that, when present, can be treated (e.g., attention-deficit/hyperactivity disorder). Treatment of the coexisting disorder may itself reduce fire-setting behavior. Next, the parents need to be taught consistent but nonpunitive methods of discipline. Family therapy may help in dealing with the broader issue of family dysfunction often found in patients with pyromania. The patient needs to understand the dangerousness and significance of the fire setting. A visit to a burn unit or scene of a fire may help to make patients particularly aware of the consequences of their behavior. Patients also need to learn alternative ways of coping with the stressful situations to decrease reliance on fire setting as an outlet.

Pathological Gambling

Pathological gambling is characterized by a continuous or periodic loss of control over gambling. The diagnostic criteria are patterned after those used for substance dependencies because many superficial similarities exist (e.g., preoccupation with gambling, repeated efforts to stop gambling). For this reason, many persons consider gambling an *addiction*. The disorder is easily diagnosed, particularly in advanced cases, despite the patient's denial, which is also typical of the substance abuser.

Pathological gambling affects about 2% of the general population. The prevalence is lower in locations with limited gambling opportunities. About one-third of gamblers are women, who generally start gambling later in life than men do. In men, the disorder typically begins in adolescence, and a few people become "hooked" almost from their first bet. More men who present for help will have had the problem for decades, whereas women usually have been ill for only a few years. Others may have a more insidious onset following years of social gambling. Pathological gambling is associated with significant psychiatric comorbidity, particularly mood and substance use disorders.

Although many different treatments have been described, few have been carefully studied. For many, the treatment of pathological gambling will involve total abstinence. Referral to Gamblers Anonymous, a 12-step program similar to Alcoholics Anonymous, may be helpful, although 75%–90% of attendees drop out in the first year, and reported success rates at 1- and 2-year follow-up are low (8% and 7%, respectively). Inpatient treatment and rehabilitation programs similar to those for substance use disorders may be helpful for some patients.

Other patients will benefit from individual psychotherapy geared toward helping them understand why they gamble and assisting them in dealing with feelings of hopelessness, depression, and guilt. Cognitive restructuring techniques can be used to address the irrational perceptions associated with pathological gambling ("I'll win big with the next bet"). Relapse prevention needs to focus on knowledge of specific triggers that lead to gambling and teaching patients how to deal more appropriately with these triggers. Family therapy is often crucial and offers the gambler an opportunity to make amends, to learn better communication skills, and to repair the rifts that gambling inevitably creates in families.

Little research has been done on the use of medication to treat pathological gambling. In an early report, three gamblers were reported to improve with lithium carbonate. More recently, both an open-label trial and a randomized controlled trial showed that patients improved with fluvoxamine, a serotonin reuptake inhibitor.

Trichotillomania

Trichotillomania is characterized by recurrent pulling out of one's hair that results in noticeable hair loss. This is usually associated with an increasing sense of tension before pulling out the hair and pleasure, gratification, or relief when pulling out the hair. Persons with trichotillomania usually report substantial subjective distress or develop other evidence of impairment.

The disorder is generally chronic, although it tends to wax and wane in symptom severity. It can affect any site where hair grows, including the scalp, eyelids, eyebrows, body, and axillary and pubic regions. In clinic samples, 70%–90% of hairpullers are female, and most report a childhood onset. Surveys show that it affects up to 1% of adolescents and college students. Compulsive hairpullers frequently have comorbid mood and anxiety disorders, other impulse-control disorders, or personality disorders. In one study, 41% of 22 subjects had a lifetime history of a mood disorder, 55% had an anxiety disorder, and 18% had a substance use disorder. More than 50% met criteria for a personality disorder, mainly from the "anxious" cluster.

The diagnosis is easily made once alternative diagnoses and medical conditions have been ruled out. Most patients have no obvious balding, but they may have small, easily disguised bald spots or patches or missing eyebrows and eyelashes. A typical patient seen in our clinic is described below:

> Shirley, a 42-year-old married homemaker, presented for evaluation of compulsive hairpulling. She had recently learned of a new medication (clomipramine) that might be helpful and wanted to try it.
>
> Shirley grew up in a small midwestern farming community. Her childhood was relatively happy, and her family life was harmonious. As a young girl, she began to twist and twirl her hair and later, before age 10, began to pull out scalp, eyebrow, and eyelash hair.
>
> The amount of hairpulling had fluctuated over the years, but she had never been free of it. The pulling was sometimes automatic, such as when she was reading or watching television, but at other times, it was more deliberate. Shirley reported that she had tried to stop pulling her hair, but her many attempts had failed.
>
> During her interview, Shirley mentioned that she was wearing a wig. She removed it, revealing an essentially bald scalp except for a fringe around the top. She had no eyebrows or eyelashes, which she disguised with makeup and eyeglasses. She admitted to feeling embarrassed and ashamed by her problem and tearfully remembered how classmates had made fun or her as a child. Over the years, she received many medical and dermatological evaluations. Ointments and solutions had been prescribed, all without benefit.
>
> She was given clomipramine up to 150 mg/day, which appeared to reduce her urge to pull, but it was not helpful cosmetically. A trial of fluoxetine was unhelpful, and she declined referral for behavior therapy. Supportive psychotherapy helped her to accept her disorder and to develop improved self-esteem.

Treatment generally involves both behavior therapy and medication. Nevertheless, a recent survey of 123 hairpullers found that most had never been treated; of those who sought treatment, most reported minimal benefit. With behavior therapy, patients are taught to identify when their hairpulling occurs (it is often automatic) and to substitute other, more benign behaviors (e.g., squeezing a ball). These techniques are often referred to as *habit reversal*. Some patients also will benefit from learning to apply barriers to prevent hairpulling, such as wearing gloves or a hat. In a controlled trial of habit reversal compared with negative practice (in which a patient is taught to go through the motions of hair pulling but to stop short of pulling it), 74% of patients receiving habit reversal reported no hairpulling at 4 months, and 75% of those contacted at 22 months reported no hair pulling. Comparable figures for subjects receiving negative practice were 33% and 25%, respectively.

Medication has been helpful in some patients. In an early study, clomipramine was more effective than desipramine in reducing hair-pulling behavior. Experience with serotonin reuptake inhibitors to treat trichotillomania has been mixed. For example, open, but not controlled, trials of fluoxetine in patients with trichotillomania have shown benefit. Some patients will benefit from cognitive-behavioral psychotherapy that aims at upgrading their often low self-esteem, addressing relationship and family issues, and helping to correct faulty cognitions (e.g., "No one likes me because my eyebrows are missing"). Topical steroids may be helpful to patients who describe localized itching that prompts hairpulling. Hypnosis also has been used and is reported to benefit some persons.

Other Disorders

Compulsive buying or shopping is another disorder of impulse control, but it is not specifically listed in DSM-IV-TR. The disorder was originally described by Kraepelin, a German psychiatrist best known for his work with schizophrenia and manic-depressive illness. Compulsive buying is characterized by an irresistible urge to buy items that are either unneeded or unwanted. Like trichotillomania, the person usually has a feeling of tension before buying, followed by a sense of gratification or relief with buying. A feeling of guilt or remorse may follow. Persons with compulsive shopping feel unable to control their behavior, which can lead to accumulating considerable debt, personal bankruptcy, and marital and family strife.

The disorder is chronic and typically has an onset in the late teens or early 20s, corresponding to the age when most persons become emancipated

Recommendations for management of impulse-control disorders

1. Intermittent explosive disorder may respond to one of the mood stabilizers (e.g., lithium, carbamazepine, valproate) or propranolol.

   • Patients must know that they are responsible for the consequences of their behavior.

   • Individual psychotherapy may be useful in identifying stressors that trigger outbursts, which patients should be taught to defuse.

2. Persons with kleptomania may benefit from serotonin reuptake inhibitors (e.g., fluoxetine, paroxetine).

   • A self-imposed shopping ban may be the best strategy to forestall stealing.

3. Pathological gambling may respond to serotonin reuptake inhibitors (e.g., fluvoxamine, 200–300 mg/day).

   • Persons with pathological gambling may benefit from cognitive-behavioral therapy to help counter the distorted thinking that often develops ("I'll win the next time!").

   • Patients should be referred to a local Gamblers Anonymous chapter.

   • Because pathological gambling can affect the individual's marriage and family life, marriage and/or family therapy may be important.

4. Trichotillomania probably responds best to combined treatment strategies.

   • Serotonin reuptake inhibitors may reduce the urge to pull (e.g., clomipramine, 150–250 mg/day).

   • Behavior therapy using habit reversal techniques may be helpful.

   • Topical steroids to reduce itching may help those with localized itching (e.g., 2% fluocinolone solution).

   • For patients with extensive hair loss, wigs and other forms of hair replacement may be the most sensible solution to restore self-esteem and boost morale.

5. Patients with compulsive buying or spending may benefit from serotonin reuptake inhibitors but also need to be counseled to give up credit cards and other means to gain easy credit access.

   • Patients should be encouraged to find other meaningful ways to spend their time.

   • Consumer credit counseling may be beneficial.

from their families and obtain credit cards. Most compulsive buyers are young women who spend excessive amounts on clothing, shoes, and make-up. Many have co-occurring psychiatric disorders, including depression, anxiety disorders, substance abuse, or eating disorders. Many have other impulse-control disorders as well, such as pathological gambling.

Treatment of this condition has not been established, although individual psychotherapy may be helpful in exploring the significance of the compulsive buying and in helping the patient to recognize and learn how to avoid situations that lead to shopping episodes. Case reports suggest that serotonin reuptake inhibitors may be helpful in reducing the behavior, although two small, controlled trials with fluvoxamine showed no difference from placebo. Family and marital therapy may be helpful in patients whose marriages or family life has been disrupted by this disorder.

Compulsive sexual behavior ("sex addiction") has achieved notoriety, and although it has no formal definition, most experts feel that this disorder is characterized by uncontrolled sexual behavior that causes impairment in social or occupational functioning. Common manifestations include multiple partners (i.e., the Don Juan syndrome), compulsive masturbation, preoccupation with pornography, unsafe sexual encounters, and telephone or internet sex (e.g., "900" numbers). Most persons with compulsive sexual behavior are male and many meet criteria for specific paraphilias (see Chapter 17).

Management of Impulse Control Disorders

Recommendations for the clinical management of impulse control disorders are summarized in the box.

Bibliography

American Psychiatric Association: Diagnostic and Statistical Manual of Mental Disorders, 4th Edition. Washington, DC, American Psychiatric Association, 1994

American Psychiatric Association: Diagnostic and Statistical Manual of Mental Disorders, 4th Edition Text Revision. Washington, DC, American Psychiatric Association, 2000

Black DW: Compulsive disorder: definition, assessment, epidemiology, and clinical management. CNS Drugs 15:17–27, 2001

Black DW, Kehrberg LLD, Flumerfelt DL, et al: Characteristics of 36 subjects reporting compulsive sexual behavior. Am J Psychiatry 154:243–247, 1997

Black DW, Gabel J, Hansen J, et al: A double-blind comparison of fluvoxamine versus placebo in the treatment of compulsive buying disorder. Ann Clin Psychiatry 12:205–211, 2000

Christenson GA, Mackenzie TB, Mitchell JE: Characteristics of 60 adult chronic hair-pullers. Am J Psychiatry 148:365–370, 1991

Goldman MJ: Kleptomania: making sense of the nonsensical. Am J Psychiatry 148:986–996, 1991

Hollander E, DeCaria C, Finkell JN, et al: A randomized double-blind fluvoxamine/placebo crossover trial in pathological gambling. Biol Psychiatry 47:813–817, 2000

Keuthen NJ, O'Sullivan RL, Goodchild P, et al: Retrospective review of treatment outcome for 63 patients with trichotillomania. Am J Psychiatry 155:560–561, 1998

Lion JR: The intermittent explosive disorder. Psychiatric Annals 22:64–66, 1992

McElroy SC, Pope HG, Hudson JI, et al: Kleptomania: a report of 20 cases. Am J Psychiatry 148:652–657, 1991

Petry NM, Armentano C: Prevalence, assessment, and treatment of pathological gambling: a review. Psychiatr Serv 50:1021–1027, 1999

Rosenthal RT: Pathological gambling. Psychiatric Annals 22:72–78, 1992

Roy A, Adinoff B, Roehrich L, et al: Pathological gambling: a psychobiological study. Arch Gen Psychiatry 45:369–373, 1988

Schlosser S, Black DW, Blum N, et al: The demography, phenomenology and family history of 22 persons with compulsive hairpulling. Ann Clin Psychiatry 6:147–152, 1994

Soltys SM: Pyromania and firesetting behavior. Psychiatric Annals 22:79–83, 1992

Self-Assessment Questions

1. What are the five listed impulse-control disorders?
2. Define intermittent explosive disorder. Which disorders exclude a diagnosis of intermittent explosive disorder?
3. How does the kleptomaniac differ from the ordinary shoplifter?
4. What kinds of problems do pathological gamblers develop?
5. What is trichotillomania, and how is it treated?
6. Describe compulsive buying disorder.

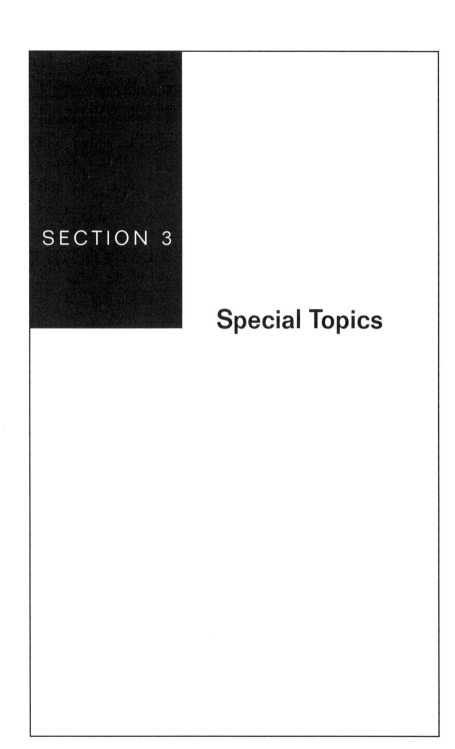

SECTION 3

Special Topics

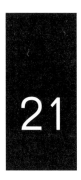

21 Suicide and Violent Behavior

> The thought of suicide is a great consolation; by means
> of it one gets successfully through many a bad night.
>
> Friedrich Nietzsche

Suicide

Suicide is a self-inflicted death that is intentional rather than accidental. It is a complex human behavior with biological, sociological, and psychological roots. It is the eighth most frequent cause of death for adults and the second leading cause of death for persons between ages 15 and 24. Nearly 30,000 suicides occur each year in the United States—about one every 18 minutes. A suicide affects not only surviving friends and family members but also the victim's physician because most people who commit suicide communicate their suicidal intentions to and see physicians before they die. For this reason, clinicians must familiarize themselves with suicide and be prepared to educate patients and family members about risk for suicide, to assess risk for suicide in their patients, and to intervene when appropriate to prevent a suicide.

The death of a presidential adviser in the early 1990s shows how suicide is widely misunderstood by the general public and the media. The adviser, a successful small-town attorney, had apparently killed himself after becoming depressed. A note revealed that he had felt hopeless about his future and responsible for the very public problems of the administration. Media reports implied that he could not tolerate the "pressure-cooker" atmosphere of our nation's capital. Clearly, job pressure may have contributed to the suicide, but little mention was made of other factors that obviously played a role, including his depressive illness and the fact that he had only recently sought treatment. The pressure of his job may have been the straw that broke the camel's back, but most people with stressful jobs do not kill themselves. The tragedy is that his depression was not recognized earlier and treated and that perhaps the stigma of mental illness prevented him from seeking help.

Epidemiology

Nearly 1% of the United States general population ultimately commit suicide, a rate of nearly 12.5 suicides per 100,000 persons. Suicide rates are specific for age, gender, and race; rates for men increase steadily with age and peak after age 75 years; rates for women are curvilinear and peak in the late 40s or early 50s. Nearly three times as many men take their lives as women, and whites are more likely than blacks to kill themselves. An alarming trend has been the rise in the suicide rate among young men and women, possibly as a result of increasing rates of drug abuse or, perhaps, the cohort effect, which is discussed later in this chapter.

About two-thirds of suicide completers are men; most tend to be older than 45, white, and separated, widowed, or divorced. Psychiatric diagnosis tends to vary with age. Suicide completers younger than 30 years are more likely to have substance abuse disorders or antisocial personality disorder; suicide completers older than 30 years tend to have mood disorders.

Suicide rates differ by geographic region as well. In the United States, rates are highest in the West and lowest in the mid-Atlantic states. In Europe, rates are highest in the former Eastern bloc countries and in Scandinavia; for example, in Hungary, the rate hovers around 40 suicides per 100,000 persons. Rates are low in Mediterranean countries, particularly those with large Catholic or Muslim populations. For reasons of religion, Catholics and Muslims are less likely than Protestants to commit suicide.

Suicide rates tend to peak during the late spring and have a smaller secondary peak in the fall. Suicides tend to be evenly distributed throughout the week, unlike homicides, which peak on Friday evening or early Saturday morning. Rates are affected by economic conditions and were very high during the Great Depression of the 1930s; they are typically low during wartime. Certain occupations are associated with a high risk for suicide. Professionals, especially physicians, are at high risk; in contrast to suicide statistics in general, female physicians are at higher risk for suicide than are male physicians. Married persons are less likely to commit suicide than are single, widowed, or divorced persons. It is not clear whether social class affects suicide rates, but some studies suggest that rates are highest in both the highest and the lowest social classes.

Etiology

Research has shown that more than 90% of suicide completers had a major psychiatric illness and that half were clinically depressed at the time of the act (see Table 21–1). Nearly one-third of suicides occur in persons with chronic alcoholism; schizophrenia, anxiety disorders, and other psychiatric disorders are less common among suicide completers. One study found drug abuse in 45% and alcoholism in 54% of the suicide completers. These findings may reflect the growing drug and alcohol abuse problem in the United States.

TABLE 21–1. Psychiatric diagnoses (in percentages) in three selected studies of suicides in the general population

| | | | Rich et al.[c] | |
Diagnosis	Robins et al.[a] (n=134)	Barraclough et al.[b] (n=100)	>30 years (n=133)	>30 years (n=150)
Depression	45	80	35	52
Alcohol abuse or dependence	23	15	54	55
Drug abuse or dependence	1	4	66	26
Schizophrenia	2	3	5	2
Dementia	4	1	—	7
Personality disorder	—	—	10	1
Other disorders	19	1	—	—
Not mentally ill	2	7	4	5

[a]Data from Robins et al. 1959.

[b]Data from Barraclough et al. 1974.

[c]Data from Rich et al. 1986.

About 5% of suicide completers have serious physical illnesses at the time of suicide. Suicide rates are reported to be high in persons who have traumatic brain injuries, epilepsy, multiple sclerosis, Huntington's disease, Parkinson's disease, cancer, and acquired immunodeficiency syndrome (AIDS). The suicide rate in patients with AIDS in the United States is nearly seven times that in the general population.

A small number of persons committing suicide appear to have no evidence of mental or physical illness. Many have argued that these suicides are rational—that is, based on a logical appraisal of the need for death. An example is an elderly widower with terminal cancer who is not clinically depressed but has no hope for the future and wishes to end his physical pain. Many of these apparently rational suicides are probably irrational, but information was simply unavailable to confirm the presence of a mental illness because the person who died was socially isolated and informants were not available for interview.

The risk for suicide is much higher among psychiatric patients than in the general population. Research shows that certain psychiatric disorders are associated with high rates of suicide; for example, nearly 15% of the persons hospitalized with mood disorders, 10% of the patients with schizophrenia, and 2%–4% of the patients with chronic alcoholism will commit suicide. A few psychiatric disorders, such as obsessive-compulsive disorder, have not been linked to increased rates of suicide. Thus, although psychiatric and/or medical illnesses usually are necessary for suicide to occur, their presence is not a sufficient explanation because most mentally ill persons do not kill themselves.

Suicide runs in families. Examination of large kindreds, such as the Old Order Amish in Pennsylvania, showed that suicide tends to cluster in certain pedigrees—pedigrees that are also filled with mood disorders. Twin studies have reported higher concordance for suicide among identical twins than nonidentical twins, suggesting that suicide may be genetic as well as familial. One large adoption study found a higher prevalence of suicide among biological relatives of probands who had killed themselves than among the relatives of control probands, providing further evidence of a hereditary contribution to suicide.

Methods of Suicide

Firearms are the most common method used to commit suicide in the United States, perhaps because firearms are readily available and are immediately lethal. Firearms are followed in frequency by poisoning (i.e., a drug overdose), hanging, cutting, jumping, and other methods. Men are more likely than women to use violent methods, such as firearms or hanging, a tendency that may explain why men are more successful in killing themselves. Women tend to use less violent means, such as poisoning by overdose. Women are beginning to choose more lethal methods, a trend that may ultimately lead to higher suicide rates.

Biology of Suicide

Low levels of cerebrospinal fluid (CSF) 5-hydroxyindoleacetic acid (5-HIAA), a serotonin metabolite, have been found in suicide completers, particularly those who died by violent means, and decreased levels of imipramine binding have been found in postmortem frontal cortex tissue samples. (Imipramine binding tends to correlate highly with plasma serotonin levels.) Follow-up studies have shown that many suicide completers had abnormal dexamethasone suppression test results, suggesting the presence of hypothalamic-pituitary-adrenal axis hyperactivity. Suicide completers also have been found to have high levels of urinary metabolites of cortisol and to have enlarged adrenal glands. All of these measures are abnormal in severe depression; therefore, they may indicate depression rather than risk for suicide.

Clinical Findings

Suicide is an act of desperation. Suicidal persons frequently convey their distress to others, and nearly two-thirds communicate their suicidal intentions to others. Their communication may be as direct as reporting their plan and the date they intend to carry it out. Other communications are less obvious; for instance, the patient may say to his relatives: "You won't have to put up with me much longer!"

Suicide can occur during all phases of a depressive episode. It is commonly believed that suicide risk is highest during the recovery phase, when a patient has regained sufficient energy to kill himself or herself. Because the suicidal urge waxes and wanes during the course of a depressive episode, the clinician should not be lulled into a false sense of security by noting the phase of a patient's illness.

Suicide completers tend to be socially isolated. Nearly 30% of suicide completers have a history of suicide attempts, and about one in six leaves a suicide note. Clinicians should be alert to behaviors that suggest suicidal intent: preparing a will, giving away possessions, or purchasing a burial plot. One of the strongest correlates of suicidal behavior is hopelessness, a finding independent of psychiatric diagnosis.

Nearly 40% of suicide completers have alcohol in their bloodstream at the time of death, suggesting that alcohol may have disinhibited them sufficiently to give them the courage to complete the act. Nearly 90% of alcoholic suicide completers have alcohol in their bloodstream at the time of death.

Patients remain at high risk for suicide after hospital discharge. Although depressed patients may appear to be significantly improved at the time of discharge, relapse can occur quickly. In a follow-up of unipolar and bipolar depressed patients, nearly 42% of 36 suicides occurred within 6 months of hospital discharge, 58% by 1 year, and 70% by 2 years. Therefore, recently discharged patients need close follow-up.

Events that appear to trigger suicide differ by age and diagnostic group. Triggering events in adolescents or young adults often include academic problems or troubled relationships with parents. In older persons, the event may be poor finances or health. More than 50% of alcoholic persons who commit suicide have a history of relationship loss (usually of a sexual partner) within the year before suicide. This is not the case among persons with major depressive disorder.

Youth Suicide

Suicide rates have been increasing in both males and females between ages 15 and 24 years. In fact, studies have shown that recent cohorts (i.e., groups of persons in the population with similar characteristics, such as being born in the same decade) have higher suicide rates than older cohorts. Why rates are increasing in younger age groups is a mystery, but other data seem to show that the prevalence of depression also is increasing in each successive cohort. Drug abuse has become a serious problem for society, especially young persons, and may be contributing to the higher rates of suicide.

Teenagers are more prone to the effects of peer pressure than are adults, and this may be reflected in suicide clusters. It has been suggested that media portrayals of suicide, such as those in television movies or documentaries, are followed by an increased rate of both suicide attempts and suicides, often by the method depicted.

Suicide Attempters Versus Suicide Completers

Suicide attempts are intentional acts of self-injury that do not result in death. They are 5–20 times as frequent as suicides, perhaps more so because most suicide attempts go unreported, and many persons who attempt suicide do not seek medical attention. Although suicide completers usually have a diagnosis of major depression or alcoholism, suicide attempters are less likely to have these disorders and frequently have other conditions, including somatization disorder and antisocial personality. More than 40% of suicide attempters are estimated to have a personality disorder.

Suicide completers carefully plan their act, use effective means (e.g., firearms, hanging), and carry out the suicide in private or make provisions to avoid discovery. They are serious about ending their lives. In contrast, suicide attempters, who are three times more likely to be women and usually younger than 35 years, act impulsively, make provisions for rescue, and use ineffective means such as drug overdoses. Suicide attempters are at risk for future attempts, and each year thereafter an estimated 1%–2% of those who have attempted suicide will complete the act—up to a total of about 10%. The differences between suicide attempters and completers are highlighted in Table 21–2.

TABLE 21–2. Differences between suicide completers and attempters

Variable	Completers	Attempters
Gender	Male	Female
Age	Older	Younger
Diagnosis	Depression, alcoholism, schizophrenia	Depression, alcoholism, personality disorder
Planning	Careful	Impulsive
Lethality	High (e.g., firearms)	Low (e.g., poisoning)
Availability of help	Low	High

Assessment of the Suicidal Patient

The assessment of suicide risk involves a thorough psychiatric history and mental status examination as well as an understanding of common risk factors. The clinician should be alert to the possibility of suicide in any psychiatric patient, especially a patient who is depressed or has a depressed affect. In these patients, the assessment will focus on vegetative signs and cognitive symptoms of depression, death wishes, suicidal ideation, and suicidal plans. Common risk factors associated with suicide are summarized in Table 21–3. Remembering these risk factors can be facilitated through the use of a simple mnemonic: SAD PERSONS. The initials stand for Sex (male gender), Age (older), Depression, Previous (suicide) attempt, Ethanol abuse, Rational thinking loss, Social support lacking, Organized plan, No spouse, Sickness.

Most suicidal patients are willing to discuss their thoughts with a physician if asked, but research shows that only one in six clinicians asks his or her patients about suicide. A common myth is that asking a patient about suicide will give the patient ideas that he or she has not already had. Yet, because suicidal thoughts are common in depression, most depressed patients will have had these thoughts. Patients are often fearful and even feel guilty about having suicidal thoughts. Giving the patient an opportunity to discuss them may itself provide relief. Specific questions that should be asked of the patient include the following:

- Are you having any thoughts that life isn't worth living?
- Are you having any thoughts about harming yourself?

TABLE 21–3. Clinical variables associated with suicide

- Being a psychiatric patient
- Being male, although the gender distinction is less important among psychiatric patients than in the general population
- Age: risk increases as men age but peaks in the middle years for women
- Race: whites are at higher risk than nonwhites
- Diagnosis: depression, alcoholism, schizophrenia
- History of suicide attempts
- Recent interpersonal loss (among alcoholic patients)
- Feelings of hopelessness and low self-esteem
- Timing: early in the post–hospital discharge period
- Adolescents: a history of drug abuse and behavior problems

- Are you having any thoughts about taking your life?
- Have you developed a plan for committing suicide? If so, what is your plan?

The physician also should assess the patient's history of suicidal behavior by asking the following questions:

- Have you ever had thoughts of killing yourself?
- Have your ever attempted suicide? If so, would you tell me about the attempt?

The physician should approach the topic of suicide in a slow and tactful manner, after having developed rapport with the patient. Because suicidal thoughts may fluctuate, physicians should reassess suicide risk at each contact with the patient. Patients who have developed well-thought-out plans and have the means to carry them out require protection, usually in a hospital on a locked psychiatric unit. When the suicidal patient refuses admission, it may be necessary to obtain a court order requiring hospitalization. Suicidal patients may plead with the doctor, family, or friends to be kept out of the hospital, but family members and friends are neither sufficiently prepared nor sufficiently educated to handle a suicidal person. Hospitalization is the only way a physician may reasonably ensure the safety of the patient.

> ## Recommendations for the management of the suicidal patient
>
> 1. Depressed patients should always be asked about suicidal thoughts and plans. The clinician will not plant ideas that were not there merely by asking.
>   - Suicidality should be reassessed at every visit with depressed patients.
> 2. Some suicidal patients should be hospitalized, even when it is against their will. Patients who do not have suicidal plans and do have supportive families who can monitor them can probably be managed at home.
> 3. In the hospital, suicide precautions should be written in the doctors' orders; one-to-one protection should be ordered if needed.
>   - Signs and symptoms must be carefully documented.
> 4. Suicidality should be frequently monitored in the outpatient, and a newer antidepressant with a high therapeutic index (e.g., fluoxetine, bupropion) should be considered.
>   - The family should remove all firearms from the home.
> 5. Even though the risk factors are known, it is not possible to predict who will commit suicide.
>   - One must simply use good clinical judgment, provide close follow-up, and prescribe effective treatments.

Managing the Suicidal Patient

In the hospital, the nursing staff will take sharp objects, belts, and other potentially lethal items from the patient. Patients at risk for elopement are carefully watched. The physician should fully document the patient's signs and symptoms of depression, along with his or her assessment of suicide risk and protective measures taken.

Once the patient's safety has been ensured, treatment of the underlying illness can begin. Treatment will depend on the diagnosis. Antidepressant medication or electroconvulsive therapy is necessary for the treatment of depression; mood stabilizers and antipsychotics are appropriate additions to the treatment of bipolar disorder and psychotic depression, respectively. Antipsychotic medications are helpful in the suicidal schizophrenic patient. Electroconvulsive therapy is often specifically recommended for the treatment of depression in the suicidal patient because it tends to have a quicker onset of action than antidepressant medication.

When the patient receives treatment as an outpatient, close follow-up is mandatory. Follow-up must include frequent physician visits (or telephone contacts) for assessment of mood and suicide risk and for psychotherapeutic support. The physician should consider prescribing antidepressants with a high therapeutic index that are unlikely to be fatal in overdose (e.g., bupropion, serotonin reuptake inhibitors). Family members can help monitor the patient's medication use. They should be instructed to remove all firearms from the home.

Recommendations for the clinical management of suicidal persons are presented in the box on page 561.

Violent Behavior

Violence is an all too common occurrence. News stories about senseless killings or assaults, drive-by shootings, and domestic disputes document these daily events. Citizens are frightened by the possibility of becoming victims of violent crime, even as crime rates have steadily dropped in the 1990s. Too often, the media have exaggerated the link between violence and mental illness, contributing to the fear felt by the public and the stigma experienced by psychiatric patients.

Although most mentally ill persons are law-abiding and nonviolent, patients with schizophrenia, mania, cognitive disorders (e.g., dementia, delirium), drug or alcohol intoxication, and mental retardation are more likely to become violent than are patients with other diagnoses or persons who are not mentally ill. Research has specifically shown that psychotic patients are more likely to commit violent acts than are nonpsychotic patients. For these reasons, and because violent behavior sometimes occurs in psychiatric hospitals and general medical wards, psychiatrists must be prepared to evaluate the risk for aggression and learn to manage violent patients.

Psychiatrists and other mental health professionals have no more skill than laypersons in predicting long-term violence. However, mental health professionals are generally in a position to predict violence in clinical settings. Certain elements of the clinical situation, including the patient's diagnosis and past behavior, can indicate the patient's potential for imminent violence, thereby allowing appropriate interventions to be made. A patient's history of violent behavior is probably the single best predictor of future dangerousness. The accuracy of predictions is improved with populations that have high base rates for violence, such as disturbed patients on a locked psychiatric inpatient unit.

Following is the case of an aggressive patient with dementia seen in our hospital:

> Donald, a 71-year-old man with advanced Alzheimer's disease, was admitted for evaluation of violent and unpredictable behavior. His wife and fam-

ily had cared for him at home during the 7-year illness. As the illness progressed, Donald became more confused and made more frequent misinterpretations of external stimuli. For example, his wife had a deep voice, which led him at times to conclude that a strange man was in the house. This was especially frightening to him and led him to threaten his wife with a knife.

Donald was observed to be disoriented and confused. He did not know the date, his location, or the situation. He required considerable assistance with his grooming and dress. At times, without apparent provocation, he would strike his nurses or would make threatening gestures, such as karate chops. This behavior was frightening because of its unpredictability.

He was given a low-potency antipsychotic (haloperidol, 2 mg/day) to reduce his paranoia and agitation. He was placed in a nursing home familiar with the care of patients with Alzheimer's disease.

Etiology

Many factors can contribute to violent behavior. One of the most common in the clinical setting is substance abuse. Alcohol is strongly associated with violence because of its well-known tendency to cause disinhibition, to decrease perceptual and cognitive alertness, and to impair judgment. Other substances of abuse, including amphetamines, cocaine, hallucinogens, phencyclidine, and sedative-hypnotics, also have been associated with violent behavior. Of course, much of the violence in society is indirectly related to drug abuse, primarily through activities involved in obtaining the drugs.

Other factors are also involved in violence. One of the strongest predictors of adult violence is childhood aggression. Childhood abuse also leads to a greater likelihood of being physically abusive as an adult. Age and maturity level are associated with violent acts in persons with conduct or personality disorders, such as antisocial personality disorder; with advancing age and maturity, persons with these disorders are less likely to act out. Persons of low socioeconomic status are more likely to be both perpetrators and victims of violence, perhaps because of the alienation, discrimination, family breakdown, and general sense of frustration that the poor experience. The presence of readily available firearms in our society has contributed to the general level of violence because they can turn what would be an assault into a murder.

At a physiological level, aggressive behavior has been correlated with low CSF 5-HIAA levels, as has suicidal behavior. Low CSF 5-HIAA may be a marker of impulsivity rather than of any specific tendency toward violence, however. Violence is sometimes blamed on partial complex seizures, although aggressive acts by patients with epilepsy are rare.

Assessing Risk for Violence

Risk assessment for violent behavior involves a review of pertinent clinical variables and requires a thorough psychiatric history and careful mental status examination. Even in routine assessments, patients should be asked

1. whether they have ever thought of harming someone else,
2. whether they have ever seriously injured another person,
3. what the most violent thing they have ever done was.

Some researchers have used a "weather forecast" model because assessment of the risk of violence, like weather forecasting, becomes progressively less accurate beyond the short term (i.e., 24–48 hours). Risk assessment, like weather forecasts, should be updated frequently. Clinical variables associated with violence are summarized in Table 21–4.

TABLE 21–4.   Clinical variables associated with violence

- A history of violent acts
- Inability to control anger
- History of impulsive behavior (e.g., recklessness)
- Paranoid ideation or frank psychosis
- Command hallucinations in psychotic patients
- The stated desire to hurt or kill another person
- Presence of an acting-out personality disorder (e.g., antisocial personality disorder, borderline personality disorder)
- Presence of a dementia, delirium, or alcohol or drug intoxication

---

A careful differential diagnosis should be made using the history, mental status examination, and, in some cases, laboratory findings, because interventions are generally based on the diagnosis. A violent schizophrenic patient will need treatment with antipsychotic medication. A violent manic patient will probably require a combination of a mood stabilizer and an antipsychotic.

When interviewing the violent or threatening patient, the clinician should remain calm and speak softly. Comments or questions should appear nonjudgmental, such as "You seem upset; maybe you can tell me why you feel that way." The interviewer should always have an easy escape route in case the patient becomes aggressive and should avoid towering over the patient. If possible, both patient and clinician should be seated, allowing personal distance between the two. Direct eye contact should be avoided, and the interviewer should try to project a sense of empathy and concern. Family members, friends, police, and others who have pertinent information on the patient should be interviewed.

Managing the Violent Patient

In the hospital or clinic setting, the violent patient presents an emergency. To ensure the safety of the patient and others, it is important that the staff be sufficient in number and well trained in seclusion and restraint techniques. Remember that seclusion or restraint is considered an emergency safety measure to prevent injury to the patient and others and is never used for punishment or as a convenience for the staff.

Once a decision has been made to restrain or to seclude the patient, a staff member, backed up by at least four other team members, should approach the patient, after first clearing the area of other patients. The patient should be told that he or she is being secluded or restrained because of uncontrolled behavior and should be asked to walk quietly to the seclusion area. If the patient does not cooperate, staff members should each take a limb in a plan agreed to beforehand. At this point, restraints should be applied; or if the patient is taken to the seclusion room, staff members should take the patient's legs and arms around the elbow with underarm support.

Once secluded, the patient should be thoroughly searched. Belts, pins, and other potentially dangerous items should be removed, and the patient should be dressed in a hospital gown. If tranquilizing medication is needed, it can be injected or taken orally if the patient is cooperative. With agitated patients, the best strategy is to combine a high-potency antipsychotic with a benzodiazepine (e.g., haloperidol, 2–5 mg; lorazepam, 1–2 mg). The dose of both agents can be repeated every 30 minutes until the patient has calmed down. One-on-one observation by nursing staff is generally mandatory for secluded or restrained patients.

Although rules differ from hospital to hospital, the clinician needs to carefully document the reasons for seclusion or restraint (e.g., harm to self or others, threatening gestures), the condition of the patient, any laboratory investigations being pursued (e.g., urine drug screen), medication being administered, type of restraint to be used, and the criteria for discontinuation of restraints.

Recommendations for the clinical management of violent persons are summarized in the box.

Recommendations for management of the violent patient

1. The patient should be approached in a slow and tactful manner.

   • The clinician should not appear threatening or provocative.

   • The clinician should use a soft voice, appear passive, and maintain interpersonal distance.

2. The clinician should ask the patient what is wrong or why he or she feels angry.

   • Most patients are willing to disclose their feelings.

3. Violent psychiatric patients need to be in the hospital, where their safety and the safety of others can be assured.

4. Orders for violence precautions and seclusion or restraint orders should be written, when applicable.

   • The risk of violence and the presence of assaultive behaviors should be monitored.

   • The clinician should carefully document the assessment and plan.

5. For outpatients, the risk of violent behaviors should be monitored at each contact; the patient (or family) should remove all firearms from the home.

6. The underlying condition should be vigorously treated.

7. Predicting violent behavior is difficult, even under the best of circumstances.

Bibliography

Barraclough B, Bunch J, Nelson B, et al: A hundred cases of suicide: clinical aspects. Br J Psychiatry 125:355–373, 1974

Beck AT, Steer RA, Kovacs M, et al: Hopelessness and eventual suicide. Am J Psychiatry 142:559–563, 1985

Black DW, Winokur G: Suicide and psychiatric diagnosis, in Suicide Over the Life Cycle. Edited by Blumenthal S, Kupfer D. Washington, DC, American Psychiatric Press, 1990, pp 135–153

Coté TR, Biggar RJ, Dannenberg AL: Rick of suicide among persons with AIDS: a national assessment. JAMA 268:2066–2068, 1992

Egeland JA, Sussex JN: Suicide and family loading for affective disorder. JAMA 254:915–918, 1985

Fawcett TJ, Scheftner W, Clark D, et al: Clinical predictors of suicide in patients with major affective disorders: a controlled prospective study. Am J Psychiatry 144:35–40, 1987

Goldstein R, Black DW, Winokur G, et al: The prediction of suicide: sensitivity, specificity, and predictive value of a multivariate model applied to suicide in 1,906 affectively ill patients. Arch Gen Psychiatry 48:418–422, 1991

Gould MS, Fisher F, Parides M, et al: Psychosocial risk factors of child and adolescent completed suicide. Arch Gen Psychiatry 53:1155–1162, 1996

Key NS, Soreff SM: Psychiatrist role responses and responsibilities when the patient commits suicide. Am J Psychiatry 148:739–743, 1991

Lidz CW, Mulvey EP, Gardner W: The accuracy of prediction of violence to others. JAMA 269:1007–1011, 1993

Mann JJ, Waternaux C, Haas GL, et al: Toward a clinical model of suicidal behavior in psychiatric patients. Am J Psychiatry 156:181–189, 1999

Marzuk PM, Leon AC, Tardiff K, et al: The effect of access to lethal methods of injury on suicide rates. Arch Gen Psychiatry 49:451–458, 1992

Miller RJ, Zadolinnyj K, Hafner RJ: Profiles and predictors of assaultiveness for different ward populations. Am J Psychiatry 150:1368–1373, 1993

Murphy GE, Wetzel RD, Robins E, et al: Multiple risk factors predict suicide in alcoholism. Arch Gen Psychiatry 49:459–463, 1992

Patterson WM, Dohn HH, Bird J, et al: Evaluation of suicidal patients: the SAD PERSONS scale. Psychosomatics 24:343–349, 1983

Phillips DP, Carstonson LL: Clustering of teenage suicides after television news stories about suicide. N Engl J Med 55:685–689, 1986

Rich CL, Young D, Fowler RC: San Diego suicide study, I: young versus old subjects. Arch Gen Psychiatry 43:577–582, 1986

Robins E, Murphy GE, Wilkinson RH, et al: Some clinical considerations in the prevention of suicide based on a study of 134 successful suicides. Am J Public Health 49:888–899, 1959

Shafii M, Steltz-Lenarsky J, Derrick AM, et al: Comorbidity of mental disorders in the post-mortem diagnoses of completed suicide in children and adolescents. J Affect Disord 15:227–233, 1988

Swartz MS, Swanson JW, Hiday VA, et al: Violence and severe mental illness: the effects of substance abuse and non-adherence to medication. Am J Psychiatry 155:226–231, 1998

Tardiff K: The Psychiatric Uses of Seclusion and Restraint. Washington, DC, American Psychiatric Press, 1984

Tardiff K, Marzuk PM, Leon AC, et al: Violence by patients admitted to a private psychiatric hospital. Am J Psychiatry 154:88–93, 1997

Winokur G, Black DW: Suicide: what can be done? N Engl J Med 327:490–491, 1992

Self-Assessment Questions

1. Why is suicide a major health problem?
2. What are the common risk factors for suicide?
3. How do completed suicides differ from attempted suicides?
4. What is a rational suicide?
5. Are there different risk factors for suicide among youth?
6. How should the suicidal patient be managed in the hospital? As an outpatient?
7. What are the risk factors for violent behavior?
8. How is the violent or potentially violent patient assessed?
9. What are the indications for seclusion and restraint? How are seclusion and restraint orders implemented?

22 Psychiatric Aspects of HIV Infection

And I looked, and behold a pale horse: and his name
that sat on him was Death, and Hell followed with him.

Revelations 6:8

One of the most fascinating—and alarming—stories in medicine during the past century has been the rise of the acquired immunodeficiency syndrome (AIDS). Although the syndrome was first identified in the early 1980s, it may have existed in the United States for up to two decades before its recognition. From the physician's perspective, a unique aspect of the epidemic is that we have been able to watch a serious new disease evolve over a short period. Because the disease is nearly always fatal and has such striking social and economic costs, AIDS has gained far more attention than other relatively new epidemics, such as genital herpes. Although the incidence (i.e., new cases) of AIDS appears to have peaked in the early 1990s, the prevalence continues to grow as the known cases accumulate. By late 1998, nearly 700,000 cases of AIDS had been reported in the United States, and more than 400,000 persons nationwide had died of AIDS. The number of persons infected with the human immunodeficiency virus (HIV) may now exceed 40 million worldwide. In the United States, AIDS is currently the number-one killer of men between ages 25 and 44 years and is straining budgets everywhere, especially because treatments are allowing these patients to live longer.

Epidemiology

In the United States, homosexual men are the largest risk group for HIV infection and constitute about two-thirds of the reported cases. In African countries, heterosexual transmission is more common. Injection drug users account for the next largest group. Heterosexual persons infected through sexual intercourse, newborns infected via placental transmission, and recipients of HIV-contaminated blood transfusions, including persons with hemophilia, make up the rest. Since the late 1980s, the face of the HIV epidemic in the United States has shifted as the percentage of HIV-infected gay and bisexual men has decreased and the number of heterosexual transmissions has increased. By 1998, gay men accounted for only 35% of the new cases, and the virus was spreading more rapidly among women, African Americans, Latinos, injection drug users, and adolescents.

Etiology and Pathophysiology

HIV is a retrovirus that specifically binds to receptors on the surface of cells of the immune system. Once bound, the virus gains entry to the cell, where the enzyme reverse transcriptase copies the viral RNA into DNA, which then inserts itself into the chromosomal DNA of the human cell. HIV infects several human cells, but its hallmark is the progressive destruction of helper, or CD4, T lymphocytes.

HIV can remain latent for months or years after incorporation into the human cell genome. During this time, infected cells produce no viral proteins and are able to elude immunological detection. After a period of latency, the virus becomes active, multiplies rapidly, and spreads throughout the body. Various target tissues are infected through cell-to-cell contact, or cell fusion, which may be one of the mechanisms by which HIV evades destruction by the immune system. As CD4 cell counts decline, the immune system is eventually paralyzed, and patients become progressively more susceptible to opportunistic infections, including *Pneumocystis carinii* and toxoplasmosis, or certain types of cancer, such as Kaposi's sarcoma. Besides its devastating effect on the immune system, HIV is neurotropic. Early on, HIV enters the central nervous system (CNS), probably carried there by macrophages that cross the blood-brain barrier.

The virus is transmitted through exchange of body fluids, such as semen and blood, and through intravenous use of contaminated syringes and needles. The virus is not transmitted through casual contact, such as touching, hugging, kissing, or sharing the same dishes.

The serum test used to detect HIV is known as the enzyme-linked immunosorbent assay (ELISA). When the result is positive, the serum is then subjected to the more accurate Western blot test. Because false-positive results may occur with the ELISA, individuals should not be notified of a positive result until the Western blot has been performed. Both assays test for antibodies to HIV; many infected patients will have a negative test result until they have synthesized antibodies to HIV. Evidence of antibodies will be present in about 90% of patients within 6 months of infection. When diagnostic uncertainty persists, polymerase chain reaction amplification of viral RNA can be used to detect circulating HIV, and some laboratories use viral culture as a supplemental test. Positive results are reported to public health authorities in some states, and AIDS registries have been established. In some countries, such as Cuba, HIV-infected persons are quarantined.

Diagnosis

The diagnosis of AIDS is made when an HIV-seropositive person develops an opportunistic infection such as *P. carinii, Toxoplasma gondii*, or Kaposi's sarcoma (see Table 22–1). The case definition of AIDS was expanded in the early 1990s to include all HIV-infected persons with CD4 cell counts of less than 200 cells/mm^3 or a percentage of less than 14%. Pulmonary tuberculosis, recurrent pneumonia, and invasive cervical cancer were added to the list of clinical conditions contained in the 1987 definition.

Clinical Findings

A broad range of clinical manifestations occur in persons infected with HIV. Symptoms vary depending on the stage of illness and organ involvement. The *initial* or *acute phase* of infection—the period between infection and the development of detectable antibodies—lasts from weeks to months but averages 2 months. Some persons experience a transient flulike syndrome or an acute clinical or subclinical meningoencephalitis. Because recently infected patients are not yet immunocompromised, they are able to recover and contain the virus. The *silent* or *latent phase*—the period between the onset of seropositivity and the onset of clinical symptoms—typically lasts from 5 to 7 years. Persons are infectious during this stage but have no HIV-related medical problems. The *symptomatic phase*—the period between the onset of clinical symptoms and death—lasts from several months to years, depending on the specific complications that develop and their response to treatment.

Patients who have yet to develop an AIDS-defining infection, such as
P. carinii, often have persistent lymphadenopathy, fatigue, night sweats, oral
candidiasis, and unexplained weight loss. In the past, this condition was
called *AIDS-related complex* (ARC), a term no longer used because the
distinction between AIDS and ARC was often arbitrary. Additionally, the
presence of ARC was not as predictive of clinical outcome as the CD4 T-
lymphocyte count.

P. carinii pneumonia is the most common initial opportunistic infectious disease in AIDS patients and typically occurs in about 75% of patients.
Symptoms include the gradual onset of a nonproductive cough, low-grade
fevers, and chest pain. Kaposi's sarcoma is the most common HIV-related
malignancy. It is particularly virulent, leading to rapid spread and death,
usually within 2 years.

The Centers for Disease Control and Prevention has established stages
for HIV-related illness. The importance of the CD4 T-lymphocyte count has
been recognized in the revised case definition, as reflected in Table 22–2.
Long-term studies, which are now available, suggest that almost all persons
who become infected will eventually deteriorate to clinical category C,
which indicates a diagnosis of AIDS. Thus, the natural history of HIV disease
is a reflection of the ability of HIV to damage the immune system, especially
the CD4 T lymphocyte, which plays a key role in directing the immune response to foreign invaders, including viruses, fungi, and protozoa. Although
the period between infection and the development of AIDS ranges from 2 to
15 years, the mean is about 9 years.

Research has led to a rapid growth in the number of potent therapies
that have contributed to a remarkable decline in hospitalization rates, morbidity, and mortality in areas where the drugs are available. The drugs also
help alleviate or reverse HIV-related cognitive impairment. The approved
drugs all fight HIV replication and include six reverse transcriptase inhibitors: zidovudine, didanosine, zalcitabine, lamivudine, stavudine, and aba-
cavir; five protease inhibitors: ritonavir, indinavir, nelfinavir, saquinavir, and
amprenavir; and three nonnucleoside reverse transcriptase inhibitors: nevirapine, delavirdine, and efavirenz. Several investigational drugs should be
available soon. The three groups of drugs use different mechanisms to inhibit virus replication and reduce HIV RNA levels (viral load). Combination
regimens are used to reduce the development of viral resistance, which is an
ongoing problem in HIV management. In general, combinations involve one
protease inhibitor and two reverse transcriptase inhibitors.

Therapy is generally recommended for HIV-seropositive patients with a
viral load greater than 5,000–10,000 copies/mL. Therapy is also recom-

TABLE 22–1. Conditions included in the 1993 AIDS surveillance case definition

Bacterial infections, multiple or recurrent[a]

Candidiasis of bronchi, trachea, or lungs

Candidiasis, esophageal

Cervical cancer, invasive[b]

Coccidioidomycosis, disseminated or extrapulmonary

Cryptococcosis, extrapulmonary

Cryptosporidiosis, chronic intestinal (more than 1 month duration)

Cytomegalovirus disease (other than liver, spleen, or nodes)

Cytomegalovirus retinitis (with loss of vision)

Encephalopathy, HIV-related

Herpes simplex, chronic ulcer(s) (more than 1 month duration) or bronchitis, pneumonitis, or esophagitis

Histoplasmosis, disseminated or extrapulmonary

Isosporiasis, chronic intestinal (more than 1 month duration)

Kaposi's sarcoma

Lymphoid interstitial pneumonia and/or pulmonary lymphoid hyperplasia[a]

Lymphoma, Burkitt's (or equivalent term)

Lymphoma, immunoblastic (or equivalent term)

Lymphoma, primary, of brain

Mycobacterium avium complex or *Mycobacterium kansaii*, disseminated or extrapulmonary

Mycobacterium tuberculosis, any site (pulmonary[b] or extrapulmonary)

Mycobacterium, other species or unidentified species, disseminated or extrapulmonary

Pneumocystis carinii pneumonia

Pneumonia, recurrent[b]

Progressive multifocal leukoencephalopathy

Salmonella septicemia, recurrent

Toxoplasmosis of the brain

Wasting syndrome due to HIV

[a]Children < 13 years old.
[b]Added in the 1993 expansion of the AIDS surveillance case definition for adolescents and adults.

TABLE 22–2.   Centers for Disease Control and Prevention classification of HIV infection

CD4+ T-lymphocyte cell category	Clinical category		
	A[a] (asymptomatic, acute HIV infection or persistent generalized lymphadenopathy)	B[b] (symptomatic, but not with category A or C conditions)	C[c] (AIDS indicator conditions)
>500/mm^3	A1	B1	C1
200–499/mm^3	A2	B2	C2
<200/mm^3	A3	B3	C3

[a]Category A: consists of one or more of the conditions listed below in an adolescent or adult (≥13 years) with documented HIV infection. Conditions listed in categories B and C must not have occurred.
• Asymptomatic HIV infection
• Persistent generalized lymphadenopathy
• Acute (primary) HIV infection with accompanying illness or history of acute HIV infection
[b]Category B: consists of symptomatic conditions in an HIV-infected adolescent or adult that are not included among conditions listed in clinical category C and that meet at least one of the following criteria: 1) the conditions are attributed to HIV infection or are indicative of a defect in cell-mediated immunity; or 2) the conditions are considered by physicians to have a clinical course or to require management that is complicated by HIV infection. Examples of conditions in clinical category B include, but are not limited to
• Bacillary angiomatosis
• Candidiasis, oropharyngeal (thrush)
• Candidiasis, vulvovaginal; persistent, frequent, or poorly responsive to therapy
• Cervical dysplasia (moderate or severe)/cervical carcinoma in situ
• Constitutional symptoms, such as fever (38.5°C) or diarrhea lasting longer than 1 month
• Hairy leukoplakia, oral
• Herpes zoster (shingles) involving at least two distinct episodes or more than one dermatome
• Idiopathic thrombocytopenia purpura
• Listeriosis
• Pelvic inflammatory disease, particularly if complicated by tuboovarian abscess
• Peripheral neuropathy
• For classification purposes, category B conditions take precedence over those in category A. For example, someone previously treated for oral or persistent vaginal candidiasis (who has not developed a category C disease) but who is not asymptomatic should be classified in category B.
[c]Category C: includes the clinical conditions listed in the AIDS surveillance case definitions. For classification purposes, once a category C condition has developed, the person remains in category C.

Source.   Adapted from Centers for Disease Control 1992.

mended for asymptomatic patients who have low viral loads (<5,000–10,000 copies/mL) but who also have low CD4 cell counts (e.g., <200 cells/mm^3). Use of antiviral therapy represents a long-term commitment, and its benefits are rapidly lost when patients are noncompliant.

Neuropsychiatric Manifestations of HIV Disease

Early explanations of psychiatric morbidity among HIV-seropositive and AIDS patients emphasized the emotional repercussions of developing AIDS. The focus soon turned to the destructive effects of HIV itself because it became clear that the CNS is a prime target of the virus, particularly areas below and connected to the cerebral cortex. Thus, persons infected with HIV are susceptible to the direct effects of the virus, as well as the effects of opportunistic infections on the CNS.

Postmortem brain findings in HIV-infected patients are variable and reflect the markedly different clinical presentations that occur. In about one-third of patients, the presence of HIV is demonstrable in CNS tissue. There is a relative sparing of the cortex, and the most prominent changes are seen in subcortical regions, including the central white matter and the deep gray structures, such as the basal ganglia, thalamus, and brain stem (hence, the term *subcortical dementia*). White matter pallor may be accompanied by marked atrophy and an astrocytic reaction. Loss of oligodendrocytes and neurons is not characteristic. The spinal cord also may be involved and shows vacuolation caused by swelling within the layers of the myelin sheath.

Initial symptoms of HIV infection are often subtle; for instance, during the latent phase, before clinical evidence of AIDS is seen, some HIV-infected adults develop a sense of mental slowing or forgetfulness without significant intellectual decline. In one study, 44% of otherwise asymptomatic HIV-seropositive persons had evidence of neuropsychological impairment, compared with 87% of persons with full-blown AIDS. HIV-infected children manifest a delay in reaching motor or intellectual milestones, also suggesting that HIV has direct effects on the CNS.

Many persons infected with HIV develop significant CNS involvement, which has been called the *AIDS dementia complex*. Because no single pathological process underlies the dementia and because symptoms may occur before AIDS has developed, it may be more appropriate to use the phrase *HIV-related brain disease*. The dementia also may result from the sequelae of delirium, as well as primary infection with HIV, the effects of secondary infections such as *Cryptococcus*, or the effects of treatment.

The early diagnosis of dementia may be difficult. Symptoms are vague, and detectable neuropsychological impairment is relatively difficult to identify. As the dementia advances, symptoms become more obvious; patients may be aware of their diminishing mental functioning and admit that they are forgetful. Patients may have trouble concentrating, feel overwhelmed by organizational tasks, and easily lose their train of thought. Motoric involvement (i.e., the "complex" part of the dementia) may include ataxia, leg weakness, tremors, and impaired eye movements. As the dementia progresses, intellectual impairment becomes more severe and affects nearly all spheres of mental functioning. Late in the illness, incontinence, incoordination, parkinsonian symptoms, seizures, muteness, and coma may occur, leading eventually to death. In DSM-IV-TR, HIV-related dementia is diagnosed on Axis I as dementia due to HIV disease; HIV disease should also be coded on Axis III. The clinical manifestations of HIV-related dementia are shown in Table 22–3.

Patients infected with HIV occasionally develop new-onset psychotic symptoms, such as vivid hallucinations, bizarre delusions, and disorganized speech and behavior. The prevalence of new-onset psychosis in patients with HIV disease may be as high as 15%. In one study, patients had been psychotic from several days to several months before presentation, and the most common symptom was a persecutory, grandiose, or somatic delusion. Auditory hallucinations also were common in this study, as were anxiety, agitation, formal thought disorder, mood disturbance, bizarre behavior, and cognitive impairment. In fact, most patients with new-onset HIV-related psychosis have substantial mood symptoms, including euphoria, depression, or mood lability. Therefore, patients with new-onset mental status changes who have one or more risk factors for AIDS need to have HIV ruled out as a cause of their symptoms.

On initial neurological examination, nearly one-half of HIV-seropositive patients show minor motor disturbances, such as hyperreflexia, increased tone, tremor, and mild ataxia. Cerebrospinal fluid examination tends to be normal unless mental changes are due to treatable CNS tumors or infections (e.g., increased number of cells, positive India ink test for *Cryptococcus*). Brain imaging is normal in most patients at the time of initial evaluation; the remainder have evidence of cortical atrophy or ventricular enlargement on computed tomography or small focal signal hyperintensity or unidentified bright objects on magnetic resonance imaging. Abnormal electroencephalogram findings, consisting of predominantly diffuse cortical slowing, are common, even in patients without clinical evidence of mental changes or neurological impairment. Patients with evidence of CNS involvement follow a more rapidly progressive downhill course.

TABLE 22–3. Clinical manifestations of HIV-related dementia

Cognitive impairments	**Generalized systemic symptoms**
Short-term memory deficit; forgetfulness rather than amnesia	Fatigue, sleep changes (hypersomnia)
	Anorexia, weight loss
Decreased concentration and attention	Enuresis
Confusion and disorientation	Hypersensitivity to medications and alcohol
Overall intellectual ability generally well preserved until late	
Visuospatial perception deficits	**Cognitive symptoms associated with advanced dementia**
	Global cognitive impairment
Changes in personality or behavior	Rudimentary social functioning
Apathy, decreased interest	Disorientation
Impaired judgment, erratic behavior	Psychomotor retardation, decreased spontaneity
Social withdrawal	
Rigidity of thought	Agitation, sundowning (e.g., nighttime delusions)
Speech impairment; slowing, dysarthria, hypophonia; difficulty in following other speakers	Mutism, vacant stare
	Coma
Psychotic symptoms	
Hallucinations	**Motor symptoms associated with advanced dementia**
Suspiciousness and delusions	Ataxia
Agitation and inappropriate behavior	Spastic weakness
	Paraplegia, quadriparesis
Motor symptoms	Hyperreflexia, myoclonus, seizures
Ataxia, loss of coordination	Bladder and bowel incontinence
Tremors	

Psychological Aspects of HIV Disease

Psychological aspects of HIV disease extend to homosexual and bisexual men and persons in other risk groups who have not had symptoms of AIDS but who are at risk for the disease. Many of the "worried well" develop signs of significant psychological distress, including anxiety, depression, and interpersonal problems. Because of their risk for illness, some persons become preoccupied with their physical condition. Like hypochondriacal persons, these patients misinterpret normal bodily sensations and seek tests but experience little relief of their anxiety with reassurance and normal test results. At this stage, the physician can be most helpful by providing regular contact with patients to examine them for new signs of illness, to explain symptoms, and to offer reassurance. Couples, both hetero- and homosexual, may need counseling, and safe sex practices should be discussed at every opportunity, as well as the importance of the proper use of condoms. In this setting, the physician can correct misinformation about AIDS and discuss the appropriateness of HIV testing, the transmission of HIV, and the relative degree of HIV susceptibility associated with various sexual practices (see Table 22–4).

TABLE 22–4. Relative degree of AIDS susceptibility associated with various sexual practices

Probably safe	Possibly safe	Unsafe
Mutual masturbation	Anal or vaginal intercourse with a condom	Anal or vaginal intercourse without a condom
Social kissing	Fellatio interruptus	Fellatio to orgasm
Body massage, hugging	Mouth-to-mouth kissing	Activities that involve bruising or bleeding
Body-to-body rubbing	Oral-vaginal contact	
Use of own sex toys		

Persons at low risk for HIV disease sometimes become unnecessarily fearful or phobic about HIV; these irrational concerns can foster discrimination against persons with HIV disease or against those in high-risk categories (e.g., homosexual men, drug-addicted persons). The appearance of HIV disease in the early 1980s seems to have led to a backsliding of public opinion about the gay-rights movement because many persons came to believe that the epidemic represented God's retribution for immoral behavior (despite the irony that lesbians are at very low risk for contracting HIV). One survey showed, for instance, that 27% of the respondents disagreed with the statement that persons with AIDS should be treated with compassion. In another survey, only 19% of the respondents said that a group home for AIDS patients would be welcome in their neighborhood; only factories, garbage landfills, and prisons ranked lower in desirability.

The effect of HIV testing can itself be traumatic because the implications of a positive result are so potentially devastating. In many states, patients must give informed consent before testing and undergo both pre- and posttest counseling. Pretest counseling involves discussion of the different tests, their usefulness, and their limitations. The session also gives the physician an opportunity to assess the patient's motives for having the test and how he or she might respond to the test results. Posttest counseling is necessary to reinforce the lessons about HIV, the testing procedures, and the implications of positive results, as well as to explain ways to prevent transmission.

Patients who receive negative results generally express relief; those who learn they are seropositive often experience a variety of emotions: withdrawal, anger, aggression, dysphoria, or anxiety. Some persons will feel guilt about their sexual orientation, drug addiction, or having infected others. Others will face the real or perceived loss of support by parents, family, friends, and employers. Some persons, particularly those with a preexisting personality disorder, may deny the positive results and escalate their self-destructive behavior through unsafe sex practices or increased use of drugs or alcohol. Although most persons eventually adjust to the news, apathy and denial can persist for many. The risk of depression and suicidal behavior typically increases after adjusting to the initial shock of learning that one is HIV seropositive.

Depression is relatively common in people with HIV disease and serves to worsen the patient's functional capabilities, independent of the underlying medical condition. The degree to which functional impairment is due to depression may be difficult to determine because many symptoms of major depression are also characteristic of the symptoms of early HIV-related dementia. Depression can interfere with the patient's ability to cope intellectually and emotionally with the complicated information and medical procedures often required to manage the illness. A frequent symptom of depression in HIV disease is social withdrawal. This withdrawal may stem from the individual's perceived rejection by others, his or her growing sense of helplessness, and his or her fear of a rapid and disfiguring death. Regardless of the cause of the patient's depression, treatment should not be delayed. The patient should be counseled to accept the reality of the illness and to work on the issues of social rejection and loss, disfigurement, the specter of declining health, and impending death. Antidepressant medication is helpful for many patients, but careful dosing and close monitoring for adverse effects are imperative.

Although some degree of anxiety is common in persons with HIV disease, the full spectrum of signs and symptoms may occur, including phobias, panic attacks, and generalized anxiety. The most frequent anxiety disorder results from the acute reaction to learning of the diagnosis, which in DSM-IV-TR is called *adjustment disorder with anxiety*. Depending on the severity of the anxiety, the patient may show a variety of autonomic symptoms (e.g., diarrhea, nausea, vomiting), which could easily be mistaken for evidence of an opportunistic infection or neurological involvement. The proper management of anxiety involves giving the patient emotional support, recommending the use of relaxation training or biofeedback, having the patient restrict the intake of caffeine, and prescribing benzodiazepines judiciously.

Patients with HIV disease are understandably concerned about their physical well-being. This concern may escalate into an unhealthy preoccupation, leading to frequent checking of the body for signs of illness, frequent requests for laboratory tests, or an obsessive concern about appearance. Patients should be reassured that their concerns are being taken seriously and that their symptoms will be carefully monitored. Having a single physician provide care can help the patient avoid the unnecessary tests and procedures associated with doctor shopping.

Other psychiatric disorders in persons with HIV are less common and perhaps are no more frequent than in the general population (e.g., schizophrenia, schizoaffective disorder, or bipolar disorder). One of the more bizarre aspects of the AIDS epidemic has been reported cases of factitious AIDS, in which persons deliberately fabricate the diagnosis and seek medical attention. (See Chapter 12 on factitious disorders and malingering.)

The following case example illustrates some of the problems seen in an HIV-seropositive patient treated in our hospital:

> Lynn, a 23-year-old man, was admitted after a diazepam overdose. Lynn lived with his parents, and after taking the pills, he told his mother, who brought him to the hospital emergency room. Lynn's stomach was lavaged, and he was taken to an inpatient psychiatric unit.
>
> Lynn had grown up in a small midwestern farming community. He had been effeminate as a boy and was picked on by his peers, but he otherwise developed normally, had friends, and behaved in school. Although he had always been attracted to the other boys and had always felt that he was homosexual, Lynn had come out of the closet only recently. In the past, Lynn had hidden his sexual orientation from his friends and family members and had even dated girls. After his coming out, he tried to fit in with what he thought was a gay lifestyle by dressing colorfully, wearing an earring, and frequenting gay bars in nearby communities. He had had a series of brief affairs and an assortment of sexual experiences with dozens of young men.
>
> A year before his hospitalization, Lynn had sought HIV testing and learned that he was seropositive. He was devastated by this knowledge, became acutely depressed, and felt hopeless about his future. Lynn sought individual counseling and began to see a therapist on a regular basis. He also joined a local support group for persons with AIDS or HIV-related illnesses. These measures helped, but Lynn was constantly reminded of what his future held as members of the support group would stop coming, and he and the others would later learn that these members had died. He also read widely about AIDS and knew of its devastating effects. Lynn was an attractive young man and had always worked out and felt physically fit. He did not want to think of himself as deformed or debilitated.
>
> On the night before admission, Lynn had been feeling particularly sor-

ry for himself and had been out with several friends. After returning home, he began ruminating about his HIV seropositivity and how alone and isolated he felt. He worried about potentially devastating complications. He knew his mother had been treated for anxiety in the past and found a bottle containing diazepam that had been prescribed for her. Lynn knew it was a tranquilizer and swallowed the contents of the bottle, believing that it would kill him. Within a few minutes, he had a change of mind, told his parents what he had done, and was brought to the hospital.

Lynn admitted that he had adjusted poorly to the knowledge of his HIV seropositivity and that he initially had denied the test results. To prove that he was healthy, he had engaged in several sexual affairs, which he now regretted, knowing that he had placed these men at risk for HIV infection. He admitted that he had become overly concerned about somatic symptoms and had constantly sought reassurance from his doctors. Despite his current dysphoria, he had no vegetative symptoms of depression, such as weight loss, anorexia, or fatigue.

Lynn was given a diagnosis of an adjustment disorder with depressed mood. He received brief supportive counseling in the hospital. He rapidly returned to his usual level of functioning.

The potential therapeutic interventions for the psychiatric sequelae of HIV infection are summarized in Table 22–5.

Clinical Management

Monitoring of mental status and evaluating signs of cognitive impairment are important parts of the overall management of HIV infection, in view of the common psychiatric and CNS sequelae. When HIV-related dementia is suspected, neuropsychological testing should be done. The results may show more or less impairment than was subjectively observed and will be helpful in treatment planning. Neuropsychological testing also can help to distinguish dementia from depression or anxiety. Depressive symptoms and suicide risk need to be assessed at each visit, especially because the rate of suicide in persons with AIDS is more than seven times higher than that in the general population.

Many patients benefit from supportive psychotherapy, in which issues such as guilt associated with previous sexual practices or drug abuse, social isolation, and acknowledgment of the illness (along with associated fear or anger) can be addressed. Stress management, including relaxation training and problem-solving techniques, also may benefit these patients. Cognitive-behavioral therapy may help to correct the distorted thinking that patients with HIV disease often develop (e.g., "No one likes me because I am HIV positive").

Patients who develop specific psychiatric syndromes can benefit from medication. Benzodiazepines may be helpful to patients with generalized

TABLE 22–5.   Therapeutic interventions for psychiatric sequelae of HIV
infection

Problem	Potential intervention
Worried well	Assessment of HIV risk and infection status
	Diagnosis and treatment of possible underlying psychiatric disorder
	Reassurance and counseling
Acute adjustment reaction to positive test results (or diagnosis)	Assessment and intervention for possible shock and/or suicide potential
	Provision of accurate medical and prognostic information
	Coordination of psychosocial care and treatment or referral for depression and anxiety
	Introduction to community support organizations
	Early diagnosis and treatment of any central nervous system disease
Anxiety	Assessment for use of caffeine, alcohol, and prescribed or illicit drugs
	Counseling of patient and patient's family or friends
	Introduction to community support organizations
	Pharmacological treatment for generalized anxiety disorder or adjustment disorder with anxiety
Depression	Workup to rule out depression due to medical illness or drugs, appropriate treatment if indicated
	Supportive or cognitive-behavioral psychotherapy
	Pharmacological treatment for moderate to severe depression with low dose of antidepressant
Hypochondriasis	Evaluation and treatment for underlying depressive, anxiety, or somatoform disorder
	Provision of reassurance and accurate medical information
	Behavior therapy, including relaxation training, desensitization, and avoidance conditioning
Psychosis	Evaluation and treatment for potential drug-induced or HIV-related brain disorder
	Evaluation and treatment for potential bipolar disorder
	Atypical antipsychotics for psychotic state
	Behavioral management to reduce stimulation and to minimize agitation
	Support and counseling for patient's family or lover, or both

Source.   Adapted from Miller 1990.

anxiety disorder or an adjustment disorder with anxiety. Patients with major depression or panic disorder may benefit from serotonin reuptake inhibitor antidepressants, which are generally effective and well tolerated. The older tricyclic and monoamine oxidase inhibitor antidepressants, with their many side effects, are not as well tolerated by patients with HIV-related illness. Monoamine oxidase inhibitors have the additional problems of having a high likelihood of drug interactions and requiring dietary restrictions. Some investigators have used low-dose psychostimulants to treat depression in AIDS patients (e.g., methylphenidate, 10–40 mg/day in divided doses). Psychostimulants are especially worth considering when lethargy and cognitive slowing are a major component of the depression. Antipsychotics are helpful in patients who develop hallucinations or delusions; atypical antipsychotics are the preferred agents because they are well tolerated (e.g., risperidone, 0.5 mg/day). Electroconvulsive therapy is useful in depressed or manic AIDS patients whose symptoms do not respond to medication.

The clinician should be aware of the potential for adverse drug interactions when prescribing a psychotropic agent for a patient with HIV-related disease who is taking one or more antiretroviral drugs. All of the protease inhibitors are metabolized primarily by the cytochrome P450 oxidative enzyme system, but only ritonavir significantly inhibits the cytochrome P450 3A3/4 isoenzymes and other isoenzymes to a lesser extent. Of the nonprotease inhibitors, nevirapine has been shown to be a moderate inhibitor of cytochrome P450 3A3/4, and delavirdine is a potent inhibitor of this enzyme. Less is known about the enzymes involved in the metabolism of the other antiretrovirals. Table 22–6 presents general guidelines about drug interactions with the protease inhibitors.

Patient management also should include providing education about HIV, information about its modes of transmission, and practical precautions regarding safe sex and safe needle use by drug abusers. Support groups organized by local AIDS outreach organizations (e.g., Shanti) can be helpful in boosting social support. Physicians need to work with public health agencies to help patients obtain needed financial and physical assistance.

Caring for the Patient With HIV-Related Disease

The problems of caring for patients infected with HIV extend beyond the medical and psychiatric complications of the disease. The medically complex nature of caring for these patients and their disorders is time-consuming, physically demanding, and emotionally draining. Many caregivers develop symptoms of depression and anxiety, leading some to burn out.

TABLE 22–6. Psychotropic drug interactions with protease inhibitors

Contraindicated with ritonavir

Anxiolytics/sedatives

  Alprazolam

  Clorazepate

  Diazepam

  Estazolam

  Flurazepam

  Midazolam

  Triazolam

  Zolpidem

Antidepressants

  Bupropion

Neuroleptics

  Clozapine

  Pimozide

Analgesics

  Meperidine

  Propoxyphene

  Piroxicam

Possible toxicities with ritonavir

Antidepressants

  Nefazodone

  Trazodone

  Fluvoxamine

  Tricyclics

Neuroleptics

Analgesics

  Methadone

  Fentanyl

  Oxycodone

Anticonvulsants

  Carbamazepine

  Clonazepam

Not recommended for use with other protease inhibitors

Potential for psychotropic toxicity

  Alprazolam

  Triazolam

  Midazolam

Potential for protease inhibitor toxicity

  Nefazodone

  Fluvoxamine

Potential for subtherapeutic levels of protease inhibitors

  Barbiturates

  Carbamazepine

  Phenytoin

Source. From *Psychiatric Care of the Medical Patient*, second edition, edited by Alan Stoudemire, Barry S. Fogel, and Donna Greenberg, copyright 2000 by Oxford University Press, Inc. Used by permission of Oxford University Press, Inc.

Additionally, many health care workers feel conflicted about caring for patients whose lifestyle, they believe, has contributed to their contracting the illness. Group discussions among caregivers to ventilate their feelings and frustrations can be helpful. Health care workers also need to confront their own prejudices toward the high-risk groups because these negative attitudes can adversely affect their ability to offer appropriate care. Many physicians still believe that HIV-infected patients are responsible for their illness and are less deserving of sympathy than are other patients. These views should not be tolerated.

Recommendations for the clinical management of HIV-related disease are summarized in the box.

Recommendations for management of patients with HIV

1. Acceptance and a nonjudgmental attitude are essential in the care of patients infected with HIV.

   • There is no excuse for blaming or belittling patients for their illness.

   • Health care workers need to separate their personal negative beliefs about the patient's lifestyle (e.g., homosexuality, drug abuse) from their care of the patient.

2. The clinician should be alert to neuropsychiatric symptoms that may signal involvement of the central nervous system, including neurological signs (e.g., tingling, numbness, weakness) and psychiatric symptoms (e.g., depression, mania, confusion).

3. AIDS patients need much emotional support, especially because many will have lost their traditional supports after having revealed simultaneously their homosexuality (or drug addiction) and their development of a communicable and ultimately fatal illness.

   • Many patients need practical assistance in solving everyday problems. Many will need to be referred to social service agencies.

   • The therapist also must help the patient deal with issues of death and dying in a realistic and humane way.

   • Support groups are available in most communities for HIV-seropositive patients and the worried well.

4. Many patients will benefit from specific treatment for depression, anxiety, or psychosis (e.g., antidepressants, anxiolytics, antipsychotics).

5. The clinician should educate himself or herself, other staff members, and the patient about AIDS and its transmission.

   • Despite great publicity and public educational efforts, some persons (including medical personnel) stubbornly cling to inaccurate beliefs (e.g., HIV can be transmitted by casual contact).

Bibliography

American Psychiatric Association: Practice guidelines for the treatment of patients with HIV/AIDS. Am J Psychiatry 157 (suppl 11):1–62, 2000

Atkinson JH, Grant I, Kennedy CJ, et al: Prevalence of psychiatric disorders among men infected with human immunodeficiency virus. Arch Gen Psychiatry 45:859–864, 1988

Blendon RJ, Donelan K, Knox RA: Public opinion and AIDS: lessons for the second decade. JAMA 267:981–986, 1992

Bozzette SA, Berry SH, Duan N, et al: The care of HIV-infected adults in the United States. N Engl J Med 339:1897–1904, 1998

Burack JH, Barrett DC, Stall RD, et al: Depressive symptoms and CD4+ lymphocyte decline among HIV-infected men. JAMA 270:2568–2573, 1993

Carpenter CC, Fischl M, Hanuner SM, et al: Antiretroviral therapy for HIV infection in 1998: updated recommendations of the International AIDS society–USA Panel. JAMA 280:78–86, 1998

Centers for Disease Control: 1993 revised classification system for HIV infection and expanded surveillance case definition for AIDS among adolescents and adults. MMWR Morbid Mortal Wkly Rep 41(RR-17):1–19, 1992

Coté TR, Biggar RJ, Dannenberg AL: Risk of suicide among persons with AIDS: a national assessment. JAMA 268:2066–2068, 1992

Dilley JW, Ochitill HN, Pearl M, et al: Findings in psychiatric consultations with patients with acquired immune deficiency syndrome. Am J Psychiatry 142:82–86, 1985

Faulstich ME: Psychiatric aspects of AIDS. Am J Psychiatry 144:551–556, 1987

Heaton RK, Velin RA, McCutchan JA, et al: Neuropsychological impairment in human immunodeficiency virus-infection: implications for employment. Psychosom Med 56:8–17, 1994

Johnson J, Williams JBW, Goetz RR, et al: Personality disorders predict onset of Axis I disorder and impaired functioning among homosexual men with and at risk of HIV infection. Arch Gen Psychiatry 53:350–357, 1996

Lyketsos CG, Hoover DR, Guccione M, et al: Depressive symptoms as "predictors of medical outcomes in HIV infection." JAMA 270:2563–2567, 1993

Markowitz JC, Kocsis JH, Fishman B, et al: Treatment of depressive symptoms in human immunodeficiency virus–positive patients. Arch Gen Psychiatry 55:452–457, 1998

Miller D: Diagnosis and treatment of acute psychological problems related to AIDS, in Behavioral Aspects of AIDS. Edited by Ostrow DJ. New York, Plenum, 1990, pp 187–206

Navia BA, Choo ES, Petito CK: The AIDS dementia complex, II: neuropathology. Ann Neurol 19:525–535, 1986a

Navia BA, Jordan BD, Price RW: The AIDS dementia complex, I: clinical features. Ann Neurol 19:517–524, 1986b

Perry SW: Organic mental disorders caused by HIV: update on early diagnosis and treatment. Am J Psychiatry 147:696–710, 1990

Perry SW, Markowitz JC: Counseling for HIV testing. Hosp Community Psychiatry 39:731–739, 1988

Rabkin JG, Wagner HGJ, Rabkin G: Fluoxetine treatment for depression in patients with HIV and AIDS: a randomized, placebo-controlled trial. Am J Psychiatry 156:101–107, 1999

Schmitt FA, Bigley JW, McKinnis R, et al: Neuropsychological outcome of zidovudine (AZT) treatment of patients with AIDS and AIDS-related complex. N Engl J Med 319:1573–1578, 1988

Sewell DD, Jeste DV, Atkinson JH, et al: HIV associated psychosis: a study of 20 cases. Am J Psychiatry 151:237–242, 1994

Self-Assessment Questions

1. How is HIV transmitted?
2. What are the major risk groups for HIV, and how have they changed over the years?
3. What are the diagnostic criteria for AIDS? How is HIV disease staged?
4. What are the testing procedures for HIV?
5. What neuropsychiatric symptoms have been reported in cases of AIDS?
6. What symptoms affect the worried well?
7. What are the common psychiatric disorders that affect persons with HIV?
8. How does prejudice affect the caregiver?

23 Disorders of Childhood and Adolescence

Children sweeten labors, but they make misfortunes more bitter. They increase the cares of life, but they mitigate the remembrance of death.

Francis Bacon

As any 17-year-old will attest, the distinction between childhood and adulthood is arbitrary, often ludicrous, and frequently fluctuating in response to the needs of the person invoking the distinction. Psychiatric nosology and classification are no exception to this rule. Many of the disorders described in other chapters (not classified among childhood disorders in DSM-IV-TR) occur frequently in children. Mood disorders and anxiety disorders are especially common. Schizophrenia often arises during adolescence and occasionally during childhood. In inner cities, crack cocaine is traded on the grade school playground. Children and adolescents show signs and symptoms of personality disorder. Indeed, apart from dementias such as Alzheimer's disease, there is probably no "adult" disorder from which children are exempt. Furthermore, childhood disorders such as mental retardation, autism, or even attention-deficit/hyperactivity disorder (ADHD) may be diagnosed in adults.

Nevertheless, DSM-IV-TR has set aside a group of disorders that are considered to be relatively specific to children and adolescents, in that they typically *arise* during that period of life rather than simply *occur* during childhood and adolescence. The overall summary of this group of disorders appears in Table 23–1, and a more detailed overview has been provided in Chapter 2. These disorders are both diverse and numerous. Some are not very common (e.g., communication disorders such as selective mutism), and some are seen more frequently in pediatric clinics than in child psychiatry clinics (e.g., elimination disorders such as encopresis and enuresis). To permit more complete coverage of the most important disorders, we selectively review only some of them in this chapter, focusing on those that are most frequently seen in child psychiatry clinics or in a family practice setting. These include mental retardation, learning disorder, autistic disorder, ADHD, conduct disorder, oppositional defiant disorder, Tourette's disorder, and separation anxiety disorder. In addition, a brief overview is provided of those adult disorders that are commonly seen in children (e.g., mood disorders, schizophrenia) and of physical, emotional, and sexual abuse.

TABLE 23–1. Disorders usually first diagnosed in infancy, childhood, or adolescence

Mental retardation	Attention-deficit and disruptive behavior disorders
Mild	
Moderate	Attention-deficit/hyperactivity disorder
Severe	Conduct disorder
Profound	Oppositional defiant disorder
Learning disorders	Feeding and eating disorders of infancy or early childhood
Reading	
Mathematics	Tic disorders
Written expression	Tourette's disorder
Motor skills	Other disorders
Communication disorders	Separation anxiety disorder
Pervasive developmental disorders	

Child psychiatry is one of the most challenging and interesting areas of specialization within psychiatry. Because it requires working with multiple individuals and groups (e.g., the child, the parents, the school system), it is in many respects a primary care specialty. Because the child psychiatrist must know a great deal about other childhood illnesses, maturational processes, and developmental disorders, it is also closely allied with pediatrics and requires a good knowledge of general medicine. Because cognitive development is an important aspect of child psychiatry as well, child psychiatry is tied to cognitive psychology. Furthermore, the clinician working in child psychiatry has an opportunity to catch disorders at their earliest; because children are adaptable, fresh in outlook, and pleasantly unpredictable, working with them and helping them overcome their problems can be particularly rewarding. Finally, childhood mental disorders are quite common. Estimates of prevalence vary depending on breadth or narrowness of definition, but it is probably a reasonable estimate that 5%–15% of children will experience an illness that is sufficiently severe to require treatment or to impair their functioning during the course of a year.

Special Aspects of the Assessment of Children

Although there are many continuities between adult and child psychiatry, there are also important differences in emphasis and approach. These differences include techniques of assessment, the importance of flexible norms or criteria, an involvement of family or significant others, an increased role of nonphysicians in the health care team, and the frequent occurrence of psychiatric comorbidity. These aspects of assessment must be kept in mind as the clinician attempts to evaluate the presence or absence of the various disorders listed in Table 23–1.

Trajectories of Development

Although the lives of adults change with time and are affected by surrounding life situations, the pace of change and the effect of life events are much greater in children. Consequently, in working with children, it is important to emphasize a longitudinal and developmental approach rather than the cross-sectional approaches that are typically used in assessing adults. This developmental approach must take into account the growth and maturational processes that all children undergo, assessing them in the light of each particular child's life situation and strengths and weaknesses. Any mental illness that arises in children must be treated within this context. Each child has a natural trajectory of development that will be completed through the process of passing from infancy to adulthood. The development of mental illness and the experience of environmental stressors will have very different effects depending on the place where a given child is in that trajectory of development. As each child is evaluated, the clinician must ask the following questions:

- What level of emotional and intellectual maturity does this child have?
- What are his or her particular strengths?
- How do they provide a protective and healing element?

- What particular weaknesses are present?
- What stresses are affecting the child?
- How do those stresses affect him or her at this particular stage of life?
- How do gender-specific challenges affect the expression of illness and its treatment?

For example, parental divorce or even abandonment has become an all-too-common experience for children, at least in the United States. What difference does it make if the father walks out or the mother walks out? If the parent walks out or dies? What is the difference in effect if the child is a boy or a girl? What difference does it make if the child is 2, 10, or 16 years old? What difference does it make if the remaining parent is strong and capable versus weak and immature? What effect does the child's place in a sibship have on him or her? How much success and self-esteem has the child achieved up to this time?

Obviously, maternal death would have a very different effect on each child in a family of five children, the oldest of whom is a 16-year-old girl (who is likely to assume the maternal role) and the youngest of whom is 2 years old. The effect would be different for the children whose surviving father is unemployed and alcoholic than it would be for the children whose surviving father is a high-functioning blue- or white-collar worker. The effect also would be different depending on whether the eldest child is herself highly functional or has some mental illness, such as autism or conduct disorder. The effect on each child would vary depending on the availability of other social supports, such as an extended family with grandparents, a good or a weak school system, and a safe environment or one characterized by crime, violence, and drug use. All things being constant, a 2-year-old will have a very different understanding of parental loss or abandonment than will an older child because the younger child will have had little time to build either a self-image incorporating that parent or a conceptual structure that can be used to comprehend parental loss.

Who Is the Patient?

Children rarely pick up the telephone and make an appointment to see a child psychiatrist. Usually they are brought in at someone else's request. Invariably, someone else is paying the bill. All these things make child psychiatry a different ball game than adult psychiatry. The child may be unwilling, noncompliant, distrusting, or resentful. In this instance, the assessment is likely to be particularly challenging because the clinician must win the child's trust. Even when the child is the identified patient, the parents usually are interviewed and evaluated as well. Sometimes it becomes clear that the parents themselves have serious problems, which they have ignored or projected onto the child. In this instance, it may be necessary to reassess and to suggest treatment of the parents in addition to (or even instead of) the child. Furthermore, in child psychiatry, as in few other medical specialties, the clinician is likely to feel ambivalent and confused from time to time about the appropriate role to play. Extraordinary maturity is required on the part of a good child psychiatrist, who typically has chosen this specialty because of a liking for children and who will feel frustrated at the lack of astuteness toward the patient shown by parents, teachers, or others. The child usually will be the identified patient, even though others may be in greater need of intervention and yet do not seek or accept it.

The Assessment of Children

Childhood disorders can be diagnosed in individuals ranging from infants through people in their late teens or early 20s. Obviously, standard approaches to interviewing and assessment, described in Chapter 3, do not apply well to infants, children, or young teenagers. Standard techniques for the psychiatric assessment of adults, which may be applicable to patients in their late teens and are applicable to patients in their early 20s, emphasize the use of questioning, self-report, and introspection. These approaches require verbal skills not yet achieved in the maturational process of children, the capacity to separate and step back from oneself to describe feelings and behavior, and the ability to form abstractions about cognition, behavior, or emotions. For example, young children may not be able to respond to questions about concepts such as depression, loneliness, or anger. The interviewer often needs to talk to children at a much more concrete level, asking questions such as

- Do you feel like crying?
- What kinds of things make you feel like crying?
- Do you ever want to hit people?
- Whom do you feel like hitting?
- Who are your best friends?
- How often do you see them?
- What kinds of things do you do together?
- Do they like you?

In addition to interviewing, playing games with the child often gives the clinician some insight into the child's ability to function interpersonally, to tolerate frustration, or to focus his or her attention. Imaginative play, using dolls that can represent important figures in the child's life, also may give some sense as to his or her feelings toward and relationships with others. Taking turns in telling stories also may elicit interesting information. For example, if the clinician suspects that the child may be feeling anxious about something, he or she may tell a story about "how Jimmy is afraid of going to school because the other children make fun of him." When the child then tells his or her own story, he or she may be able to describe his or her own fears in this indirect manner. Direct observation of activity level, motor skills, verbal expression, and vocabulary is also a fundamental component of assessment.

Application of Norms and Criteria

In assessing children, the clinician must have a good sense of what is normal for a given child at a given age, as well as an awareness that norms may vary widely. Younger clinicians who are completing medical school or a residency usually have not had the experience of rearing their own children or of watching a large number of younger siblings develop. Thus, they must get their sense of norms from reading textbooks, from observing large numbers of children, or from recalling their own experiences in the process of growing up. The latter approach may be particularly helpful in the assessment of teenagers, although the average medical student or physician must recognize that he or she is likely to be much more uptight, obsessional, and compliant with authority than the average child. Nevertheless, remembering one's own "growing pains" often helps to increase empathy with the frustrations and struggles that many adolescents experience and seek help for.

Having a sense of what is normal or abnormal for a given child, in a given family, and in a given social and intellectual environment can be extremely difficult. For example, a typical normal 10-year-old has an IQ of 100, is able to read at a fourth-grade level, is able to perform addition and subtraction and some multiplication, and is able to throw, catch, and kick a ball with at least some accuracy. Some normal children have an IQ of only 85, however, whereas some have an IQ of 160. These children will clearly differ from one another a great deal in their school performance. Boys and girls also have quite different levels of maturation both physically and mentally, and these differences are especially pronounced in younger children. Boys and girls also have different maturational tasks as they go through puberty and enter adolescence, and consequently, they experience different stresses. Success and failure also mean different things to an inner-city child than to a child from an affluent background.

Clinicians are likely to be asked over and over, "Is this child normal?" or "Is this behavior normal?" In answering these questions, most clinicians will experience some doubt, ambiguity, and difficulty about what constitutes normality. Making facile judgments about normality is probably an indication that the clinician has not been thinking hard enough or has too simple and authoritarian a notion of what constitutes normality. Extreme cases are simple, of course, but most are likely to be in the murky middle.

Involvement of Family and Significant Others

Clinicians who work with children usually need to work with their families and significant others as well. The degree of family involvement varies, of course, depending on the age of the child. In the case of very young children, the parents are likely to be the primary informants and important recipients of treatment as well because they will probably need both psychological support and assistance in learning behavioral techniques to manage their child's behavior. For grade school children, involvement of family members is essential, but the child becomes an increasingly important protagonist in both assessment and treatment. Teenagers, who are going through important maturational changes as they move into adulthood, usually are brought to the forefront of the assessment and treatment process, although the family also will provide resources much of the time.

Deciding whether to maintain complete confidentiality or to share information becomes a critical issue in the assessment of teenagers. In general, teenagers should be assured that what they tell the clinician will end there, unless the teenager gives permission to share the information or can be encouraged to bring it out in a family or group setting. The assurance of confidentiality is important in establishing a bond of trust between teenager and clinician because the patient otherwise is likely to see the therapist as a potentially antagonistic authority figure. Although this advice may seem easy in principle, it places a great burden of responsibility on the clinician because he or she is likely to hear about things that parents would want to know about and that the clinician instinctively feels he or she should discuss with them, such as suicidal thinking, sexual experimentation, lying, cheating, or drug use.

Only in situations dangerous to the child, such as a clear risk of suicide, should the rule of confidentiality be broken. This rule should be explained to the parents in a tactful manner so that they do not feel excluded. Depending on circumstances, the clinician also may choose to see the parents independently. Alternatively, he or she may refer the parents to another psychiatrist, psychologist, or social worker with whom he or she has a good working relationship. If the parents are referred elsewhere, maintaining some liaison in the continuing assessment and treatment process is quite important.

Involvement of Nonphysicians in the Health Care Team

Depending on the specific problem, the evaluation and treatment of children may require more knowledge and input than a single psychiatrist can provide. Child psychiatry is more difficult and complicated than adult psychiatry because the problems of children tend to impinge on many different aspects of their lives, and treatment often involves many of these different aspects. Children with some particular childhood disorder, such as ADHD, are likely to have difficulty with their parents, their siblings, their school performance, and their relationships with their peers. Most people who interact with children who have ADHD are likely to find their high level of impulsivity, distractibility, and physical activity annoying and disruptive. The children themselves have a poor self-concept, produced in part by a sense of frustration and failure in all spheres of their lives.

In such instances, assessment involves determining how well the child is functioning in these various domains. That is, the clinician needs to talk to and observe the child. In addition, however, the clinician needs to talk to the parents and perhaps the entire family. With the permission of the child and family, the clinician may need to talk to the child's teacher and to obtain some assessment of his or her performance in the classroom. School records, as well as the child's scores on tests of educational achievement, are important aspects of assessment. Parents or teachers also may need to provide information about the child's interaction with his or her peers.

Because of the diversity of the domains involved, many clinicians working in the area of child psychiatry like to operate in the context of a health care team. This team may be relatively small, involving a psychologist or social worker in addition to the psychiatrist. In larger settings, however, it includes a psychiatrist (who works primarily with the child in psychotherapy and the prescription of medication), a social worker (who works primarily with the family), an educational specialist (who assesses the child's educational achievement and assists in designing a nonfrustrating remedial program as needed), and a psychologist (who develops programs for behavioral management, may do psychotherapy as needed, and may work with child, family, and school system as needed).

Psychiatric Comorbidity

Comorbidity, or the simultaneous occurrence of two or more diagnoses in the same patient, tends to be the norm rather than the exception in children. For example, children with ADHD often have impairment in academic skills, such as specific disabilities in reading or arithmetic. They also may show symptoms of conduct disorder, oppositional defiant disorder, or anxiety disorder.

Clinicians must remain very alert to the likelihood of multiple problems and design their assessment and treatment plan accordingly. This aspect of child psychiatry also makes it somewhat more complex and difficult than adult psychiatry. On the positive side, however, is the hope that early intervention will prevent larger problems from developing or the addition of new diagnoses (e.g., substance abuse in addition to ADHD).

Testing in Child Psychiatry

Because of the complexity and ambiguity of child psychiatry, some selected objective assessment measures may be quite useful. Psychological tests, such as IQ tests, may be helpful in determining a child's specific areas of strength and weakness, as well as the level of academic performance that he or she can be expected to achieve. Some diagnoses in child psychiatry, such as mental retardation or learning disorders, depend on knowledge of the child's IQ. Some disorders of childhood, such as Tourette's disorder or autism, have an organic quality to them that suggests a need to rule out an associated or underlying medical or neurological disorder, such as seizures. Other disorders, such as mental retardation, are often accompanied by a variety of medical problems (e.g., seizures, congenital anomalies, metabolic disorders). In these instances, laboratory tests are useful either in diagnosing the accompanying organic disorders or in monitoring their progress.

Psychological and Educational Testing in Child Psychiatry

Psychological and educational testing often play a central role in the evaluation of children. Several tests that are commonly used in child psychiatry are listed in Table 23–2.

TABLE 23–2. Cognitive, psychological, and educational tests used in child psychiatry

Factor	Test
Intelligence	Stanford-Binet Intelligence Scale, Wechsler Intelligence Scale for Children—Revised (WISC-R), Peabody Picture Vocabulary, Kaufman ABC, Wechsler Preschool and Primary Scale of Intelligence (WPPSI)
Education and achievement	Iowa Test of Basic Skills (ITBS), Iowa Test of Educational Development (ITED), Wide Range Achievement Test—Revised (WRAT-R), Woodcock-Johnson Psychoeducational Battery
Adaptive behavior	Vineland Adaptive Behavior Scales, Iowa Conner's Teacher Rating Scale
Perceptual-motor abilities	Draw-a-Person, Bender-Gestalt, Benton Visual Retention Test, Purdue Pegboard Test, Beery Developmental Test of Visual-Motor Integration
Personality	Thematic Apperception Test, Rorschach Test

General Intelligence

General intelligence may be assessed with the Stanford-Binet Intelligence Scale, the Wechsler Intelligence Scale for Children—Revised (WISC-R), and other well-validated instruments. The Stanford-Binet Intelligence Scale was one of the earliest IQ tests to be developed, and it is still appropriate for relatively young children because its bottom threshold is lower and does not require extensive acquisition of knowledge. The Kaufman ABC and the Wechsler Preschool and Primary Scale of Intelligence (WPPSI) are appropriate for assessing young children.

The WISC-R has become established as the standard test for assessing the intelligence of school-aged children. Like the Wechsler Adult Intelligence Scale—Revised (WAIS-R), the WISC-R consists of a group of verbal scales (information, vocabulary, similarities, arithmetic, and comprehension, plus digit span) and a set of performance tests (picture completion, picture arrangement, block design, object assembly, coding, and mazes). Thus, verbal and performance IQs can be derived separately, as well as a full-scale IQ.

Examining the scores on individual WISC-R subtests gives clinicians a sense of the child's overall intellectual skills and weaknesses. The test is scaled to have a mean of 100 and a standard deviation of 15. Sixty-seven percent of children have IQs that fall between 85 and 115, whereas 95% have IQs that fall between 70 and 130. Children from middle-class and culturally advantaged backgrounds tend to perform better on these tests. In such instances, the performance scales of the test may give a somewhat better indication of the child's "culture-free intelligence," although this clearly will not be helpful for those children who have performance deficits for some reason (e.g., visual-motor and/or perception difficulties). Interpretation of the WISC-R must be made within the context of each child's social background and educational opportunities.

The Peabody Picture Vocabulary Test is a simpler and cruder test that is sometimes used to give a simple global measure of intelligence. The test uses pictures to provide a measure of oral language comprehension, from which verbal intelligence can be inferred. In general, IQ based on the Peabody test tends to be an overestimate.

Educational Achievement

Several standardized educational achievement tests are often used in the public school systems. Two of the most widely used are the Iowa Test of Basic Skills (ITBS) and the Iowa Test of Educational Development (ITED). The former is typically used for younger children, whereas versions of the latter are available for assessment until completion of high school. For the ITBS and the ITED, national, state, and school-specific norms are available, so that the child's achievement can be assessed within his or her specific environmental context. These achievement tests provide scores for specific areas such as reading, language arts, study skills, arithmetic, and social studies. Evaluating the pattern of achievement can provide some index as to whether the child has a learning disorder.

The ITBS and ITED are group tests. When a specific concern is present, the child also may be referred for individual testing by an educational specialist, which often involves the Wide Range Achievement Test—Revised (WRAT-R). The Woodcock-Johnson Psychoeducational Battery is another widely used individual test to assess skills such as reading and arithmetic. Children may perform poorly on group tests because of inattention or other problems; therefore, group tests may underestimate the child's true abilities.

Adaptive Behavior

Various standard questionnaires can be used to assess adaptive behavior. The Vineland Adaptive Behavior Scales were originally developed to evaluate children with mental retardation, but they are now widely used to provide a standardized measure of adaptive skills for children with a broader range of problems, including those with normal intelligence. The Iowa Conners' Teacher Rating Scale was developed to assess the child's behavior in the classroom. It is specifically targeted to assessing behavior that tends to be associated with ADHD, such as impulsivity, physical activity, or impaired attention. It also has subscales to assess social withdrawal and aggressive behavior.

Perceptual-Motor Skills

Various standardized tests are used to assess perceptual-motor skills. In the assessment of young children, the Draw-a-Person Test is one of the most popular. The complexity and detail of the person drawn give a crude indication of the child's maturity, whereas the drawing skills shown allow assessment of the child's ability to translate his or her thoughts into a visual representation. The Bender-Gestalt and Benton Visual Retention Test assess the ability to copy a design and to recall it later, which are also fundamental aspects of perceptual-motor skills. The Purdue Pegboard Test is a somewhat pure test of manual dexterity, assessing the child's ability to place pegs in appropriate slots. The Beery Developmental Test of Visual-Motor Integration is popular with school systems.

Personality Style and Social Adjustment

Personality style and social adjustment are typically evaluated in children through projective tests. The Thematic Apperception Test uses a series of cards depicting obscure figures in ambiguous situations; the child is asked to describe what is happening and tell a story about it. The Rorschach Test is the famous inkblot test. In this test, the child is shown cards containing inkblots that have ambiguous and suggestive shapes. The child is asked to identify and label what he or she sees (e.g., two men dancing) and to indicate the basis for his or her perception. Although semistandardized scores can be applied, one of the most common applications of these tests is to provide a standardized structured stimulus to the child, using his or her response as an indication of interpersonal experiences, anxieties, fears, drives, and other important psychological components.

Other Tests

Other laboratory tests also may be useful in the assessment of children. The decision to order these tests will depend on the child's history and the clinician's index of suspicion for finding an abnormality. For example, there is often comorbidity between seizure disorders and other childhood disorders, such as autism or mental retardation, and children with these diagnoses should probably be evaluated with an electroencephalogram (EEG). For other disorders in which seizures sometimes occur or in which EEG abnormalities have been noted, such as conduct disorders or ADHD, an EEG may be appropriate when the history indicates a possibility of seizures.

Evaluation of children with mental retardation typically includes an assessment for possible causes of the mental retardation. Karyotyping may be used to evaluate for the fragile X syndrome, Down's syndrome, or XYY. Computed tomography (CT) or magnetic resonance imaging (MRI) may be appropriate in such patients, as well as in patients with autism or Tourette's disorder.

Physical Examination

A careful physical examination, incorporating some simple standardized neuropsychological tests, is an important part of the evaluation. In addition to the standard physical examination, the clinician should carefully inspect the child for indications of congenital anomalies, such as a high-arched palate, low-set ears, single palmar creases, unusual carrying angle, webbing, abnormalities of the genitalia, and neuroectodermal anomalies. It is well recognized that congenital anomalies tend to occur together and that midline or neuroectodermal anomalies are more likely to be associated with central nervous system anomalies. The observation of any such anomalies is an indication for CT or MRI.

The clinician should be attentive to assessment of neurological soft signs in children as well. A standardized repertoire should be developed for assessing graphesthesia, left-right discrimination, motor coordination, and simple perceptual-motor skills that can be evaluated at the bedside. For example, left-right discrimination can be examined systematically through a graded series of questions such as the following: "Hold up your right hand. Hold up your left foot. Put your right forefinger on your nose. Use your left forefinger to point to your right foot. Point my right hand. Use your left forefinger to point to my left hand." Tongue twisters such as "Methodist-Episcopal" or "Luke Luck likes lakes" may be used to assess oral-motor coordination, whereas hopping, tandeming, and rapid alternating movements are used to evaluate other motor skills. Fine motor skills are evaluated through drawing and writing. After the clinician has assessed many children across a wide range of ages, he or she will gradually develop a sense of what constitutes normal performance on such tests of neurological soft signs for a given child at a given age. Extensive neurological soft signs may serve as an indicator for ordering a more extensive laboratory workup, involving an EEG or a brain scan.

Mental Retardation

Mental retardation is characterized by subnormal intelligence, as measured by IQ, accompanied by deficits in adaptive functioning. IQ is defined as mental age (as assessed by a standard test such as the WISC-R) divided by chronological age and multiplied by 100. Thus, a child with an IQ of 50 might have a mental age of 5 years and a chronological age of 10 years; in other words, he or she would be performing with the intellectual skills of a 5-year-old. The specific IQ cutoff point used to define mental retardation is 70. Persons with an IQ below 70 are more than 2 standard deviations below the population mean. IQs between 70 and 85 (1 standard deviation below the mean) are considered to indicate *borderline intellectual functioning*—that is, the border between normal intelligence and mental retardation. The criteria also require that the individual have problems in coping with social and economic demands or abnormalities in interpersonal adjustment.

The DSM-IV-TR criteria for mental retardation (Table 23–3) summarize this definition. They also require an onset before age 18 years. In general, mental retardation is typically observed and diagnosed long before age 18 and usually is considered to be present from very early in life. For example, a 13-year-old who sustains a head injury in a car accident and subsequently has a marked decrement in IQ is considered to have a dementia induced by trauma rather than mental retardation. In the DSM-IV-TR system, mental retardation is coded on Axis II.

Mental retardation is divided into four broad categories: mild, moderate, severe, and profound. Children with *mild mental retardation* have IQs between 50 and 70. They represent the majority of cases of mental retardation, constituting approximately 85% of the individuals with IQs below 70. Children with IQs in this range are considered educable, and they usually are able to attend special classes and to work toward the long-term goal of being able to function in the community and to hold some type of job. They usually can learn to read, write, and perform simple arithmetical calculations. Children with *moderate mental retardation* have IQs ranging from 35 to 50 (between 3 and 4 standard deviations below the population mean) and constitute approximately 10% of the mentally retarded population. They are considered trainable, in that they can learn to talk, to recognize their name and other simple words, to perform activities of self-care such as bathing or

TABLE 23–3. DSM-IV-TR diagnostic criteria for mental retardation

A. Significantly subaverage intellectual functioning: an IQ of approximately 70 or below on an individually administered IQ test (for infants, a clinical judgment of significantly subaverage intellectual functioning).

B. Concurrent deficits or impairments in present adaptive functioning (i.e., the person's effectiveness in meeting the standards expected for his or her age by his or her cultural group) in at least two of the following areas: communication, self-care, home living, social/interpersonal skills, use of community resources, self-direction, functional academic skills, work, leisure, health, and safety.

C. The onset is before age 18 years.

Code based on degree of severity reflecting level of intellectual impairment:

317	**Mild Mental Retardation:**	IQ level 50–55 to approximately 70
318.0	**Moderate Mental Retardation:**	IQ level 35–40 to 50–55
318.1	**Severe Mental Retardation:**	IQ level 20–25 to 35–40
318.2	**Profound Mental Retardation:**	IQ level below 20 or 25
319	**Mental Retardation, Severity Unspecified:**	when there is strong presumption of Mental Retardation but the person's intelligence is untestable by standard tests

doing their laundry, and to handle small change. They require management and treatment in special education classes. The ideal long-term goal for these individuals is care in a sheltered environment, such as a group home. The severely and profoundly mentally retarded children constitute the smallest groups. *Severe mental retardation* is defined as an IQ between 20 and 35, and *profound mental retardation* is defined as an IQ below 20. Individuals with IQs in this range almost invariably require care in institutionalized settings, usually beginning relatively early in life.

Epidemiology

Mental retardation is very common, affecting 1%–2% of the population. Mental retardation is more common in males, with a male-to-female ratio of approximately 2:1. Mild mental retardation is more common in lower social classes, but moderate, severe, and profound mental retardation are equally common among all social classes.

Etiology and Pathophysiology

The etiology and pathophysiology of mental retardation are heterogeneous. Mental retardation is almost certainly a syndrome that represents a final common pathway produced by a variety of factors that injure the brain and affect its normal development. Individuals with IQs below 55 often have an identifiable cause for their mental retardation, whereas those above 55 often do not and probably develop their mental retardation through some complex multifactorial and polygenetic combination. Down's syndrome is the most common cause of mental retardation. Fragile X syndrome is the most common heritable form of mental retardation and is second only to Down's syndrome in frequency. The fragile X gene has been discovered; it contains an unstable segment that expands as it is passed through generations and affects children differently depending on whether it is passed through fathers or mothers (imprinting). Inborn errors of metabolism account for a small percentage of cases; examples include Tay-Sachs disease and untreated phenylketonuria.

In addition to these clearly defined genetic causes, a substantial proportion of cases of mental retardation probably also reflect polygenic inheritance, possibly interacting with a variety of nongenetic factors such as nutrition and psychosocial nurturance. Many prenatal factors also may affect fetal development and lead to neurodevelopmental anomalies. The high rate of Down's syndrome (trisomy 21) in children born to older mothers is a prime example. Other prenatal factors that may affect fetal development include maternal nutrition or substance abuse, exposure to mutagens such as radiation, or maternal illnesses such as diabetes, toxemia, or rubella. Perinatal and early postnatal factors also may contribute. Examples include traumatic deliveries that cause brain injury, malnutrition, exposure to toxins, infections such as encephalitis, or head injuries occurring during infancy or early childhood. Psychosocial factors obviously contribute to some of these biological factors, and some psychosocial factors also may contribute independently. Malnutrition, exposure to toxins such as lead, increased likelihood of maternal infection because of inadequate immunization, and poor prenatal and perinatal care are more likely to occur in children born in impoverished environments.

Course and Outcome

The long-term outcome of mental retardation is variable. Some severe and profound forms may be characterized by progressive physical deterioration and ultimately premature death, as early as the teens or early 20s (e.g., Tay-Sachs disease). Individuals with mild and moderate forms of mental retardation have a somewhat reduced life expectancy, but active intervention may enhance their quality of life. Like all children, children with mental retardation grow and develop, and they may show maturational spurts that could not be predicted at an earlier age. Typically, mentally retarded children progress through normal milestones, such as sitting, standing, talking, and learning numbers and letters, in a pattern similar to that of nonretarded children but at a slower rate. The educable and trainable mentally retarded children are able to learn to read, write, and calculate at some level, as long as appropriately structured educational settings are provided.

Differential Diagnosis

As in other childhood disorders, the differential diagnosis of mental retardation (particularly mild mental retardation) can be complex because of the frequent comorbidity of childhood disorders. The differential diagnosis includes ADHD, learning disorders, autism, and childhood psychoses or mood disorders, but all these conditions can occur with mental retardation. Seizure disorders also are very common in children with mental retardation. Children in whom mental retardation is suspected should be thoroughly evaluated with a careful physical and neurological examination, EEG, and CT (or MRI if available), as well as IQ testing.

Clinical Management

The clinical management of mental retardation is similar to that of other serious chronic childhood disorders such as autism. After a thorough evaluation, a comprehensive program should be developed to determine the best situation in which to place and treat the child, taking the needs and abilities of both the child and the parents into account. Decisions may range from care in the home (supplemented by family support and special education), to placement in a foster or group home, to long-term institutionalization. Because most mentally retarded children are mildly retarded, the majority will remain at home, at least initially. Because the parents of some of these children themselves have mental retardation, ongoing evaluation through social service agencies may be helpful and even necessary to ensure that the child's needs are being adequately met.

Whatever their own intellectual resources, the parents of mentally retarded children are confronted with a host of burdens and stresses and will benefit from both supportive counseling and training in behavioral techniques to help manage their child's behavior problems. Comorbid conditions such as seizures require medical management. Intellectual evaluation will help to determine the appropriate educational placement for the child, but this should be subjected to periodic review. At this stage, it is still not clear whether mildly mentally retarded children benefit more from placement in regular school programs (mainstreaming) or from placement in special settings where education is tailored to their specific needs. To a large extent, however, mainstreaming is currently the dominant trend.

Learning Disorders

The learning disorders are characterized by an inability to achieve in a specific area of learning (reading, writing, or arithmetic) at a level consistent with the person's overall IQ. Typically, individuals with these disorders have normal intelligence (although it may be borderline or high) but have a specific inability to learn at least one of these academic skills and sometimes several.

The DSM-IV-TR criteria for *reading disorder* appear in Table 23–4. The definitions for *mathematics disorder* and *disorder of written expression* are similar. In each case, the diagnosis is made on the basis of educational testing that indicates that the individual is performing markedly below a level expected on the basis of the person's IQ. For example, a 14-year-old with reading disorder (developmental dyslexia) may have an IQ of 110 and be reading at a third-grade level.

TABLE 23–4.   DSM-IV-TR diagnostic criteria for reading disorder

A. Reading achievement, as measured by individually administered standardized tests of reading accuracy or comprehension, is substantially below that expected given the person's chronological age, measured intelligence, and age-appropriate education.
B. The disturbance in Criterion A significantly interferes with academic achievement or activities of daily living that require reading skills.
C. If a sensory deficit is present, the reading difficulties are in excess of those usually associated with it.
Coding note: If a general medical (e.g., neurological) condition or sensory deficit is present, code the condition on Axis III.

These disorders are relatively common. A specific disability in reading affects 2%–8% of school-aged children. The rates for writing and mathematics disabilities are unknown, but they are probably high as well. These disorders are from two to four times as common in boys as in girls.

Specific learning disabilities tend to be familial, but not uniformly or consistently so. They are assumed to represent a neurodevelopmental defect or cerebral injury affecting the particular brain region involved in developing the academic skill. For example, in the case of some developmental reading or writing disorders, the language regions in the brain (i.e., Broca's area,

Wernicke's area, or the left hemisphere) are thought to be affected.

If not diagnosed and treated early and aggressively, learning disorders are extremely handicapping. Although children with these disorders typically have normal intelligence, they quickly come to view themselves as failures because of their inability to progress academically in a particular area. They may come to regard themselves as stupid and feel rejected by their peers.

The frustration associated with an impairment in academic skills can lead to a variety of complications, such as truancy, school refusal, conduct disorder, mood disorder, or substance abuse. Consequently, it is important to identify the condition early and treat it aggressively. Rather than being causal, learning disorders may be comorbid with these conditions, as well as with ADHD. In this instance, it is important to recognize the multiple disorders and to treat both (or all) of them appropriately.

Educational intervention proceeds on two fronts. Children or teenagers usually need remedial instruction to shore up skill deficits, as well as instruction in developing "attack" skills that will assist them in learning strategies to compensate for the neural deficits that underlie their condition. With steady, sympathetic educational support, most children with these specific learning disabilities are able to develop acceptable skills in reading, writing, and arithmetic.

Autistic Disorder and Asperger's Disorder

Autistic Disorder

Autistic disorder is the most important among the *pervasive developmental disorders.* The film *Rain Man,* through its sympathetic portrayal of a person with autism, has done much to help increase public understanding of this particular disorder. Although Raymond Babbit is not a perfectly typical autistic person because he is cognitively very gifted in specific isolated areas, he is not atypical. He shows all the characteristic features of autism: impaired social interactions, impaired ability to communicate, and a restricted repertoire of activities and interests.

Individuals with autism are usually noted to be developing abnormally relatively soon after birth. Within the first 3–6 months of these children's lives, their parents may note that they do not develop a normal pattern of smiling or responding to cuddling. The first clear sign of abnormality is usually in the area of language. As they grow older, they do not progress through developmental milestones such as learning to say words and speak sentences. They seem aloof, withdrawn, and detached. Instead of developing patterns of relating warmly to their parents, they may instead engage in self-stimulating behavior, such as rocking or head banging. By age 2 or 3 years, it is usually clear that there is something severely wrong, and the features of the disorder continue to become more obvious over time as the child fails to develop normal verbal and interpersonal communication. Children with this disorder are referred to as autistic because they appear to be withdrawn and self-absorbed. Most of the defining features of autistic disorder reflect this autistic pattern of thinking, speaking, feeling, and behaving.

The DSM-IV-TR criteria for autistic disorder appear in Table 23–5. The criteria require that at least 6 of 12 items be present. The items cover the three major domains involved in autism (i.e., social interaction, communication, and behavioral repertoire). The criteria provide an excellent comprehensive description of the symptoms of this disorder.

The impairment in social interaction is one of the first signs of the disorder. Autistic children appear to lack the ability to bond with their parents or with others. In severe cases, these children seem totally withdrawn. In milder cases, they have some interaction but lack warmth, sensitivity, and awareness. Interactions, when they occur, tend to have a detached and mechanical quality to them. Displays of love and affection do not occur, and autistic children (or autistic adults) do not appear to respond to such displays from others.

The failure to develop spoken language is usually the first thing that leads parents to realize the gravity of the problem and eventually to seek medical attention. The verbal impairments range from the complete absence of verbal speech to mildly deviant speech and language patterns. Even in patients who develop good facility in verbal expression, the speech has an empty, repetitive quality to it, and intonations may be singsong and monotonous. Autistic children and adults seem to lack the capacity to engage in conversation with others, sometimes talking spontaneously without an audience and at other times replying irrelevantly or inappropriately.

Finally, the behavioral repertoire is impaired. There is an intense and rigid commitment to maintaining specific routines, and autistic children tend to become quite distressed if routines are interrupted. They may have to sit in a particular chair, dress in a particular way, or eat particular foods.

Most autistic individuals (70%) show some evidence of mental retardation, but others have normal intelligence, and some have very specific talents or abilities, particularly in the areas of music and mathematics. IQ testing tends to show considerable scatter, and patients with autism tend to perform better on performance scales than on verbal scales.

Children who present with symptoms suggestive of autism should re-

TABLE 23–5. DSM-IV-TR diagnostic criteria for autistic disorder

A. A total of six (or more) items from (1), (2), and (3), with at least two from (1), and one each from (2) and (3):

    (1) qualitative impairment in social interaction, as manifested by at least two of the following:

        (a) marked impairment in the use of multiple nonverbal behaviors such as eye-to-eye gaze, facial expression, body postures, and gestures to regulate social interaction

        (b) failure to develop peer relationships appropriate to developmental level

        (c) a lack of spontaneous seeking to share enjoyment, interests, or achievements with other people (e.g., by a lack of showing, bringing, or pointing out objects of interest)

        (d) lack of social or emotional reciprocity

    (2) qualitative impairments in communication as manifested by at least one of the following:

        (a) delay in, or total lack of, the development of spoken language (not accompanied by an attempt to compensate through alternative modes of communication such as gesture or mime)

        (b) in individuals with adequate speech, marked impairment in the ability to initiate or sustain a conversation with others

        (c) stereotyped and repetitive use of language or idiosyncratic language

        (d) lack of varied, spontaneous make-believe play or social imitative play appropriate to developmental level

    (3) restricted repetitive and stereotyped patterns of behavior, interests, and activities, as manifested by at least one of the following:

        (a) encompassing preoccupation with one or more stereotyped and restricted patterns of interest that is abnormal in either intensity or focus

        (b) apparently inflexible adherence to specific, nonfunctional routines or rituals

        (c) stereotyped and repetitive motor mannerisms (e.g., hand or finger flapping or twisting, or complex whole-body movements)

        (d) persistent preoccupation with parts of objects

B. Delays or abnormal functioning in at least one of the following areas, with onset prior to age 3 years: (1) social interaction, (2) language as used in social communication, or (3) symbolic or imaginative play.

C. The disturbance is not better accounted for by Rett's Disorder or Childhood Disintegrative Disorder.

ceive comprehensive psychiatric and physical examinations, with emphasis on neurological evaluation as well. Children should be screened for metabolic disorders such as phenylketonuria, and karyotyping also should be done. Because these children present with profound social withdrawal, hearing and vision should be checked to rule out sensory defects as a cause. Many children with autism have a comorbid seizure disorder (25%) or eventually develop one. For that reason, an EEG also should be obtained. IQ testing will help assess the child's intellectual strengths and weaknesses.

Epidemiology

Autism is relatively rare and has a prevalence of approximately 10–15 per 10,000 individuals. It is more common in males than in females, with a ratio of 3:1 or 4:1. The onset of autism usually occurs in early childhood, and problems are typically noted during the first or second year of life.

Etiology and Pathophysiology

Autism is a neurodevelopmental disorder that manifests shortly after birth, but the etiology for the neurodevelopmental abnormality is as yet unknown. Twin studies have shown a monozygotic-to-dizygotic ratio of 36:0, making autism perhaps the most genetic of all mental illnesses (e.g., the same ratio for schizophrenia is 4:1). Family studies also support a genetic role. The siblings of autistic children have an increased rate of both autistic disorder (2% vs. the population rate of 0.01%) and mental retardation and speech and language disorders. The illness does not appear to follow any classic mendelian patterns of transmission, however, suggesting that autism, like most mental illnesses, is probably a complex polygenic and multifactorial disorder.

Imaging studies have been used in an attempt to identify the nature of the neurodevelopmental abnormality. Various findings have been reported. In autism, unlike in most mental illnesses, children have been found to have large brain size relative to body size, with some evidence for gyral malformation (polymicrogyria). The large cerebral size has been interpreted as reflecting a failure to achieve normal pruning, the process by which neurons are systematically eliminated or "pruned" back. Abnormalities in the cerebellum (particularly the vermis), the temporal lobes, the hippocampal complex, and cerebral asymmetries also have been reported. Functional imaging studies support the occurrence of temporal lobe abnormalities (hypoperfusion), as well as decreased metabolic activity in the anterior cingulate gyrus. The most consistent finding noted with neuroimaging has been ventricular enlargement. Neuropathological studies have reported small, densely packed (and presumably immature) cells in limbic structures in the cerebellum. Physically, autistic children have a variety of soft neurological signs and primitive reflexes, an excess of non-right-handedness, and an apparent failure to achieve normal cerebral dominance of language functions in the left hemisphere. All of these observations are consistent with a pathophysiology that affects multiple brain regions and a failure to achieve normal cerebral asymmetry.

Course and Outcome

Autism is associated with relatively severe morbidity. It is a chronic, lifelong disorder. Some children do show some improvement as they mature, although others may in fact worsen. Very few individuals with autism (2%–3%) are able to progress normally through school or to live independently. Follow-up studies of a group of autistic individuals who received diagnoses in childhood and were reevaluated in adulthood indicated that most autistic persons show some improvement in social interaction over time, but even the most functional never achieve normality. Nearly all of the defining features of the disorder, including social aloofness, language abnormalities, and rigid and ritualistic behavior, tend to persist into adulthood. Good prognostic features include higher IQ and better language and social skills.

Differential Diagnosis

The major differential diagnoses include childhood psychosis, mental retardation, and congenital deafness, blindness, or language disorders. The most important distinctions are between autism and mental retardation or language disorders such as selective mutism and expressive language disorder. These distinctions can be quite difficult, and the differential turns largely on the quality of the social interactions (in the context of the individual's particular intellectual abilities). Mentally retarded children also typically have pervasive intellectual impairments, whereas autistic children tend to have a much more uneven profile of functional intellectual abilities on the WISC-R and may be normal to superior in some areas. The major distinction between autism and childhood-onset schizophrenia is the presence or absence of overt psychotic symptoms (delusions and hallucinations), which typically do not occur in autism but are difficult to assess in the noncommunicative child.

Clinical Management

The clinical management of autism requires assistance and support in the many different areas of functioning in which these children are impaired. Once the diagnosis is made, the disorder should be described and explained to the parents, making it clear that their child has a neurodevelopmental disease and not a psychological disturbance that they caused through poor parenting. Guidelines for behavioral management should be provided, so that the parents can help reduce the rigid and stereotyped behaviors and improve language and social skills. Children with autism usually require special education or specialized day care programs that also emphasize improvement in social and language skills. Medications are often used as adjuncts to these supportive and behavioral approaches. Children who have seizures require anticonvulsants. Among other medications, both conventional antipsychotics (e.g., haloperidol) and atypical antipsychotics (e.g., risperidone) have been empirically observed to decrease aggressive and self-stimulating behavior. Other medications that have been found to be empirically helpful in some cases include clomipramine, naltrexone, fluoxetine, and carbamazepine.

Asperger's Disorder

Asperger's disorder is closely related to autism and is considered by some to be simply a milder version of autistic disorder (also referred to as *high-functioning autism*). Children with Asperger's disorder have a similar early onset of impairment in social interaction and abnormal behavior such as stereotypies and rituals, but they have normal language functions and usually have normal intelligence as well. The criteria for Asperger's disorder are shown in Table 23–6.

Asperger's disorder is relatively new, in that its first description in a standardized nomenclature occurred in DSM-IV. Although it was believed to be relatively rare, it now appears that the disorder is more common than previously thought, and Asperger's disorder is diagnosed at least as frequently as autism. Whether it is a different disorder or a milder version of autistic disorder on a continuum of severity remains a matter of debate.

Because Asperger's disorder is relatively new, very little is known about its epidemiology, etiology, or pathophysiology. Because of the relative normality of intelligence and language, children with Asperger's disorder perform better in school and appear to have a better long-term outcome than do children with autistic disorder. Some are able to complete college and have normal careers.

Management strategies for Asperger's disorder are similar to those for autistic disorder, but higher expectations can be set.

Attention-Deficit and Disruptive Behavior Disorders

The attention-deficit and disruptive behavior disorders are the staples of child psychiatry. Children with these disorders are experienced as difficult

TABLE 23–6. DSM-IV-TR diagnostic criteria for Asperger's disorder

A. Qualitative impairment in social interaction, as manifested by at least two of the following:

    (1) marked impairment in the use of multiple nonverbal behaviors such as eye-to-eye gaze, facial expression, body postures, and gestures to regulate social interaction

    (2) failure to develop peer relationships appropriate to developmental level

    (3) a lack of spontaneous seeking to share enjoyment, interests, or achievements with other people (e.g., by a lack of showing, bringing, or pointing out objects of interest to other people)

    (4) lack of social or emotional reciprocity

B. Restricted repetitive and stereotyped patterns of behavior, interests, and activities, as manifested by at least one of the following:

    (1) encompassing preoccupation with one or more stereotyped and restricted patterns of interest that is abnormal in either intensity or focus

    (2) apparently inflexible adherence to specific, nonfunctional routines or rituals

    (3) stereotyped and repetitive motor mannerisms (e.g., hand or finger flapping or twisting, or complex whole-body movements)

    (4) persistent preoccupation with parts of objects

C. The disturbance causes clinically significant impairment in social, occupational, or other important areas of functioning.

D. There is no clinically significant general delay in language (e.g., single words used by age 2 years, communicative phrases used by age 3 years).

E. There is no clinically significant delay in cognitive development or in the development of age-appropriate self-help skills, adaptive behavior (other than in social interaction), and curiosity about the environment in childhood.

F. Criteria are not met for another specific Pervasive Developmental Disorder or Schizophrenia.

to manage and therefore disruptive by those around them, including parents, teachers, and often peers. Sometimes this group of disorders is referred to as involving acting-out behavior, meaning that the child expresses his or her problems outwardly rather than holding them within. This group of behavior disorders is contrasted with the internalizing disorders, such as the anxiety disorders, in which the child is considered to turn his or her suffering inward. Although closer contact with many of the children who manifest disruptive behavior makes it clear that they too may suffer a great deal internally and also may experience considerable anxiety, this aspect of the disorder is not immediately obvious to those who must deal with these children on a day-to-day basis. On superficial contact, these children may seem hard to love and even hard to like. The three major classes of disruptive behavior disorders include ADHD, conduct disorder, and oppositional defiant disorder.

Attention-Deficit/Hyperactivity Disorder

ADHD has been recognized under various names for many years—probably for many centuries. Children with this disorder are a caricature of the active child. They are physically overactive, distractible, inattentive, impulsive, and difficult to manage. They may have soft neurological signs and indices of slight delay in reaching developmental milestones. ADHD is typically evident early in childhood, with signs of increased activity being noted very early (e.g., "As soon as he could crawl, he got into everything"; "He never seemed to sleep and kicked constantly, even before he was born"). Although the disorder improves with maturation, in many individuals it persists into adulthood. Adult ADHD has become an increasingly common diagnosis.

ADHD is defined by two broad groups of symptoms: 1) difficulty focusing and maintaining attention and 2) hyperactivity and impulsivity. The DSM-IV-TR criteria for ADHD are summarized in Table 23–7. They require that at least 12 of 18 symptoms (6 from the domain of attention and 6 from the domain of hyperactivity-impulsivity) be present for at least 6 months. Subtypes can be specified to indicate whether the presentation is predominantly inattentive, predominantly hyperactive-impulsive, or mixed.

The actual manifestation of these symptoms will vary depending on the age of the child. Younger children (in the 4- to 6-year age range) are "little terrors." They run from one part of the room to another, hop on furniture, knock objects off tables, explore the contents of visitors' handbags, talk incessantly, run outside without telling their parents where they are going, have difficulty learning to look both ways before crossing the street, lose and break toys, stay up late, wake up early, and generally exhaust their parents. When these children enter school and begin the task of learning, the difficulties in focusing attention become more obvious. They may miss things that the teacher says, be unable to finish assignments, forget their pencils or notebooks, and answer the teacher's questions without holding up a hand and often without even waiting to have the question completed. They may annoy their schoolmates by pushing ahead in line, grabbing equipment on the playground, or violating the rules of games without seeming to be aware of them. These children may begin to fall behind their peers in school and to develop a poor concept of themselves. Teachers may complain about their behavior to their parents and request that help be sought.

The following is a relatively typical case history of a patient with ADHD:

TABLE 23–7. DSM-IV-TR diagnostic criteria for attention-deficit/hyperactivity disorder

A. Either (1) or (2):

    (1) six (or more) of the following symptoms of inattention have persisted for at least 6 months to a degree that is maladaptive and inconsistent with developmental level:

    Inattention

        (a) often fails to give close attention to details or makes careless mistakes in schoolwork, work, or other activities

        (b) often has difficulty sustaining attention in tasks or play activities

        (c) often does not seem to listen when spoken to directly

        (d) often does not follow through on instructions and fails to finish schoolwork, chores, or duties in the workplace (not due to oppositional behavior or failure to understand instructions)

        (e) often has difficulty organizing tasks and activities

        (f) often avoids, dislikes, or is reluctant to engage in tasks that require sustained mental effort (such as schoolwork or homework)

        (g) often loses things necessary for tasks or activities (e.g., toys, school assignments, pencils, books, or tools)

        (h) is often easily distracted by extraneous stimuli

        (i) is often forgetful in daily activities

    (2) six (or more) of the following symptoms of hyperactivity-impulsivity have persisted for at least 6 months to a degree that is maladaptive and inconsistent with developmental level:

    Hyperactivity

        (a) often fidgets with hands or feet or squirms in seat

        (b) often leaves seat in classroom or in other situations in which remaining seated is expected

        (c) often runs about or climbs excessively in situations in which it is inappropriate (in adolescents or adults, may be limited to subjective feelings of restlessness)

        (d) often has difficulty playing or engaging in leisure activities quietly

        (e) is often "on the go" or often acts as if "driven by a motor"

        (f) often talks excessively

    Impulsivity

        (g) often blurts out answers before questions have been completed

        (h) often has difficulty awaiting turn

        (i) often interrupts or intrudes on others (e.g., butts into conversations or games)

TABLE 23–7.   DSM-IV-TR diagnostic criteria for attention-deficit/hyperactivity disorder *(continued)*

B. Some hyperactive-impulsive or inattentive symptoms that caused impairment were present before age 7 years.
C. Some impairment from the symptoms is present in two or more settings (e.g., at school [or work] and at home).
D. There must be clear evidence of clinically significant impairment in social, academic, or occupational functioning.
E. The symptoms do not occur exclusively during the course of a Pervasive Developmental Disorder, Schizophrenia, or other Psychotic Disorder and are not better accounted for by another mental disorder (e.g., Mood Disorder, Anxiety Disorder, Dissociative Disorder, or a Personality Disorder).

Code based on type:

314.01   **Attention-Deficit/Hyperactivity Disorder, Combined Type:** if both Criteria A1 and A2 are met for the past 6 months

314.00   **Attention-Deficit/Hyperactivity Disorder, Predominantly Inattentive Type:** if Criterion A1 is met but Criterion A2 is not met for the past 6 months

314.01   **Attention-Deficit/Hyperactivity Disorder, Predominantly Hyperactive-Impulsive Type:** if Criterion A2 is met but Criterion A1 is not met for the past 6 months

Coding note: For individuals (especially adolescents and adults) who currently have symptoms that no longer meet full criteria, "In Partial Remission" should be specified.

Charlie, a 6-year-old boy, was brought in by his mother after a recent school conference in which it was pointed out that he seemed to be having difficulty in adjusting to first grade.

Charlie's mother described that he had always been a somewhat difficult child. He was the second of two, and his older sister Mary (age 9) had always been much quieter and more pliable. Charlie's mother had assumed that much of Charlie's disruptive behavior was because "little boys tend to be more active." Whereas Mary had responded well to encouragement to put her toys away each evening and had kept their various components intact (e.g., puzzles in their boxes, Lincoln Logs in their containers), Charlie never seemed to be able to keep track of anything or put it away. He had been a whiny infant who had had colic. Even as an infant, he was irritable and overactive. He learned to crawl at 7 months and was soon exploring the entire house, leaving a wake of emptied wastepaper baskets and disrupted cupboards behind him. He did not seem to be able to remember or follow through with parental instructions that he should keep his feet off the furniture, not walk on the tops of tables, and not run through the living room carrying melting chocolate popsicles. As he learned to talk, he seemed to talk incessantly and to be continuously in need of attention from his parents. Attempts to ignore his attention-seeking behavior seemed to have little effect on him. His parents complained that he was a "perpetual-motion machine."

He began to attend preschool at age 4 years. His teachers at that time complained that he was disruptive and impulsive, seeming to have little consideration for the other children in the school. The same noisy, attention-seeking behavior that occurred at home was noticed at the preschool. Similar complaints were registered by his teacher when he entered kindergarten the following year. After 3 months of first grade, the patience of the public school system was already exhausted. Charlie's teacher complained that it was difficult to even get through a routine class day because of Charlie's behavior. He would not sit in his seat like the other children and would often get up and run around the room. He could not work on an assignment for more than 5 minutes without being distracted. He would also distract his classmates by talking to them when they were supposed to be working quietly. None of the teacher's efforts seemed to be effective in quieting or calming Charlie.

On initial evaluation, Charlie was noted to be quite active. He entered the doctor's office with a firm, aggressive step. He jumped on his chair rather than sitting down, finally squirming himself into a sitting position, which he maintained for only 2 or 3 minutes. He then jumped up and began pulling books off the bookshelves, asking what they were for in a somewhat immature, whiny-sounding tone of voice. When told that they belonged to the doctor and should be placed back on the shelf, he threw one or two on the floor and proceeded to the doctor's desk to examine the pens, pencils, and paperweights. Charlie's mother looked embarrassed and exasperated and tried to get him to sit back down.

An individual evaluation with Charlie alone, involving an attempt to put a puzzle together, indicated that Charlie indeed did have problems focusing his attention on a relatively simple task. He was given a five-piece puzzle that the average 6-year-old can complete quickly. Charlie put one piece in place and then lost interest, instead pounding another puzzle piece on the floor and then throwing the remainder across the room. He was unable to perform any tests of graphesthesia. After five tries, when asked to write the first six letters of the alphabet, he completed four with one letter reversal and then lost interest. He also reversed the letter "r" when writing his name. He could not distinguish between right and left at any level. Otherwise, his physical examination was totally normal.

The clinician decided to prescribe methylphenidate. Within 1 week, his mother related that the effects were "amazing." Almost immediately, Charlie's behavior improved, and he showed a distinct increase in his ability to focus attention and a decrease in impulsive, overactive behavior. His teacher also noticed a distinct difference. He was able to complete the first grade with only minimal difficulty and was considered to have appropriate progress for his age in basic skills of learning to read and to do very simple arithmetic.

Although ADHD was originally defined as a childhood disorder, increasing numbers of adults also have been given diagnoses of ADHD during the past few years. The rising incidence of adult ADHD has raised concerns about overdiagnosis, risks of substance abuse because the disorder is treated with psychostimulants, and propensity for secondary gain. DSM-IV-TR is very explicit in requiring that ADHD cannot be diagnosed in adults without documentation of a childhood diagnosis, and the clinician should exert great care in documenting evidence of a childhood onset. Individuals with adult ADHD may present with difficulties at work caused by inattentiveness as their chief complaint. Alternatively, they may seek treatment because of problems with impulsive behavior that is troublesome. Because the disorder is covered by the Americans With Disabilities Act, some individuals with adult ADHD may request special treatment at work. Furthermore, because the disorder is treated with psychostimulants such as methylphenidate or amphetamine and because comorbid substance abuse is not uncommon even in childhood or adolescent ADHD, careful assessment is also needed to rule out the possibility that the patient is simply attempting to obtain illegal drugs through a legal mechanism. Obviously, however, some cases of adult ADHD are quite legitimate. Therefore, issues around the diagnosis and treatment of adult ADHD are currently very controversial.

Epidemiology

Because the definition of ADHD has changed over time, its prevalence is uncertain, but it is definitely common in young and school-aged children. Estimates range from 3% to 10%. It is far more common in boys than in girls, with a male-to-female ratio of approximately 3:1.

Etiology and Pathophysiology

The etiology and pathophysiology of ADHD are uncertain, but substantial strides have been made in the past decade in studies of the pathophysiology and etiology of ADHD. Genetic, environmental, neurobiological, and social explanations have been proposed. It is well documented that ADHD runs in families, based principally on family studies. Not only does ADHD itself show a familial aggregation, particularly in males, but other psychiatric disorders aggregate with it as well. There is an association with mood disorder, learning disorders, substance abuse, and antisocial personality disorder. There may be a gender threshold effect, in that girls with ADHD have a stronger family history of ADHD than do boys.

Genetic studies have begun to identify the underlying mechanisms for familial transmission. Because dopamine mediates brain reward systems and because the treatments used for ADHD (i.e., psychostimulants) may work through the dopamine system, genes related to dopamine have received special attention. In particular, the dopamine D_4 receptor, which is prominent in limbic regions and associated with novelty-seeking behavior, has been implicated. The gene for D_4 has a mutation involving a 48-bp repeat sequence that is seen more frequently in children with ADHD, suggesting a link between D_4 receptor pathology and ADHD. A mutation in the gene for the dopamine transporter has been identified in 55% of the patients with ADHD, as compared with 8% of the control subjects.

Nongenetic factors also may be important in the development of ADHD. Initial descriptions of ADHD referred to the disorder as *minimal brain dysfunction.* Most nongenetic explanations have stressed the role of perinatal problems such as maternal substance abuse, obstetrical complications during delivery, maternal nutrition, exposure to toxins, and viral infections. The possible role of such nongenetic factors is consistent with the higher prevalence of ADHD in males, as well as the gender threshold effect, because male children are more vulnerable to prenatal and perinatal injury. Children with well-documented perinatal problems, such as those with fetal alcohol syndrome, tend to have prominent behavior problems that include inattention, hyperactivity, and impulsivity.

In vivo neuroimaging has added to our knowledge of the neural mechanisms of ADHD. Although clinical CT and MRI scans are typically normal, more focused research studies have indicated various abnormalities in children and adults with ADHD. Quantitative MRI studies indicate that the prefrontal cortex, basal ganglia, and cerebellum either are reduced in size or have abnormalities in asymmetry in ADHD. These findings correlate well with neuropsychological data, which indicate that individuals with ADHD have difficulties in response inhibition, executive functions mediated through the prefrontal cortex, or timing functions mediated through the cerebellum. Functional imaging studies with positron emission tomography (PET) and MRI also have examined abnormalities in blood flow and metabolism in ADHD. These studies are generally consistent with the structural and anatomical studies, in that they have shown hypoperfusion in prefrontal and basal ganglia regions that may be reversible with psychostimulant treatment.

Neuropsychological studies have examined the cognitive mechanisms that may explain the clinical symptoms of ADHD. It is not surprising that tests of executive functions mediated through the prefrontal cortex are impaired, such as formulating an abstract plan, structuring and organizing the narration of a story, and multitasking. Working memory, another prefrontal function, is impaired in ADHD. Because encoding is a key component in working memory, and because encoding is closely linked to the ability to focus attention, this deficit may explain some symptoms of the disorder. Furthermore, children and adults with ADHD have difficulty inhibiting inappropriate responses that may be selected impulsively rather than through the guidance of executive prefrontal mechanisms. Response inhibition is tested through a variety of neuropsychological tests, such as the Stroop Test and the Wisconsin Card Sorting Test (see Chapter 4).

Psychosocial explanations for ADHD stress the role of parental anxiety and inexperience, as well as failure to extinguish undesirable behavior by ignoring it (often difficult to do with hyperactive children). Parents may become uncertain of their parenting skills when faced with a child who seems so difficult to control or shape, thereby conveying uncertainty or anxiety to him or her.

Course and Outcome

The long-term course and outcome of ADHD are variable. Approximately one-half of the children with this disorder have a good outcome, completing school on schedule with acceptable grades consistent with their family background and family expectations. For a time, it was assumed that most children with ADHD would grow out of it. This does not seem to be the case in many individuals, however, and approximately half of the patients who are given the diagnosis of ADHD during childhood continue to show some problems with attention and impulsivity as adults.

Some patients with ADHD have a relatively poor outcome. Twenty-five percent subsequently meet criteria for antisocial personality disorder as adults. Children given this diagnosis also have higher rates of substance abuse, more arrests, more suicide attempts, and more car accidents, and they complete fewer years of school than children without ADHD. Problems with confidence and self-esteem may be prominent because the disorder invites rejection by both parents and peers.

Differential Diagnosis

The differential diagnosis of ADHD includes a wide variety of disorders. In making a differential diagnosis, the clinician must be aware that a child with this disorder may have comorbidity with other disorders common in childhood, such as seizure disorders, other disruptive behavior disorders (e.g., conduct disorder and oppositional defiant disorder), and learning disorders.

When any of these disorders is present, it is often difficult to distinguish which is primary and which is secondary. Other disorders that may present with similar symptoms include childhood bipolar disorder, childhood depression, conduct disorder, a normal response to a pathological or abusive home environment (e.g., physical abuse or neglect by the parents), or a neuroendocrine abnormality, such as thyroid disorder.

Clinical Management

The clinical management of ADHD often involves a combination of somatic therapy and behavioral management.

Most children respond favorably to psychostimulants. Methylphenidate in a dose of 10–60 mg/day usually is the first line of treatment, followed by D-amphetamine in a dose of 5–40 mg/day. If neither of these succeeds, pemoline (another psychostimulant), tricyclic antidepressants (e.g., imipramine), or bupropion may be used. In general, methylphenidate and D-amphetamine offer short-term effects, lasting 4–6 hours, whereas the effects of the antidepressants tend to last longer. Further information about the rational use of psychostimulants is found in Chapter 27.

Behavioral and environmental management are also important. Parents will benefit from learning basic techniques of behavioral management, such as the value of positive reinforcement and firm, nonpunitive limit setting. They can also be taught techniques for reducing stimulation, thereby diminishing distractibility and inattentiveness. For example, young hyperactive children do better playing with only one friend rather than in groups. Noisy or complex toys should be avoided, as should toys that encourage impulsivity and aggression. The parent may want to work closely with the child in completing homework tasks and to teach him or her the value of working on tasks in the single, small increments that are best suited to the child's relatively short attention span, mastering one completely before going on to another.

Conduct Disorder

Conduct disorder is characterized by a pattern of behavior that violates the rights of others, such as stealing, lying, or cheating. In terms of both behavior and diagnostic criteria, conduct disorder can be considered to be a forerunner of antisocial personality disorder in adults because it involves similar antisocial behavior. Nevertheless, not all children who manifest conduct disorder develop antisocial personality disorder as adults. With appropriate treatment and rehabilitation, many of these children go on to lead acceptable and normal adult lives.

The DSM-IV-TR criteria for conduct disorder appear in Table 23–8. The criteria require the presence of at least 3 of 15 antisocial behaviors in the past 12 months (with at least 1 criterion present in the past 6 months). The criteria define four major domains of relevant behavior: aggression toward people and animals, destruction of property, deceitfulness or theft, and serious violations of rules. Individuals who manifest this delinquent behavior are further subdivided into two different types. The *childhood-onset type* begins before age 10 years and probably has a more guarded prognosis, whereas the *adolescent-onset type* begins after age 10 years and is more likely to have a better outcome.

As is the case for antisocial personality disorder (the adult equivalent of conduct disorder), the DSM-IV-TR criteria stress behavior in the definition of conduct disorder, as opposed to values, motives, or attitudes. Although the objective behavioral definition clearly improves reliability, some critics have expressed the concern that these behavioral definitions ignore the true core phenomena of delinquency and antisocial personality: shallowness of relationships and attachments, an inability to feel for others, and an impaired capacity to feel guilt. A distinction between group delinquency and solitary aggressive behavior has been used to refine the definition by stressing that young delinquents who commit antisocial acts as part of a gang are able to form some ties to others. Recent episodes of "wilding" make it clear, however, that group delinquents can commit senseless acts of violence that also seem to indicate a fundamental and severe lack of moral sense.

Children and adolescents who present with signs and symptoms of conduct disorder are a very mixed group, and most clinicians regard this category as fundamentally quite heterogeneous, with respect to both etiology and outcome. The child seen in a psychiatry clinic for conduct disorder is usually brought in at someone else's request after he or she has committed some kind of socially unacceptable behavior, such as lying, cheating, stealing, fighting, or assaulting others. Some children come from families in which this type of behavior is not unusual, but others perform these acts in a more middle-class context, thereby shocking and dismaying their parents. The degree of parental support for the child, and assistance in modifying his or her behavior, will vary substantially.

Children or adolescents with conduct disorder typically are angry, sullen, and resentful when placed in the context of the adult world, with its pressures to conform, stay in school, and persist in conspicuously dull activities. School performance usually is average to poor. These children or adolescents typically consider their schoolwork irrelevant or uninteresting, do not complete homework, and often cut class to joyride with buddies, smoke

TABLE 23–8. DSM-IV-TR diagnostic criteria for conduct disorder

A. A repetitive and persistent pattern of behavior in which the basic rights of others or major age-appropriate societal norms or rules are violated, as manifested by the presence of three (or more) of the following criteria in the past 12 months, with at least one criterion present in the past 6 months:

Aggression to people and animals

(1) often bullies, threatens, or intimidates others

(2) often initiates physical fights

(3) has used a weapon that can cause serious physical harm to others (e.g., a bat, brick, broken bottle, knife, gun)

(4) has been physically cruel to people

(5) has been physically cruel to animals

(6) has stolen while confronting a victim (e.g., mugging, purse snatching, extortion, armed robbery)

(7) has forced someone into sexual activity

Destruction of property

(8) has deliberately engaged in fire setting with the intention of causing serious damage

(9) has deliberately destroyed others' property (other than by fire setting)

Deceitfulness or theft

(10) has broken into someone else's house, building, or car

(11) often lies to obtain goods or favors or to avoid obligations (i.e., "cons" others)

(12) has stolen items of nontrivial value without confronting a victim (e.g., shoplifting, but without breaking and entering; forgery)

Serious violations of rules

(13) often stays out at night despite parental prohibitions, beginning before age 13 years

(14) has run away from home overnight at least twice while living in parental or parental surrogate home (or once without returning for a lengthy period)

(15) is often truant from school, beginning before age 13 years

B. The disturbance in behavior causes clinically significant impairment in social, academic, or occupational functioning.

C. If the individual is age 18 years or older, criteria are not met for Antisocial Personality Disorder.

TABLE 23–8.   DSM-IV-TR diagnostic criteria for conduct disorder (*continued*)

Code based on age at onset:
   312.81   **Conduct Disorder, Childhood-Onset Type:**   onset of at least one criterion characteristic of Conduct Disorder prior to age 10 years
   312.82   **Conduct Disorder, Adolescent-Onset Type:**   absence of any criteria characteristic of Conduct Disorder prior to age 10 years
   312.89   **Conduct Disorder, Unspecified Onset:**   age at onset is not known

Specify severity:

Mild: few if any conduct problems in excess of those required to make the diagnosis **and** conduct problems cause only minor harm to others

Moderate: number of conduct problems and effect on others intermediate between "mild" and "severe"

Severe: many conduct problems in excess of those required to make the diagnosis or conduct problems cause considerable harm to others

pot, or drink beer. When with their peers, their anger and sullenness often disappear, and they seem to be having a good time. Beneath the veneer of anger, toughness, and rebellion, however, they often have profound feelings of self-doubt and worthlessness, although they may be reluctant to discuss these feelings with either adults or their peers. Some children with conduct disorder have been either physically or sexually abused by their parents.

The following is a representative case history of a child with conduct disorder:

> Heather, a 14-year-old girl, was brought to the child psychiatry clinic by her mother with the complaint that "Heather is getting out of hand. I just can't seem to discipline her anymore." Heather was the youngest of four children and the only girl in the family. She was the product of a normal pregnancy and delivery and had completed her developmental milestones on schedule. She had been an average student but had taken a particular interest in sports as a child. Her three older siblings were all boys, and she tended to tag along after them and play with them and their friends whenever they would permit. Her brother Tom, with whom she was closest, was 3 years older. Heather was noted to be somewhat stubborn and moody as a child and was occasionally defiant but otherwise had seemed completely normal.
>
> Heather's father was a truck driver and was often away from the family, leaving the mother to rear the four children largely by herself. Heather's mother remained at home with the children until Heather was in second grade and then took a job as a clerk in a store. Both parents had completed high school and had similar expectations for their children. Although the two oldest boys had some problems with drinking, using drugs, and truancy, both were able to complete high school. Both obtained jobs, married,

and settled down. Tom, a high school senior, was currently showing behavior similar to that of his older brothers, but his school performance was adequate, and he appeared to be due for graduation in the spring, with plans to join the military thereafter.

Heather's parents had separated and divorced 3 years earlier. This appeared to bother Heather much more than the boys because she had always been "her father's little girl." Her father had developed a relationship with a woman in another city, had moved away, saw the children infrequently, and was not dependable in child support payments. Heather had not told her sixth-grade friends about the separation and divorce for many months because she felt embarrassed and ashamed.

Heather's behavior problems began when she entered junior high school. She began to enter puberty in sixth grade, and by seventh grade, her body was markedly feminized. Her mother reported that she seemed to react to this by "acting tougher instead of more like a girl." She started to hang out more with boys her own age or slightly older and began to smoke cigarettes secretly (although the evidence was smelled all over the house and on her clothes). Her grades, previously average, began to drop steadily. She also showed signs of increasingly devious behavior, lying to her mother about where she was going, returning at night well past predefined deadlines, and staying home "sick" without telling her mother (having called the school herself to report the "illness" in her mother's guise). Items that Heather could not afford, such as expensive costume jewelry and cosmetics, began to appear in the house. Heather's mother suspected her of having stolen these things, but Heather insisted that they were gifts from friends. Several times, her mother found marijuana in Heather's room. Whenever Heather's mother confronted her, Heather became angry and ran out of the house. Several times she stayed away overnight without telling her mother of her whereabouts.

When interviewed alone, Heather was initially evasive and defensive, looking at the floor and answering questions very briefly. She was an attractive, slightly overweight, dark-haired girl attired in conventional teenage garb with a slightly punk touch (multiple earrings in her ears, leather boots, sleeveless T-shirt showing a nude couple embracing and bearing and obscene logo). Eventually she admitted to most of the conduct abnormalities that her mother had described.

As a consequence of this assessment, it was concluded that Heather was having difficulties but that she had many strengths as well: a relatively intact childhood, normal intelligence, a history of adequate school performance, and a mother who appeared to genuinely care about her. Heather was seen in individual therapy on a weekly basis for 3–4 months, with a primary emphasis on supportive and relationship approaches. Heather responded well to this therapy and began to talk freely about her difficulties in adjusting to the loss of her father, her experience of entering puberty, and her confusion about whether it was better to relate to her male peers (from whom she desperately desired love and approval) as a "tough girl" or a "sexy girl." With Heather's permission, she was also seen jointly with her mother in family therapy, and on several occasions, her older brother joined as well. Tom was able to assist his mother by assuming the role of a surrogate father and encouraging his "little sis" to be more honest, to attend school regularly, and to behave in ways that he and his older brothers could be proud of. Heather responded well to this increased attention and support, and it was possible to terminate the therapy successfully at the end of the school year.

Epidemiology

Approximately 10% of males and 2% of females younger than 18 meet criteria for conduct disorder. The rate in females may be increasing.

Etiology and Pathophysiology

The etiology and pathophysiology of conduct disorder are almost certainly multifactorial. Family studies indicate that children with conduct disorder tend to come from families that have increased prevalence rates of antisocial personality disorder, mood disorder, substance abuse, and learning disorders. Adopted children may have higher rates of conduct disorder, consistent with reports that the adopted offspring of female felons have a high rate of antisocial behavior, such as traffic violations or arrests for robbery, which suggests that there may be at least some genetic component to conduct disorder. Apart from a possible genetic component, no specific neurobiological factors have been identified in children with conduct disorders to any consistent degree, although a slight increase in neurological soft signs and psychomotor seizures has been observed.

Psychosocial factors probably play a major role in the development of conduct disorders. Psychosocial factors that have been shown to have some relation to conduct disorders include parental separation or divorce; parental substance abuse; forms of poor parenting such as rejection, abandonment, abuse, inadequate supervision, and inconsistent or excessively harsh discipline; and association with a delinquent peer group.

Course and Outcome

The long-term course and outcome of conduct disorders are variable, although about 40% of the boys and 25% of the girls with conduct disorder will develop adult antisocial personality disorder. To some extent, outcome depends on the degree of socialization and aggressiveness. Children with the "socialized" types of conduct disorder tend to have a much better outcome, as do children who are less aggressive. As children get older, the severity of the conduct disorder worsens in that teenagers or young adults get into increasingly serious problems that may eventually lead to incarceration.

Differential Diagnosis

Conduct disorders have considerable comorbidity with other childhood disorders. Among those that often coexist with conduct disorder are learning disorders, ADHD, and mood disorders. The clinician often will encounter these disorders in the differential diagnosis of conduct disorder because these disorders most commonly must be distinguished from conduct disorder. From 60% to 70% of the children who present with ADHD also meet criteria for conduct disorder. At least 10% of the children with conduct disorder have specific learning disorders. In general, the greater the comorbidity, the more complicated the case, and the worse the outcome.

Clinical Management

The clinical management of conduct disorders varies greatly, depending on the age of the child, the symptoms with which he or she presents, the extent of comorbidity, the availability of family supports, and the child's intellectual and social assets. A relatively mild case of conduct disorder, such as was represented by Heather in the case history earlier in this chapter, typically is treated with individual and family therapy. At the opposite extreme are those cases in which the child comes from a highly deviant family and engages in repeated antisocial acts that bring him or her to legal attention; such cases may require removal from the home and placement in a group home or perhaps even in a juvenile detention facility. In some situations, an important part of managing the child with a conduct disorder involves training his or her parents to become more effective as parents. Parental effectiveness training involves instructing parents on how best to communicate with their child, apply appropriate and consistent discipline, monitor the child's whereabouts, and steer the child away from bad peers. Early reports suggest that this approach may offer the best hope for the errant child.

Children and adolescents with conduct disorder who have comorbid disorders such as hyperactivity or seizures will benefit from medication to treat the comorbid disorder. Apart from such indications, however, medications are not typically used to treat conduct disorder. Nevertheless, both lithium carbonate and haloperidol have been shown to reduce aggression in children who are out of control.

Oppositional Defiant Disorder

Oppositional defiant disorder is a relatively new diagnosis that attempts to provide a category for children and adolescents with difficult behavior but not full-blown conduct disorder. As this category has been increasingly used, it has become apparent that many youngsters who would have received diagnoses of good-prognosis or mild conduct disorder in DSM-III are now being placed in this category. The criteria for oppositional defiant disorder are summarized in Table 23–9.

TABLE 23–9. DSM-IV-TR diagnostic criteria for oppositional defiant disorder

A. A pattern of negativistic, hostile, and defiant behavior lasting at least 6 months, during which four (or more) of the following are present:
 (1) often loses temper
 (2) often argues with adults
 (3) often actively defies or refuses to comply with adults' requests or rules
 (4) often deliberately annoys people
 (5) often blames others for his or her mistakes or misbehavior
 (6) is often touchy or easily annoyed by others
 (7) is often angry and resentful
 (8) is often spiteful or vindictive
 Note: Consider a criterion met only if the behavior occurs more frequently than is typically observed in individuals of comparable age and developmental level.
B. The disturbance in behavior causes clinically significant impairment in social, academic, or occupational functioning.
C. The behaviors do not occur exclusively during the course of a Psychotic or Mood Disorder.
D. Criteria are not met for Conduct Disorder, and, if the individual is age 18 years or older, criteria are not met for Antisocial Personality Disorder.

There is clearly a fine line between normal naughtiness and oppositional defiant disorder. Most children at times lose their tempers, argue with their parents, refuse to clean their rooms, or fail to obey a curfew. Thus, the proviso is added that these behaviors must be more frequent than those of most people at the same mental age. Clearly, however, there will be great variation in the definition of *more frequent,* depending on who is rendering the judgment. Religiously conservative or authoritarian families are likely to be less tolerant of opposition and defiance than are families with a background of behavioral abnormalities. Thus, to some extent, the appearance of children with this diagnosis in child psychiatry clinics may partially reflect a given family's threshold for accepting defiant behavior, which must be considered in treatment planning. Unlike conduct disorders, which specify that the child must have violated personal rights and social rules (thereby making it more likely that the child's deviant behavior has come to the attention of people outside the immediate family), oppositional defiant disorder is defined almost totally on the basis of annoying, difficult, and disruptive behavior.

Because this is a new disorder, very little is known about its epidemiology, etiology, pathophysiology, comorbidity, or treatment. By definition, it cannot coexist with conduct disorder, but it may coexist with ADHD. Common sense dictates that management will emphasize individual and family counseling, with treatment of comorbid hyperactivity (or possibly mood disorder) with medications as needed.

Tourette's Disorder

Tourette's disorder is a fascinating syndrome characterized by a tendency to produce vocal and motor tics. The vocal tics are typically somewhat socially offensive, such as making loud grunting or barking noises or shouting words. The words are sometimes obscenities such as "shit." The person is aware that he or she is producing the vocal tics, is able to exert a mild degree of control over them, but ultimately has to submit to them. Because people with Tourette's disorder are aware that their tics are socially inappropriate, they find them embarrassing. Motor tics occurring in Tourette's disorder are also often odd or offensive behaviors, such as tongue protrusion, sniffing, hopping, squatting, blinking, or nodding. Because most of the general public is unaware of the nature of Tourette's disorder, the behavior is seen as inappropriate or bizarre. The criteria for Tourette's disorder appear in Table 23–10.

TABLE 23–10. DSM-IV-TR diagnostic criteria for Tourette's disorder

---

A. Both multiple motor and one or more vocal tics have been present at some time during the illness, although not necessarily concurrently. (A *tic* is a sudden, rapid, recurrent, nonrhythmic, stereotyped motor movement or vocalization.)

B. The tics occur many times a day (usually in bouts) nearly every day or intermittently throughout a period of more than 1 year, and during this period there was never a tic-free period of more than 3 consecutive months.

C. The onset is before age 18 years.

D. The disturbance is not due to the direct physiological effects of a substance (e.g., stimulants) or a general medical condition (e.g., Huntington's disease or postviral encephalitis).

Tourette's disorder usually begins during childhood or early adolescence, and motor tics usually antedate vocal tics. Thus, grade school–aged children may show motor tics and some barks or grunts. During late grade school or early junior high school, vocalization of obscenities (coprolalia) begins to appear. Twenty percent have a remission of motor and vocal tics during their third decade, and most of the remaining patients with Tourette's disorder have a significant decrease in their symptoms as they grow older. Patients with Tourette's disorder may experience shame and embarrassment about their disorder, which may lead them to avoid public or social situations or even close interpersonal relationships.

Epidemiology

Tourette's disorder is relatively rare, affecting 0.4% of the population. It is more common in males than in females, with a ratio of 3:1. As with ADHD, a gender threshold effect has been observed; that is, female patients with Tourette's disorder appear to have higher genetic loading than male patients with Tourette's disorder, suggesting that there is a lower penetrance for the disorder in females.

Etiology and Pathophysiology

Research on Tourette's disorder suggests that several different mechanisms may explain the onset and occurrence of this syndrome.

One clue arises from patterns of familial aggregation. Tourette's disorder is both highly familial and comorbid with obsessive-compulsive disorder (OCD). Clinically, tics and compulsions have a superficial resemblance to each other, suggesting that these symptoms may be on a continuum with each other. Two-thirds of the first-degree relatives of patients with Tourette's disorder have tics, and a substantial number also have OCD.

Some children with Tourette's disorder have their onset of symptoms after infection with group A β-hemolytic *Streptococcus*. Streptococcal infections are a well-known cause of Sydenham's chorea, and it now appears that Tourette's disorder is a related condition. This group of syndromes is now referred to as a pediatric autoimmune neuropsychiatric disorder associated with streptococcal infections (PANDAS). Children with PANDAS have choreiform movements, obsessions, compulsions, and tics, as well as emotional lability, anxiety, and other emotional and behavioral symptoms. The mechanism behind PANDAS, and also behind at least some cases of Tourette's disorder, is the production of antistreptococcal antibodies that also have antineuronal properties and that attach to the basal ganglia.

For two decades, it has been clear that the symptoms of Tourette's disorder can be markedly improved through treatment with antipsychotic medication. Because antipsychotics exert a primary effect by blocking dopaminergic pathways in the brain, abnormalities in dopamine transmission are the most commonly hypothesized neurochemical abnormality. Because Tourette's disorder has a prominent motor component, investigators suspect that its primary abnormalities may lie within nigrostriatal projections, but (given the complex feedback loops of the dopamine system, as described in Chapter 5) many other localizations are also possible.

Differential Diagnosis

The evaluation of a patient presenting with Tourette's disorder should include a comprehensive neurological evaluation to rule out other possible causes of the tics. The patient should be examined for stigmata of Wilson's disease, and a family history should be obtained to evaluate the possibility of Huntington's disease. The patient also should be evaluated for other psychiatric conditions. Comorbidity with ADHD may occur, as may symptoms of mood disorder, anxiety disorders, or OCD.

Clinical Management

The clinical management of Tourette's disorder primarily stresses the use of antipsychotics. Haloperidol has been used for many years as the first-line treatment; doses are lower than those used to treat psychosis and tend to range from 1 to 5 mg/day. Pimozide, used for decades in Europe, also is effective; doses of 8–10 mg/day are used (maximum dose is 0.3 mg/kg/day, or a total of 20 mg/day). More recently, Tourette's disorder has been effectively treated with the atypical antipsychotics, such as risperidone. Although the treatment of Tourette's disorder stresses the use of medications, it is also important to educate the family about the disorder and to assist them in providing psychological support to the patient. Because of the social embarrassment that it produces, Tourette's disorder has a potential for serious long-term social complications, and supportive psychotherapy for the patient or family may help minimize these problems.

Separation Anxiety Disorder

Separation anxiety disorder represents a more severe and disabling form of a maturational experience that all children normally have. Most infants and children experience fear at the possibility (or reality) of being separated from their parents. Once infants learn to recognize maternal and paternal faces and shapes, they also learn to cry when the parent leaves the room or hands them to a stranger. No doubt this pattern of behavior reflects some type of primal fear of loss or fear of the unknown. As the child grows older, he or she also experiences natural fears of being left with a babysitter, being sent to preschool, or entering kindergarten. Crying, tenseness, or physical complaints may appear and last for minutes, hours, or days in such situations.

As specified in the DSM-IV-TR criteria (see Table 23–11), separation anxiety disorder is defined largely by the persistence of such symptoms for a long enough duration to be considered pathological. At least three of eight characteristic symptoms must be present for at least 4 weeks. The characteristic symptoms include three types of distress or worry (distress at being separated from home, worry that some harm will come to the parents, and worry that the child will be lost or somehow separated from them), three types of behaviors (school refusal, sleep refusal, and clinging), and two physiological symptoms (nightmares and physical complaints such as headache or nausea).

Another clinically significant anxiety disorder observed in children is variously referred to as *school phobia, school refusal,* or *school absenteeism.* Although this particular anxiety disorder is classified in DSM-IV-TR among the adult disorders as a type of social phobia, it is an important and common childhood anxiety disorder. In some cases, it may be related to separation anxiety disorder. Children with this problem develop a fear of going to school. It may begin with attendance at preschool or kindergarten, but more typically it develops during grade school or junior high school. Typically, a child who has previously been going to school (albeit with some anxiety) begins to develop methods for staying home. He or she may have repeated episodes of "illness" such as headache or nausea. Such children may be truant, leaving home with the appearance of going to school and then returning home without their parents' knowledge or going to some other environment that they experience as safe. They may simply refuse to go to school and give only some vague explanation such as "I don't like it." These various reasons explain why the problem is variously referred to as a phobia, absenteeism, or refusal. There is some controversy among child psychiatrists as to whether school refusal should be considered strictly a subset of separation anxiety disorder or should be defined more broadly to include all children who do not attend school, for whatever reason (e.g., truancy secondary to conduct disorder, avoidance of school as a complication of mood disorder, school avoidance secondary to a psychosis).

Once discovered, school avoidance should be thoroughly evaluated and

TABLE 23–11. DSM-IV-TR diagnostic criteria for separation anxiety disorder

A. Developmentally inappropriate and excessive anxiety concerning separation from home or from those to whom the individual is attached, as evidenced by three (or more) of the following:

    (1) recurrent excessive distress when separation from home or major attachment figures occurs or is anticipated

    (2) persistent and excessive worry about losing, or about possible harm befalling, major attachment figures

    (3) persistent and excessive worry that an untoward event will lead to separation from a major attachment figure (e.g., getting lost or being kidnapped)

    (4) persistent reluctance or refusal to go to school or elsewhere because of fear of separation

    (5) persistently and excessively fearful or reluctant to be alone or without major attachment figures at home or without significant adults in other settings

    (6) persistent reluctance or refusal to go to sleep without being near a major attachment figure or to sleep away from home

    (7) repeated nightmares involving the theme of separation

    (8) repeated complaints of physical symptoms (such as headaches, stomachaches, nausea, or vomiting) when separation from major attachment figures occurs or is anticipated

B. The duration of the disturbance is at least 4 weeks.

C. The onset is before age 18 years.

D. The disturbance causes clinically significant distress or impairment in social, academic (occupational), or other important areas of functioning.

E. The disturbance does not occur exclusively during the course of a Pervasive Developmental Disorder, Schizophrenia, or other Psychotic Disorder and, in adolescents and adults, is not better accounted for by Panic Disorder With Agoraphobia.

Specify if:

    Early Onset: if onset occurs before age 6 years

treated as quickly as possible to prevent personal, social, and academic complications. The clinician should attempt to determine why the child does not want to go to school. These reasons may be expressed overtly (e.g., "The kids make fun of me because I'm stupid," "I'm afraid that Jimmy Taylor will beat me up"), but often considerable investigation is needed. The child's intellectual and school performance should be evaluated to determine whether the child has some problem with academic skills, which may make him or her feel inferior and avoidant. Teachers and parents should be consulted about the child's relationships with his or her peers, and a specific effort should be made to determine whether a problem with teasing or bullying exists.

Other situations that children often find stressful may occur on the playground, in the gym, or in the school lunchroom. Young teenagers may be embarrassed about the appearance of their bodies, or they may be afraid that others will not sit with them in the lunchroom or on the bus. Clearly, the child's own self-esteem and self-concept need to be examined, and parental behavior needs to be explored to determine whether it is contributing to the child's problem or even causing it. Anxious, fearful, controlling parents may be communicating their own fears about separation to the child. They may be setting academic or social expectations so high that the child feels doomed to failure at school.

Treatment of school avoidance depends on the cause that has been identified. Often, the child will need encouragement and support from several directions: at home, at school, and from the clinician. If specific problems with academic skills are identified, remedial training should be initiated. Similar training may be appropriate for problems with athletic or social skills. Whatever the cause, however, it is important to impress on both the child and the family that the child must attend school regularly and that absenteeism or refusal will not be tolerated.

Other "Adult" Disorders Frequently Seen in Children

Several other common adult disorders may have their first onset during childhood or adolescence. Because these are syndromally similar across all ages, they are classified among the adult disorders. Two common examples are schizophrenia and mood disorder. In general, children with these disorders meet the criteria that have been defined for adults. There may be subtle differences in presentation and management, however.

Schizophrenia often presents initially during adolescence, but in rare instances the onset is during childhood. Schizophrenia in adolescents often begins insidiously, with apathy, a change in personal hygiene, and withdrawal. Schizophrenia may be particularly difficult to distinguish from depression, and it is usually preferable to make an initial diagnosis of depression if there is any doubt; after an unsuccessful trial of several different antidepressants, the diagnosis of schizophrenia is more certain. The major challenge in assessing childhood schizophrenia involves determining the difference between normal childhood fantasies and frank delusions and hallucinations. In addition, the symptoms of disorganization of speech and behavior must be distinguished from abnormalities of speech and behavior that are simply due to developmental slowness or frank mental retardation. Children with a definite diagnosis of schizophrenia usually are given antipsychotic medications, but the dose is typically lower than that in adults.

Depression in adolescents is extremely common, and it is also more common in children than was thought several decades ago. A major difference between the two ages at onset is in suicide risk: the risk is high in adolescents but much lower in children. In both age groups, the patient may present initially with physical complaints rather than the psychological complaint of depression. In young children, the complaints may be abdominal pain, nightmares, or trouble sleeping. In teenagers, complaints of fatigue, insomnia or hypersomnia, headache, or tension are common. Depression also may present initially as a disruptive behavior disorder. The somatic treatment of depression in children and adolescents is similar to that in adults, but the need for psychotherapy or family therapy is much greater.

Physical, Emotional, and Sexual Abuse

Attitudes toward the abuse of children have evolved dramatically during the past several decades. The variability in attitudes toward the rights of children versus those of adults is a striking example of the extent to which the definitions of both mental illnesses and general medical disorders are culture bound. Until the twentieth century, few adults anywhere in the world considered the possibility that children (or women, for that matter) might have any rights at all. Disciplining children through whipping and beating was considered to be good for them and to build character. Corporal punishment was routine not only at home but also within the schools. At present, the climate has changed—and is still changing—so rapidly that corporal punishment *even by parents* has been outlawed in Sweden, and teachers, physicians, and social workers in the United States are trained to be alert for signs of physical and emotional abuse in the children they see.

Within Western society, sexual activity in children was considered abnormal and was vigorously repressed until very recently. ("Masturbation will lead to blindness," as children and teenagers were sometimes taught as recently as 40 or 50 years ago.) At the other extreme, initiation into sexuality at the time of puberty, often by an older relative, has been and is still the norm in some non-Western societies. Thus, it is difficult to formulate absolute and immutable rules as to what constitutes physical, emotional, and sexual abuse and how this abuse should be assessed and treated. Nevertheless, these forms of abuse are a matter of increasing concern to psychiatrists and primary care providers, who often must assume front-line responsibility for recognizing and managing them.

Given the problems of definition, the epidemiology of physical and emotional abuse is at best uncertain. Nevertheless, this abuse is common, and it may be increasing rather than decreasing. The National Center on Child Abuse estimated that 2%–3% of children have been abused; approximately two-thirds of the cases involved neglect, and approximately one-quarter involved physical abuse.

Children who have been physically or emotionally abused are more likely to present with physical than with psychological symptoms. At the furthest extreme is the child who has obvious signs of physical abuse—broken bones, cigarette burns, bruises, scars, and open wounds. The signs of physical neglect or emotional abuse may be more subtle—failure to thrive; somatic complaints such as abdominal pain, sleep disturbances, and nightmares; or marked anxiety and exaggerated startle responses. The physician who notices such signs and suspects abuse must proceed both carefully and appropriately; excessive vigilance in either overdiagnosing or underdiagnosing can lead to problems. The child should be carefully evaluated on several consecutive appointments, accompanied by tactful interviewing of both child and parents or caregivers concerning behavioral difficulties, disciplining practices, feeding and bathing routines, and other key aspects of parent-child interactions. If the evidence of physical or emotional abuse is consistent and clear, then social service agencies should be contacted to conduct further investigations.

The treatment of abuse varies depending on its nature. In extreme cases, the child is removed from the home and placed in foster care. Ideally, such children and their foster parents should be provided with supportive individual and family therapy to assist in recovery from the consequences of the abuse. Those cases involving milder forms of abuse, with the child remaining in the home, should receive careful follow-up. Parents may need evaluation and treatment for problems that they are experiencing (e.g., depression, alcoholism, drug abuse), and family or marital therapy may assist in identifying interpersonal problems that trigger the abuse. Depending on the child's age and the nature of the problems, the child also will benefit from individual therapy that focuses on building confidence and coping with problems in feeling basic trust.

Sexual abuse is perhaps an even murkier area than physical and emotional abuse. Guidelines for norms in this area are also steadily evolving. On the one hand, in some subcultures, incest between siblings or between parents and children is common and is conveniently overlooked. On the other hand, some grandfathers are beginning to worry about being accused of child sexual abuse if they kiss and cuddle with their grandchildren. The definition of what constitutes sexual abuse is unclear on many fronts. Rape of a stepdaughter by a stepfather is obvious. So is seduction of a child by a teacher that involves sexual intercourse. So is a sex or prostitution ring organized by a "friendly neighbor" who frequently invites the neighborhood girls or boys to his house and rewards them with small gifts such as cosmetics, compact disc players, or drugs. But how many of the following also constitute child sexual abuse: frequent exposing of genitalia by a parent or stepparent of the opposite sex, children and parents getting into bed together on Sunday morning and reading together, taking children into opposite-sex locker rooms at a swimming pool after age 3, and intercourse between a 21-year-old male and a 16-year-old (or 12-year-old) female?

The epidemiology of sexual abuse is also unclear. Variable definitions obviously affect prevalence rates. Depending on the definition and the methods for assessment, lifetime prevalence rates range from 15% to as high as 70%. It is clear, however, that girls are more frequently victims than boys are, with a ratio of approximately 5:1.

The assessment of sexual abuse in children involves careful history taking, accompanied by a physical examination. The methods for history taking will vary depending on the age of the child and the way that he or she has come to attention. If a mother brings in a child complaining about abuse by a stepfather, the situation may be relatively straightforward (although one must be cautious about being caught in marital or other interpersonal cross fire even in such "obvious" situations). Younger children may lack the concepts or vocabulary to discuss their experiences but can explain them through storytelling or the use of anatomically explicit dolls. Older children usually can describe their experiences more directly. A physical examination should be conducted (with the child's permission), and the child may be able to explain what has happened more easily in the context of this examination. Unfortunately, the examination will not necessarily confirm the diagnosis unless obvious evidence (e.g., semen) is found.

Although it was once safe to assume that a child would not make up allegations of abuse, media attention to this issue and the ugly quarrels that may occur in divorce cases have made it clear that the clinician must approach the stories of both adults and children with some caution and skepticism.

The long-term emotional effect of childhood sexual abuse is not clear. Reports of posttraumatic stress disorders and various personality disorders secondary to childhood sexual abuse are steadily increasing. One must remember the early experience of Freud in relation to reports of childhood

Recommendations for management of disorders in children and adolescents

1. In assessing children and adolescents, the clinician should be imaginative and meet each patient on his or her own terms.
   - Problem-solving and motor skills can be evaluated by playing games.
   - Dolls and toys should be used with young children to create pretend situations that will provide insight about personal and social interactions.
2. Normal maturational levels are highly variable in children and adolescents.
3. Children and adolescents often do not have a level of cognitive development suitable for the insight-oriented and introspective approaches used with adults.
4. Establishing rapport with adolescents is difficult but may be crucial to creating a therapeutic alliance.
   - The therapist should find out what the patient is interested in and relate to him or her through these interests.
5. The clinician must not preach or judge.
6. The basic maturational task of adolescents is to disengage themselves from their parents, become independent, and define their own identities; reliance on peers is an important crutch for adolescents in this transitional period.
7. The therapist should remain neutral and try not to criticize either parents or peers.
8. Most work with adolescents will carry an inevitable transference component; the adolescent's first reaction will be to see the therapist as a parent. The therapist should try to use this transference to a therapeutic advantage, or at least to prevent it from being a therapeutic handicap.
9. It is best to strike a balance between being perceived as a good parent and being perceived as a good peer, but this balance cannot and should not (usually) be achieved by attacking the real parent or real peer.
10. Because the parents and peers of adolescents may vary in quality, the therapist needs to be flexible, insightful, and creative in dealing with transference components.
11. The clinician must be aware of the pervasiveness of comorbidity in childhood and adolescent disorders.

sexuality; originally, he believed the accounts of parental seduction that his patients reported, but he later realized that he was often hearing wish-fulfilling fantasies rather than actual experiences. Nevertheless, children who are clearly the victims of obvious and/or repeated abuse are likely to be significantly traumatized. Treatment varies depending on the situation. Most of the guidelines outlined above for physical and emotional abuse also apply to sexual abuse.

Management of Child and Adolescent Disorders

General suggestions for the management of disorders occurring in children and adolescents appear in the box.

Bibliography

Bailey AJ, Bolton P, Butler L, et al: Prevalence of the fragile X anomaly amongst autistic twins and singletons. J Child Psychol Psychiatry 34:673–688, 1993

Biederman J, Munir K, Knee D, et al: High rate of affective disorders in probands with attention deficit disorder and in their relatives: a controlled family study. Am J Psychiatry 144:330–333, 1987

Black DW: Bad Boys, Bad Men: Confronting Antisocial Personality Disorder. New York, Oxford University Press, 1999

Cantwell DP, Baker L: Developmental Speech and Language Disorders. New York, Guilford, 1987

Cohen DJ, Volkmar FR: Handbook of Autism and Pervasive Developmental Disorders, 2nd Edition. New York, Wiley, 1997

Cohen D, Bruun R, Leckman J: Tourette's Syndrome. New York, Wiley, 1988

Gemelli R: Normal Child and Adolescent Development. Washington, DC, American Psychiatric Press, 1996

Gillberg C, Coleman M (eds): The Biology of the Autistic Syndromes, 2nd Edition. New York, Cambridge University Press, 1992

Gittleman R: Anxiety Disorders of Childhood. New York, Guilford, 1986

Kanner L: Autistic disturbances of affective contact. Nerv Child 2:217–250, 1943

Kelso J, Stewart MA: Factors which predict the persistence of aggressive conduct disorder. J Child Psychol Psychiatry 27:77–86, 1986

Klin A, Sparrow SS, Volkmar FR: Asperger Syndrome. New York, Guilford, 2000

Krishnan KRR, Doraiswamy PM (eds): Brain Imaging in Clinical Psychiatry. New York, Marcel Dekker, 1997

March JS: Anxiety Disorders in Children and Adolescents. New York, Guilford, 1995

Mash EJ, Barkley RA (eds): Child Psychopathology. New York, Guilford, 1996

Pauls DL, Leckman JF: The inheritance of Gilles de la Tourette's syndrome and associated behaviors. N Engl J Med 315:993–997, 1986

Piven J, Nehme E, Siman J, et al: Magnetic resonance imaging in autism: measurement of the cerebellum, pons, and fourth ventricle. Biol Psychiatry 31:491–504, 1992

Popper CW, West SA: Disorders usually first diagnosed in infancy, childhood, or adolescence, in The American Psychiatric Press Textbook of Psychiatry, 3rd Edition. Edited by Hales RE, Yudofsky SC, Talbot JA. Washington, DC, American Psychiatric Press, 1999, pp 825–954

Rumsey JM, Andreasen NC, Rapoport JL: Thought, language, communication, and affective flattening in autistic adults. Arch Gen Psychiatry 43:771–777, 1986

Rutter M: Pathways from childhood to adult life. J Child Psychol Psychiatry 8:1–11, 1989

Rutter M, Taylor E, Hersov L: Child and Adolescent Psychiatry, 3rd Edition. Oxford, UK, Blackwell Scientific, 1994

Shapiro E, Shapiro AK, Fulop G, et al: Controlled study of haloperidol, pimozide, and placebo for the treatment of Gilles de la Tourette's syndrome. Arch Gen Psychiatry 46:722–730, 1989

Silver LB: Attention-Deficit/Hyperactivity Disorder: A Clinical Guide to Diagnosis and Treatment for Health and Mental Health Professionals, 2nd Edition. Washington, DC, American Psychiatric Press, 1999

Swedo SE: Sydenham's chorea: a model for childhood autoimmune neuropsychiatric disorders. JAMA 272:1788–1791, 1994

Swedo SE, Leonard HL, Garvey M, et al: Pediatric autoimmune neuropsychiatric disorders associated with streptococcal infections: clinical description of the first 50 cases. Am J Psychiatry 154:264–271, 1998

Volkmar F (ed): Psychoses and Pervasive Developmental Disorders in Childhood and Adolescence. Washington, DC, American Psychiatric Press, 1996

Volkmar F, Klin A, Schultz RT, et al: Asperger's disorder. Am J Psychiatry 157:262–267, 2000

Yu S, Pritchard M, Kremer E, et al: Fragile X genotype characterized by an unstable region of DNA. Science 252:1179–1181, 1991

Self-Assessment Questions

1. Describe some techniques that are useful in assessing younger children and establishing rapport with them.
2. Describe some techniques that are useful in assessing adolescents and establishing rapport with them.
3. List and describe the various types of nonphysician clinicians who may be helpful in assessing and managing children and adolescents.
4. Give four examples of psychiatric conditions that often are comorbid in children and adolescents.
5. What IQ range defines children within 1 standard deviation of the population mean of 100? What percentage of children fall in this range?

What IQ range encompasses children between 1 and 2 standard deviations from the mean? What percentage of the population falls in this range? List the IQ levels that are used to define borderline intelligence and mild, moderate, severe, and profound mental retardation. Discuss the distinction between autism, mental retardation, and learning disorders. List three well-recognized causes of mental retardation.

6. Why is it important to obtain IQ testing and educational testing in some children and adolescents? Give three examples in which the use of such testing may be crucial either to establishing a diagnosis or to planning treatment.

7. List three disorders of childhood or adolescence that may be comorbid with a seizure disorder and for which an EEG may be a useful laboratory assessment procedure.

8. List three disorders of childhood or adolescence for which karyotyping may be useful.

9. Describe four simple tests to assess soft neurological signs in children.

10. Define learning disorder, and list the three skills that are commonly affected.

11. Describe the three major domains that are abnormal in autism, and give examples of signs and symptoms within these domains. How common is autism? What are its long-term course and outcome? What methods are used to treat it?

12. List the two broad categories of symptoms used to define ADHD, and give several examples of each. Describe the long-term course and outcome of ADHD. Identify two medications commonly used to treat ADHD and specify the appropriate dose range.

13. Describe the symptoms of conduct disorder. What are the prevalence and gender ratio for conduct disorder? What are the long-term course and outcome of conduct disorder? Give two different case vignettes of conduct disorder, and describe appropriate treatment for each.

14. Describe the clinical features of Tourette's disorder. What are the hypothesized pathophysiology and etiology of this disorder? How common is it? Describe two pharmacological strategies for treating Tourette's disorder.

15. Describe oppositional defiant disorder and discuss its relation to conduct disorder.

16. Describe separation anxiety disorder and discuss its relation to school refusal (phobia, avoidance). List three factors that may predispose to the development of school avoidance. Describe three approaches to treating school avoidance.

17. Why do you think most disorders of childhood and adolescence are more common in boys than in girls? (The answer to this question is not really included in the chapter, and if you can come up with a definitive answer, you may be on your way to winning a Nobel Prize!)

24 Sleep Disorders

The woods are lovely, dark and deep.
But I have promises to keep,
and miles to go before I sleep.

Robert Frost

Sleep disorders are among the most common complaints that people report to their physicians. More than 60 million Americans have sleep-related complaints, and about 20% of patients consulting a general practitioner report sleep disturbances. Insomnia is the most common sleep disorder; each year, between 20% and 50% of adults report difficulty sleeping, and about 17% consider the problem serious. Because sleep disorders are so common, it is important for clinicians to be familiar with them.

The classification and management of sleep disorders have evolved as physicians and researchers have learned more about them. DSM-IV-TR divides the sleep disorders into two major subgroups: the *dyssomnias* and the *parasomnias*. The predominant disturbance in dyssomnias is in initiating and maintaining sleep. The predominant disturbance in parasomnias is an abnormal event occurring during sleep. A category exists for *sleep disorders related to another mental disorder*, such as major depression or borderline personality disorder. A residual category also exists for other sleep disorders that may result from the effects of a general medical condition or the physiological effects of a substance. The sleep disorders are listed in Table 24–1.

TABLE 24–1. DSM-IV-TR sleep disorders

Dyssomnias

    Primary insomnia

    Primary hypersomnia

    Narcolepsy

    Breathing-related sleep disorder

    Circadian rhythm sleep disorder

    Dyssomnia not otherwise specified

Parasomnias

    Nightmare disorder

    Sleep terror disorder

    Sleepwalking disorder

    Parasomnia not otherwise specified

Sleep disorders related to another mental disorder

    Insomnia related to an Axis I or Axis II disorder

    Hypersomnia related to an Axis I or Axis II disorder

Other sleep disorders

    Sleep disorder due to a general medical condition

    Substance-induced sleep disorder

Although the diagnostic criteria do not include data from laboratory procedures such as polysomnography (a procedure in which electroencephalographic, electrooculographic, and electromyographic tracings are recorded during sleep), these data may be necessary in some patients to thoroughly investigate their disorder. Polysomnography provides data on sleep continuity, sleep architecture, rapid eye movement (REM) physiology, sleep-related breathing impairment, oxygen desaturation, cardiac arrhythmias, and periodic movements. The Multiple Sleep Latency Test (MSLT) often is used to measure excessive sleepiness. With the MSLT, the patient is given an opportunity to fall asleep in a darkened room for five 20-minute periods in 2-hour intervals across the patient's usual period of wakefulness. The average latency to sleep onset, measured polysomnographically, is a measure of the tendency to fall asleep. An average sleep latency of less than 5 minutes indicates the presence of pathological sleepiness.

Normal Sleep and Sleep Architecture

The average healthy adult requires about 7½ hours of sleep per night, although some persons require more and some less to feel sufficiently rested. Normal sleep is influenced by many factors; for example, young persons tend to sleep more than the elderly, whose total sleep time is decreased because of various factors associated with aging. Furthermore, the longer a person has been awake, the more quickly he or she falls asleep (i.e., sleep latency).

In the adult, sleep stages are divided into REM and non-REM (NREM) sleep. These two stages of sleep alternate in a cycle that lasts between 70 and 120 minutes. Generally, four to six NREM-REM cycles occur nightly. The first REM period lasts from 5 to 10 minutes; as the night progresses, REM periods tend to become longer and closer together and show progressively greater density of rapid eye movements. (Figure 24–1 depicts a polysomnographic recording during the various sleep stages.)

The normal sleep stages of an adult are as follows:

- *Stage 0* is a period of wakefulness with eyes closed, which occurs just before sleep onset. The electroencephalogram (EEG) mainly shows sinusoidal alpha waves over the occiput, which have a frequency of 8–12 cycles/sec and a fairly low amplitude (or voltage). Muscle tone tends to be increased. Alpha activity decreases with increasing drowsiness.
- *Stage 1* is called the sleep-onset stage, or drowsiness, because it provides a brief transition from wakefulness to sleep. Alpha activity diminishes to less than 50% of the EEG recording. There is a low-amplitude, mixed-frequency signal, composed mostly of beta and the slower theta (4–7 cycles/sec) activity. Stage 1 accounts for about 5% of the total sleep period.
- *Stage 2* is dominated by theta activity and is characterized by the appearance of sleep spindles and K complexes. *Sleep spindles* are brief bursts of rhythmic (12–14 cycles/sec) waves with a duration of 500–1500 msec. *K complexes* are sharp, negative, high-voltage EEG waves, followed by slower, positive activity, with a duration of 500 msec. They are thought to represent a CNS response to internal stimuli; they also can be elicited during sleep with external stimuli, such as a loud noise. Stage 2 usually accounts for between 45% and 55% of the total sleep time.
- *Stage 3* is characterized by 20%–50% high-voltage delta wave activity, with a frequency of 1–2 cycles/sec. Like Stage 2, muscle tone is increased, but eye movements are absent.
- *Stage 4* occurs when delta waves compose more than 50% of the EEG re-

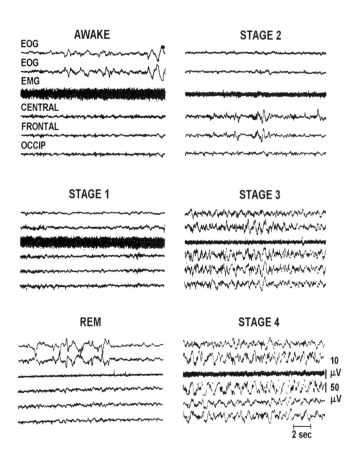

FIGURE 24–1.   Polysomnographic recording during the various stages of sleep. Notice the high electromyogram (EMG) and eye movements during wakefulness, the slow eye movements but absence of rapid eye movements (REMs) during descending Stage 1, and REMs with low EMG during stage REM. Stages 2, 3, and 4 are characterized by the slowing of frequency and an increase in amplitude of the electroencephalogram.

EOG = electrooculogram; OCCIP = occipital.

Source.   Reprinted from Bixler EO, Vela-Bueno A: "Normal Sleep: Physiological, Behavioral, and Clinical Correlates." *Psychiatric Annals* 17:437–445, 1987. Used with permission.

cording. Stages 3 and 4 are often indistinguishable and are collectively referred to as *slow-wave sleep, delta sleep,* or *deep sleep*. These stages together account for about 15%–20% of the total sleep time.

- *REM sleep* is characterized by an EEG recording similar to that seen in Stage 1, along with a burst of rapid conjugate eye movements and a reduced level of muscle tone. REM periods occur in phasic bursts and are accompanied by fluctuations in respiratory and cardiac rate, as well as engorgement of the penis and clitoris. This stage constitutes between 20% and 25% of the total sleep period and is also known as *desynchronized* sleep.

A normal young adult goes from waking into a period of NREM sleep lasting approximately 90 minutes before the first REM period; this portion of NREM sleep is referred to as *REM latency*. The sequence of sleep stages during an early sleep cycle is as follows: NREM Stages 1, 2, 3, 4, 3, and 2; then, an REM period occurs. The number of sleep cycles with REM varies from four to six per night depending on the length of sleep. In young adults, REM sleep constitutes about 25% of the total sleep time but may exceed 50% in newborns.

The sleep cycle (REM time to REM time) is shorter in infants than in adults. REM periods emerge every 50–60 minutes during the sleep of infants and gradually increase to the adult sleep cycle length of 70–100 minutes during adolescence. At birth, REM and NREM periods are equally dispersed throughout the sleep period; as an individual ages, REM periods are typically confined to the final third of the night. Figure 24–2 depicts typical sleep architecture and shows the effects of age on the different sleep stages.

Serotonin-containing nuclei and pathways play an important role in regulating NREM sleep. Noradrenergic systems are principally involved in the control of REM sleep. The serotonin-containing neurons are mainly located in the group of nuclei in the lower midbrain and upper pons, referred to as the *raphe nuclei*. Activation of these neurons regulates NREM sleep. This knowledge is based on animal models in which destruction of the raphe nuclei induced total insomnia and on models in which animals were injected with parachlorophenylalanine, which inhibits serotonin synthesis.

Noradrenergic neurons are found throughout the brain stem. They achieve their highest concentration in the *locus coeruleus* in the pons, which is thought to regulate REM sleep; this inference is primarily based on animal research in which lesions of neurons in the *locus coeruleus* abolished REM sleep and led to hyperactive behavior. REM suppression is brought about by injecting animals with α-methylparatyrosine, a substance that inhibits the synthesis of norepinephrine.

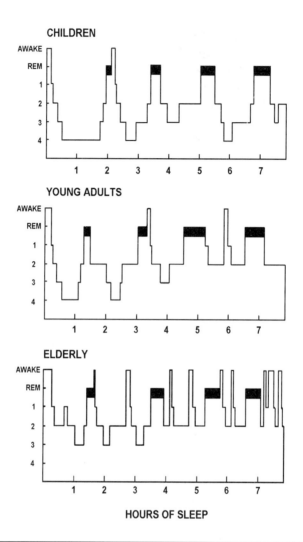

FIGURE 24–2.   The effects of age on the various stages of sleep. Rapid eye movement (REM) sleep (**shaded area**) occurs cyclically throughout the night at intervals of approximately 90 minutes in all age groups. REM sleep shows little variation in the different age groups, whereas Stage 4 sleep decreases with age. In addition, the elderly have frequent awakenings and a marked increase in total wake time.

Source.   Reprinted from Bixler EO, Vela-Bueno A: "Normal Sleep: Physiological, Behavioral, and Clinical Correlates." *Psychiatric Annals* 17:437–445, 1987. Used with permission.

Acetylcholine also plays a major role in sleep, and the reciprocal interaction between serotonergic and noradrenergic systems on the one hand and cholinergic systems on the other may underlie the basic oscillation of the NREM-REM cycle.

Dyssomnias

The essential feature of the dyssomnias is a disturbance in the amount, quality, or timing of sleep. These disorders include the *insomnias,* which are disorders of initiating or maintaining sleep or of not feeling rested after sleep; *hypersomnias,* or disorders of excessive daytime sleepiness or sleep attacks; *breathing-related sleep disorder;* and *circadian rhythm sleep disorder,* in which there is a mismatch between the person's sleep-wake pattern and the pattern that is normal for his or her environment. The category *dyssomnia not otherwise specified* is used when a dyssomnia is present but cannot be better classified.

Primary Insomnia

Primary insomnia is characterized by difficulty initiating or maintaining sleep or having nonrestorative or nonrestful sleep that lasts for at least 1 month and is not due to another mental disorder, a general medical condition, or the effects of a substance (see Table 24–2). The subjective report of poor or nonrefreshing sleep may or may not be associated with any objective sleep disturbance and may not accurately reflect the magnitude of the objective sleep disturbances when present. The objective evidence is often relatively minor because subjective estimates of sleep latency and total sleep time tend to exaggerate the degree of any disturbance present. Many people with primary insomnia are anxious worriers who are overaroused and hyperalert.

As indicated earlier, insomnia is relatively common in the general population and is even more common among psychiatric patients; however, only a small proportion of persons with insomnia consult a physician. Sleep difficulty occurs more frequently among the elderly, in women, among individuals with limited education and lower socioeconomic status, and persons with chronic (or multiple) medical problems.

The duration of insomnia is the most helpful factor in evaluating the patient's problem. Transient insomnia (no more than a few nights) typically occurs in persons who usually sleep normally. This form of insomnia occurs at times of acute psychological stress, such as during bereavement. Other situ-

TABLE 24–2.   DSM-IV-TR diagnostic criteria for primary insomnia

A. The predominant complaint is difficulty initiating or maintaining sleep, or non-restorative sleep, for at least 1 month.

B. The sleep disturbance (or associated daytime fatigue) causes clinically significant distress or impairment in social, occupational, or other important areas of functioning.

C. The sleep disturbance does not occur exclusively during the course of Narcolepsy, Breathing-Related Sleep Disorder, Circadian Rhythm Sleep Disorder, or a Parasomnia.

D. The disturbance does not occur exclusively during the course of another mental disorder (e.g., Major Depressive Disorder, Generalized Anxiety Disorder, a delirium).

E. The disturbance is not due to the direct physiological effects of a substance (e.g., a drug of abuse, a medication) or a general medical condition.

ations associated with transient insomnia include a hospital admission, a public speaking engagement, or a scheduled examination. In these situations, insomnia is rarely brought to medical attention because it is not regarded as pathological and tends to correct itself.

Primary insomnia lasts more than 4 weeks and is more likely to come to a physician's attention. An estimated one-third to one-half of the patients with chronic insomnia have an underlying psychiatric disorder that is responsible for the disturbance; therefore, these individuals do not have primary insomnia. (Sleep disorders associated with specific mental disorders are discussed later in the chapter.)

The patient with primary insomnia should receive a thorough medical and psychiatric assessment (see Table 24–3). The medical history should include a careful review of drug and medication use. Patients should be asked to maintain a sleep log, in which they record their bedtime, sleep latency (estimated time required to fall asleep), awake time, number of awakenings, daytime naps, and use of drugs or medications. Interviewing the patient's bed partner to learn about the presence of snoring, breathing difficulties, or leg jerks can be helpful.

"Sleep hygiene" measures have been developed for patients with chronic insomnia. These measures include the following:

• Waking up and going to bed at the same time every day, even on weekends
• Avoiding long periods of wakefulness in bed
• Not using the bed as a place to read, watch television, or work

---

TABLE 24–3. Sleep history outline

Obtain data from patient, chart, and nursing staff. Review medication history, including illicit drugs, alcohol, and use of hypnotic medication. Obtain information on the following sleep characteristics:

- Usual sleep pattern
- Characteristics of disturbed sleep (for insomnia, difficulty falling asleep, difficulty staying asleep, or early-morning awakenings)
- The clinical course: onset, duration, frequency, severity, and precipitating and relieving factors
- 24-hour sleep-wake cycle (corroborate with staff and chart)
- History of sleep disturbances, including childhood sleep pattern and pattern of sleep when under stress
- Family history of sleep disorders
- Personal history of other sleep disorders
- Sleep pattern at home as described by bed partner

- Leaving the bed and not returning until drowsy if sleep does not begin within a set period (such as 20–30 minutes)
- Avoiding napping
- Exercising at least three or four times a week (but not in the evening if this interferes with sleep)
- Discontinuing or reducing the consumption of alcoholic beverages, beverages containing caffeine, cigarettes, and sedative-hypnotic drugs

Some aspects of the program may be difficult for the patient, such as quitting smoking; withdrawal of caffeine could cause temporary headaches and sluggishness. Nonetheless, many patients who are motivated to improve their daytime functioning are willing to make an effort to follow these simple measures.

Although sedative-hypnotic medications (i.e., sleeping pills) do not cure insomnia, they can provide dramatic temporary relief. They should be used mainly to treat transient and short-term insomnia, in combination with the sleep hygiene measures just outlined. Long-term benefits are difficult to document, and some patients become dependent on these medications. Traditionally, the benzodiazepines have been the first choice for reasons of safety and efficacy. Tolerance to their sleep-promoting effects appears to develop less often than it does with barbiturates, barbiturate-like compounds, and antihistamines. Benzodiazepines marketed as sleeping aids include estazolam, 1–2 mg nightly; flurazepam, 15–30 mg nightly; quazepam, 7.5–15 mg nightly; temazepam, 15–30 mg nightly; and triazolam, 0.25–0.5 mg nightly. Nonbenzodiazepine alternatives are zolpidem, 5–10 mg nightly, and zaleplon, 10–20 mg nightly; both agents appear to have little abuse potential, produce little tolerance, and tend not to cause daytime somnolence, unlike the benzodiazepines. Further details about the rational use of these drugs are found in Chapter 27.

Other drugs frequently used as sleeping aids include chloral hydrate (500–2,000 mg), a nonbarbiturate sedative-hypnotic known more for the fact that it is markedly potentiated by alcohol and forms the basis for "knockout drops" (also known as a Mickey Finn), and the antihistamines diphenhydramine (25–100 mg) and doxylamine (25–100 mg), which are often used as hypnotic agents but are not as potent as the benzodiazepines. Sedating antidepressants such as trazodone (50–200 mg) are often used in low doses as hypnotic agents for patients with primary insomnia. Most over-the-counter sleeping aids are not very effective. They contain an anticholinergic agent or an antihistamine and often produce a variety of side effects.

Primary Hypersomnia

Although excessive daytime somnolence is less common than insomnia, it affects about 5% of the adult population, including similar numbers of men and women. According to DSM-IV-TR, the excessive sleepiness lasts at least 1 month, as evidenced by either prolonged sleep episodes or daytime sleep episodes occurring almost daily; the excessive sleepiness causes significant impairment or distress; and the excessive sleepiness is not accounted for by another sleep disorder, a medical condition, or the effects of a substance (see Table 24–4).

Primary hypersomnia usually involves prolonged nocturnal sleep and continual daytime drowsiness. Nearly one-half of the patients report sleep drunkenness (i.e., excessive grogginess) on awakening, which may last several hours. Patients may report taking one or two naps daily (which can each last more than an hour), unlike the short naps typical of narcoleptic patients.

Polysomnographic studies have shown diminished delta sleep, increased number of awakenings, and reduced REM latency in patients with primary hypersomnia. The MSLT is used to document the short sleep latency. Primary hypersomnia is considered a diagnosis of exclusion, and other more specific disorders should be ruled out, such as narcolepsy.

Treatment of primary hypersomnia involves a combination of sleep hygiene measures, stimulant drugs, and naps for some patients. Stimulants can

---

TABLE 24–4. DSM-IV-TR diagnostic criteria for primary hypersomnia

A. The predominant complaint is excessive sleepiness for at least 1 month (or less if recurrent) as evidenced by either prolonged sleep episodes or daytime sleep episodes that occur almost daily.

B. The excessive sleepiness causes clinically significant distress or impairment in social, occupational, or other important areas of functioning.

C. The excessive sleepiness is not better accounted for by insomnia and does not occur exclusively during the course of another Sleep Disorder (e.g., Narcolepsy, Breathing-Related Sleep Disorder, Circadian Rhythm Sleep Disorder, or a Parasomnia) and cannot be accounted for by an inadequate amount of sleep.

D. The disturbance does not occur exclusively during the course of another mental disorder.

E. The disturbance is not due to the direct physiological effects of a substance (e.g., a drug of abuse, a medication) or a general medical condition.

Specify if:

   Recurrent: if there are periods of excessive sleepiness that last at least 3 days occurring several times a year for at least 2 years

---

help maintain wakefulness; dextroamphetamine and methylphenidate both have relatively short half-lives and are taken in multiple divided doses. Pemoline, a longer-acting stimulant, also can be used. Modafinil, which is used to treat narcolepsy (see next section), can be used to treat primary hypersomnia as an alternative to the stimulants. Nonsedating tricyclic antidepressants (e.g., protriptyline) also are reported to be helpful. Because stimulants have substantial abuse potential, their use should be carefully monitored.

The following case example describes one of our patients who had primary hypersomnia:

> Chris, a 24-year-old college student, was being treated for obsessive-compulsive disorder (OCD), consisting mainly of intrusive and unwanted thoughts of harming others. His symptoms were well controlled with paroxetine, a serotonin reuptake inhibitor.
>
> His mother, who usually accompanied him to the clinic, felt that his excessive sleeping and napping were even more of a problem than his OCD. She described how Chris would sleep 12–14 hours nightly and take afternoon naps. Chris admitted that he was frequently late for class and often fell asleep in class. He complained that he was too sleepy to study in the evening. All of these symptoms predated his treatment for OCD.
>
> Chris was referred to a sleep disorders clinic; his polysomnograph was unremarkable. Because there was no evidence of sleep attacks, cataplexy, sleep paralysis, or hypnagogic hallucinations, he received a diagnosis of primary hypersomnia and began treatment with methylphenidate. On this

regimen, Chris was able to remain awake and alert during the day without napping. He was more alert in class, and his academic performance improved.

Narcolepsy

Narcolepsy is characterized by excessive sleepiness associated with irresistible sleep attacks that occur either as the only symptoms or in combination with one or more auxiliary symptoms of cataplexy, sleep paralysis, or hypnagogic hallucinations. This disorder affects about 1 in 2,000 persons; men and women are equally likely to develop narcolepsy. Narcolepsy may have a hereditary basis because up to half of the patients with narcolepsy have a first-degree relative with the disorder.

The symptoms of narcolepsy are striking; sleep attacks can last from seconds to 30 minutes or longer; they may be precipitated by sedentary and monotonous activity, such as watching television. Narcoleptic patients also may experience sleep attacks at work, during conversations, or under other circumstances normally considered stimulating, such as having sexual intercourse. Up to 80% of narcoleptic patients experience episodes of cataplexy, in which sudden loss of muscle control occurs. This may cause the person to collapse (as if fainting) without loss of consciousness. This loss of muscle tone characteristically occurs in response to strong emotions, such as experiencing laughter or a surprise.

Sleep paralysis and hypnagogic hallucinations occur less frequently than cataplexy. Sleep paralysis causes a temporary loss of muscle tone with a resulting inability to move. Hypnagogic hallucinations are vivid hallucinatory perceptions, usually visual or auditory, that occur while the person is falling asleep. (Hypnopompic hallucinations occur just after awakening.) Although these symptoms sometimes occur in nonnarcoleptic persons, individuals with narcolepsy can experience them as often as several times a week. These auxiliary symptoms generally appear several years after the onset of sleep attacks. Their exact mechanism is unknown, but sleep attacks and other narcoleptic symptoms appear to be closely related to the neurophysiological mechanisms underlying REM sleep.

A careful sleep history is helpful in making the diagnosis of narcolepsy, as are descriptions provided by parents, spouses, and bed partners. The diagnosis is relatively easy to make when auxiliary symptoms (e.g., cataplexy) are present. Polysomnography with MSLT is used to diagnose narcolepsy and allows the clinician to rule out other sleep disorders such as a breathing-related sleep disorder (sleep apnea). Persons with narcolepsy tend to enter REM sleep at sleep onset rather than after the more typical 90–120 minutes and during daytime naps. Patients often develop psychological problems, which are probably a consequence of the adverse effects of the disorder on their family lives, job situations, and social interactions; these problems need to be explored.

The clinical management of narcolepsy involves different treatments for the sleep attacks and the auxiliary symptoms. Stimulants are the preferred drugs for treating sleep attacks because of their rapid onset and relative lack of side effects. For example, methylphenidate is prescribed in multiple divided dosages starting with 5 mg; the dose may be gradually increased to a total daily dose of 60 mg. Dextroamphetamine can be prescribed in similar dosages. Pemoline is prescribed in doses ranging from 18.75 to 150 mg, typically in divided doses. Modafinil, recently approved by the U.S. Food and Drug Administration for the treatment of narcolepsy, is an effective alternative to the stimulants. It is well tolerated and has minimal cardiovascular effects; the daily dose ranges from 200 to 400 mg. Tricyclic antidepressants are often used to treat cataplexy or sleep paralysis but have little effect on sleep attacks; the dose used to control these symptoms is much lower than that used for treating depression (e.g., imipramine, 10–75 mg nightly).

The physician should explain the nature of the disorder to the patient and his or her family. Social acquaintances and employers also may need education to understand that the symptoms of narcolepsy are outside the patient's volitional control. The cooperation of an employer can be enormously helpful because one or two brief daily naps may reduce job difficulties and help lower the dosage requirement for stimulant medication. Patients must be warned that an occurrence of symptoms while driving or engaging in activities requiring constant alertness could be dangerous, just as epileptic patients need to be warned.

Breathing-Related Sleep Disorder

Disturbed breathing mechanisms can disrupt sleep and lead to potentially serious medical, social, and psychological consequences. This form of sleep disorder is generally called *sleep apnea*. Sleep apnea is characterized as central, obstructive, or of mixed origin. Central apnea results from a failure of the respiratory center to initiate sufficient peripheral respiratory effort. In obstructive apnea, respiratory efforts persist but are compromised by upper-airway blockage. Obstructive apnea is more common than central apnea.

In an adult, *breathing-related sleep disorder* is characterized by episodes of breathing cessation for 10 seconds or more during sleep, with a frequency of 10 or more events per hour and with significant oxygen desaturation. Other

nocturnal signs include snoring, gasping and snorting sounds, gastroesoph-
ageal reflux, nocturia, excessive body movements, night sweats, and morning
headaches. Daytime symptoms frequently include excessive sleepiness or
sleep attacks. The disorder can have serious psychological consequences, including a general slowing of thought processes, memory impairment, and inattention. Patients often report anxiety, dysphoric mood, or multiple physical
complaints. The typical patient with sleep apnea is an overweight, middle-
aged man, yet persons of all ages and women may be affected.

A thorough medical assessment is necessary and may include a sleep
laboratory evaluation with recording of respiration and monitoring of nocturnal oxygen desaturation. Obese patients are counseled to reduce their
weight, which in some cases may be sufficient to relieve the apnea. Tricyclic
antidepressants (e.g., protriptyline, 10–60 mg nightly) have been used, and
reports indicate that buspirone and fluoxetine also may be beneficial. Benzodiazepines should not be used because of their tendency to inhibit alerting
responses and to depress respiration at higher dosages.

Continuous positive airway pressure (CPAP) is the most widely used
treatment. Room air is blown into the nose through a nasal mask or cush-
ioned cannulae. Some patients do not tolerate CPAP well, but compliance
will be enhanced with careful follow-up. The major surgical alternative is
uvulopalatopharyngoplasty, which is reserved for patients with redundant
oropharyngeal tissue. Tracheostomy is reserved for life-threatening situations in patients whose condition does not respond to CPAP and uvulopalatopharyngoplasty.

Circadian Rhythm Sleep Disorder (Sleep-Wake Schedule Disorder)

Disrupted sleep may result when the sleep-wake cycle is not correctly syn-
chronized with a person's daily schedule. For example, persons with night
shift work or who frequently change their work shift (e.g., nurses, factory
workers) may develop *circadian rhythm sleep disorder*. Persons who travel frequently and cross time zones also develop disrupted sleep, known as *jet lag*.
Persons with these disorders may never feel fully rested. When they want to
sleep, they cannot, and when they are expected to be awake and alert, they
are sleepy and drowsy.

The best way to avoid these problems is to forego shift work. Industrial
plants have gradually become more aware of these problems, and many have
redesigned their schedules, finding that productivity increases and personnel turnover decreases. Some persons will always be intolerant to shifting

work schedules; these individuals should probably seek other types of employment.

The person who travels frequently probably cannot avoid jet lag. Because of the human circadian time-keeping system, it is usually easier for persons to adjust when the cycle is lengthened rather than shortened, traveling west rather than east.

The treatment for jet lag, other than tincture of time, involves the recommendation that usual sleep hours be maintained in the new time zone. Conventional wisdom is that in most adults it takes about 1 day to adjust to each eastward time zone crossed and slightly less after westward travel. Travelers may minimize the loss of sleep by judicious use of hypnotic agents (e.g., zolpidem, 5–10 mg at bedtime) and by avoiding alcohol and other substances that interfere with sleep. Melatonin, recently touted as a cure for jet lag, has not been shown effective in controlled trials.

Parasomnias

Parasomnias consist of nightmares, sleep terrors, and sleepwalking (or somnambulism). All three disorders are relatively common in children but rarely lead to medical attention unless they are frequent and severe. These disorders generally resolve by late adolescence but can persist into adulthood.

Nightmare Disorder (Dream Anxiety)

Nightmare disorder consists of repeated awakenings with detailed recall of extended and frightening dreams, often involving threats to survival, security, and self-esteem (see Table 24–5). The awakenings usually occur during the second half of the sleep period. On awakening, the individual rapidly becomes alert and oriented. This condition affects as many as 5% of the general population and can become chronic.

Nightmares tend to occur during REM sleep. They may occur at any time during the night but are more frequent during the second half, when REM cycles are increased in frequency and duration. In childhood, nightmares are often related to specific developmental phases and are particularly common during the preschool and early school years. In that age group, children may be unable to distinguish reality from dream content.

Nightmares also have been associated with febrile illness and delirium, particularly in elderly and chronically ill persons. Withdrawal from certain drugs, such as the benzodiazepines, also may result in nightmares. The increase in REM sleep after withdrawal of barbiturates or alcohol may be

TABLE 24–5.   DSM-IV-TR diagnostic criteria for nightmare disorder

A. Repeated awakenings from the major sleep period or naps with detailed recall of extended and extremely frightening dreams, usually involving threats to survival, security, or self-esteem. The awakenings generally occur during the second half of the sleep period.

B. On awakening from the frightening dreams, the person rapidly becomes oriented and alert (in contrast to the confusion and disorientation seen in Sleep Terror Disorder and some forms of epilepsy).

C. The dream experience, or the sleep disturbance resulting from the awakening, causes clinically significant distress or impairment in social, occupational, or other important areas of functioning.

D. The nightmares do not occur exclusively during the course of another mental disorder (e.g., a delirium, Posttraumatic Stress Disorder) and are not due to the direct physiological effects of a substance (e.g., a drug of abuse, a medication) or a general medical condition.

associated with a temporary increase in the intensity of dreaming and nightmares. More recently, the use of serotonin reuptake inhibitors (e.g., citalopram, fluoxetine, fluvoxamine, paroxetine, sertraline) and their withdrawal have been linked to vivid dreams or nightmares.

The main differential diagnoses for nightmare disorder are a major psychiatric illness that could lead to nightmares (e.g., major depression), the effects of a medication, or withdrawal from a drug or alcohol. When the psychiatric disorder is diagnosed and treated, the nightmares may resolve. Nightmares caused by psychologically traumatic events may resolve with short-term counseling or the judicious use of sedative-hypnotics.

Sleep Terror Disorder

Night terrors, or *pavor nocturnus,* are a sudden partial arousal from delta sleep associated with screaming and frantic motor activity. These episodes occur during the first third of the sleep episode and often begin with a terrifying scream followed by intense anxiety and signs of autonomic hyperarousal, such as tachycardia and rapid breathing (see Table 24–6). Persons with night terrors may not fully awaken after an episode and usually have no detailed recall of the event the following morning. Any attempt to restrain the person may result in injury to the person experiencing the terrors or to the person attempting the restraint.

The cause of night terrors is unknown, but they often co-occur with sleepwalking, which is discussed in the next section. Both conditions are familial, begin in childhood, and resolve by late adolescence. When the epi-

TABLE 24–6. DSM-IV-TR diagnostic criteria for sleep terror disorder

A. Recurrent episodes of abrupt awakening from sleep, usually occurring during the first third of the major sleep episode and beginning with a panicky scream.

B. Intense fear and signs of autonomic arousal, such as tachycardia, rapid breathing, and sweating, during each episode.

C. Relative unresponsiveness to efforts of others to comfort the person during the episode.

D. No detailed dream is recalled and there is amnesia for the episode.

E. The episodes cause clinically significant distress or impairment in social, occupational, or other important areas of functioning.

F. The disturbance is not due to the direct physiological effects of a substance (e.g., a drug of abuse, a medication) or a general medical condition.

sodes occur very frequently or persist into late adolescence or adulthood, an underlying psychiatric disturbance may be present.

Sleepwalking (Somnambulism)

Sleepwalking is defined as repeated episodes of arising from sleep and walking about (see Table 24–7). It usually occurs during the first third of the sleep episode. During sleepwalking, the person generally has a blank stare, is relatively unresponsive to the efforts of others to communicate, and can only be awakened with great difficulty. On awakening, the person has amnesia for the episode and is generally alert and oriented within minutes. The episodes of sleepwalking and night terrors generally occur within 3 hours of falling asleep. EEG recordings show high-amplitude slow waves preceding the muscular activation that triggers the attack; sleepwalking occurs during Stages 3 and 4 NREM sleep.

Sleepwalking episodes typically last less than 10 minutes. Persons may move about without purpose in a clumsy way and are indifferent to their environment. Sleepwalkers usually have the ability to maneuver around objects and perform simple tasks such as opening doors or windows, a fact that makes sleepwalking potentially dangerous.

The most important consideration in managing patients with sleepwalking or night terror episodes is protection from injury. Attempts to actively interrupt episodes should be avoided because intervention may confuse or frighten the patient. Special precautions may include placing latches on bedroom windows, installing alarms on doors, and having the patient sleep on the first level of the home.

The disorder is more likely to occur in children than in adults. Nearly 15% of children have had at least one episode of sleepwalking, whereas few-

TABLE 24–7.   DSM-IV-TR diagnostic criteria for sleepwalking disorder

A. Repeated episodes of rising from bed during sleep and walking about, usually occurring during the first third of the major sleep episode.

B. While sleepwalking, the person has a blank, staring face, is relatively unresponsive to the efforts of others to communicate with him or her, and can be awakened only with great difficulty.

C. On awakening (either from the sleepwalking episode or the next morning), the person has amnesia for the episode.

D. Within several minutes after awakening from the sleepwalking episode, there is no impairment of mental activity or behavior (although there may initially be a short period of confusion or disorientation).

E. The sleepwalking causes clinically significant distress or impairment in social, occupational, or other important areas of functioning.

F. The disturbance is not due to the direct physiological effects of a substance (e.g., a drug of abuse, a medication) or a general medical condition.

er than 3% have experienced night terrors. Fewer than 5% of healthy adults report a history of sleepwalking. Parents need to be told that their child's problem will probably be outgrown by late adolescence. In adults, sleep-walking is frequently associated with the presence of a major psychiatric disorder, such as depression.

Drugs that suppress Stages 3 and 4 sleep, such as the benzodiazepines (e.g., diazepam, 5–20 mg nightly), may be prescribed for adults with sleep-walking or night terrors. Relapse is likely when the drugs are discontinued or at times of stress. Tricyclic antidepressants (e.g., imipramine, 50–100 mg nightly) also may be effective in reducing the frequency of sleepwalking and night terror episodes. The drugs can also be given to children, although lower doses are used. Improved sleep hygiene may lead to the resolution of mild disorders.

Sleep Disorders Related to Another Mental Disorder

The category *sleep disorders related to another mental disorder* was created to acknowledge that sleep disorders are regularly associated with specific mental disorders, including psychotic, mood, and anxiety disorders. Sleep disorders also may be related to a general medical condition or to the direct physiological effects of a substance (e.g., a drug of abuse, a medication). When a relation can be identified, the patient should receive a diagnosis of *sleep disorder related to another mental disorder* or *other sleep disorder* if the disorder is related to a general medical condition or substance use. A summary of typical sleep disorders related to other conditions follows (see Table 24–8).

TABLE 24–8. Common electroencephalogram sleep characteristics in mental disorders

Diagnosis	General sleep findings
Psychoses	
Schizophrenia	Marked variability in sleep continuity
	Reduced REM sleep after REM sleep deprivation
	Reduced slow-wave sleep
Mood disorders	Sleep continuity disturbances
	Reduced slow-wave sleep
	Shifting of REM sleep to earlier in the night
Anxiety disorders	Difficulty falling asleep
	Difficulty staying asleep
	Reduced total sleep time
Panic disorder	Difficulty falling asleep
	Difficulty staying asleep
	Reduced total sleep time
	Sleep "panic attacks" may occur during Stages 2 or 3 sleep
Alcoholism	
Acute use	Reduced wakefulness and REM sleep, with increased delta sleep in first half of night, rebound of REM sleep, and increased wakefulness in second half of the night
Chronic use	Fragmented sleep with frequent arousals
Abstinence	Continued fragmentation and reduced slow-wave sleep
Personality disorders	
Borderline	REM sleep changes may be related to concurrent mood disorder
Dementia	Sleep continuity disruptions
	Polyphasic sleep-wake schedule

Note. REM=rapid eye movement.
Source. Adapted from Nofzinger et al. 1993.

Psychotic Disorders

The primary sleep disturbances in psychotic patients are insomnia and excessive sleepiness. Schizophrenic patients, for instance, may experience severe disruption of their sleep during psychotic episodes. Changes include reduced total sleep time, variability in REM time, and increased REM density. A reduction in Stage 4 NREM sleep is the most frequently replicated finding.

Mood Disorders

The insomnia of depression is typically described as early-morning awakening (i.e., waking earlier than usual and being unable to fall back to sleep). Hypersomnia is sometimes observed, particularly in patients with bipolar depression or dysthymia. Manic and hypomanic patients may go without sleep or have shorter sleep durations because of their reduced need for sleep.

Polysomnographic changes in sleep in depressed patients include prolonged sleep latency, increased nocturnal awakenings, and early-morning awakenings; diminished slow-wave sleep (Stages 3 and 4); and changes in REM sleep, including the occurrence of REM sleep earlier in the night (i.e., shortened REM latency) and increased frequency of eye movements during REM sleep.

Anxiety Disorders

Anxiety disorders are frequently associated with delayed sleep onset or trouble remaining asleep. Polysomnographic features include nonspecific changes in sleep latency, decreased sleep efficiency, increased amounts of Stages 1 and 2 sleep, and decreased slow-wave sleep.

Posttraumatic stress disorder may lead to insomnia and disturbing dreams, but polysomnographic changes are not specific. Panic disorder may be associated with sudden awakenings from sleep, which is often the patient's main complaint. Polysomnographic features include marginally increased sleep latency and decreased sleep efficiency.

Alcohol Abuse or Dependence

Alcohol dependence may lead to insomnia or excessive sleepiness. The effects of alcohol differ depending on use. Acute use induces sleepiness and reduces wakefulness for the first 3–4 hours of sleep, with subsequent increases in wakefulness and anxiety-related dreams in the latter half of the

---

Recommendations for management of sleep disorders

1. For accurate diagnosis, a thorough sleep history is essential, including

   • Drug use pattern

   • Use of caffeine

   • An interview with the patient's bed partner

2. For patients with insomnia, the sleep hygiene measures outlined in this chapter are the simplest and most overlooked strategy.

3. Complaints of disturbed sleep should alert the clinician to the possibility of a major psychiatric illness. Depression and alcoholism are probably the most common causes of sleep disturbance.

4. Prescribing sedative-hypnotics for patients with sleep complaints is inappropriate without having first made a diagnosis. For primary insomnia, patients should be told that the sleeping pills are for temporary use only.

5. Temazepam and estazolam have probably the best therapeutic properties for a benzodiazepine hypnotic: rapid absorption, lack of metabolites, and an intermediate half-life that will allow a full night's sleep. Zolipidem and zaleplon are excellent alternatives.

6. Some clinicians consider methylphenidate the drug of choice for patients with narcolepsy or primary hypersomnia. It should be titrated up to 60 mg/day. The clinician should keep track of pill use because some patients may be tempted to abuse them. Modafinil is a newer alternative to the stimulants.

7. If patients have unusual sleep complaints or disorder, a referral should be made to a sleep disorders clinic for a more thorough evaluation, which may include polysomnography.

---

night. With chronic alcohol use, sleep becomes fragmented, with short periods of deep sleep interrupted by brief arousal periods. With abstinence, sleep is initially disrupted; insomnia and nightmares may occur. Sleep improves over time, but light sleep and increased vulnerability to other sleep-disrupting factors may persist even after 2 weeks of abstinence.

Other Psychiatric Disturbances

Delirium may lead to agitation, combativeness, and wandering during early evening or nighttime hours. Clinically, sleep may be fragmented with frequent awakenings, initial insomnia, or early-morning awakenings. The polysomnographic findings include sleep fragmentation, lower sleep efficiency, decreased Stages 3 and 4 sleep, and a decreased percentage of REM sleep.

Sleep Disorder Due to a General Medical Condition or Substance Other Than Alcohol

A variety of medical and neurological conditions may lead to disturbed or disrupted sleep. Examples include hypertension or cardiovascular insufficiency, hyperthyroidism, rheumatological conditions, Parkinson's disease, esophageal reflux, asthma, and head injury. Patients with coronary artery disease may report that anginal pain and breathing problems disrupt their sleep; patients with arthritis may report that a painful joint prevents them from sleeping well. Pregnant women may experience difficulty sleeping because of urinary frequency, fetal movements, and trouble finding a comfortable position.

TABLE 24–9. Medical and neurological conditions and substances associated with sleep disorders

Medical and neurological disorders	Substances
Alzheimer's disease	Alcohol
Angina	Anticonvulsants
Asthma	Antidepressants
Coronary artery disease	Antipsychotics
Diabetes mellitus	Lithium
Eczema	Opioids
Gastrointestinal reflux	Psychostimulants
Hypertension	Sedative-hypnotics
Hyperthyroidism	
Muscular dystrophy	
Myotonic dystrophy	
Obstructive lung disease	
Pain syndromes	
Paroxysmal nocturnal hemoglobinuria	
Peptic ulcer disease	
Pregnancy	
Progressive supranuclear palsy	
Shy-Drager syndrome	
Uremia	

A variety of substances, both legal and illegal, have the ability to disturb sleep. For example, persons who abuse stimulants (e.g., cocaine) may have difficulty falling or remaining asleep. Prescription medication also may lead to sleep disturbance; for example, a patient with a seizure disorder who is taking carbamazepine may report excessive sleep. A list of the more common medical conditions and substances that can cause sleep disturbances appears in Table 24–9.

Management of Sleep Disorders

Recommendations for the clinical management of sleep disorders are summarized in the box on page 663.

Bibliography

Dahl RE: The pharmacologic treatment of sleep disorders. Psychiatr Clin North Am 15:161–178, 1992

Dashevsky BA, Kramer M: Behavioral treatment of chronic insomnia in psychiatrically ill patients. J Clin Psychiatry 59:693–699, 1998

Driver HS, Shapiro CM: ABC of sleep disorders and parasomnias. BMJ 306:921–923, 1993

Ford DE, Kamerow DB: Epidemiologic study of sleep disturbances and psychiatric disorders: an opportunity for prevention? JAMA 262:1479–1484, 1989

Jacobs EA, Reynolds CF, Kupfer DJ, et al: The role of polysomnography in the differential diagnosis of chronic insomnia. Am J Psychiatry 145:346–349, 1988

Morin CM, Culbert JP, Schwartz SM: Non-pharmacological interventions for insomnia: a meta-analysis for treatment efficacy. Am J Psychiatry 151:1172–1180, 1994

Morin CM, Colecchi C, Stone J, et al: Behavioral and pharmacological therapies of late-life insomnia. JAMA 281:991–999, 1999

Nofzinger EA, Buysse DJ, Reynolds CF, et al: Sleep disorders related to another mental disorder: a DSM-IV literature review. J Clin Psychiatry 54:244–255, 1993

Nowell PD, Buysse DJ, Reynolds CF, et al: Clinical factors contributing to the differential diagnosis of primary insomnia and insomnia related to mental disorders. Am J Psychiatry 154:1412–1416, 1997

Ohayon MM, Caulet M, Lemoine P: Comorbidity of mental and insomnia disorders in the general population. Compr Psychiatry 39:185–197, 1998

Regestein QR, Monk TH: Is the poor sleep of shift workers a disorder? Am J Psychiatry 148:1487–1493, 1991

Regestein QR, Dambrosia J, Hallett HM, et al: Daytime alertness in patients with primary insomnia. Am J Psychiatry 150:1529–1534, 1993

Reynolds CF, Kupfer D (eds): Sleep disorders, in American Psychiatric Press Review of Psychiatry, Vol 13. Edited by Oldham J, Riba M. Washington, DC, American Psychiatric Press, 1994, pp 619–777

Roberts RE, Shema SJ, Kaplan GA, et al: Sleep complaints and depression in an aging cohort: a prospective perspective. Am J Psychiatry 157:81–88, 2000

Salin-Pascuel RJ, Roehrs TA, Merlott LA, et al: Long-term study of the sleep of insomnia patients with sleep state misperceptions and other insomnia patients. Am J Psychiatry 149:904–908, 1992

Shapiro CM, Flanigan MJ: ABC of sleep disorders: function of sleep. BMJ 306:383–385, 1993

Simon GE, VonKorff M: Prevalence, burden, and treatment of insomnia in primary care. Am J Psychiatry 154:1417–1423, 1997

Walsh JK, Fry J, Erwin CW, et al: Efficacy and tolerability of 14-day administration of zaleplon 5 mg and 10 mg for the treatment of primary insomnia. Clinical Drug Investigation 16:347–354, 1998

Waterhouse J: ABC of sleep disorders: circadian rhythms. BMJ 306:448–451, 1993

Young T, Palta M, Dempsey J, et al: The occurrence of sleep disordered breathing among middle-aged adults. N Engl J Med 328:1230–1235, 1993

Self-Assessment Questions

1. What are the major categories of sleep disorders?
2. Describe the different dyssomnias.
3. What are sleep hygiene measures?
4. What are the REM and NREM stages? What is their significance?
5. Describe the appropriate use of hypnotic agents. Which are preferred?
6. Distinguish between nightmare disorder and sleep terrors.
7. Does sleepwalking have the same significance in a child that it does in an adult? Describe simple measures that can be taken to reduce the chance of injury in the sleepwalker.
8. How is hypersomnia managed?
9. Do other psychiatric disorders, such as depression, disrupt sleep? What about general medical conditions or substances?

25 Legal Issues in Psychiatry

> Lawsuit, n. a machine which you go into as a pig and come out as a sausage.
>
> Ambrose Bierce, *Devil's Dictionary*

P sychiatrists have a unique role among medical specialists regarding the law because they have regular contact with lawyers, courts, and legal issues. Whether they like it or not, psychiatrists must regularly confront sensitive legal issues. Should this patient be committed to the hospital for treatment against his or her will? Should this patient be forcibly medicated? Can I release information to my patient's parents without his or her permission? These are examples of situations that nonpsychiatric physicians rarely encounter.

Because our society values individual freedom and civil liberties, questions about involuntary hospitalization, the right to treatment (or the right to refuse treatment), confidentiality, and other legal issues have no easy answers. What may seem right may not be legally permissible. What may be legal may not make any practical sense. The right of a man with schizophrenia to live on the streets, for instance, loses its meaning when he clearly has lost his capacity to make important decisions. Thus, the psychiatrist often gets caught in the middle between what may be legally right (i.e., leaving the schizophrenic patient to fend for himself on the streets) and what may be ethically right (i.e., bringing the schizophrenic patient to the hospital for proper care). Because of this interface with the law, physicians who treat psychiatric patients need to have an understanding of fundamental legal issues and the typical problems they will face as practitioners.

Legal issues pertaining to mental illness are best conceptualized by dividing them into three broad categories: civil, criminal, and personal issues (see Table 25–1). *Civil issues* have primarily to do with involuntary hospitalization, the right that patients have to treatment (as well as the right to refuse treatment), and a patient's competency to assist in treatment decisions. *Criminal issues* tend to focus on a patient's competency to stand trial or to bear criminal responsibility (i.e., whether the person accused of a crime is legally competent or insane). *Personal issues* involve a wide range of problems that have to do with the doctor-patient relationship and include confidentiality, informed consent, and malpractice.

TABLE 25–1.   Categories of legal issues affecting psychiatrists

Civil

    Involuntary hospitalization

    Right to treatment

    Right to refuse treatment

Criminal

    Competency to stand trial

    Competency to bear criminal responsibility

Personal

    Physician-patient relationship

    Confidentiality

    Informed consent

    Malpractice

In this chapter, we focus primarily on civil and personal issues because these are the problems that physicians are most likely to encounter in their day-to-day work. Although we touch on criminal issues, persons seeking comprehensive information are referred to *Clinical Psychiatry and the Law.* Forensic psychiatry, a subspecialty within psychiatry, focuses on the interface between psychiatry and the law. Psychiatrists working in this area devote a great deal of their time to criminal issues, including testifying in court and examining persons to determine criminal responsibility.

Although general legal principles and concepts are universal across the United States, specific laws differ from state to state and even from region to region within a state, depending on how the law is interpreted. Furthermore, laws are always being changed by legislatures or being reinterpreted by courts. Therefore, it is essential for psychiatrists to become familiar with relevant laws that apply in their own regions.

Civil Law

Psychiatrists have a responsibility to provide for the safety of both their patients and others who may be affected by them. Therefore, when a patient is thought to be a threat to self or others and refuses hospitalization, the psychiatrist will have to seek a court order for involuntary hospitalization. In the past, it was relatively easy for a psychiatrist to obtain a civil commitment, usually with a signature or a telephone call. Legislatures and courts have gradually backed away from the once freewheeling nature of mental health commitment. In response to the civil rights movement, which included recognizing the rights of mentally ill persons, most states now carefully regulate civil commitment. The appropriateness of this emphasis on civil rights over the right to humane care has been hotly debated. It is sometimes said that the homeless are being allowed to "die with their rights on."

Most commitment laws employ the concepts of mental illness, dangerousness, and disability. For civil commitment, these laws require the presence of mental illness, although the precise definition of *mental illness* differs from place to place. A diagnosis of personality disorder, for example, may be insufficient for commitment in some areas; a diagnosis of alcoholism or substance abuse may not be accepted in other areas. The law may specify that the mental illness be treatable, which may complicate matters because many disorders are only partially treatable, and some untreatable disorders are still very dangerous. The concept of *dangerousness* usually requires that persons be an imminent danger to themselves or others. An example is a patient thought likely to commit suicide or homicide within the next 24 hours if not hospitalized. (Evidence of past dangerousness usually is insufficient for commitment.) Because physicians are unable to accurately predict dangerousness except in the most obvious of situations, this requirement can be difficult to apply. The third concept, *disability,* is a measure of the patient's inability to properly care for himself or herself because of mental illness. Some states use the phrase *gravely disabled* (or similar language) to imply that individuals are unable to take care of their personal grooming and dress, to maintain adequate hydration, and to feed themselves. Clearly, persons who are gravely disabled may not be in imminent danger of harming themselves, but they still need hospitalization and treatment.

Most states allow for patients to be hospitalized on an emergency basis to provide short-term intervention; this period may range from 1 to 20 days depending on the statute. Civil commitments either after the emergency hospitalization or on direct petition from the community provide for a longer period of involuntary hospitalization. These commitments are done with judicial approval and due process protection. A variety of due process protections for mentally ill persons are standard in most states. These include an adequate notice of legal action, the right to a timely hearing, the right to appear at all legal proceedings, the right to be represented by an attorney, formal rules of evidence, and privilege against self-incrimination. The burden of proof is placed on the state to establish the reason for commitment, and the patient is guaranteed the right to appeal. These requirements contribute to the tension between the individual's need for legal protection and the desire of society to provide necessary treatment.

These due process protections differ substantially among the states. In many areas, hearsay testimony is admissible, and hearings are closed to the public and conducted in treatment facilities; a hearing officer may be used rather than a judge or jury. In Iowa, for example, civil commitment hearings are conducted informally at the hospital, and formal rules of evidence do not apply. The case for commitment is made by a county attorney to a hospitalization magistrate, who makes a decision based on "clear and convincing evidence," not the more strict standard of "beyond a reasonable doubt." The hearing is not considered adversarial, and the decision is intended to favor the best interests of the patient. Once committed, the patient is judged incapable of making mental health decisions, which the physicians are then empowered to make on his or her behalf.

Outpatient commitment, now permitted in many states, is generally reserved for chronically noncompliant patients, most of whom are severely mentally ill. Because treatment noncompliance can result in rehospitalization, patients have an incentive to follow through on treatment plans. Outpatient commitments can be enormously helpful in the care of patients who are otherwise chronically noncompliant and can reduce the frequency of their hospitalizations.

In the past, many patients were involuntarily hospitalized, and there was no explicit right to receive treatment. Although most patients can be helped, a substantial number of involuntarily hospitalized patients are unlikely to improve with any treatment. The person with antisocial personality disorder, for example, may be mentally ill and dangerous, but there are no proven treatments for the condition. Paralleling the decisions about the right to receive treatment have been legal decisions about the right to refuse treatment. Under some state laws, a person can be involuntarily hospitalized and still be judged capable of refusing certain treatments. Psychiatrists find this situation particularly frustrating and ironic; an ill and dangerous person may be involuntarily hospitalized and under their care, yet they are powerless to provide needed treatment.

Much litigation has concerned the right of civilly committed patients to refuse psychotropic medication in nonemergency situations. (Voluntarily hospitalized patients have almost always been allowed to refuse medication except in emergency situations.) Antipsychotic medication has been the major focus of this litigation because of the potential risk of serious side effects such as tardive dyskinesia. Unfortunately, some courts have emphasized the potential risk of treatment rather than its potential benefits; some have even elevated treatment with antipsychotic medication to the status of an "extraordinary" form of medical treatment requiring special judicial scrutiny. In some states, a patient retains the right to refuse medication until the medical treatment team has petitioned the local court to declare the patient incompetent to consent to or refuse medication. In other states, such as Iowa, physicians are allowed to medicate patients on the basis of the commitment hearing alone.

As a practical matter, when should the clinician decide to involuntarily hospitalize a patient? In the most typical scenario, a law enforcement officer brings a person thought to be mentally ill to an emergency room. The psychiatrist is contacted and asked to assess the individual and to make an appropriate decision about disposition. When the person is deemed mentally ill, dangerous, and/or disabled and refuses hospitalization, the decision is relatively easy to make: the hospitalization magistrate is contacted, and an order for involuntary hospitalization is sought. From the physician's perspective, it is probably better to err on the side of safety than to allow someone who is potentially dangerous to self or others to leave the emergency room.

Another common scenario occurs when a patient admitted voluntarily requests discharge but is believed to present an ongoing danger to self or others (e.g., a person who has admitted to having suicidal plans). In these situations, a court order should be sought for continued hospitalization.

Personal Issues

Confidentiality

Maintaining confidentiality is one of the most important obligations psychiatrists have to their patients. What passes between doctor and patient should remain private and should not be divulged without the patient's consent. Indiscriminate disclosure could be socially embarrassing or harmful and represents a breach of the fiduciary relationship between doctor and patient. As a practical matter, this means that before information is given to a third party, the patient must provide written consent.

In rare instances, a psychiatrist is required to breach confidentiality to protect a person from being harmed by the patient. In the course of treating a patient, a psychiatrist may learn of potential harm to a third party. In these situations, the psychiatrist has a legal responsibility to break confidentiality and warn the third party. This *duty to protect* is referred to as the *Tarasoff* rule, named after a 1976 decision by a California court. A therapist was held responsible for harm committed to a third party by his patient because it had been revealed that the therapist was aware of the potential threat.

How the *Tarasoff* rule should be implemented by psychiatrists and other mental health professionals has been debated. In practice, once the psychiatrist believes that a patient will become violent, hospitalization is the best course. If violence is believed to be a distinct possibility, but is not imminent, the best course is to warn the intended victim.

Once a decision has been made to warn the intended victim, a telephone call is appropriate because it allows him or her to ask questions. Sometimes psychiatrists will phone in the patient's presence, which may help alleviate suspicions about the psychiatrist going behind the patient's back. A trusted third party may sometimes act as a go-between for the psychiatrist and the intended victim (e.g., a law enforcement officer). The psychiatrist should always discuss the warning with the patient before giving it.

Although a psychiatrist may need to repair the damage done to the therapeutic relationship by the breach of confidentiality, some patients may actually feel relieved. It also may have a deterrent effect; a patient who is ambivalent about harming another person may decide not to carry out the threat after learning that the intended victim has been warned.

Confidentiality can be waived for other reasons as well. In some states, mental health providers have the right to disclose confidential information to close family members without consent when it is thought to be in the best interest of the patient. Further, utilization review groups and third-party payers often demand access to hospital charts. When signing into the hospital, a patient will waive his or her right to confidentiality, so as to allow these bodies to review the records.

Informed Consent

Informed consent should be obtained from all patients before any psychiatric treatment, although formal written consent is probably necessary only before electroconvulsive therapy (ECT). Many hospitals now require written informed consent before administration of medications, especially antipsychotics because they carry the potential risk of tardive dyskinesia. Patients should be informed of the indications and contraindications for the treatment, possible adverse effects, and alternative therapies (if applicable). The physician should carefully document that the patient has given consent. One problem with informed consent arises when the patient is not capable of giving consent. In these situations, the patient should have a court-appointed guardian who can make health care decisions on his or her behalf.

Malpractice

Malpractice is negligence in the conduct of one's professional duties. The number of malpractice suits filed in the United States seems to climb each year. It has been estimated that every physician will experience at least one malpractice lawsuit during his or her professional lifetime.

Psychiatrists are sued less frequently than other physicians. One reason is that psychiatrists, by virtue of the disorders treated and the types of treatments provided, are less likely to physically harm a patient; a surgeon, for example, has the potential to maim or kill. Psychiatric patients are also reluctant to publicize their mental disorders and treatments, and there are typically no witnesses to the alleged mistreatment.

Suicide is the most common reason that psychiatrists are sued, even though no study has ever shown that they are able to predict suicides. Nonetheless, the courts and the public tend to blame the psychiatrist for failing to predict or prevent a patient's self-injury or death. Suicides that occur during hospitalization are probably the ones most likely to result in litigation because they are seen as entirely preventable; suicidal behavior may, in fact, be the reason the patient was in the hospital. Potential errors by a psychiatrist include his or her failure to take an adequate history of suicidal behavior, failure to provide adequate protection in the hospital (e.g., one-to-one supervision), or failure to communicate changes in the patient's condition to other doctors and nurses.

Sexual activity with current or former patients has become a relatively common reason for malpractice litigation. In addition to legal sanctions, a psychiatrist may be expelled from professional associations and have his or her license suspended or revoked. The American Psychiatric Association has made it clear that sexual contact with current or previous patients is inappropriate and unethical. There is never a good excuse for a sexual relationship with a patient, regardless of how seductive the patient is or how much time has elapsed since the physician treated the patient.

Psychiatrists also are sued because of failure to obtain informed consent. Patients may claim that the information provided to them was inadequate, that alternatives were omitted, or that the consent was never obtained. It behooves the clinician to maintain careful records about what happens during an appointment, particularly as it pertains to obtaining consent and providing information.

Psychiatrists are occasionally sued by patients who sustain injuries from psychotropic medications. Situations that have led to claims include failure to disclose relevant information to the patient about adverse effects, failure to obtain an adequate history, and prescription of a drug or drug combination when it is not indicated or when potentially harmful drug interactions might occur. The development of tardive dyskinesia is one of the major complications that results in litigation. It is generally recommended that prescribing physicians regularly monitor patients for the presence and severity of tardive dyskinesia and repeatedly educate the patient and family members (or guardian) about the risks of treatment as well as the continuing need for antipsychotic medication. For these reasons, psychiatrists may wish to consider prescribing one of the newer atypical antipsychotics (e.g., risperidone, olanzapine), which have less potential to induce tardive dyskinesia.

Psychiatrists are sometimes sued for abandonment, defined as improperly terminating a doctor-patient relationship despite the continuing need for treatment. Abandonment can give rise to actions for both negligence and breach of contract. Termination may occur because a patient fails to cooperate with treatment, fails to pay bills, threatens or assaults the psychiatrist, or presents a difficult management problem.

Claims involving ECT are relatively rare but do occur and involve allegations of failure to obtained informed consent, inappropriate or improper treatment, or injury resulting from treatment, such as memory loss. Liability can be minimized by using ECT in accordance with accepted standards and monitoring and supervising patients carefully between treatments. The consent process should be fully documented and preferably witnessed.

Criminal Issues

Situations involving criminal law as it applies to psychiatry are rarely encountered by most practicing psychiatrists. The two main criminal issues are *competency to stand trial* and *criminal responsibility*. To receive a fair trial, a person must be able to understand the nature of the charges against him or her, the possible penalty, and the legal issues and procedures; he or she also must be able to work with the attorney to participate in preparing the defense. Competency is a legal distinction, not a medical one; in most regions, it is decided by a judge, who may base his or her decision on expert testimony. When the court determines that the defendant is incompetent to stand trial, the defendant is typically transferred to a psychiatric hospital. The goal of treatment is to restore the defendant to a competent state. Once competency has been restored, the defendant is returned to court to stand trial.

Defendants determined by the courts to be incompetent to be sentenced (or executed) are managed in the same way as those who are alleged or determined to be incompetent to stand trial; they may be referred for psychiatric treatment for the purpose of restoring competency. This, of course, presents the ironic situation of a person sent for psychiatric treatment that on his or her improvement will lead to execution.

The presence of a psychiatric disorder, even a severe psychosis, generally does not render a defendant incompetent to stand trial. Most patients referred for competency evaluation are able to understand the nature and quality of their acts and to participate in their own defense, the usual measures for determining legal competence to stand trial.

Criminal responsibility has to do with the subject's state of mind at the time of a crime. Under our current system, criminal responsibility occurs only in the presence of blameworthy state of mind.

Evidence of a psychiatric condition is used in three categories of traditional criminal defense. First, evidence of a psychiatric disorder at the time of the alleged offense can be used to negate the requirement for criminal intent. Second, the defense may claim that the defendant's mental condition at the time of the act relieves him or her of criminal responsibility through the special verdict of not guilty by reason of insanity. According to the *M'Naghten* rule used in many states, defendants can establish an insanity defense when, at the time of the alleged offense, they were laboring under such defective reasoning caused by a disease of the mind that they did not know the nature and quality of the criminal act. The rule is named after Daniel M'Naghten, who in 1843 shot and killed Edward Drummond, private secretary to the prime minister Sir Robert Peel, the intended victim. M'Naghten had had delusions for many years and believed that he was being persecuted by the Tory Party and their leader Peel.

The American Law Institute standard is used in many states and incorporates a volitional test: a person is not held responsible for criminal conduct if at the time of such conduct and as a result of mental disease the person "lacks substantial capacity to appreciate the criminality of his [or her] conduct, or to conform his [or her] conduct to the requirements of the law."

The third traditional criminal defense acknowledges that the defendant is guilty but was mentally ill at the time of the act. Defendants found "guilty but mentally ill" are usually referred to correctional facilities where psychiatric treatment can be given.

A guilty but mentally ill verdict has become more popular since John Hinckley's not guilty verdict for his shooting of President Ronald Reagan. Critics have charged that excusing Hinkley and others from responsibility lessens society's ability to deal with potentially dangerous persons and knowingly encourages the inappropriate use of the insanity defense, which they feel makes a mockery of our system of justice. Nonetheless, the verdict of guilty but mentally ill recognizes the obvious in certain cases: although a crime was committed and a person was found guilty of that crime, the person was mentally ill at the time of the act.

Management of Legal Situations

Recommendations for handling legal situations are summarized in the box.

Recommendations for handling legal situations

1. When seeking involuntary hospitalization, there must be evidence of a treatable mental illness, recent (or potential for) harm to self or others, or grave disability.

   • The clinician must know the state laws.

   • The clinician should know the local magistrate who handles civil commitments.

   • Outpatient commitments are useful in patients who tend to be noncompliant with treatment and are a nuisance to the community.

2. The clinician should understand his or her state laws on confidentiality and informed consent.

3. Breaking confidentiality under the *Tarasoff* rule may involve contacting the threatened party (or the police).

   • Although breaking confidentiality may harm the doctor-patient relationship, many patients will feel a sense of relief.

4. Malpractice lawsuits are common in our litigious society; adequate insurance is essential.

   • The best defense against claims of malpractice is to maintain proper records and documentation.

5. Most psychiatrists do not routinely conduct competency evaluations to determine whether a patient can stand trial. Psychiatrists should become familiar with the forensic psychiatrists in their region.

Bibliography

American Medical Association Board of Trustees: Insanity defense in criminal trials and limitation of psychiatric testimony. JAMA 251:2967–2981, 1984

Appelbaum PS: Tarasoff and the clinician: problems in fulfilling the duty to protect. Am J Psychiatry 142:425–429, 1985

Appelbaum PS, Roth LH: Clinical issues in the assessment of competency. Am J Psychiatry 138:1462–1467, 1981

Applebaum PS, Zoltek-Jick R: Psychotherapists' duties to third parties: Ramona and beyond. Am J Psychiatry 153:457–465, 1996

Drane JF: Competency to give informed consent: a model for making clinical assessments. JAMA 252:925–927, 1984

Faust D, Ziskin J: The expert witness in psychology and psychiatry. Science 241:31–35, 1988

Guthiel TG, Appelbaum PS: Clinical Handbook of Psychiatry and the Law. New York, McGraw-Hill, 1982

Guthiel TG, Gabbard GO: Misuses and misunderstandings of boundary theory in clinical and regulatory settings. Am J Psychiatry 155:409–414, 1998

Lamb HR: Incompetency to stand trial. Arch Gen Psychiatry 44:754–758, 1987

Leang GB, Eth S, Silva JA: The psychotherapist as witness for the prosecution: the criminalization of Tarasoff. Am J Psychiatry 149:1011–1015, 1992

McNeil DE, Binder RL, Fulton FM: Management of threats of violence under California's duty-to-protect statute. Am J Psychiatry 155:1097–1101, 1998

Miller RD: Need for treatment criteria for involuntary civil commitment: impact on practice. Am J Psychiatry 149:1380–1384, 1992

Simon RI: Clinical Psychiatry and the Law. Washington, DC, American Psychiatric Press, 1992

Simon RI, Sadoff RL: Psychiatric Malpractice: Cases and Comments for Clinicians. Washington, DC, American Psychiatric Press, 1992

Self-Assessment Questions

1. What is forensic psychiatry?
2. What are the three main categories of legal issues psychiatrists face?
3. What are the major concepts that most civil commitment laws contain?
4. Explain both the right to treatment and the right to refuse treatment. Why is the latter so frustrating to psychiatrists?
5. Explain the *Tarasoff* ruling and the duty to protect.
6. Why is confidentiality important? List several situations in which it can be waived.

7. What are the usual reasons behind malpractice lawsuits filed against psychiatrists?
8. How may a psychotic patient be competent to stand trial?
9. Explain the *M'Naghten* standard.
10. What is the guilty but mentally ill verdict about?

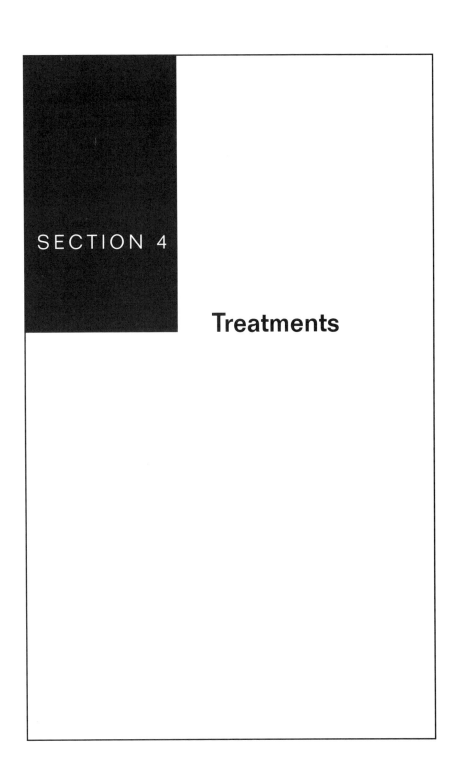

SECTION 4

Treatments

26 Psychosocial Treatments

The mind is its own place, and can make
A hell of heaven, a heaven of hell

John Milton, *Paradise Lost*

B ecause psychiatrists deal with diseases that are especially human, involving thoughts, feelings, and relationships, it is essential that they maintain a humanistic, empathic, and caring attitude toward their patients and that they become skilled in using therapies directed at the mind in addition to the brain. Although the empathic relationship that is used in many types of psychotherapy is in principle not different from that also used by a caring and involved family practitioner or medical specialist, an empathic relationship is more prominent and pervasive in psychiatric practice because of the nature of the illnesses that are being diagnosed and treated.

In the layperson's mind, psychiatry and psychotherapy are closely intertwined. Many people think of a psychiatrist as a person who is not necessarily even a physician and who treats patients (or clients) by listening, talking, and counseling. As this textbook has shown throughout, however, the modern psychiatrist is in fact a well-trained physician who understands his or her patients on multiple levels simultaneously. The twenty-first century psychiatrist moves freely from an understanding of the normal or abnormal mind/brain to thinking about disruptions in neural circuits and neurochemistry. At the same time, he or she thinks about how the effects of medication can relieve the symptoms of mental illness by reversing the effects of disordered brain chemistry, circuits, and systems.

Because the use of medication has become an increasingly important tool in psychiatric care, the role of psychotherapy has diminished. Psychiatry in the twenty-first century is confronting two interacting trends that are working at cross-purposes with each other: reduction of the use of psychotherapy by psychiatrists and a rapid growth in the understanding of the biological mechanisms that make psychotherapy an effective treatment.

On the one hand, changes in health care delivery and economics have reduced the role of psychotherapy in psychiatry, increasingly transferring nonpharmacological care to the hands of psychologists, nurses, and social workers. In many health maintenance organizations and other medical systems, the psychiatrist is asked to function as a diagnostician and psychopharmacologist. The effects of this economic trend are unfortunate, and they run counter to the essence of psychiatry.

On the other hand, paradoxically, the economic trends pushing psychiatry away from the use of psychotherapy are occurring exactly when we are beginning to understand the neural mechanisms by which psychotherapy exerts its effects. Although the psychotherapies do not use medications to effect change, they do cause biological changes in the brain and mind that are just as real and physical as those produced by medications. Increasingly, psychiatrists and other neuroscientists recognize that psychotherapies capitalize on the fact of brain plasticity and produce long-term changes at the neural level. They do so by training the brain to form new neural associative networks that help the individual respond in ways that are more adaptive and healthy. The observations indicate that psychotherapy is as biologically based as pharmacotherapy.

Because writing a prescription is easier and more obviously medical than performing psychotherapy, beginning students often wonder whether there is any need to do psychotherapy at all. Such disinterest in psychosocial treatments is unwarranted. In addition to the growing neuroscience base illuminating the biological mechanisms by which psychotherapy works, a substantial empirical base has confirmed the effectiveness of psychosocial treatments. For some disorders (e.g., eating disorders), they are first-line treatments, and they have been repeatedly shown to produce good outcomes. For many other disorders (e.g., schizophrenia, mood and anxiety disorders), they have been shown to be an important adjunct to medications by dealing with issues such as encouraging compliance, educating patients about symptoms and expected outcome, and providing insight or support to deal with the psychological consequences of a severe illness.

In this chapter, we provide a brief overview of the major classes of psychotherapy that are used by specialists who care for mentally ill patients. Some of these psychosocial treatments require extensive experience and training, on a scale that is outside the range of description of a single chapter. Students who want to explore specific types of psychosocial treatments in more detail may want to read material cited in the Bibliography at the end of this chapter. The various psychosocial treatments that are often used for major mental illnesses include behavior therapy, cognitive-behavioral therapy (CBT), the individual psychotherapies that draw on psychodynamic principles, group therapy, marital and family therapy, and social skills training. The major classes of psychosocial treatments are summarized in Table 26–1.

TABLE 26–1. Types of psychosocial therapy

Behavior therapy

Cognitive-behavioral therapy (CBT)

Individual therapy

    Classical psychoanalysis

    Psychodynamic psychotherapy

    Insight-oriented psychotherapy

    Relationship psychotherapy

    Interpersonal psychotherapy

    Supportive psychotherapy

Group therapy

Marital therapy

Family therapy

Social skills training

Behavior Therapy

The theoretical underpinnings of behavior therapy derive from British empiricism, Pavlov's studies of conditioning, and subsequent research on stimulus-response relationships conducted by other leading behaviorists such as Skinner, Wolpe, and Eysenck. Behaviorists stress the importance of working with objective, observable phenomena, usually referred to as *behavior*, including physical activities such as eating, drinking, talking, and completing the serial-sequential activities that lead to habit formations and social interactions. In contrast to psychodynamic psychotherapies, discussed later in this chapter, behavioral techniques do not necessarily help the patient to understand his or her emotions or motivations. Instead of working on the patient's thoughts and feelings, the behavior therapist works on *what the patient does*. Indeed, some clinicians who use behavioral approaches argue that changing a patient's behavior may lead to substantial changes in how the patient thinks and feels and that correcting pathological behavior may be more effective than correcting pathological emotions. The motto for this approach is "Change the behavior, and the feelings will follow."

Behavior therapies are particularly effective for disorders that are associated with clearly abnormal behavioral patterns in need of correction. These disorders include alcohol and drug abuse, eating disorders, anxiety disorders, and particularly phobias and obsessive-compulsive behavior. A general knowledge of the principles of behaviorism may be useful in dealing with a broad range of patients, however, including patients with dementias, psychoses, adjustment disorders, childhood disorders, and personality disorders.

The concept of *conditioning* is fundamental to the various behavior therapies. Two types of conditioning have been described: classical (Pavlovian) and operant. Early in the twentieth century, the Russian physiologist Pavlov described the first controlled experiments with conditioning. He demonstrated that by pairing stimuli, such as striking a bell at the same time that dogs were given food, he could eventually produce a conditioned reflex in the animals in the absence of the original triggering stimulus. For example, if the two stimuli (food and the ringing of a bell) were paired frequently enough, the dog would eventually learn to salivate when it heard the bell alone. In this model, the food is regarded as the unconditioned stimulus, the bell as the conditioned stimulus, and salivation in response to the bell the conditioned reflex.

The concept of stimulus pairing can obviously be used both to explain the development of psychopathology and to create behavior therapies through conditioning patients to alter their response patterns.

The study and use of *operant conditioning* involve examining responses that are produced within the subject rather than produced by some outside stimulus. A therapist who uses operant conditioning seeks to understand the forces that trigger and modify specific behaviors rather than beginning with a predetermined conditioned stimulus. Operant responses, in contrast to conditioned reflexes, are voluntary. For example, a young child sitting in a high chair quickly learns that banging a spoon on his or her tray gets his or her mother's attention and is likely to produce gratification of some desire, such as more milk in his or her cup or another piece of toast. By varying the amount of banging, he or she also may learn that if he or she bangs too much, his or her mother may become annoyed, take away his or her spoon, and remove him or her from the high chair before a dessert is provided. Thus, the child learns to change both his or her behavior and his or her environment in relation to the responses that the behavior elicits in a manner that is under his or her voluntary control.

The study of operant conditioning has created an enormous experimental literature that explores the various ways that learning occurs and that behaviors are reinforced or extinguished. The concepts of positive and negative reinforcement are fundamental. A *positive reinforcer* (e.g., giving a reward) strengthens the response, whereas a *negative reinforcer* (e.g., giving a punishment) diminishes the response. An extensive behavioral literature now suggests that positive reinforcement is more effective in sustaining behavior than negative reinforcement, that failure to provide reinforcements usually will extinguish a behavior, and that variable and unpredictable schedules of reinforcement may be more effective in maintaining behavior than fixed, regular reinforcements. For example, pathological gamblers receive the positive reinforcement of winning only occasionally, but they continue to gamble and are rarely deterred by threats of punishment or even by punishment itself, such as loss of their financial assets or even incarceration. If they won every time they gambled, they would very likely lose interest eventually, and, likewise, they would lose interest if they never won at all.

Some of the established forms of behavior therapy that use these principles are listed in Table 26–2. They include relaxation training, systematic desensitization, flooding, and behavior modification. These principles also can be used to shape the behavior of patients (and one's children, colleagues, or friends) in spontaneous and creative ways.

TABLE 26–2. Established forms of behavior therapy

Relaxation training

Systematic desensitization

Flooding

Behavior modification techniques

Relaxation Training

Relaxation training is used to teach patients control over their bodies and mental states. Relaxation training is a simple and straightforward procedure; the patient is instructed to move through the muscle groups of the body and make them tense and then completely relaxed. Through this procedure, patients learn how to achieve voluntary control over feelings of tension and relaxation. Relaxation training can be done simply by providing patients with an instructional audiotape that they can listen to in order to practice the techniques on their own. Relaxation training can be used alone to help patients who have anxiety or various problems involving pain (e.g., headache, low back pain), or it can be used in conjunction with systematic desensitization.

Systematic Desensitization

Systematic desensitization is a behavioral technique that involves teaching the patient how to reduce or control the fear elicited by specific stimuli. This technique is particularly useful for patients with specific fears, such as agoraphobia or the various social phobias. The therapist may use any one of a variety of techniques to train the patient to reduce his or her tense and anxious response to the feared stimulus. For example, the therapist may ask the agoraphobic patient to imagine what it is like to leave his or her house and visit the shopping mall where he or she typically develops panic attacks, thereby leading the patient to experience the panic attack. The patient is then encouraged to use relaxation techniques to diminish the sensation of panic and place it under voluntary control. The patient will gradually become able to enter the feared situation—that is, actually going to the shopping mall—and use relaxation techniques while in the feared setting. In complex and difficult situations, the therapist may need to lead the patient gradually to a sense of control, by developing a hierarchy of stimuli that increasingly approximate the feared stimulus (e.g., moving from imagination to photographs to photographs plus recorded noises and finally to the actual situation itself).

Flooding

Flooding involves teaching patients to extinguish anxiety produced by a feared stimulus through placing them in continuous contact with the stimulus and helping them learn that the stimulus does not in fact lead to any feared consequences. For example, a patient with a disabling fear of riding on airplanes may be forced to take repeated flights until the fear is extinguished. The patient with a fear of snakes may be requested to go to the zoo and stand in front of the snake cage until his or her anxiety is completely gone.

Behavior Modification Techniques

Behavior modification techniques tend to use the concept of reinforcement as a way of shaping behavior—in particular, to reduce or eliminate undesirable behavior and to replace it with healthier behaviors or habits. Behavior modification techniques are especially appropriate for disorders characterized by poor impulse control, such as alcohol or other substance abuse, eating disorders, and conduct disorders.

Individual programs must be designed to suit the particular patient by using stimuli that are specific positive and negative reinforcers for that individual. For example, the long-term goal for a patient with anorexia nervosa is weight gain. Intermediate goals are to become less preoccupied with food and body image. Patients with anorexia nervosa typically enjoy exercise. A particular patient with anorexia also may enjoy reading mystery novels and chewing gum. A specific program would be developed for such a patient in which she would be provided with three regular, well-balanced meals per day and told that access to her specific preferred pleasures would be contingent on going to the dining room for meals, eating them, and demonstrating a regular pattern of weight gain. A schedule of reinforcers would be developed to encourage her compliance with eating regularly. For example, she might be restricted to her room initially between meals and given no access to exercise, mystery novels, or chewing gum. After she gains 5 pounds, she will be allowed to leave her room. After she gains an additional 5 pounds, she will be given access to mystery novels. After the gain of another 5 pounds, she will be allowed access to chewing gum. After she reaches her desired target weight (involving a total weight gain of 20 pounds), she will be allowed to exercise regularly. To be permitted to continue exercising, however, she must maintain her target weight for 2 weeks while exercising as much as she desires. If her weight drops, positive reinforcers will gradually be removed until the weight gain is reestablished. In such a program, negative reinforcers, such as tube feeding, also may be built in. As mentioned above, however, it is well recognized that these negative reinforcers are much less effective than are the positive reinforcers.

Different mixtures of behavior modification techniques are required for different disorders. For example, a program similar to the one above, but involving a different schedule of reinforcers and different targets, might be appropriate for the obese patient. Behavior modification programs for patients with substance abuse are more likely to stress teaching the patient the various stimuli that tend to trigger his or her craving, such as diminishing the pent-up irritation of a long day at work by dropping by the bar and socializing with friends. The patient would be taught instead to substitute other positive reinforcers in their place, such as dropping by a health club and releasing his or her hostility by hitting a punching bag, followed by drinking copious amounts of his or her favorite nonalcoholic beverage with a new set of friends developed through contacts with Alcoholics Anonymous (AA).

Combining Therapies

Originally, proponents of behavior therapy were purists, and they tended to denigrate mixing behavior therapy with other types of psychotherapy or with the use of medications. Increasingly, however, various types of therapy are being combined. Thus, the treatment of panic disorder and agoraphobia may involve the use of a serotonin reuptake inhibitor along with systematic desensitization. Behavior therapy also may be combined with psychodynamic psychotherapy; for example, a patient with anorexia nervosa may benefit from a behavior modification program and from efforts to help her understand the underlying fears that make her seek a bodily appearance that most people find quite unattractive. A patient with comorbid anxiety and depression may benefit from a program of relaxation training, cognitive therapy, and antidepressant medication.

Cognitive-Behavioral Therapy

The theoretical support for CBT derives from a variety of sources, including cognitive psychology, Freudian psychodynamic theory, and some aspects of behaviorism. The theory and techniques of CBT have been developed principally by Aaron Beck. The techniques of CBT are based on the assumption that *cognitive structures* or *schemas* shape the way people react and adapt to a variety of situations that they encounter in their lives. An individual's particular cognitive structures derive from a variety of constitutional and experiential factors (e.g., physical appearance, loss of a parent early in life, previous achievements or failures at school or with friends). Each person has his or her own specific set of cognitive structures that determines how he or she will react to any given stressor in any particular situation. A person develops a psychiatric syndrome, such as anxiety or depression, when these schemas become overactive and predispose him or her to developing a pathological or negative response.

The most widespread use of CBT is for the treatment of depression. In this instance, the individual is typically found to have schemas that lead to negative interpretations. Beck designated the three major cognitive patterns observed in depression as the *cognitive triad*: a negative view of oneself, a negative interpretation of experience, and a negative view of the future. Patients with these cognitive patterns are predisposed to react to situations by interpreting them in the light of these three negative sets. For example, a woman who applied for a highly competitive job and did not receive it, and whose perceptions are shaped by such negative sets, may conclude, "I didn't get it because I'm not really bright, in spite of my good school record, and the employer was able to figure that out" (negative view of self). "Trying to find a decent job is so hopeless that I might as well just give up trying" (negative view of experience). "I'm always going to be a failure. I'll never succeed at anything" (negative view of the future).

The techniques of CBT focus on teaching patients new ways to change these pathological schemas. CBT tends to be relatively short term and highly structured. Its goal is to help patients restructure their negative cognitions so that they can perceive reality in a less distorted way and learn to react accordingly.

The actual practice of CBT combines a group of behavioral techniques with a group of cognitive restructuring techniques. The behavioral techniques include a variety of homework assignments and a graded program of activities designed to teach patients that their negative schemas are incorrect and that they are in fact able to achieve small successes and interpret them as such.

For example, the woman who failed to obtain the job, described earlier in this section, might be asked to keep a record of her daily activities during the course of a week. Together, the therapist and patient would then review this diary and (in the context of other information about her) develop a set of assignments to be completed during the ensuing week. The diary of activities might indicate a very limited range of social contacts, based on the patient's fear and expectation of rejection. The patient might be assigned to make at least five social contacts during the course of the week by talking to neighbors, phoning friends, and going out on at least one social engagement. These activities also would be recorded in a diary and reviewed the following week with the therapist, including the patient's notes about her responses to the various contacts. She would be helped to see that she tended to initiate each contact with a negative hypothesis or expectation, which typically was disconfirmed by her actual experience. In fact, the contacts were largely affirmative. As therapy progresses and confidence builds, the assignments would gradually be made more difficult, until the patient achieved an essentially normal level of behavior and expectation. The diary would serve as a comforting reminder to the patient that, based on experience, negative hypotheses are typically disconfirmed. The patient would, of course, have some negative experiences; the therapist would assist her in understanding that such negative experiences are not a consequence of her own deficiencies and that even negative experiences can be surmounted.

These behavioral techniques are complemented with a variety of cognitive techniques that help the patient identify and correct the dysfunctional schemas that shape the patient's perception of reality. These techniques involve identifying a variety of cognitive distortions that the patient is prone to make and *automatic thoughts* that intrude into the patient's consciousness and produce negative attitudes. Six typical cognitive distortions, identified by Beck, are listed in Table 26–3.

TABLE 26–3. Typical cognitive distortions treated through cognitive-behavioral therapy

Distortion	Definition
Arbitrary inference	Drawing an erroneous conclusion from an experience
Selective abstraction	Taking a detail out of context and using it to denigrate the entire experience
Overgeneralization	Making general conclusions about overall experiences and relationships based on a single instance
Magnification and minimization	Altering the significance of specific events in a way that is structured by negative interpretations
Personalization	Interpreting events as reflecting on the patient when they have no relation to him or her
Dichotomous thinking	Seeing things in an all-or-none way

Arbitrary inference involves drawing an erroneous conclusion from an experience. For example, if the patient's hairdresser suggests that she may want to try a new hairstyle, the patient assumes that the hairdresser believes that the patient is becoming older-appearing and unattractive. *Selective ab-*

straction involves taking a detail out of context and using it to denigrate the entire experience. For example, while playing tennis, the patient may hit the ball out of the court, losing it in a grassy area, and reach the conclusion "That just proves I'm a lousy tennis player." *Overgeneralization* involves making general conclusions about overall experiences and relationships based on a single interaction. For example, after a disagreement with another employee at his or her current (less desirable) job, the patient concludes, "I'm a failure. I can't get along with anybody." *Magnification and minimization* involve altering the significance of specific small events in a way that is structured by negative interpretations. For example, the significance of a success may be minimized (a good grade on an examination is considered trivial because the examination was easy), and the significance of a failure may be maximized (losing a tennis game is seen as indicating that the patient will never succeed at anything). *Personalization* involves interpreting events as reflecting on the patient when they in fact have no specific relation to him or her. For example, a frown from a grouchy traffic policeman is seen as recognition of the patient's overall lack of skill as a driver and general worthlessness. *Dichotomous thinking* represents a tendency to see things in an all-or-none way. For example, an A– student with high expectations receives a B in a course and concludes, "That just proves it. I'm really a terrible student after all."

In addition to these erroneous interpretations, patients are often troubled with a variety of automatic thoughts that spontaneously intrude into the patient's flow of consciousness. The specific automatic thoughts vary from one individual to another but involve negative themes of self-denigration and failure (e.g., "You're so stupid," "You never do anything right," "People wouldn't want to talk to you"). These thoughts intrude spontaneously and produce an accompanying dysphoria. Patients are encouraged to identify these automatic thoughts and to learn ways to counteract them. Such techniques include replacing the automatic thoughts with positive counterthoughts, testing the hypotheses embedded in the thoughts through behavioral techniques as described above, and identifying and testing the assumptions behind the thoughts.

The goal of the cognitive component of CBT is to identify and restructure the various negative schemas that shape the patient's perceptions. The cognitive goal is achieved like the behavioral goals: the patient is encouraged to do homework, to complete assignments that identify the occurrence of dysfunctional cognitions, and to steadily test and correct these cognitions. The therapist also reviews these aspects of the patient's diary and helps formulate an organized program for restructuring the dysfunctional cognitive sets, providing ample empathy and positive reinforcement.

CBT is particularly effective for patients with depression. Its techniques also can be adapted to treat various anxiety disorders through identifying cognitive schemas characterized by fear. It may be used either alone for the treatment of relatively mild disorders or in conjunction with medications for patients with more severe disorders.

Individual Psychotherapy

The term *individual psychotherapy* covers a broad range of psychotherapeutic techniques. Both behavior therapy and cognitive therapy usually are done individually (i.e., a single therapist working with a single patient). The historical roots of individual psychodynamic psychotherapy derive from Freudian psychodynamic approaches. In addition, however, simpler, briefer approaches to individual psychotherapy have been developed, which may draw either directly or indirectly on psychodynamic approaches. Countless schools of psychotherapy offer a variety of approaches. The description below provides a simplified and selective overview.

The various psychotherapies do share some common elements. These include the following, which are characteristic of all psychotherapies:

- Based on an interpersonal relationship
- Use of verbal communication between two (or more) people as a healing element
- Specific expertise on the part of the therapist in using communication and relationships in a healing way
- Based on a rationale or conceptual structure that is used to understand the patient's problems
- Use of a specific procedure in the relationship that is linked to the rationale
- Structured relationship (e.g., contact time, frequency, and duration are prespecified)
- Expectation of improvement

Classical Psychoanalysis and Psychodynamic Psychotherapy

Psychoanalysis was originally developed by Sigmund Freud during the early twentieth century. This technique arose from Freud's experience in attempting to treat patients with hysterical conversion symptoms, such as pains and paralyses. Following the lead of Charcot, his initial efforts involved the use of hypnosis. He observed, however, that this treatment was not always effective and that there was a high recurrence and relapse rate. He began to suspect that these conversion symptoms reflected some sort of painful early psychological experience that had been repressed. Instead of hypnosis, he began to experiment with the technique of having the patient lie down and relax while he placed his hand on his or her forehead and encouraged him or her to talk about whatever came into his or her mind and to release the repressed thoughts.

This treatment developed at a time when Victorian Puritanism and hypocrisy still reigned supreme, and even Freud must have been astonished at the thoughts that flowed from his patients' minds, covering a variety of sexual fantasies and experiences. Based on his many years of experience in applying this approach, initially to conversion symptoms but subsequently to a range of symptoms including anxiety disorders and even psychoses, Freud developed a systematic theory to describe the structure and operations of the human psyche. Basic concepts include stages of psychosexual development (oral, anal, phallic, and genital), the structure of conscious and unconscious thoughts (primary vs. secondary process thinking), the structure of drives and motivations (id, ego, and superego), the symbolism inherent in dreams, theories of infant sexuality, and a host of other concepts that the layperson associates with Freudianism.

Subsequent psychoanalysts elaborated and modified Freud's original work in various ways, such as developing theories of ego psychology and expanding understanding of the mental mechanisms involved in defense, coping, and adaptation. These various ideas and theories are major resources for clinicians trained in either psychoanalysis or psychodynamic psychotherapy. Use of these approaches requires extensive experience and training under the supervision of a qualified psychoanalyst.

Classical psychoanalysis is now used only in relatively special situations and settings. The form of treatment is best adapted to individuals who are fundamentally healthy (both psychologically and financially) and who have sufficient adaptive resources to go through the intensive process of self-scrutiny required by psychoanalysis. Typical reasons for seeking psychoanalysis include difficulties in relationships and persistent and recurrent anxiety, although neither should be so severe as to be incapacitating.

The core component of classical psychoanalysis is the development of a *transference neurosis*. That is, the patient transfers to the therapist all the thoughts and feelings that he or she experienced during early life; through this transference, he or she is able to make conscious the various unconscious drives and emotions that are troubling him or her and ultimately to modify and heal them, as the analyst makes appropriate interpretations during the course of the psychoanalysis.

The patient is typically asked to lie on a couch and to free-associate, saying whatever comes into his or her mind without any type of censorship. The analyst sits behind the patient, remaining a relatively shadowy and neutral figure to encourage the development of transference. (If the analyst becomes too human or "real," then transference cannot develop.) To maintain an appropriate level of intensity, the patient must be seen four to five times per week for 50-minute sessions. The process typically requires 2–3 years. Because the analyst becomes a repository of large quantities of intimate and highly personal information, he or she must be both psychologically and ethically trustworthy. Analysts must go through an extensive period of psychoanalysis themselves to understand their own psychological vulnerabilities and, in particular, the nature of the countertransference that they are likely to develop in relation to their patients.

Psychodynamic psychotherapy uses many of the concepts embodied in psychoanalytic theory, but these concepts are used in ways that make them more suitable for the treatment of larger numbers of patients. Treatment is not necessarily less intensive, in the sense of attempting to focus on and correct problems, but it does not involve the relatively rigidly defined techniques (e.g., use of the couch) that characterize classical psychoanalysis.

Psychodynamic psychotherapy is used to treat patients with a variety of problems, including personality disorders, sexual dysfunctions, somatoform disorders, anxiety disorders, and mild depression. Psychodynamic psychotherapy is typically conducted face to face. Depending on the frequency and duration of therapy, a transference neurosis may or may not occur. The therapist attempts to help the patient in a neutral but empathic way. The patient is encouraged to review early relationships with parents and significant others but also may focus on the here and now. As in classical psychoanalysis, the patient is expected to do most of the talking, while the psychodynamic psychotherapist occasionally interjects clarifications to help the patient understand the underlying dynamics that shape his or her behavior. Psychodynamic psychotherapy typically involves sessions one to two times a week and may involve 2–5 years of treatment.

Insight-Oriented and Relationship Psychotherapy

Insight-oriented psychotherapy and relationship psychotherapy are two other variants of individual psychotherapy that may be somewhat less intensive or long term.

Insight-oriented psychotherapy draws on many basic psychodynamic concepts but focuses even more on interpersonal relationships and here-and-now situations than does purely psychodynamic psychotherapy. Patients are typically seen once a week for 50 minutes. During the sessions, they are encouraged to review and discuss relationships, attitudes toward themselves, and early life experiences. The therapist maintains an involved and supportive attitude and occasionally assists patients with interpretations that will help them achieve insights. This form of psychotherapy does not encourage transference, regression, and abreaction. Instead of reexperiencing and reliving, patients are encouraged to achieve an intellectual understanding of the mainsprings of their behavior that will help them change their behavior as needed.

In *relationship psychotherapy,* the therapist assumes a more active role. The stress is on achieving a corrective emotional experience, with the therapist serving as a loving and trustworthy surrogate parent who assists the patient in confronting unrecognized needs and unresolved drives.

The patient is typically seen once per week, and the therapy may last from 6 months to several years, depending on the patient's problems and level of maturity. As in insight-oriented psychotherapy, the content of the sessions focuses primarily on current situations and relationships, with some looking backward to early life experiences. Although the patient may achieve insight, the most important component of this type of psychotherapy is the empathic and caring attitude of the therapist.

Interpersonal Therapy

Interpersonal therapy (IPT) is a specific type of psychotherapy that was developed for the treatment of depression, although it is also potentially useful for the treatment of other conditions, such as personality disorders. Drawing on the ideas of thinkers such as Harry Stack Sullivan, who stressed that mental illnesses may reflect and be expressed in problems in relationships (as opposed to intrapsychic conflict stressed by psychodynamic approaches), IPT emphasizes working on improving interpersonal relationships during the process of psychotherapy.

During IPT, the emphasis is on the here and now rather than on the past. During a process of exploration, the therapist helps the patient identify specific problem areas that may be interfering with self-esteem and interpersonal interactions. These usually involve four general domains: grief, interpersonal disputes, role transitions, and interpersonal deficits. After the exploration and identification process, the therapist works systematically with the patient to facilitate the learning of new adaptive behaviors and communication styles.

IPT is usually conducted in weekly sessions, and the overall course of therapy lasts from 3 to 4 months. It is one of the few forms of psychotherapy that has been subjected to rigorous empirical testing of its efficacy. In well-controlled acute and maintenance studies of depression, it has been shown to be superior to no active treatment and to medication alone when used in combination with amitriptyline. IPT also has been used with some success in treating depressed adolescents and persons with bulimia.

Supportive Psychotherapy

Supportive psychotherapy is used to help patients get through difficult situations. Components of supportive psychotherapy may be incorporated into any of the other types of psychotherapy described in this section, with the exception of classical psychoanalysis.

In conducting supportive psychotherapy, the therapist maintains an attitude of sympathy, interest, and concern. Patients describe and discuss the various problems they are confronting, which could range from marital discord to psychotic experiences such as persecutory delusions. Supportive psychotherapy is appropriate for the full spectrum of psychiatric disorders, ranging from adjustment disorders through the psychoses and even dementia.

As in relationship psychotherapy, the therapist may function much like a healthy and loving parent who provides the patient with encouragement and direction as needed. The goal of supportive therapy is to help the patient cope with difficult situations, experiences, or periods of adjustment. Patients typically describe their problems, and the therapist counters with encouragement and even specific advice. The therapist may suggest specific techniques that patients can use in coping with their problems, such as developing new interests or hobbies, trying new activities that may expand their range of social contacts, achieving emancipation from their parents by moving into independent living circumstances, and developing more organized study habits to improve their school performance. Psychotic patients may be taught to refrain from discussing their delusional ideas, except with the therapist. Alcoholic patients may receive praise and encouragement for refraining from drinking, as well as suggestions about ways to increase their self-esteem by achieving mastery and control, such as through improving their skills in a particular sport or developing a new creative hobby. As these examples indicate, the clinician involved in conducting supportive therapy needs to tailor the therapy sessions to the individual needs of each particular patient.

Supportive psychotherapy is typically done weekly. It is often done in conjunction with other treatments, particularly the somatic therapies. It may be relatively brief, as when it is used for crisis intervention in patients with adjustment disorders. Conversely, it may be very long term (although it may be less frequent than weekly) when it is used as a treatment modality for patients with more chronic or protracted mental illnesses, such as schizophrenia, recurrent mania or depression, and various anxiety disorders.

Defense and Coping Mechanisms

Defense and coping mechanisms are techniques that both patients and psychiatrically normal people use to help themselves deal with difficult situations or emotional experiences. These techniques are divided into *defense mechanisms* (which are considered less mature and more primitive and therefore less healthy) and *coping mechanisms* (which represent a higher adaptive level and are considered mature ways to cope with life's stresses and problems) (See Table 26–4). The clinician can observe these mechanisms in operation in a variety of medical settings, ranging from the emergency room to the recovery room. Understanding these mechanisms assists the clinician in providing most types of psychosocial treatments for psychiatric patients and in providing general medical care.

TABLE 26–4. Some common defense and coping mechanisms

Defense mechanisms (immature)	Coping mechanisms (mature)
Denial	Sublimation
Projection	Religiousness
Regression	Humor
Repression	Altruism
Splitting	Mastery and control
Reaction formation	
Undoing	
Isolation	
Displacement	

Defense Mechanisms

Defense mechanisms are used to ward off or avoid painful feelings and thoughts that are difficult to confront. They are usually considered to be neurotic and immature.

Denial is characterized by ignoring an undesirable situation or piece of information and behaving as though it did not exist. For example, a man with established coronary artery disease may insist that he feels fine and refuse to comply with instructions to diet, lose weight, stop smoking, and exercise. A patient with recurrent mania may refuse to admit the presence of periods of pathological euphoria.

Projection involves attributing to others unwanted ideas or feelings that are experienced within oneself. This mechanism involves attributing to others the negative emotions that one has toward them; for example, a paranoid patient who feels angry with her doctor (an unacceptable emotion) believes instead that the doctor is angry with her and is tormenting her by insisting that she take medication. On a more everyday level, projection is often seen as a mechanism by which patients refuse to accept responsibility for their own mistakes and instead place the blame on others. For example, a person who is having difficulty at work because of procrastination and failure to meet deadlines says to himself, "It isn't my fault. They're all being too demanding. If only my co-workers would be more helpful, I'd be able to get my work done."

Regression is withdrawal to a more primitive level of adaptation in response to some overwhelming stressor. For example, a woman with a mild dementia may be able to cope at a minimal but acceptable level but regresses into an infantile state characterized by inability to feed herself or maintain her toilet habits when confronted with the death of the husband who has supported her for the past 50 years. A 40-year-old woman in intensive psychotherapy may relate to her therapist in a childlike, dependent way, treating the therapist as if he is a father (a regression that may be appropriate in the context of intensive psychodynamic therapy).

Repression involves suppressing from awareness emotions and memories that are experienced as painful. For example, a patient dying from cancer may go through a period when he feels quite cheerful, even though he is consciously aware that his illness is terminal, simply because he feels an uncontrollable need to ward off the recognition of his inevitable and impending death.

Splitting involves keeping emotions and past experiences in stereotyped univalent logic-tight compartments, preventing recognition and integration of the nuances and complexities of relationships and experiences (i.e., everything is either good or bad). For example, a woman who feels angry with her mother for divorcing her father and remarrying may be unable to develop a much-needed reconciliation because she has split away the good affects (based on the genuine periods of happiness that she shared with her mother) and can recognize only the bad affects of anger and estrangement.

Reaction formation involves substituting an opposite attitude and experience for one that is experienced as psychologically painful. For example, a patient with hemophilia may take up motorcycle racing and skydiving as a way of counteracting the painful fact of his or her disease. A patient with obsessive-compulsive personality disorder, who feels angry that his or her boss does not recognize his or her meticulousness and diligence, may maintain an air of affection and cheerfulness toward the boss.

Undoing involves the substitution of one behavior for another, in an effort to change or modify the initial behavior. It is particularly common in patients with obsessive-compulsive disorder and is thought to reflect the patient's basic ambivalence and indecisiveness. For example, a person may become angry with a supervisor or teacher and express this anger by making a critical comment. Later, he or she may try to undo this behavior by performing an opposite one, such as giving the supervisor or teacher a small gift or praising him or her in some way.

Isolation (intellectualization) is a defense technique for coping with painful affects. The affect is separated from its content, often by treating it objectively rather than experientially. Thus, a patient who is in fact prone to experience intense anxiety about some topic, such as sexuality or emotional intimacy, will avoid placing himself or herself in situations in which he or she will be forced to confront this anxiety. Instead, he or she may pursue research on the mating habits of frogs or bees. In a clinical therapy setting, this defense is most commonly noted when the patient talks about his or her problems in an intellectual, overly abstract manner and has difficulty describing, recalling, or experiencing his or her actual feelings.

Displacement involves the resolution of a conflict about some particular relationship or event by shifting the emotion attached to it onto some other relationship or event. For example, a woman who feels intense anger toward her father or her husband because of neglect or mistreatment may direct her anger toward her young male child (or even her female child) because she perceives her husband or father as more powerful than she is and thus feels unable to express her anger directly.

Coping Mechanisms

Coping mechanisms are considered to be on a somewhat higher adaptational level than defense mechanisms. Although coping mechanisms also may ward off unpleasant or unconscious emotions and experiences, they are usually productive and helpful to both the patient and those around him or her.

Sublimation involves using past traumatic or unpleasant experiences or emotions as well as basic "id drives" in a way that both reduces anxiety and is not injurious to society. For example, a person with high levels of sexual energy may choose to work long hours.

Religiousness involves making painful past experiences more acceptable by experiencing them as part of God's will. For example, a dying patient may come to terms with impending death by seeing it as simply part of a universal pattern ordained by God.

Humor involves counteracting painful affects by seeing the comic side of the human situation. Sometimes the comedy may be black, but other times it may be light and positive. Jokes made in the anatomy laboratory, the operating room, and the military trenches are all examples.

Altruism involves taking a negative experience and turning it into a socially useful or positive one. For example, a reformed alcoholic person may obtain great satisfaction by helping others in the context of AA.

Mastery and control involve gaining a sense of control over a painful situation by confronting it directly and developing techniques that prevent the person from feeling overwhelmed. For example, a medical student confronted with an enormous mass of information and responsibility (which makes the student feel psychologically threatened and powerless) will throw himself or herself intensively into work, eventually reducing anxiety and increasing his or her sense of self-worth and internal strength by learning as much as possible. Some individuals choose to go into medicine as a way of gaining mastery and control; having experienced illness or death within their immediate families, they may seek to gain control over it by choosing a profession that involves working toward reducing illness and death.

Group Therapy

Group therapy provides a highly effective way for clinicians to follow up with and monitor relatively large numbers of patients. It also provides patients with a social environment or even surrogate peer group that will help them learn new and constructive ways to interact with others in a controlled and supportive environment.

Irving Yalom, one of the major leaders of the group therapy movement in the United States, enumerated a variety of factors that summarize the therapeutic mechanisms that occur during the process of group therapy. These include instilling hope, developing socializing skills, using imitative behavior, experiencing catharsis, imparting information, behaving altruistically by attempting to help other members of the group, experiencing a corrective recapitulation of the primary family group, developing a sense of group cohesiveness, diminishing feelings of isolation (universality), and learning through feedback how one's behavior affects others (interpersonal learning).

There are many different kinds of group therapy. The types vary depending on the individuals who compose the group, the problems or disorders that they are confronting, the setting in which the group meets, the type of role that the group leader takes, and the therapeutic goals that have been established.

In many hospital settings, a group therapy program is established for inpatients. Such groups are typically led by a physician, a nurse, a social worker, or some combination thereof. In very large inpatient hospital settings, several groups may run concurrently and be composed of patients with similar types of problems. For example, one group might consist of relatively high-functioning individuals with personality problems or depression. Another group might consist of patients with severe mood and psychotic disorders, and yet another group might consist of individuals with eating disorders. Such groups provide patients with a forum to share their problems, diminish their sense of isolation and loneliness, enable them to learn new techniques to cope with their problems either through other patients or through the group leader, and provide support, inspiration, and hope. Such groups also may help patients improve interpersonal and social skills. For example, patients with schizophrenia and other psychoses may improve their social skills in relating to others, and patients with personality disorders may receive useful feedback from other group members about counterproductive behavior.

In many clinical settings, such inpatient groups are supplemented by outpatient or aftercare groups, where patients receive continued follow-up, pursuing goals similar to those described above but in the more stressful environment of the real world. These outpatient groups represent an attempt to consolidate and support the learning and skills that have already been developed in the inpatient setting.

Some groups are oriented largely toward providing support. Such groups may or may not have a professional leader. Examples of such support groups include AA meetings, family support groups such as those organized by chapters of the Alliance for the Mentally Ill (an organization composed of the family members of patients with serious mental illnesses), support groups for individuals who conceive of themselves as minorities in a particular setting (e.g., women professionals, women medical students, black students), groups composed of Persian Gulf War veterans, or groups composed of individuals who have experienced some serious medical illness or difficult surgery (e.g., patients with diabetes, women who have had mastectomies, individuals receiving dialysis). Such groups provide a forum for sharing information, giving encouragement and support, and instilling hope through diminishing feelings of isolation.

Groups are also created to conduct group psychotherapy. Such groups are typically led by therapists with extensive experience in group psychotherapy and are often conducted with a cotherapist. These groups aim to achieve goals similar to those of insight-oriented and interpersonal psychotherapy or cognitive therapy within the context of a group setting. Psychotherapy groups are typically more highly structured than the other types of groups described above. The group leaders take an active role in organizing each session, often prescribe exercises within the session, establish ground rules for membership within the group (e.g., no tardiness, regular attendance), resolve conflicts between members of the group, and assume responsibility for providing summaries of each session and access to videotapes of the sessions. Patients are typically carefully screened before being admitted to a psychotherapy group to ensure that they will be able to participate effectively. Such groups are particularly helpful for individuals with the same type of problems that led them into individual psychotherapy, such as interpersonal and relationship problems, anxiety, mild depression, and personality disorders.

Marital Therapy and Family Therapy

Some problems for which patients seek treatment clearly involve other people. A man may present with feelings of depression and inadequacy because his wife has returned to work and is requesting that he assume his fair share of household duties and child care, a situation that he finds demeaning and inappropriate. A young teenager may present with mild symptoms of acting-out behavior, such as truancy from school and experimenting with alcohol, and indicate that she is seeking support from peers because she is having difficulty coping with her parents' inappropriately high expectations and overprotective smothering. In such situations, although the patient may come in initially as an individual case, the clinician usually will rapidly determine that he or she needs to be seen within the context of the larger family unit, which might be husband and wife in the first example (marital counseling) and the parents and child in the second example (family therapy).

These two types of therapy may be done by psychiatrists but are also often done by psychologists, social workers, or nurses. Depending on the specific problems of the presenting individual, family therapy or marital counseling may be done in addition to individual therapy and medication management. Both of these types of therapy are usually relatively short term, lasting from weeks to months, and both are oriented toward identifying and resolving specific and clearly identifiable problems as quickly as possible. All physicians should have at least a superficial familiarity with these types of therapy because they must recognize that nearly all their patients live within the context of a family. In specific instances, the internist, pediatrician, or family physician must be able to recognize the need for marital counseling or family therapy and to refer the patient appropriately (usually through additional screening and assessment by a psychiatrist, who will evaluate the need for a referral and may conduct the treatment).

Marital Therapy

Marital therapy involves working with two people who see themselves as partners in a marital relationship to help them stabilize and improve their relationship. This therapy once involved seeing a husband and wife. In contemporary society, the partners seeking treatment may be unmarried, gay, or lesbian. Depending on the commitment of the two partners, marital therapy has many variations. Ideally, both partners are willing and cooperative participants who are anxious to initiate change. Sometimes, however, marital therapy is sought because of a crisis: one of the partners may have lost interest in the relationship (and may or may not want to get out), whereas the other is hanging on tight and trying to save the relationship. In the latter instance, one possible outcome might be the eventual decision to end the relationship, and therapy might become divorce mediation and counseling. If children are involved, then what began as marital therapy might turn into family therapy as the couple attempts to work out an equitable arrangement in the context of the larger number of people who will be affected. In some instances, a dysfunctional sexual relationship between the couple will become apparent, and the couple may want referral to a sex therapy clinic for treatment of impotence or anorgasmia. (The treatment of sexual disorders is described in Chapter 17.)

An individual conducting marital therapy must take care to maintain an atmosphere of fairness, neutrality, and impartiality. Either partner will be particularly sensitive to the possibility that the therapist may take sides and treat him or her unfairly. The gender of the therapist may seem quite significant to either partner, even though the therapist may feel quite comfortable with his or her ability to be impartial. Women may believe that only a female therapist is able to understand their point of view and may feel quite defensive if asked to work with a male therapist. Male partners may have similar attitudes or problems.

Marital counseling typically begins with identifying the specific problem. Each partner is asked to identify specific areas in which he or she would like to see change in the other. The therapist attempts to assist the couple in implementing changes in a gradual, graded way, attacking one problem at a time. Typically, in the early sessions, a single, salient problem is the focus of attention. For example, a wife may express feelings of being ignored, whereas a husband may complain of his wife's whining expressions of dependency. Each will identify specific target behaviors in the other that need modification. They then contract with each other to modify these behaviors. Subsequent marital sessions focus on the steps they have taken to achieve improvement and on continuing work in new areas of concern.

This type of graded behavior change is the minimum component of marital therapy. Often, couples also benefit from discussing their hopes for and expectations of each other in the context of personal values, prior family experiences (i.e., role expectations about men and women, based on the behavior of their own parents), changing social norms about the roles of men and women, and needs for both intimacy and independence that occur within the context of a relationship.

Family Therapy

Family therapy tends to focus on the larger family unit—at a minimum, one parent and the child (in single-parent families), but more typically both parents and the child (or a parent and stepparent, two separated parents, other parental pairings depending on the family environment in which the child lives), or one or more parents and the child plus siblings. Typically, the child is brought in initially for treatment of a specific problem, such as school difficulties, hyperactivity, delinquency, or aggressive behavior. Often, it rapidly becomes clear that these problems exist in the overall context of the family setting. The family should not necessarily be regarded as dysfunctional, however. Because of changing circumstances or demands (e.g., a recent move), the parents may have difficulty in determining methods for coping with the child's behavior or understanding why it is occurring.

As in marital therapy, it is important for the therapist to be fair and impartial in family therapy. In this instance, however, the therapist is not dealing with two potential equals but rather with a hierarchy in which parents are expected to assume some authority and responsibility for the behavior of their child. The degree of hierarchy in the family will vary, depending on the age of the child. For adolescents and teenagers, one important problem may be the challenge that the "child's" growing independence is adding to this hierarchical structure.

As in marital therapy, behavioral approaches are a mainstay of family therapy. The therapist usually begins by focusing on here-and-now problems. Parents and child discuss openly the nature of the problem that has brought about the need for therapy. For example, a 12-year-old boy may be intermittently truant from school, tell lies about his activities, and seek out parties on the weekends where he has been known to drink beer occasionally. The child may complain of parental pressure and repeated criticism, whereas the parents may express their fears about the child's unreliability and poor school performance. As in marital therapy, graded areas of priority are identified, and contracts are made about changes that both parents and child will implement. Parents are given tactful but explicit suggestions about the value of positive reinforcement instead of criticism as a way of modifying behavior, and the child is led to realize that some hierarchy and structure will remain in his or her life, although to a gradually lessening degree as he or she shows mature and dependable behavior.

Family therapy also may be used to help families in which at least one member has a relatively serious mental illness, such as schizophrenia, bipolar disorder, or recurrent depression. In this type of family therapy, it is important to work firmly within the medical model and to emphasize that the patient has an illness for which neither the patient nor the family can be considered responsible. This approach minimizes guilt, scapegoating, and castigation, and it permits both patient and family members to seek more consoling and constructive methods for coping with the symptoms of the illness. A young schizophrenic patient living at home may need some assistance from his or her family in developing social skills (see "Social Skills Training" later in this chapter), whereas family members may need assistance in learning ways to cope with outbursts of anger or periods of emotional disengagement and withdrawal. Families with high levels of involvement (referred to as high "expressed emotion") may need counseling on ways to be less intensely involved because it has been shown that in some instances, high levels of expressed emotion may be experienced as stressful by the schizophrenic patient and lead to relapse. Thus, families may need assistance in finding the right balance between providing needed support and encouragement and setting up excessively high expectations. Education about the symptoms of the illness is also an important component of family therapy for both the patient and the family members.

Social Skills Training

Social skills training is a specific type of psychotherapy that focuses primarily on developing abilities in relating to others and in coping with the demands of daily life. It is used primarily for patients with severe mental illnesses, such as schizophrenia, which are often accompanied by marked impairments in social skills.

Social skills training may be done initially on an inpatient basis, but the bulk of the effort is typically done with outpatients because the long-term goal of social skills training is to assist patients in learning to live in the real world. Social skills training is typically done by nurses, social workers, or psychologists. It may be done individually, but it more typically is accompanied by some group work as well, and it may occur in the context of day hospitals or sheltered workshops.

The techniques of social skills training also are primarily behavioral. Specific problems are identified and addressed in a sequentially integrated manner. Severely disabled patients may need assistance initially in grooming and hygiene. They may need encouragement in learning to shave or bathe daily, to keep their clothes laundered, and to eat regular meals. They also may need help in learning how to approach other people and to talk with them appropriately. At higher levels of functioning, they may need assistance in learning how to apply for a job, complete job interviews, and relate to employers and co-workers. Because long-term institutional care is no longer available to most patients with psychotic illnesses, these individuals are literally being forced to learn to live in the community. Many cannot do so without receiving training and assistance in activities of daily living, such as grooming, managing money, and achieving at least a minimal level of social interaction with others. Although the development of such skills may seem elementary or minimal, for some patients it can lead to a substantial improvement in their quality of life.

Bibliography

Beck AT, Rush AJ, Shaw BF, et al: Cognitive Therapy of Depression. New York, Guilford, 1979

Beck AT, Emery G, Greenberg BL: Anxiety Disorders and Phobias: A Cognitive Perspective. New York, Basic Books, 1985

Davanloo H (ed): Short-Term Dynamic Psychotherapy. New York, Jason Aronson, 1980

Emery RE: Marriage, Divorce, and Children's Adjustment, 2nd Edition. London, UK, Sage Publications, 1999

Fenichel O: The Psychoanalytic Theory of Neurosis. New York, WW Norton, 1945

Freud A: The Ego and the Mechanisms of Defense. New York, International Universities Press, 1965

Freud S: The dynamics of transference (1912), in The Standard Edition of the Complete Psychological Works of Sigmund Freud, Vol 12. Translated and edited by Strachey J. London, UK, Hogarth Press, 1958, pp 97–108

Freud S: On beginning the treatment (1913), in The Standard Edition of the Complete Psychological Works of Sigmund Freud, Vol 12. Translated and edited by Strachey J. London, UK, Hogarth Press, 1958, pp 121–144

Gabbard GO: Psychodynamic Psychiatry in Clinical Practice, 3rd Edition. Washington, DC, American Psychiatric Press, 2000

Glick ID, Berman EM, Clarkin JF, et al: Marital and Family Therapy, 4th Edition. Washington, DC, American Psychiatric Press, 2000

Gunderson JG, Gabbard GO: Psychotherapy for Personality Disorders. Washington, DC, American Psychiatric Press, 2000

Gurman AS, Messer SB (eds): Essential Psychotherapies: Theory and Practice. New York, Guilford, 1995

Kandel ER: Biology and the future of psychoanalysis: a new intellectual framework for psychiatry. Am J Psychiatry 156:505–524, 1999

Kingdon DG, Turkington D: Cognitive-Behavioral Therapy of Depression. New York, Guilford, 1994

Klerman GL, Weissman MM, Rounsaville BJ, et al: Interpersonal Psychotherapy of Depression. New York, Basic Books, 1984

Moore BE, Fine BD (eds): Psychoanalysis: The Major Concepts. New Haven, CT, Yale University Press, 1999

Nichols M: Family Therapy: Concepts and Methods. New York, Gardner, 1984

Perris C: Cognitive Therapy With Schizophrenic Patients. New York, Guilford, 1989

Reid WH: A Clinician's Guide to Legal Issues in Psychotherapy. Phoenix, AZ, Zieg & Tucker, 1999

Richards PS, Bergin AE (eds): Handbook of Psychotherapy and Religious Diversity. Washington, DC, American Psychological Association, 2000

Sharpe SA: The Ways We Love: A Developmental Approach to Treating Couples. New York, Guilford, 2000

Vaillant GE: Theoretical hierarchy of adaptive ego mechanisms. Arch Gen Psychiatry 24:107–118, 1971

Vaillant GE: Adaptation to Life. New York, Little, Brown, 1977

Vaillant GE: An empirically derived hierarchy of adaptive mechanisms and its usefulness as a potential diagnostic axis, in Diagnosis and Classification in Psychiatry: A Critical Appraisal of DSM-III. Edited by Tischler G. New York, Cambridge University Press, 1987, pp 464–476

Vaillant GE, Bond M, Vaillant CO: An empirically validated hierarchy of defense mechanisms. Arch Gen Psychiatry 43:786–794, 1986

Weiner M: Practical Psychotherapy. New York, Brunner/Mazel, 1986

Yalom ID: The Theory and Practice of Group Psychotherapy, 3rd Edition. New York, Basic Books, 1985

Self-Assessment Questions

1. What is the difference between classical conditioning and operant conditioning?
2. What is the definition of a positive reinforcer? A negative reinforcer?
3. Describe four common techniques for conducting behavior therapy.
4. Describe CBT. What is the cognitive triad? What are automatic thoughts?
5. Describe classical psychoanalysis. How does it differ from psychodynamic psychotherapy? What is transference?
6. Describe the concept of a corrective emotional experience in psychotherapy.
7. Describe two different types of group therapy, and enumerate some situations in which they would be appropriate.
8. Describe the role of the therapist in marital and family therapy.

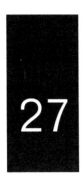

27 Somatic Treatments

> The desire to take medicine is perhaps the greatest feature that distinguishes man from animals.
>
> Sir William Osler

The modern treatment era in psychiatry began with the introduction of effective psychotropic medication in the early 1950s. Until that time, the mainstay of treatment was psychotherapy, although prefrontal lobotomy and electroconvulsive therapy (ECT) had been recently introduced—each accompanied by the excitement that any new treatment generates. Their limitations soon became apparent, and after the introduction of antipsychotic and antidepressant medications, lobotomy fell into disuse, and the use of ECT became limited to a relatively small group of patients with severe illnesses, such as major depression.

Before the availability of these new somatic treatments, psychiatrists were greatly limited in their ability to help patients, and overcrowded mental hospitals were common. The introduction of effective medications revolutionized psychiatry and led to the era of deinstitutionalization, a period in which mental patients were released from state hospitals in large numbers to be cared for in the community. The wisdom of this movement is now being critically assessed because promised community resources were often poorly funded or unavailable, and many patients ended up on the streets.

Antipsychotics

Chlorpromazine was introduced in 1952 by two French psychiatrists, Jean Delay and Pierre Deniker, after it was recognized that the drug had powerful calming effects on agitated psychotic patients. Delay and Deniker soon discovered that the drug was especially effective in patients with schizophrenia. Not only were agitated patients calmed, but the new drug seemed to diminish their terrifying hallucinations and troubling delusional thoughts.

Many antipsychotics have been developed and marketed since chlorpromazine was introduced and are similar in action and efficacy. Although these drugs are effective in controlling psychotic symptoms and diminishing the patient's disturbed thought processes, they are not curative. Improvement can be dramatic, and medication effectiveness is generally sustained over years or decades. Nonetheless, from 10% to 40% of patients respond poorly to conventional antipsychotics, and the quality of response varies from patient to patient. Furthermore, these drugs do little for negative symptoms of schizophrenia such as apathy and avolition. Recently, a new generation of antipsychotic drugs was introduced, beginning with clozapine and later joined by risperidone, olanzapine, quetiapine, and ziprasidone, with additional drugs in the pipeline. Both the older—or typical—antipsychotics and the newer atypical antipsychotics ameliorate the symptoms of psychotic illnesses, including hallucinations, delusions, bizarre behavior, disordered thinking, and agitation. The atypical antipsychotics have fewer side effects, are better tolerated, and may be more effective than the older typical antipsychotics. Although they are collectively referred to as *major tranquilizers,* this term is a misnomer because antipsychotic drugs do not produce a state of tranquillity in nonpsychotic or psychotic persons. The term *antipsychotic* is more appropriate in that the drugs are helpful in ameliorating symptoms of psychoses.

There are 13 classes of antipsychotics, each differing in molecular structure (see Table 27–1). The phenothiazines, the oldest class, have a three-ring nucleus, but the subtypes differ by nature of the side chains joined to the nitrogen atom in the middle ring. The three phenothiazine subtypes are the aliphatics (e.g., chlorpromazine), the piperidines (e.g., thioridazine), and the piperazines (e.g., trifluoperazine). Other classes of antipsychotics include the thioxanthenes (e.g., thiothixene), the dibenzoxazepines (e.g., loxapine), the butyrophenones (e.g., haloperidol), the dihydroindolones (e.g., molindone), the dibenzodiazepines (e.g., clozapine), the benzamides (e.g., sulpiride, not available in the United States), the benzisoxazoles (e.g., risperidone), the dibenzothiazepines (e.g., quetiapine), the thienbenzodiaz-

TABLE 27–1. Common antipsychotic agents

Category	Drug (trade name)	Sedation	Orthostatic hypotension	Anticholinergic effects	Extrapyramidal effects	Equivalent dosage, mg	Dosage range, mg/day
Conventional agents							
Phenothiazines							
Aliphatics	Chlorpromazine (Thorazine)	H	H	M	M	100	50–1,200
Piperidines	Mesoridazine (Serentil)	H	H	H	L	50	50–400
	Thioridazine (Mellaril)	H	H	H	L	95	50–800
Piperazines	Fluphenazine (Prolixin)	L	L	L	VH	2	2–20
	Fluphenazine decanoate	L	L	L	VH	—[a]	12.5–50 mg q 2 wk
	Perphenazine (Trilafon)	L	L	L	H	10	12–64
	Trifluoperazine (Stelazine)	L	L	L	H	5	5–40
Thioxanthenes	Thiothixene (Navane)	L	L	L	H	5	5–60
Dibenzoxazepines	Loxapine (Loxitane)	M	M	L	H	15	20–250
Butyrophenones	Haloperidol (Haldol)	L	L	L	VH	2	2–60
	Haloperidol decanoate	L	L	L	VH	—[a]	50–250 mg q 4 wk
Dihydroindolones	Molindone (Moban)	VL	L	L	H	10	50–400

TABLE 27–1. Common antipsychotic agents (*continued*)

Category	Drug (trade name)	Sedation	Orthostatic hypotension	Anticholinergic effects	Extrapyramidal effects	Equivalent dosage, mg	Dosage range, mg/day
Atypical agents							
Benzisothiazolyls	Ziprasidone (Geodon)	M	L	VL	VL	30	80–160
Dibenzodiazepines	Clozapine (Clozaril)	VH	H	VH	VL	50	200–900
Benzisoxazoles	Risperidone (Risperdal)	L	M	VL	VL	1	2–6
Dibenzothiazepines	Quetiapine (Seroquel)	M	M	VL	VL	100	150–800
Thienbenzodiazepines	Olanzapine (Zyprexa)	M	L	L	VL	2–3	10–20

[a]Long-acting ester; dosage is not directly comparable with that of standard compounds.
H = high; L = low; M = moderate; VH = very high; VL = very low.

epines (e.g., olanzapine), the benzisothiazolyls (e.g., ziprasidone), the rauwolfia alkaloids (e.g., reserpine, no longer used to treat psychoses), and the diphenylbutylpiperidines (e.g., pimozide, used to treat Tourette's disorder).

Indications for Antipsychotics

The use of antipsychotic drugs is primarily limited to schizophrenia and other psychotic disorders (e.g., schizophreniform disorder, schizoaffective disorder), but they are also prescribed to psychotic patients with mood disorders and to patients whose psychoses are medically induced or due to drugs of abuse. Antipsychotics are used to control aggressive behavior in mentally retarded patients, autistic patients, patients with borderline personality disorder, and patients with delirium or dementia. They also are prescribed to patients with Tourette's disorder to diminish the frequency and severity of vocal and motor tics. The atypical antipsychotic olanzapine recently has received an indication as monotherapy for the treatment of acute mania.

Mechanism of Action of Antipsychotics

The potency of conventional antipsychotic drugs correlates closely with their affinity for the dopamine 2 (D_2) receptor, blocking the effect of endogenous dopamine at this site. The pharmacological profile of the newer atypical antipsychotics differs from that of the conventional antipsychotics in that they are weaker D_2 receptor antagonists but are potent serotonin type 2A (5-HT_{2A}) receptor antagonists and have significant anticholinergic and antihistaminic activity as well. Central 5-HT_{2A} receptor antagonism is believed to broaden the therapeutic effect of the drug, while reducing the incidence of extrapyramidal side effects (EPS) associated with D_2 antagonists.

Antipsychotics appear to exert their influence at mesocortical and mesolimbic dopaminergic pathways. Positron emission tomography (PET) studies show that antipsychotics block these receptors almost immediately, yet onset of action takes weeks to develop. Furthermore, although all antipsychotics block these same receptors, a patient may respond preferentially to one antipsychotic but not to another. These observations suggest that these drugs have other effects in the brain that may actually be responsible for their antipsychotic properties, such as an action on second-messenger systems. Although many drug side effects can be linked to their dopamine-blocking properties (e.g., EPS), these drugs also block noradrenergic, cholinergic, and histaminic receptors to differing degrees, accounting for the unique side effect profile of each agent.

Pharmacokinetics of Antipsychotics

Absorption of orally administered antipsychotics is variable, but their clinical effects (e.g., mainly sedation) generally appear within 30–60 minutes. Intramuscular administration produces effects within 10 minutes because injectable antipsychotics have much greater bioavailability than oral medication. For example, intramuscular chlorpromazine is 4–10 times more bioavailable than an equivalent oral dose. Metabolism occurs mostly in the liver, largely by oxidation, so that these highly lipid-soluble agents are converted to water-soluble metabolites and excreted in the urine and feces. Excretion of antipsychotics tends to be slow because of drug accumulation in fatty tissue. Most antipsychotics have a half-life of 24 hours or longer and have many active metabolites with longer half-lives; depot formulations have even longer elimination half-lives. For this reason, it has been difficult to correlate blood levels with therapeutic response. As a result, no definitive dose-response curve has been demonstrated for most of the antipsychotics.

Measuring plasma levels can be helpful in selected cases, but there is little reason for routine monitoring, with the exception of haloperidol and clozapine. Plasma concentrations can be measured reliably for many antipsychotic drugs, but studies attempting to correlate plasma level with response have been inconsistent. Haloperidol and clozapine blood levels appear to correlate with clinical response. Haloperidol may have a therapeutic window between 5 and 18 ng/mL. Clozapine levels greater than 350 ng/mL appear to be effective for most patients. The other situations in which plasma levels are useful to obtain include the following:

- When patients' symptoms have not responded to conventional doses
- When antipsychotic medications are combined with drugs that can affect their pharmacokinetics (e.g., carbamazepine)
- When patient compliance must be assessed

Use of Antipsychotics in Acute Psychosis

A high-potency conventional antipsychotic such as haloperidol (5–10 mg/day), risperidone (4–6 mg/day), olanzapine (10–20 mg/day), quetiapine (150–800 mg/day), or ziprasidone (80–160 mg/day) is recommended as an initial choice for the treatment of acute psychosis. An adequate trial should last from 4 to 6 weeks. The trial should be extended for another 4–6 weeks when the patient shows a partial response to the initial antipsychotic. If no response occurs after 4–6 weeks, then another drug should be tried. Clozapine is a second-line choice because of its expense and propensity to cause agranulocytosis.

Highly agitated patients who are out of control require rapid control of their symptoms and should be given frequent, equally spaced doses of an antipsychotic drug. High-potency antipsychotics (e.g., haloperidol) can be given every 30–120 minutes orally or intramuscularly until agitation has subsided. A combination of an antipsychotic and a benzodiazepine may work even better in calming the patient (e.g., haloperidol, 5 mg, plus lorazepam, 4 mg), repeating the doses every 30 minutes until tranquilization is achieved. Intramuscular droperidol (5–10 mg) is an effective alternative but may cause tachycardia and orthostatic hypotension.

Maintenance Treatment With Antipsychotics

Patients benefiting from short-term treatment with antipsychotic drugs are candidates for long-term prophylactic treatment, which has as its goal the sustained control of psychotic symptoms. To minimize the risk of side effects, particularly tardive dyskinesia, an often irreversible movement disorder, the lowest effective antipsychotic dose should be used. The general rule with conventional antipsychotics is that the maintenance dose can be as low as one-third to one-half of the treatment dose, achieved by reducing the antipsychotic dose 20% every 6 months until the maintenance dose is reached. Dosing recommendations with atypical antipsychotics are less certain, although doses need to be individually adjusted.

The following guidelines regarding relapse prevention were developed at an international conference:

1. Prevention of relapse is more important than risk of side effects because most side effects are reversible, and the consequences of relapse may be irreversible.
2. At least 1–2 years of treatment are recommended following the initial episode because of the high risk of relapse and the possibility of social deterioration from further relapses.
3. At least 5 years of treatment are indicated for multiepisode patients. Chronic, or ongoing, treatment is recommended for patients who pose a danger to themselves or to others.

Maintenance treatment with antipsychotics is effective in preventing relapse. Numerous studies have consistently shown that about 30% of those continuing to take medications relapse, whereas about 65% of those taking placebo do so. When well-stabilized patients are taken off of their medication, about 75% relapse within 6–24 months.

Patients with schizoaffective disorder generally receive maintenance treatment with an antipsychotic and a mood stabilizer when the patient has the bipolar type or an antipsychotic and an antidepressant when the patient has the depressed type. Antipsychotics usually are unnecessary as maintenance treatment for psychotic mood disorders. Instead, antidepressants or a mood stabilizer should be used. Some patients with psychotic mood disorders will need ongoing antipsychotic treatment, but the decision to use antipsychotics for maintenance must be based on clinical judgment.

Long-acting antipsychotic preparations are available for patients who are unable to take oral medication on a regular basis or who are noncompliant. There is no universally accepted method for converting a patient from oral to long-acting dosage forms, and dosing with sustained-release preparations (e.g., fluphenazine decanoate, haloperidol decanoate) must be individualized. A patient can be started on a dose of 6.25 mg of fluphenazine decanoate intramuscularly every 2 weeks, and the dose is titrated upward or downward based on the patient's therapeutic response and side effects. For haloperidol, a 400-mg loading dose in the first month, followed by a maintenance dose of 250 mg/month, produces a blood level of 10 ng/mL (the middle of the therapeutic range), and a dose of 150 mg/month produces a blood level between 5 and 6 ng/mL.

Further information about the use of antipsychotics in the treatment of schizophrenia can be found in Chapter 7.

Adverse Effects of Antipsychotics

Despite their effectiveness in treating psychotic syndromes, antipsychotics have the potential to induce a variety of troublesome side effects. The severity of these effects differs from drug to drug and corresponds with the drug's ability to affect a particular neurotransmitter system (e.g., dopaminergic, noradrenergic, cholinergic, histaminic). Because of their blockade of 5-HT$_{2A}$ receptors, atypical antipsychotics are less likely to induce EPS than are conventional antipsychotics. Side effect profiles of the antipsychotics are shown in Table 27–1.

Patients receiving long-term treatment with antipsychotic medication should be regularly monitored for the development of *tardive dyskinesia* (TD), a condition that consists of abnormal involuntary movements usually involving the mouth and tongue. Other parts of the body, including the trunk and extremities, may become affected. TD is believed to result when postsynaptic dopamine receptors develop a supersensitivity to dopamine following prolonged receptor blockade from antipsychotics.

The movements of TD are generally mild and tolerable, but perhaps 10% of patients with TD develop a more malignant form of the disorder that can be totally disabling. Elderly patients, women, and patients with mood disorders appear more susceptible to developing TD, and it has a reported incidence of 5% per year of exposure in young persons and 30% after 1 year of treatment in the elderly. (The Abnormal Involuntary Movement Scale [AIMS] has been developed to help clinicians and researchers rate the severity of TD. A copy of this scale is included in the Appendix.)

Patients with TD present special problems because the treatment of choice is to stop the offending antipsychotic. Many patients will choose to continue taking the drug regardless of the TD because their life may be intolerable without medication and the TD may be mild. One option is to switch the patient to an atypical antipsychotic, which will help mask the symptoms and will probably not worsen the TD. Vitamin E (i.e., 1,600 IU/day) may help alleviate the abnormal movements to some extent, although the data are not conclusive. If patients do not benefit from a 3-month trial, vitamin E should be discontinued.

Antipsychotic medications are also frequently associated with the development of *pseudoparkinsonism*. This side effect usually takes 3 or more weeks to develop. Patients develop symptoms typical of Parkinson's disease, including tremor, rigidity, and hypokinesia. *Akathisia* is another side effect that may appear in the first few weeks of antipsychotic treatment. This condition causes subjective feelings of anxiety and tension and objective fidgetiness and agitation. Patients may feel compelled to pace, move around in their chairs, or tap their feet. Treatment for both pseudoparkinsonism and akathisia generally consists of reducing the dose of the antipsychotic drug whenever possible and/or adding an antiparkinsonian agent to the medication regimen. Akathisia has been treated with β-blockers (e.g., propranolol, 40–160 mg/day in divided doses) or amantadine, a drug that potentiates the release of dopamine in the basal ganglia. Benzodiazepines are also helpful in relieving the symptoms of akathisia. Clonidine has been successfully used to treat akathisia, but it may cause sedation and orthostatic hypotension.

Another potential neurological side effect is the *acute dystonic reaction,* which usually occurs during the first 4 days of treatment with antipsychotics. A dystonia is a sustained contraction of the muscles of the neck, mouth, tongue, or occasionally other muscle groups that is subjectively distressing and often painful. Acute dystonias typically respond within 5 minutes to intravenous benztropine (i.e., 1–2 mg) or diphenhydramine (i.e., 25–50 mg). These drugs can be administered intramuscularly as well, but symptom resolution is slower. After the dystonia resolves, a 2-week course of benztropine

(2 mg twice daily) or another antiparkinsonian drug usually prevents recurrences. Patients with a history of dystonic reactions can benefit from a week of prophylactic benztropine when antipsychotic medications are restarted.

Antipsychotics, particularly low-potency compounds such as chlorpromazine, commonly cause anticholinergic side effects. These effects include dry mouth, urinary retention, blurry vision, constipation, and exacerbation of narrow-angle glaucoma. These side effects are best treated by reducing the dose of the drug or switching to a more potent agent (e.g., haloperidol) or to an atypical antipsychotic. Antiparkinsonian drugs commonly used to treat EPS, such as benztropine, can worsen these side effects. If urinary retention continues to be a problem, bethanechol (i.e., 15 mg three times daily) may help the patient empty his or her bladder more efficiently. Bulk laxatives will help with constipation.

The most common cardiovascular side effect of the antipsychotics is *orthostatic hypotension,* mediated by α-adrenergic blockade. This side effect is caused more frequently by low-potency compounds (e.g., chlorpromazine, thioridazine). Antipsychotics generally do not cause arrhythmogenic effects when used in standard doses. Chlorpromazine, thioridazine, and pimozide can prolong the Q-T interval, which can be of potential concern.

Agranulocytosis is a rare side effect that is associated with the use of low-potency antipsychotics. Its incidence peaks during the first 2 months of treatment. The best preventive measure is to be alert to the appearance of malaise, fever, and sore throat early in the course of therapy; routine blood counts usually are not necessary. Because clozapine causes agranulocytosis at a higher rate than other antipsychotics (usually between weeks 6 and 24 of treatment) and is potentially fatal, patients receiving clozapine must have weekly blood counts for the first 6 months, then every 14 days as long as they take the drug.

Hyperprolactinemia, often considered an unavoidable consequence of treatment with conventional antipsychotics, can induce amenorrhea, galactorrhea, gynecomastia, and impotence. These drugs probably block dopamine receptors in the pituitary prolactin-secreting cells, preventing dopamine-induced reduction of dopamine release. Atypical antipsychotics are less likely to cause hyperprolactinemia. When the patient is unable to reduce the dose or change antipsychotics, the addition of bromocriptine may be helpful.

Other miscellaneous side effects of the antipsychotics include nonspecific skin rashes, retinitis pigmentosa (especially with doses of thioridazine >800 mg/day), fever (with clozapine), pigmentary changes in the skin (i.e., blue, gray, or tan), weight gain, cholestatic jaundice (with chlorpromazine),

Rational use of antipsychotics
1. A high-potency conventional antipsychotic (e.g., haloperidol), risperidone, olanzapine, quetiapine, or ziprasidone should be given as the first-line treatment.
• Atypical antipsychotics are effective and well tolerated, with less propensity to induce tardive dyskinesia.
2. Second-line drug choices include the other conventional antipsychotics.
3. A drug trial should last 4–6 weeks.
• The trial should be extended when there is a partial response that has not plateaued and shortened when no response occurs or side effects are intolerable or unmanageable.
• Risperidone may be the better choice in patients at risk for weight gain.
• Quetiapine may be favored when low extrapyramidal side effects and low prolactin levels are desired.
4. All antipsychotics should be started at a low dose and gradually increased to fall within a therapeutic range.
• Evidence suggests that blood levels can help guide dosage adjustments for haloperidol and clozapine.
5. Clozapine, because of its expense and risk of agranulocytosis, should be reserved for treatment-refractory patients.

reduced libido, and inhibition of ejaculation (with thioridazine). Low-potency antipsychotics are associated with a risk for seizures, especially at higher doses (e.g., >1,000 mg/day of chlorpromazine). The drugs are not contraindicated in epileptic patients as long as they receive adequate treatment with anticonvulsants. Antipsychotics are generally safe during pregnancy.

All conventional antipsychotics have the potential to cause the *neuroleptic malignant syndrome* (NMS), a rare idiosyncratic reaction that does not appear to be dose related. The newer atypical agents appear less likely to induce NMS. Usually considered a medical emergency, the syndrome is characterized by rigidity, high fever, delirium, and marked autonomic instability. Serum levels of creatinine phosphokinase and of liver enzymes are generally elevated. There is no standard approach to the treatment of NMS. Both the muscle relaxant dantrolene and the dopamine agonist bromocriptine have been successfully used to treat NMS. Merely stopping the offending antipsychotic drug and providing supportive care may be as effective. In severe cases not responding to medical management, ECT is used. Once the patient has recovered, antipsychotics may be cautiously reintroduced following a 2-week wait. Selecting an agent from a different antipsychotic class (e.g., chlorpromazine rather than haloperidol, if haloperidol caused the NMS) or switching to an atypical agent is advisable.

Antidepressants

Not long after chlorpromazine appeared in the late 1950s, the antidepressant imipramine was synthesized in an attempt by researchers to find additional compounds for the treatment of schizophrenia. It was soon learned that imipramine had little effect on hallucinations and delusions, but it alleviated depression in patients who were both psychotic and depressed. This finding led to the development of the tricyclic antidepressants (TCAs); modifications of the three-ring structure followed as additional TCAs were produced, including amitriptyline and desipramine.

At about the same time that TCAs were synthesized, the antidepressant properties of the monoamine oxidase inhibitors (MAOIs) were discovered. Iproniazid, an antibiotic used to treat tuberculosis, was found to relieve depression in tuberculosis patients. Later work showed that the drug also was effective in relieving depression in psychiatric patients. Although iproniazid is no longer used as an antidepressant, it has been succeeded by more effective MAOIs, including phenelzine and tranylcypromine.

A second and third generation of antidepressants have since been developed, some of which differ structurally from both the TCAs and the MAOIs. In the early 1980s, tetracyclic compounds with a somewhat similar structure and comparable properties were marketed, including maprotiline and amoxapine, also referred to as *heterocyclics*. Another group of antidepressants, collectively known as the *serotonin reuptake inhibitors* (SRIs), was developed in the late 1980s and early 1990s. Other antidepressants also were introduced but do not fit within any particular grouping, including bupropion, nefazodone, and mirtazapine. The antidepressants are all thought to work by altering levels of neurotransmitters in the central nervous system (CNS). All antidepressants are, with minor exceptions, equally effective and differ primarily in their potency and side effects.

Indications for Antidepressants

The primary indication for antidepressants is the treatment of major depression. The effectiveness of antidepressants is unquestioned, and approximately 65%–70% of patients receiving an antidepressant will respond within 6 weeks. (The placebo response rate in depression ranges from 25% to 40%.) Depressed patients with melancholic symptoms (e.g., diurnal variation, psychomotor agitation or retardation, terminal insomnia, pervasive anhedonia) may respond better to antidepressants, particularly TCAs, than do depressed patients without these symptoms. Secondary depressions (i.e., depressions that follow or complicate other psychiatric disorders); depressions accompanied by anxiety, somatization, or hypochondriasis; and depressions accompanied by personality disorders respond less well than do depressions without these features. Chronic forms of depression, including dysthymia, also respond to antidepressants, although treatment results are not as robust as those seen in acute forms of depression. Antidepressants also are used for maintenance therapy in major depression.

Other disorders that are treated with antidepressants include the depressed phase of bipolar disorder, panic disorder, agoraphobia, obsessive-compulsive disorder (OCD), social phobia, generalized anxiety disorder, posttraumatic stress disorder (PTSD), bulimia nervosa, and certain childhood conditions (e.g., enuresis, school phobia). Because antidepressants are used to treat a broad range of psychiatric disorders, the term *antidepressant* is a misnomer.

Tricyclic and Tetracyclic Antidepressants

TCAs are believed to work by blocking the reuptake of both norepinephrine and serotonin at the presynaptic nerve ending. The tertiary amines (e.g., amitriptyline, imipramine, doxepin) primarily block serotonin reuptake, whereas the secondary amines (e.g., desipramine, nortriptyline, protriptyline) mainly block norepinephrine reuptake. Clomipramine is an exception because it is a relatively selective serotonin reuptake inhibitor. Tetracyclic compounds (e.g., maprotiline, amoxapine) have a four-ring central structure and work in a fashion similar to that of the TCAs; for that reason, they also have similar side effects. Amoxapine is unusual in that it has a mild antipsychotic effect, but for this reason, it is associated with a risk for TD. All of these drugs also block muscarinic, histaminic, and α-adrenergic receptors. The degree of blockade corresponds with the side-effect profile of the agent as shown in Table 27–2.

In general, TCAs are well absorbed orally, undergo an enterohepatic cycle, and peak plasma levels develop 2–4 hours after ingestion. They are highly bound to plasma and tissue proteins and are fat soluble. TCAs are metabolized by the liver, and their metabolites are excreted through the kid-

TABLE 27–2. Commonly used antidepressants

Category	Drug (trade name)	Sedation	Anti-cholinergic effects	Orthostatic hypotension	Sexual dysfunc-tion	GI effects	Activation/ insomnia	Half-life, hours	Target dosage, mg	Dosage range, mg/day
Tricyclics										
Tertiary amines	Doxepin (Sinequan, Adapin)	VH	VH	VH	H	VL	None	8–25	200	50–300
	Amitriptyline (Elavil)	VH	VH	VH	H	VL	None	9–46	150	50–300
	Imipramine (Tofranil)	H	VH	VH	H	VL	None	6–28	200	50–300
	Trimipramine (Surmontil)	H	H	H	H	VL	None	16–40	150	50–300
	Clomipramine (Anafranil)	VH	VH	VH	VH	VL	None	23–122	150	50–300
Secondary amines	Protriptyline (Vivactil)	VL	VH	M	H	VL	H	54–198	30	10–60
	Nortriptyline (Pamelor)	M	M	M	H	VL	None	18–56	100	20–150
	Desipramine (Norpramin)	M	M	M	H	VL	VL	12–28	150	50–300

TABLE 27–2. Commonly used antidepressants (*continued*)

Category	Drug (trade name)	Sedation	Anticholinergic effects	Orthostatic hypotension	Sexual dysfunction	GI effects	Activation/ insomnia	Half-life, hours	Target dosage, mg	Dosage range, mg/day
Monoamine oxidase inhibitors										
	Phenelzine (Nardil)	L	M	VH	H	VL	L	—a	60	15–90
	Tranylcypromine (Parnate)	None	M	VH	L	VL	M	—a	30–40	20–90
	Isocarboxazid (Marplan)	M	L	H	H	VL	L	—a	30	10–50
Newer agents										
	Amoxapine (Asendin)	L	L	L	H	VL	None	8	200	100–600
	Maprotiline (Ludiomil)	M	M	M	M	VL	None	51	150	75–300
	Trazodone (Desyrel)	VH	VL	VH	None	M	Yes	6–11	400	300–800
	Bupropion (Wellbutrin)	None	None	None	None	M	H	12	300	150–450
	Nefazodone (Serzone)	H	None	L	None	M	VL	2–4	300	100–600

TABLE 27–2. Commonly used antidepressants (continued)

Category	Drug (trade name)	Sedation	Anti-cholinergic effects	Orthostatic hypotension	Sexual dysfunction	GI effects	Activation/ insomnia	Half-life, hours	Target dosage, mg	Dosage range, mg/day
	Venlafaxine (Effexor)	L	None	VL	H	VH	M	3–5	225	75–350
	Mirtazapine (Remeron)	H	None	None	None	VL	None	20–40	30	15–45
Serotonin reuptake inhibitors	Fluoxetine (Prozac)	None	None	None	VH	H	VH	24–72	20	20–80
	Sertraline (Zoloft)	VL	None	None	VH	VH	M	25	100	50–200
	Paroxetine (Paxil)	L	L	None	VH	H	L	20	20	20–50
	Fluvoxamine (Luvox)	M	None	None	VH	H	L	15	200	100–300
	Citalopram (Celexa)	VL	None	None	VH	H	VL	35	20	10–60

aMaximal inhibition by monoamine oxidase inhibitors is achieved in 5–10 days.

GI = gastrointestinal; H = high; L = low; M = moderate; VH = very high; VL = very low.

neys. All have active metabolites, and there is as much as a tenfold variation in steady-state plasma levels of TCAs among individuals. These differences are primarily caused by individual variations in the way the liver metabolizes the drugs. Their half-lives vary but are generally in the range of 1 day. Steady-state plasma levels are achieved after five half-lives; half-life, in turn, is dependent on metabolism of the drug by hepatic microsomal enzymes. Blood levels tend to be increased by drugs that inhibit the cytochrome P450 system, including chlorpromazine and other antipsychotics, disulfiram, cimetidine, estrogens, methylphenidate, and many of the SRIs.

The established therapeutic range for imipramine (the total for imipramine plus its metabolite desipramine) is between 175 and 350 ng/mL and for nortriptyline is between 53 and 148 ng/mL. Desipramine plasma levels greater than 116 ng/mL have been shown to correspond with clinical improvement. Plasma blood levels can be measured for the other TCAs but are not clinically meaningful. Levels should be obtained 12 hours after the last dose.

Plasma levels should not be routinely obtained, particularly if the patient is doing well. Reasons for obtaining blood levels include failure to respond adequately, significant symptoms of toxicity, cases of suspected patient noncompliance, establishment of a therapeutic window, and perhaps the presence of a significant cardiac or other medical disease, when it is desirable to keep the blood level at the lower range of the therapeutic value. Blood levels are helpful in cases of drug overdose.

TCAs commonly cause sedation, orthostatic hypotension, and anticholinergic side effects such as constipation, urinary hesitancy, dry mouth, and visual blurring. Each TCA differs in its propensity to cause these effects. Tertiary amines (e.g., amitriptyline, imipramine, doxepin) tend to cause more prominent side effects. Tolerance usually develops to anticholinergic side effects and sedation, but TCAs should be used with caution in patients with prostatic enlargement and narrow-angle glaucoma. Elderly patients should have their blood pressure carefully monitored because drug-induced hypotension can lead to falls and resultant fractures.

Antihistaminic effects include sedation and weight gain. α-Adrenergic blockade causes orthostatic hypotension and reflex tachycardia. Miscellaneous side effects of TCAs include tremors, pedal edema, myoclonus, restlessness or hyperstimulation, insomnia, nausea and vomiting, electroencephalographic changes, rashes or allergic reactions, confusion, and seizures. It is uncertain whether TCAs are teratogenic, but their use in the first trimester of pregnancy should be avoided whenever possible. Because a metabolite of amoxapine is an antipsychotic, the drug can cause EPS, akathisia, and TD. For this reason, amoxapine is not considered a first-line treatment for depression.

Cardiovascular side effects tend to be the most worrisome. All TCAs prolong cardiac conduction, much like quinidine or procainamide, and carry the risk of exacerbating existing conduction abnormalities. Patients with low-grade abnormalities such as first-degree atrioventricular (AV) block or right bundle branch block should use these medications cautiously; dosage increase should be accompanied by serial electrocardiograms. Patients with higher block (e.g., second-degree AV block) should not take TCAs. One of the newer antidepressants that does not prolong cardiac conduction (e.g., trazodone, fluoxetine) should be used in patients with cardiac conduction defects.

A withdrawal syndrome occurs in some patients who have been taking high doses of TCAs for weeks or months. Symptoms, including anxiety, insomnia, headache, myalgia, chills, malaise, and nausea, can begin within days following abrupt discontinuation of the drug. This syndrome usually can be prevented by a gradual medication taper of 25–50 mg/week. If this is not possible, small doses of an anticholinergic medication such as diphenhydramine (e.g., 25 mg two to three times daily) may help alleviate the symptoms.

Monoamine Oxidase Inhibitors

MAOIs inhibit monoamine oxidase (MAO), an enzyme responsible for the degradation of tyramine, serotonin, dopamine, and norepinephrine. Blocking this enzymatic process leads to an increase in CNS levels of these monoamines. Two types of MAO have been identified: MAO-A, found in the brain, liver, gut, and sympathetic nerves, and MAO-B, found in the brain, liver, and platelets. MAO-A acts primarily on serotonin and norepinephrine, and MAO-B acts primarily on phenylethylamine; both act on dopamine and tyramine. Inhibitors of MAO-A may be more effective as antidepressants.

The four MAOIs commonly used in the United States are isocarboxazid, phenelzine, tranylcypromine, and selegiline. Selegiline is marketed for the treatment of Parkinson's disease and is not used as an antidepressant.

MAOIs are readily absorbed when orally administered. They do not have active metabolites, and the drugs are renally excreted. MAOIs irreversibly inhibit MAO, reaching maximum inhibition after 5–10 days. It is generally thought that platelet MAO activity, which reflects MAO inhibition, needs to be reduced by 80% to achieve an antidepressant response. The body takes approximately 2 weeks after the discontinuation of MAOIs to synthesize enough new MAO to restore its baseline concentrations. Plasma levels are not measured for the MAOIs.

MAOIs are thought to be particularly effective in forms of depression accompanied by significant anxiety. They have been found effective in treating panic disorder and agoraphobia, social phobia, PTSD, and bulimia nervosa. They are thought to be particularly valuable in the treatment of atypical depression. Patients with this condition usually have a mixture of anxiety and depression, along with a reversal of diurnal variation (i.e., worse in the evening), hypersomnia, mood lability, and hyperphagia.

The MAOIs have minimal anticholinergic and antihistaminic effects. They are, however, potent α-adrenergic blockers, resulting in a high frequency of orthostatic hypotension. Other common side effects include sedation or hyperstimulation (e.g., agitation), insomnia, dry mouth, weight gain, edema, and sexual dysfunction. The most serious side effect results from the concomitant ingestion of an MAOI and substances containing tyramine, leading to severe hypertension and death or stroke in rare cases. Patients taking MAOIs must follow a special low-tyramine diet. Because these drugs can interact with sympathomimetics (e.g., amphetamines) to produce a hypertensive crisis, patients need to be aware of potential interactions with prescribed and over-the-counter medications. MAOIs also have a potentially lethal interaction with meperidine, the mechanism of which is not fully understood but may have to do with serotonin agonism. See Table 27–3 for as list of restricted foods and medications.

When symptoms of the hypertensive crisis occur (e.g., headache, nausea, or vomiting), patients should be instructed to immediately seek medical attention at a medical clinic or hospital emergency room. There, patients can be treated with intravenous phentolamine (e.g., 5 mg). Patients who do not have easy access to medical care should be advised to carry a 10-mg tablet of nifedipine with them; its α-blocking properties, which act to lower blood pressure when taken sublingually, make it a useful stopgap measure.

All physicians and dentists should be informed when their patients are taking MAOIs, especially when surgery or dental work is indicated, so that drugs that interact adversely with MAOIs can be avoided. It is advisable to wait 2 weeks after discontinuing an MAOI before resuming a normal diet or using a TCA, an SRI, or another medication that may have an adverse interaction with the MAOI.

Serotonin Reuptake Inhibitors

The SRIs have rapidly become the most widely prescribed antidepressants in the United States since fluoxetine was introduced in 1988. Five SRIs are currently marketed: citalopram, fluoxetine, fluvoxamine, paroxetine, and

TABLE 27–3.   Dietary instructions for patients taking monoamine oxidase inhibitors (MAOIs)

Foods to avoid

Cheese: all cheeses except cottage cheese, farmer cheese, and cream cheese

Meat and fish: caviar; liver; smoked, dried, pickled, cured, or preserved meats and fish

Vegetables: overripe avocados, fava beans

Fruits: overripe fruits, canned figs

Other foods: yeast extracts

Beverages: chianti wine, beers that contain yeast

Foods to use in moderation

Chocolate

Coffee

Medications to avoid

Over-the-counter pain medications except for plain aspirin, acetaminophen, and ibuprofen

Cold or allergy medications

Nasal decongestants and inhalers

Cough medications; plain guaifenesin elixir may be taken, however

Stimulants and diet pills

Sympathomimetic drugs

Meperidine

Serotonin reuptake inhibitors (e.g., fluoxetine, fluvoxamine, paroxetine, sertraline), bupropion, mirtazapine, nefazodone, trazodone, venlafaxine

Source.   Adapted from Hyman and Arana 1987.

sertraline. Although all are structurally dissimilar, they share similar pharmacological properties involving their relatively selective serotonin reuptake inhibition. They largely lack the side effects of TCAs caused by blockade of muscarinic, histaminic, and α-adrenergic receptors. Thus, SRIs are generally better tolerated than TCAs and are safer in overdose. Because they are unlikely to affect seizure threshold or cardiac conduction, SRIs are safer for patients with epilepsy or cardiac conduction defects.

The SRIs are remarkably versatile and are effective in treating major depression, panic disorder, OCD, social phobia, PTSD, bulimia nervosa, and probably other disorders as well. However, marketing strategy has led to the following U.S. Food and Drug Administration (FDA)–approved indications: citalopram, fluoxetine, paroxetine, and sertraline for major depression; fluoxetine, fluvoxamine, paroxetine, and sertraline for OCD; paroxetine and sertraline for panic disorder; sertraline for PTSD; fluoxetine for bulimia nervosa; paroxetine for social phobia; and fluoxetine for premenstrual dysphoric disorder.

All of the SRIs are metabolized by the liver, but only fluoxetine and sertraline have active metabolites. The half-life varies from drug to drug, although fluoxetine's half-life is the longest at 2–3 days, and its major metabolite, norfluoxetine, has a half-life of 4–16 days. The other SRIs have half-lives ranging from 15 to 35 hours. The active metabolite of sertraline, norsertraline, has a half-life of 2–4 days. All are well absorbed from the gut and reach peak plasma levels within 4–8 hours.

The SRIs share a similar side effect profile, although there are subtle differences among them. Commonly reported side effects include mild nausea, loose bowel movements, anxiety or hyperstimulation (which leads to jitteriness, restlessness, muscle tension, and insomnia), headache, insomnia, sedation, and increased sweating. These side effects tend to diminish over time and are largely dose related. Patients sometimes report other side effects, including weight gain or weight loss, bruxism, vivid dreams, skin rash, and amotivation.

Sexual dysfunction is relatively common in both men and women. SRIs can decrease libido in both genders; in men, they also may cause ejaculatory delay or failure, and in women, they may cause anorgasmia. Because of this side effect, SRIs are frequently prescribed to men to treat premature ejaculation. For persistent complaints of sexual dysfunction, management strategies include lowering the dose, switching to one of the newer non-SRI antidepressants (e.g., bupropion, nefazodone), or coadministering another medication as an antidote (e.g., bupropion, 75–150 mg/day, or cyproheptadine, 4–8 mg, taken 1–2 hours before sexual activity).

These side effects may diminish with time but can persist in some patients. Fluoxetine is the most likely SRI to induce these symptoms, and citalopram the least likely. When hyperstimulation is problematic, it can be managed by either lowering the dose, switching to another SRI, or switching to one of the newer non-SRI antidepressants. A β-blocker (e.g., propranolol, 10–30 mg three times daily) is often helpful in treating the feelings of jitteriness and tremor; benzodiazepines (e.g., lorazepam, 0.5–1 mg twice daily) can be prescribed to counteract this side effect as well. Because complaints of hyperstimulation may diminish over time, these adjunctive medications may not be needed long term. Trazodone (e.g., 50–150 mg at bedtime) is often effective in treating insomnia, although men should be warned of its rare propensity to cause priapism.

When SRIs are discontinued, many patients develop a withdrawal syndrome. The exception is fluoxetine, which self-tapers because of the long half-life of both the parent compound and its major metabolite. Withdrawal symptoms include nausea, headache, vivid dreams, irritability, and vertiginous sensations. These symptoms often begin within days of drug discontinuation and continue for 2 weeks or longer. These symptoms can be minimized by tapering the drug slowly over several weeks; the short-term addition of a benzodiazepine is often helpful.

Rare cases of a *serotonin syndrome* have been reported, particularly among patients who have taken two or more serotonergic drugs concurrently. Typical symptoms include lethargy, restlessness, mental confusion, flushing, diaphoresis, tremor, and myoclonic jerks. Left untreated, the serotonin syndrome can progress to hyperthermia, hypertonicity, rhabdomyolysis, renal failure, and death. Several deaths have been reported in patients taking a combination of an SRI and MAOI, presumably as a result of this syndrome. Because of the potential lethality of this combination, when a patient is switched from an SRI to an MAOI, a long enough time must pass to ensure that the SRI has been fully eliminated from the body before initiating treatment with an MAOI. With fluoxetine, for example, this means that about 6 weeks must pass.

The SRIs each inhibit one or more cytochrome P450 isoenzymes to a substantial degree and therefore have the potential to cause clinically important drug interactions. For that reason, care should be taken when prescribing adjunctive or concurrent medication metabolized through this enzyme system. This means that SRIs may induce a several-fold increase in the levels of coprescribed drugs that are dependent on the inhibited isoenzymes for their clearance. Fluoxetine, fluvoxamine, and paroxetine are the most likely to cause drug interactions, whereas citalopram and sertraline have less potential to do so. See Table 27–4 for a description of the SRIs and the isoenzyme systems inhibited and coadministered drugs affected.

SRIs appear to be safe during pregnancy, and although they are secreted in breast milk, they are unlikely to show up in an infant's serum.

Other New Antidepressants

Bupropion

Bupropion is a unicyclic aminoketone with a unique chemical structure similar to that of psychostimulants, including the amphetamines, which

TABLE 27–4. Newer antidepressants and potentially important drug interactions

Antidepressant	Enzyme system inhibited	Potential drug interactions
Fluoxetine	2D6	Secondary TCAs, haloperidol, type 1C antiarrhythmics
	2C	Phenytoin, diazepam
	3A4	Carbamazepine, alprazolam, terfenadine
Sertraline	2D6	Secondary TCAs, antipsychotics, type 1C antiarrhythmics
	2C	Tolbutamide, diazepam
	3A4	Carbamazepine
Paroxetine	2D6	Secondary TCAs, antipsychotics, type 1C antiarrhythmics, trazodone
Fluvoxamine	1A2	Theophylline, clozapine, haloperidol, amitriptyline, clomipramine, imipramine
	2C	Diazepam
	3A4	Carbamazepine, alprazolam, terfenadine, astemizole
Nefazodone	3A4	Alprazolam, triazolam, terfenadine, astemizole

Note. TCAs=tricyclic antidepressants.

Source. Adapted from Nemeroff et al. 1996.

may account for certain shared properties. Because hydroxybupropion, its main metabolite, inhibits the reuptake of dopamine and norepinephrine, the drug has been called a dopamine-norepinephrine reuptake inhibitor. Bupropion is used for the treatment of major depression but is also approved for the treatment of smoking cessation under the trade name Zyban. The drug also has been used successfully to treat attention-deficit/hyperactivity disorder (ADHD). The drug is not effective in treating panic disorder, OCD, social phobia, or other anxiety syndromes.

The drug is rapidly absorbed following oral administration, and peak concentrations are achieved within 2 hours, or 3 hours after administration of the sustained-release formulation. The drug's elimination is biphasic, with an initial phase of approximately 1.5 hours and a second phase lasting about 14 hours; the biphasic decline for the sustained-release formulation is less pronounced than that of the immediate-release formulation.

Bupropion is relatively well tolerated, having minimal effects on weight gain, cardiac conduction, or sexual functioning. The most common side effects are headache, nausea, anxiety, tremors, insomnia, and increased sweating. These symptoms generally subside with time. Restlessness and tremor can be treated with propranolol (e.g., 10 mg three times daily). The patient may benefit from short-term coadministration of benzodiazepines.

The main disadvantage of bupropion is that the incidence of seizures increases substantially at doses greater than 450 mg/day. For this reason, the drug is contraindicated in patients with a seizure disorder or an eating disorder that may be associated with a lower seizure threshold. Reports indicate that bupropion can exacerbate psychotic symptoms. The main risk of overdose is the development of seizures.

Nefazodone

Nefazodone combines blockade of the 5-HT$_2$ receptor with weak inhibition of neuronal serotonin reuptake and is structurally similar to trazodone. The drug is indicated for the treatment of major depression. Side effects include nausea, somnolence, dry mouth, dizziness, constipation, asthenia, and blurred vision. The drug is generally well tolerated, and these side effects are considered benign. Nefazodone does not appear to alter seizure threshold, does not cause weight gain, and does not impair sexual functioning. The drug has the potential to inhibit the cytochrome P450 3A3/4 isoenzyme, which can lead to drug-drug interactions when other medications metabolized by that isoenzyme are coadministered. Drawbacks include the need for twice-daily dosing and a slow dosage titration. The drug does not appear to be fatal in overdose.

Trazodone

Trazodone is a weak inhibitor of serotonin but also blocks 5-HT$_2$ receptors. The drug is a triazolopyridine derivative that shares the triazolo ring structure with alprazolam, a benzodiazepine. The drug is readily absorbed from the gastrointestinal tract, reaches peak plasma levels in 1–2 hours, and has a half-life of 6–11 hours. Trazodone is metabolized by the liver, and 75% of its metabolites are excreted in the urine. Adverse effects are partially mediated by α-adrenergic antagonism and antihistaminic activity. The drug should not be coadministered with MAOIs; concurrent use with antihypertensives may lead to hypotension.

The most common adverse effects are sedation, orthostatic hypotension, dizziness, headache, nausea, and dry mouth. These effects are mostly benign. Trazodone does not block anticholinergic receptors, so urinary retention and constipation are uncommon. The drug has no significant effect on cardiac conduction, although there are reports of increased ventricular irritability in patients with preexisting cardiac conduction defects or ventricular arrhythmias. It is unlikely to be fatal in overdose.

One concern with trazodone is that in rare cases it has been associated with priapism, which can be irreversible and require surgical intervention. Men prescribed trazodone should be warned of this side effect and be advised to report any change in the frequency or firmness of erections. The drug should be immediately discontinued if these changes occur. Immediate medical treatment should be sought for sustained erections.

Venlafaxine

Venlafaxine inhibits the neuronal uptake of serotonin at low doses and norepinephrine and dopamine at higher doses. Its main indication is for the treatment of major depression, but its slow-release formulation recently was approved for the treatment of generalized anxiety disorder. The drug is rapidly absorbed from the gut and is 98% bioavailable; its half-life is about 5 hours, and its major metabolite has a half-life of about 11 hours. Venlafaxine is metabolized by the liver and is renally excreted.

The side effect profile of venlafaxine is similar to that of the SRIs, including hyperstimulation, sexual dysfunction, and transient withdrawal symptoms. The drug does not affect cardiac conduction or lower seizure threshold and generally is not associated with sedation or weight gain. The drug is unlikely to inhibit cytochrome P450 isoenzymes, so drug-drug interactions are unlikely. Nonetheless, the drug should not be combined with MAOIs because of the risk of inducing a serotonin syndrome. The drug generally is not fatal in overdose. The main drawback with venlafaxine is that it is generally taken twice daily, although the slow-release preparation can be taken once daily. Blood pressure monitoring is recommended because of dose-dependent increases in mean diastolic blood pressure in some patients, particularly hypertensive patients.

Mirtazapine

Mirtazapine has a dual mode of action and enhances both serotonergic and noradrenergic neurotransmission but is not a reuptake inhibitor. The drug is also a potent histamine antagonist, a moderate α-adrenergic antagonist, and a moderate antagonist at muscarinic receptors. Mirtazapine is indicated for the treatment of major depression. It is well tolerated but may cause

Rational use of antidepressants

1. A serotonin reuptake inhibitor (SRI) should be used initially; tricyclic antidepressants (TCAs) and the other agents should be reserved for nonresponders.

2. Doses should be carefully adjusted, and each drug trial should last 4–8 weeks.

3. SRIs generally are given once daily. TCAs can be administered as a single dose, usually at bedtime. Monoamine oxidase inhibitors (MAOIs) usually are prescribed twice daily but not at bedtime because they can cause insomnia. Bupropion is administered in two to three divided doses to minimize its propensity to cause seizures.

4. Although adverse effects appear within days of starting a drug, therapeutic effects may require 2–4 weeks to become apparent.
   • Improvement should be monitored by following up target symptoms (e.g., mood, energy, appetite).

5. Patients with heart rhythm disturbances should be given one of the newer antidepressants that does not affect cardiac conduction (e.g., bupropion, mirtazapine, or an SRI).

6. Antidepressants are usually unnecessary in patients with grief reactions (uncomplicated bereavement) or adjustment disorders with depressed mood because these disorders are self-limiting.

7. When possible, SRIs should be tapered (except for fluoxetine because of its long half-life) because they induce withdrawal syndromes in some patients. TCAs also should be tapered slowly (e.g., weeks to months) because of their tendency to cause withdrawal reactions. No clinically significant withdrawal reaction occurs with MAOIs, but a taper over 5–7 days is sensible.

8. The coadministration of two different antidepressants does not boost efficacy and will only worsen side effects. In rare cases, the combined use of a TCA and an MAOI or a TCA and an SRI is justified, but these combinations should never be used routinely.
   • MAOIs should not be coadministered with SRIs or with any of the other new antidepressants.

prominent early sedation, weight gain, and elevation of serum lipid levels. Because of its long half-life, it needs to be taken only once daily; the drug has little effect on the cardiovascular system and minimally affects sexual functioning. Mirtazapine is unlikely to be associated with cytochrome P450–mediated drug interactions. One potential advantage is its early effect on reducing anxiety symptoms and sleep disturbance.

Somnolence occurs in more than half of the patients receiving mirtazapine, although tolerance develops after the first few weeks of treatment. Rare cases of agranulocytosis have been reported. In these cases, patients recovered after medication discontinuation. Routine laboratory monitoring is not currently recommended because this side effect is rare, but the development of fever, chills, sore throat, or other signs of infection in association with a low white blood cell count warrants close monitoring and discontinuation of the drug. The drug is unlikely to be fatal in overdose. The drug should not be used in combination with an MAOI.

Use of Antidepressants

Treatment should begin with one of the SRIs. Because these drugs are effective, well tolerated, and generally safe in overdose, they have generally replaced the TCAs as first-line therapy, when cost is not a consideration. Most patients will respond to a low dose, and frequent dosage adjustments are unnecessary. Patients with a history of cardiac conduction defects should receive one of the SRIs or another new agent (e.g., bupropion, mirtazapine). Impulsive patients or those with suicidal urges should receive an SRI or one of the newer agents that are unlikely to be fatal in overdose. When a TCA is used, nortriptyline, imipramine, or desipramine are the drugs of choice because meaningful plasma levels can be assessed. These drugs all require close titration, beginning with relatively low doses. Recommended dosage ranges for the different antidepressants are found in Table 27–2.

In patients receiving treatment for their first episode of major depression, antidepressants should be maintained for at least 16–20 weeks after achieving remission. When medication is ultimately tapered and discontinued, patients should be carefully monitored to ensure that their remission is stable. Patients who have had multiple prior episodes of depression should be considered for chronic maintenance treatment to reduce—but not eliminate—the probability of relapse.

Drug trials generally should last 4–8 weeks. When the patient's symptoms do not respond to an antidepressant after 4 weeks of treatment in the target dosage, the dose should be increased, or the patient should be switched to another antidepressant, preferably from a different class with a slightly different mechanism of action. When this regimen fails, nonresponders may benefit from the addition of lithium, which increases the likelihood of response in many patients. Response from lithium augmentation is often evident within a week with relatively low doses (e.g., 300 mg three times daily). ECT is an option in patients whose depression does not respond to medication.

Other agents have been used to augment the effect of TCAs, including triiodothyronine (e.g., 25–50 µg/day), tryptophan (e.g., 0.5–2.0 g/day), and methylphenidate (e.g., 10–40 mg/day), but the effectiveness of these agents in augmenting response has not been adequately determined.

Mood Stabilizers

Lithium carbonate, a naturally occurring salt, became available in 1970. Its first use in medicine (in the form of lithium chloride) was as a salt substitute for people with hypertension who needed a low-sodium diet, but its use was abandoned when it was found to make some people sick. In the late 1940s, Australian psychiatrist John Cade found that lithium calmed agitated psychotic patients. Later, it was discovered that lithium was particularly effective in people with mania. A Danish researcher, Mogens Schou, observed that lithium was effective in relieving the target symptoms of mania and that it also had a prophylactic effect. Lithium has since been joined by valproate, carbamazepine, and several newer anticonvulsants for the treatment of bipolar disorder. The different mood stabilizers are listed in Table 27–5. (Further information about the treatment of bipolar disorder is found in Chapter 9.)

Lithium Carbonate

The precise mechanism of action of lithium remains unknown. Lithium has effects on intracellular processes, such as inhibiting the enzyme inositol-1-phosphatase within neurons. The inhibition leads to decreased cellular responses to neurotransmitters that are linked to the phosphatidylinositol second-messenger system.

The onset of action often takes 5–7 days to become apparent. The usual plasma level of lithium for the treatment of acute mania is 0.9–1.4 mEq/L; individual patients may do well outside this range. Antipsychotics, which work more quickly, may be preferred when rapid behavioral control is needed, although benzodiazepine-induced sedation may be as effective.

Maintenance doses may be smaller, aiming for a blood level in the range of 0.45–0.60 mEq/L. Lithium has no proven role in the acute treatment of unipolar major depression, although the bipolar depressed patient or patient with a family history of bipolar illness may respond to lithium alone. Lithium also is used to augment the effect of antidepressants used in the treatment of major depression.

The most dramatic effect of lithium is in the prophylaxis of manic and depressive episodes in bipolar patients. Lithium appears to work best at re-

TABLE 27–5. Commonly used mood stabilizers

Drug (trade name)	Therapeutic plasma level	Dosage range, *mg/day*
Lithium carbonate (Eskalith, Lithobid)	0.6–1.2 mEq/L	900–2,400
Carbamazepine (Tegretol)	6–12 mg/L	400–2,400
Valproate (Depakene, Depakote)	50–120 mg/L	500–3,000

ducing the frequency and severity of manic episodes. Prevention with lithium is not absolute, and most patients will still have breakthrough episodes. Lithium has been shown to be effective in preventing recurrences of depression in patients with unipolar major depression.

Lithium is also used in the treatment of schizoaffective disorder, especially the bipolar subtype. Other uses of lithium include treatment of aggression in patients with dementia, mental retardation, and impulsive personality disorders (especially borderline and antisocial types).

Pharmacokinetics of Lithium

Lithium carbonate is administered orally but is available in liquid form as lithium citrate. Lithium carbonate is rapidly absorbed from the gut, and peak blood levels are obtained about 2 hours after ingestion. The elimination half-life is about 8–12 hours in manic patients and about 18–36 hours in euthymic patients. (Manic patients are overly active and have a higher glomerular filtration rate and therefore clear lithium from their system more rapidly.) Lithium is not protein bound and does not have metabolites. It is almost entirely excreted through the kidney but may be found in all body fluids (e.g., saliva, semen). Blood plasma levels are checked 12 hours after the last dose is given.

Slow-release preparations are available and indicated when gastrointestinal toxicity is evident or when twice-daily dosing would enhance compliance. Lithium usually is administered two or three times daily in patients with acute mania. Once-daily dosing with extended-release preparations is recommended in patients receiving the drug prophylactically. Once-daily dosing may offer some protection to the kidneys, although a single large daily dose may cause gastric irritation. Lithium carbonate usually is started at 300 mg twice daily in the average patient and is then titrated until a therapeutic blood level is achieved. Dosage may be adjusted every 3–5 days. Levels should be checked monthly for the first 3 months and every 3 months thereafter. Patients receiving chronic lithium administration can be monitored less frequently. Lithium can be safely discontinued without a taper.

Adverse Effects of Lithium

Minor side effects of lithium occur relatively soon after initiating treatment. Thirst or polyuria, tremor, diarrhea, weight gain, and edema are all relatively common side effects but tend to diminish with time. About 5%–15% of the patients undergoing long-term treatment may develop clinical signs of hypothyroidism. This side effect is more common in women and tends to occur during the first 6 months of treatment. Hypothyroidism can be managed effectively with thyroid hormone replacement. Baseline thyroid assays should be obtained before starting lithium; thyroid-stimulating hormone should be monitored on a semiannual basis or whenever there is a clinical suspicion of abnormality. Thyroid dysfunction reverses after lithium is discontinued.

Long-term lithium treatment may lead to increased levels of calcium, ionized calcium, and parathyroid hormone. High levels of calcium can cause lethargy, ataxia, and dysphoria, symptoms that may be attributed to depression rather than hypercalcemia.

Lithium is excreted through the kidneys and is reabsorbed in the proximal tubule with sodium and water. When the body has a sodium deficiency, the kidneys compensate by reabsorbing more sodium than normal in the proximal tubules. Lithium is absorbed along with sodium and poses the risk of lithium toxicity with hyponatremia. Thus, patients should be instructed to avoid becoming dehydrated from exercise, fever, or other causes of increased sweating. Sodium-depleting diuretics (e.g., thiazides) should be avoided because they may increase lithium levels.

Lithium has the potential to cause nephrogenic diabetes insipidus because lithium reduces the ability of the kidneys to concentrate urine. As a result, lithium-treated patients produce large volumes of dilute urine; this can be clinically significant for some patients, particularly if output exceeds 4 L/day. Significant polyuria may be difficult for some patients to tolerate. Amiloride (e.g., 5 mg twice daily) or hydrochlorothiazide (e.g., 50 mg twice daily) will paradoxically reduce urine output. A nephrotic syndrome caused by glomerulonephritis occurs rarely. This complication typically reverses after lithium is discontinued.

Long-term lithium use can cause a decrease in the glomerular filtration rate; significant decreases are uncommon. The decrease is presumably due to a tubulointerstitial nephropathy, perhaps caused by the patient's cumulative exposure to lithium; therefore, the lowest effective dose possible should be maintained. Serum creatinine measurement and urinalysis should be obtained at baseline and every 6–12 months thereafter. If proteinuria or an increase in creatinine is evident, additional tests should be performed.

About one-quarter of lithium-treated patients develop reversible, nonspecific T-wave changes similar to those seen with hypokalemia. Arrhythmias are uncommon, but sinus node dysfunction has been reported. Some patients develop acne, and those with acne may have an exacerbation. Psoriasis also may be worsened. Lithium has been reported to cause hair loss in some patients.

Lithium induces a reversible leukocytosis, with white blood cell counts of 13,000–15,000 mm^3. The increase is usually in neutrophils and represents a step-up of the total body count rather than demargination.

Parkinsonian-like symptoms, such as cogwheeling, hypokinesis, and rigidity, may occur in lithium-treated patients. Cognitive effects, such as distractibility, poor memory, and confusion, also can develop at therapeutic levels of lithium.

Contraindications to Lithium

Patients with a severe renal disease (e.g., glomerulonephritis, pyelonephritis, polycystic kidneys) should not receive lithium because it is renally excreted; dangerous blood levels may result when the kidneys are not functioning normally. In patients who have had myocardial infarction, lithium should be discontinued for at least 10–14 days. If treatment with lithium is necessary during the postinfarct period, low doses and periodic cardiac monitoring are recommended.

Lithium is contraindicated in the presence of myasthenia gravis because it blocks the release of acetylcholine. Lithium should be given cautiously in the presence of diabetes mellitus, ulcerative colitis, psoriasis, and senile cataracts. Because of the increased incidence of cardiovascular malformations in infants of mothers taking lithium (Ebstein's anomaly), lithium should be discontinued during the first trimester of pregnancy. Because lithium is secreted in breast milk, mothers taking the drug should not breast-feed.

Valproate

Valproate, a simple branched-chain carboxylic acid, is commonly used as an anticonvulsant. Research has shown that it is also effective for treating the manic phase of bipolar disorder and for long-term maintenance. It is considered a first-line treatment for bipolar disorder, along with lithium carbonate, although it is better tolerated.

The mechanism of its action is unknown, although it enhances CNS levels of γ-aminobutyric acid (GABA) by inhibiting its degradation and stimulating its synthesis and release. Valproate is rapidly absorbed after oral ingestion, and its bioavailability is nearly complete. Peak concentrations occur in 1–4 hours; it is rapidly distributed and highly (90%) protein bound.

The half-life of valproate ranges from 8 to 17 hours. The drug is metabolized by the liver, primarily through glucuronide conjugation. Less than 3% is excreted unchanged. Valproate does not induce its own metabolism, unlike carbamazepine. The usual custom is to aim for a plasma concentration of about 50–125 μg/mL, but this level does not correlate with antimanic activity. The response to valproate may be associated with rapid-cycling illness (more than four episodes per year), the presence of nonparoxysmal electroencephalogram abnormalities, and to a lesser extent, a history of closed head trauma occurring before the onset of the mood disorder.

Commonly reported side effects include gastrointestinal complaints (e.g., nausea, poor appetite, vomiting, diarrhea), asymptomatic serum hepatic transaminase elevation, tremor, and sedation. Less frequent side effects include rashes and hematological abnormalities. Hepatic transaminase elevation can occur in more than 40% of patients and is dose related; it generally subsides spontaneously. The enteric-coated form of valproate is generally well tolerated and has a low incidence of gastrointestinal side effects; however, it is more expensive than generic formulations.

Neural tube defects have been reported with the use of valproate during the first trimester of pregnancy; therefore, its use in pregnant women is not recommended. Coma and death have occurred from valproate overdoses with serum levels greater than 2,000 μg/mL.

Before valproate treatment is begun, the patient should have a complete blood count and a liver enzyme measurement; the latter should be done frequently (e.g., every 1–4 weeks) for the first 6 weeks and every 6–24 months thereafter. The drug is started at 250 mg three times daily and can be increased by 250 mg every 3 days. Serum levels can be obtained after 3–4 days. Most patients will need between 1,250 and 2,500 mg/day.

Carbamazepine

Carbamazepine, an anticonvulsant used to treat complex partial and tonico-clonic seizures, has a structure similar to that of the TCAs. It is used as an alternative to lithium and valproate in the treatment of acute mania and may be effective as a prophylaxis for bipolar illness.

The precise mechanism of action of carbamazepine is unknown, but the drug has multiple CNS effects. Of theoretical interest is its dampening effect on kindling, a process in which repeated biochemical or psychological stressors are thought to result in abnormal excitability of limbic neurons.

When carbamazepine is used to treat mania, there is generally a delay of 5–7 days before its effect is apparent. Carbamazepine can safely be combined with antipsychotics, especially when behavioral control is necessary. It may be more effective in patients who cycle rapidly (i.e., more than four episodes per year) and who tend not to respond well to lithium. The usual custom is to aim for typical anticonvulsant blood levels of 8–12 μg/mL; no dose-response curve has been established.

From 10% to 15% of the patients taking carbamazepine develop a skin rash, which is a cause for discontinuation. Other common side effects include impaired coordination, drowsiness, dizziness, slurred speech, and ataxia. Many of these symptoms can be avoided by increasing the dose slowly. A transient leukopenia causing as much as a 25% decrease in the white blood cell count occurs in 10% of patients. A smaller reduction in the white blood cell count may persist in some patients as long as they take the drug, but this is not a reason for discontinuation. Aplastic anemia develops in rare cases, with an estimated prevalence of fewer than 1 in 50,000 patients exposed.

Carbamazepine is typically started at a dose of 200 mg twice daily and increased to three times daily after 3–5 days. Blood levels should be determined 5 days later, 12 hours after the last dose. Most patients will need doses of 600–1,600 mg/day.

Before starting carbamazepine, the patient should have a complete blood count and an electrocardiogram. The patient should be warned about its hematological side effects; any indication of infection, anemia, or thrombocytopenia (e.g., petechiae) should be investigated, and a complete blood count should be obtained. Routine blood monitoring is unnecessary. Hyponatremia may be associated with carbamazepine; therefore, convulsions or undue drowsiness should be cause for obtaining serum electrolyte measurements. Because carbamazepine has been linked with fetal malformations similar to those seen with phenytoin, this drug should be avoided in pregnant women, especially during the first trimester. Breast-feeding by women taking this drug is not recommended.

Other Mood Stabilizers

Gabapentin and lamotrigine, both anticonvulsants, have been used with some success to treat bipolar disorder. Gabapentin is generally well tolerated

Rational use of mood stabilizers
1. Lithium or valproate should be used initially for the treatment of acute mania. Carbamazepine or other anticonvulsants are second-line treatments.
• An antipsychotic and/or a benzodiazepine should be coadministered in highly agitated patients.
2. A clinical trial of lithium or valproate should last 3 weeks at therapeutic blood levels; at this point, another drug should be added or substituted.
• Drug nonresponders may respond to electroconvulsive therapy.
3. Lithium may be given as a single dose at bedtime when the amount is less than 1,200 mg. Lithium should be given with food to minimize gastric irritation.
4. Renal function should be regularly monitored (i.e., every 6–12 months) in patients treated with lithium. Hepatic function should be regularly monitored (i.e., every 6–24 months) in patients treated with valproate.
5. Because no withdrawal syndrome occurs, mood stabilizers can be abruptly withdrawn.
6. Both valproate and carbamazepine may be safely combined with lithium and may be effective in lithium nonresponders.
• Both agents are thought to be particularly effective in rapid cyclers (i.e., more than three episodes/year).

and has few interactions with other medications. Lamotrigine also is well tolerated but has been associated with the rare, potentially life-threatening Stevens-Johnson syndrome.

Gabapentin resembles the anxiolytics in its mechanism of action because it increases the synthesis of GABA and reduces levels of the neurotransmitter glutamate. The drug is an amino acid that is not metabolized and does not bind to plasma protein. The drug can be titrated rapidly, and laboratory monitoring generally is unnecessary. Major side effects are sedation, dizziness, weight gain, nystagmus, and edema in rare cases. Several open-label trials have shown it to be effective in treating mania at doses ranging from 600 to 3,800 mg. Several case reports have shown that the drug is effective in various anxiety disorders, particularly panic disorder and social phobia.

Like many antidepressants, lamotrigine appears to inhibit serotonin reuptake. Case reports and small case series suggest that the drug is effective in bipolar disorder, particularly in rapid-cycling patients. The treatment dose ranges from 50 to 500 mg/day. The drug also has been successfully used to treat bipolar depression.

Some evidence indicates that calcium channel blockers also may be effective in the treatment of mania. The best evidence is for verapamil, although diltiazem, nifedipine, and nimodipine also may work to treat mania or rapid cycling. Verapamil dosages range from 360 to 480 mg/day in divided doses.

Anxiolytics

Anxiolytics are the most widely prescribed class of psychotropic drugs. They include the barbiturates, the nonbarbiturate sedative-hypnotics (e.g., meprobamate), the benzodiazepines, and buspirone. Currently, only the benzodiazepines and buspirone can be recommended because of their superior safety record. The use of anxiolytics probably peaked in the 1970s and has since dropped by about one-third, perhaps as a result of the increased awareness of their abuse potential. There is still a strong belief in the general population that these medications are overprescribed by psychiatrists and other physicians. Despite their reputation, benzodiazepines are generally prescribed for short periods, are prescribed for rational indications, and are not overused by most patients.

Benzodiazepines

Benzodiazepines—an important class of drugs with clear superiority over the barbiturates and nonbarbiturate sedative-hypnotics—have been marketed in the United States since 1964. They have a high therapeutic index, little toxicity, and relatively few drug-drug interactions. The benzodiazepines are indicated for the treatment of anxiety syndromes, sleep disturbances, musculoskeletal disorders, seizure disorders, and alcohol withdrawal and for inducing anesthesia. Their approved indications reflect subtle differences among them (e.g., side effects, potency) and marketing strategy. Commonly used benzodiazepines are compared in Table 27–6.

Benzodiazepines are believed to exert their effects by binding to specific benzodiazepine receptors in the brain. The receptors are intimately linked to receptors for GABA, a major inhibitory neurotransmitter. By binding to benzodiazepine receptors, the drugs potentiate the actions of GABA, leading to a direct anxiolytic effect on the limbic system.

TABLE 27–6. Commonly used benzodiazepines

Drug (trade name)	Rate of onset	Half-life, hours	Long-acting metabolite	Equivalent dosage, mg	Dosage range, mg/day
Anxiolytics					
Alprazolam (Xanax)	Fast	6–20	No	0.5	1–4
Chlordiazepoxide (Librium)	Fast	20–100	Yes	10.0	15–60
Clonazepam (Klonopin)	Moderate	30–40	No	0.25	1–6
Clorazepate (Tranxene)	Very fast	30–100	Yes	7.5	15–45
Diazepam (Valium)	Very fast	30–100	Yes	5.0	5–40
Halazepam (Paxipam)	Fast	100	Yes	20.0	60–160
Lorazepam (Ativan)	Fast	10–20	No	1.0	0.5–10
Oxazepam (Serax)	Slow	5–20	No	15.0	30–120
Prazepam (Centrax)	Slow	60–70	Yes	7.5	20–60
Hypnotics					
Estazolam (ProSom)	Very fast	10–24	No	1.0	1–2 hs
Flurazepam (Dalmane)	Very fast	50–100	Yes	30.0	15–30 hs
Quazepam (Doral)	Very fast	15–35	Yes	7.5	7.5–15 hs
Temazepam (Restoril)	Moderate	8–18	No	15.0	15–30 hs
Triazolam (Halcion)	Very fast	2–3	No	0.25	0.125–0.5 hs

Note. hs=at bedtime.

Indications for Benzodiazepines

Benzodiazepines are useful for the treatment of generalized anxiety disorder, especially when symptoms are severe. Many patients benefit when their anxiety is most acute and problematic, although these drugs generally should be given for short periods (e.g., weeks or months). Patients with mild anxiety may not need medication and can be successfully managed with behavioral interventions (e.g., progressive muscle relaxation). Further information about the treatment of generalized anxiety disorder is found in Chapter 10.

Benzodiazepines have been shown to have an antipanic effect when administered at relatively high doses (e.g., alprazolam, 4–8 mg; clonazepam, 2–4 mg). Because of the abuse potential of benzodiazepines, SRIs are recommended as the initial treatment for panic disorder.

Benzodiazepines also are effective in treating social phobia. With this disorder, patients tend to avoid social situations or endure them with great discomfort. Because SRIs effectively relieve phobic symptoms and do not have an abuse potential, they should be used initially to treat social phobia.

Anxiety frequently complicates depression. Although major depression should be treated with an antidepressant, accompanying anxiety may be more quickly relieved with a benzodiazepine. For some patients, the combination of an antidepressant with a benzodiazepine will provide rapid symptomatic relief. When the antidepressant begins to take effect, the benzodiazepine can then be withdrawn gradually.

Benzodiazepines are effective in alleviating situational anxiety. These syndromes, called *adjustment disorders with anxiety* in DSM-IV and DSM-IV-TR, are characterized by anxiety symptoms (e.g., tremors, palpitations) that occur in response to a stressful event. Adjustment disorders are generally brief; therefore, treatment with benzodiazepines is time limited.

Benzodiazepines have established efficacy in the short-term treatment of insomnia unrelated to identifiable medical or psychiatric illness. Most patients with insomnia do not require long-term treatment, and there are few hazards with well-monitored therapy of limited duration. Estazolam, flurazepam, quazepam, temazepam, and triazolam are approved by the FDA for the treatment of insomnia, although other benzodiazepines are probably as effective. Most patients with insomnia report difficulty falling asleep, so the rate of absorption is a critical determinant of the drug's efficacy. All of these agents are rapidly absorbed except temazepam. Accumulation of compounds with long half-lives increases the likelihood of continued efficacy during repeated administration and minimizes the probability that rebound insomnia will occur when the drug is discontinued. The likelihood of daytime drowsiness and impairment of performance is increased but is partly offset by clinical adaptation or tolerance. Nonaccumulating hypnotics with short half-lives, such as triazolam, are less likely to cause daytime sedation.

Alcohol withdrawal syndromes are commonly treated with benzodiazepines because benzodiazepines and alcohol are cross-tolerant. The treatment of these syndromes is described in Chapter 14.

Pharmacokinetics of Benzodiazepines

Benzodiazepines are rapidly absorbed from the gastrointestinal tract and, with the exception of lorazepam, are poorly absorbed intramuscularly. Lorazepam is available for parenteral use, and its versatility contributes to its widespread use in hospitalized patients. Midazolam is a short-acting agent used to induce anesthesia but is not available orally. Benzodiazepines are metabolized chiefly by hepatic oxidation and have active metabolites. Lorazepam, oxazepam, and temazepam, however, are metabolized by glucuronide conjugation, have no active metabolites, are relatively short acting, and are thus the preferred benzodiazepines for elderly patients.

There are differences between single-dose and steady-state kinetics. Rapid-onset drugs tend to be lipophilic, a property that facilitates rapid crossing of the blood-brain barrier. Drugs with longer elimination half-lives accumulate more slowly and take longer to reach steady state. Washout of these drugs is similarly prolonged. Drugs with shorter half-lives reach steady state more rapidly but also have less total accumulation. Drugs with long half-lives tend to have active metabolites.

Because of the differences in metabolism and half-lives, the best therapeutic results are obtained when the needs of the patient and the situation are taken into account. When prescribing, three parameters—1) half-life, 2) presence of metabolites, and 3) route of elimination—largely determine drug selection. For example, in elderly patients, the clinician should select a benzodiazepine with a short half-life, few metabolites, and renal excretion—all in an effort to reduce accumulation and side effects.

Adverse Effects of Benzodiazepines

CNS depression is common with benzodiazepines. Common symptoms include drowsiness, somnolence, reduced motor coordination, and memory impairment. These symptoms diminish with continued administration or dose reduction. However, patients should be cautioned not to drive or use machines, especially when starting these drugs.

All benzodiazepines have the potential for abuse and addiction. Because physiological dependence is more likely to occur with longer drug exposure, minimizing the duration of continuous treatment should reduce this potential. Also, benzodiazepines should not be prescribed for patients with histories of alcohol or drug abuse or for patients with unstable personalities (e.g., borderline, antisocial types). When signs of dependence appear (e.g., drug-seeking behavior, increasing the dose to get the same effect), the drug should be tapered and discontinued. Patients should be advised to avoid alcohol when taking benzodiazepines because the combination will cause greater CNS depression than either drug alone.

Discontinuation of benzodiazepine therapy after long-term treatment can lead to tremulousness, sweating, sensitivity to light and sound, insomnia, abdominal distress, and systolic hypertension. Serious withdrawal syndromes and seizures are relatively uncommon but are more likely after abrupt discontinuation. Symptom recurrence appears to have a more rapid onset after discontinuation of short-acting benzodiazepines; the effect of drug discontinuation can be minimized by gradually tapering the drug over 1–3 months. Such a slow taper is particularly important for benzodiazepines with short half-lives. When discontinuing short-acting benzodiazepines, it may be helpful to switch the patient to a long-acting medication before initiating a taper (e.g., from alprazolam to diazepam).

The benzodiazepines appear to be safe during pregnancy. Benzodiazepines are secreted in breast milk; therefore, mothers taking these drugs should be instructed not to breast-feed.

Benzodiazepines can be used safely in medically ill and elderly patients. In general, drugs that do not accumulate (e.g., lorazepam) should be used. Because benzodiazepines can cause respiratory depression, they should not be used in persons with sleep apnea, although small doses are tolerated even in patients with chronic pulmonary disease. Small doses are also indicated for the elderly, who are susceptible to the CNS depressant effects of benzodiazepines, which can contribute to memory difficulties and falls.

The least controversial aspect of benzodiazepines is their tremendous index of safety. When taken alone, even massive overdoses are rarely fatal.

Buspirone

Buspirone is used to treat generalized anxiety disorder but is ineffective in blocking panic attacks, relieving phobias, or diminishing obsessions or compulsions. Structurally unlike other anxiolytics, buspirone is relatively nonsedating, does not alter the seizure threshold, does not interact with alcohol, and is not a muscle relaxant. It does not interact with the benzodiazepine receptor and is not effective in treating alcohol withdrawal; it appears to have little abuse potential. Buspirone is well absorbed orally and is metabolized by the liver. Its half-life ranges from 2 to 11 hours. Drowsiness, headache, and dizziness are common side effects.

Buspirone's effect on chronic anxiety is equal to that of diazepam, although its effects are not apparent for 1–2 weeks. The usual dose range is 20–30 mg/day in divided doses. An alternative to buspirone for the treatment of generalized anxiety disorder is a slow-release form of venlafaxine, a commonly prescribed antidepressant.

Rational use of anxiolytics

1. The benzodiazepines should be used for limited periods (e.g., weeks to months) to avoid the problem of dependency because most conditions they are used to treat are probably self-limiting.

   - Some patients will benefit from long-term benzodiazepine administration; in these situations, patients should be periodically assessed for its continuing need.

2. The benzodiazepines have similar clinical efficacy, so the choice of a specific agent depends on its half-life, the presence of metabolites, and the route of administration.

3. Once- or twice-daily dosing is sufficient for most patients.

   - A dose given at bedtime may eliminate the need for a separate hypnotic.

   - Short-acting agents (e.g., alprazolam) are an exception because their dosing interval is determined by their half-lives.

4. Buspirone is not effective on an as-needed basis and is useful only for the treatment of chronic anxiety (e.g., generalized anxiety disorder).

5. The slow-release preparation of venlafaxine is an effective alternative to the benzodiazepines and buspirone in the treatment of generalized anxiety disorder.

Agents Used to Treat Extrapyramidal Syndromes

Anticholinergic agents closely resemble atropine in their ability to block muscarinic receptors, and all are similar in action and efficacy for alleviating antipsychotic-induced EPS, especially pseudoparkinsonism. These drugs are believed to diminish or eliminate EPS by reestablishing dopamine-acetylcholine equilibrium, which they do by blocking acetylcholine in the corpus striatum. An equilibrium of dopaminergic (inhibitory) and cholinergic (excitatory) neuronal activity in the corpus striatum is thought to be necessary for normal motor functioning. Antipsychotic medications cause dopamine re-uptake blockage and an absolute decrease in dopamine and, hence, a relative increase in interneuronal acetylcholine, which results in EPS.

The anticholinergic drug benztropine should be started at a dose of 1–2 mg/day. Smaller dosages should be used with geriatric patients. The maximum allowable dose is 6 mg/day of benztropine or its equivalent because a delirium can occur at higher doses. Benztropine can be administered once daily, preferably at bedtime because it may cause sedation. The side effects of anticholinergic medications—dry mouth, blurry vision, constipation, and urinary hesitancy—are additive with those of the antipsychotics. Most of the anticholinergics are similar in action and efficacy. Table 27–7 shows common agents used to treat EPS and their dose ranges.

TABLE 27–7. Common agents used to treat extrapyramidal syndromes

Category	Drug (trade name)	Dosage range, *mg/day*	Comments
Anticholinergics	Benztropine (Cogentin)	0.5–6	Use 1–2 mg iv of benztropine or 25–50 mg iv of diphenhydramine for acute dystonia. Anticholinergics tend to work better at relieving the tremor of pseudoparkinsonism than hypokinesia.
	Biperiden (Akineton)	2–6	
	Diphenhydramine (Benadryl)	12.5–150	
	Procyclidine (Kemadrin)	2.5–22.5	
	Trihexyphenidyl (Artane)	1–15	
Dopamine facilitators	Amantadine (Symmetrel)	100–300	Useful in situations in which anticholinergic side effects need to be avoided.
β-Blockers	Propranolol (Inderal)	10–80	Works well for treating akathisia.
α-Agonists	Clonidine (Catapres)	0.2–0.8	May cause orthostatic hypotension; therefore, dose should be increased slowly. Works well for treating akathisia

Parenteral benztropine (1–2 mg) or diphenhydramine (25–50 mg) works within minutes to alleviate acute dystonic reactions. Diazepam (5–10 mg iv) also seems to work. Benztropine is the preferred agent because it usually does not cause sedation.

Amantadine and propranolol also are commonly used to treat EPS. Amantadine acts to increase CNS concentrations of dopamine by blocking its reuptake and increasing its release from presynaptic fibers. This action is thought to restore the dopamine-acetylcholine balance in the striatum. Amantadine is primarily useful in treating the symptoms of pseudoparkinsonism, such as tremors, rigidity, and hypokinesia. One advantage of amantadine is its lack of anticholinergic effects, so that it can be safely combined with antipsychotics without concern for the development of an anticholinergic delirium. Treatment is initiated at 100 mg/day and increased to 200–300 mg/day. Onset of action occurs within 1 week. Adverse effects include orthostatic hypotension, livedo reticularis, ankle edema, gastrointestinal upset, and visual hallucinations in rare cases.

Propranolol and other β-blockers have been used to treat akathisia, which usually is not alleviated with an anticholinergic agent. Propranolol (e.g., 10–20 mg three to four times daily) or another equivalent centrally acting β-blocker seems to work well; its effect should be apparent within days. Propranolol is well tolerated, and up to 65% of the patients who take it will benefit. Discontinuation of the drug will lead to a recurrence of symptoms within 4–5 days.

Clonidine, an α_2-receptor agonist, also has been used to treat akathisia. The drug is usually given in divided doses ranging from 0.2 to 0.8 mg/day. Orthostatic hypotension and sedation are the main side effects. Clonidine should be used as a second-line agent for patients unresponsive to propranolol.

In treating any EPS, the clinician should begin by reducing the dose of the antipsychotic drug whenever possible or switching to an atypical antipsychotic with less tendency to cause EPS. When these steps fail, anticholinergics, amantadine, or propranolol can be useful adjuncts. Because EPSs are unpleasant and reduce the likelihood that the patient will remain compliant with treatment, drugs used to treat EPS can make a significant difference in the patient's subjective comfort.

Psychostimulants

Amphetamines were introduced for clinical use in the 1930s and soon were used in many different conditions. When their abuse potential became apparent, governmental regulations became highly restrictive. Their medical use today has been confined to a few specific indications (e.g., narcolepsy, childhood ADHD, refractory obesity). However, interest in their use for psychiatric patients remains strong.

Amphetamine is an indirect-acting sympathomimetic agent that exerts its action through direct neuronal release of dopamine and norepinephrine and the blockade of catecholamine reuptake. Its pharmacological effects include CNS stimulation, appetite suppression, vasoconstriction, and hypothermia. Development of tolerance has been documented for certain effects, such as anorexia, although not for CNS-stimulant properties. The D-isomer is more active than the L form, is highly lipophilic, and is rapidly absorbed from the gut. Plasma half-life is about 12 hours. Onset of clinical effects is rapid, and peak plasma levels following oral dosages are achieved in 1–3 hours. Renal excretion occurs after hepatic biotransformation.

Methylphenidate is structurally related to amphetamine and has similar pharmacological actions but is a somewhat milder stimulant. An oral dose is rapidly absorbed, peaks in the plasma in about 2 hours, and has a half-life of about 2–3 hours. Pemoline is structurally different from amphetamine and is a very mild CNS stimulant with minimal sympathomimetic activity. Its half-life is about 13 hours, and it peaks in the plasma in about 3–4 hours. Excretion is primarily renal. The drug has little or no abuse potential.

The main psychiatric indications for psychostimulants are the treatment of ADHD in children and selected sleep disorders. As noted earlier in the chapter, some psychostimulants have been used to augment the effects of TCAs in patients with refractory major depression. They have been successfully used to treat depression in elderly and medically ill patients (e.g., patients with acquired immunodeficiency syndrome). Their use in treating sleep disorders is discussed in Chapter 24.

Stimulants are highly effective in relieving the symptoms of ADHD. Parents, teachers, and clinicians rate 75% of the children with ADHD as improved while taking stimulants compared with 40% of placebo-treated children. Stimulants tend to decrease physical activity, particularly during times when children are expected to be less active, such as during school; decrease vocalization, noise, and disruptive activity; and improve handwriting. Stimulants improve compliance with adult commands, improve attention span and short-term memory, and reduce distractibility and impulsivity. (Common psychostimulants used to treat ADHD are listed in Table 27–8.)

Stimulant medication should be initiated at a low dose and titrated gradually according to response and side effects within the recommended dose range. Stimulants should be given after meals to reduce the likelihood of suppressing appetite. Starting treatment with a morning dose may be useful in assessing the drug's effect because morning and afternoon school performance then may be compared. The need for medication on weekends or after school must be determined on an individual basis. Pulse and blood pressure should be measured initially and when the dose is changed. Weight

TABLE 27–8. Common psychostimulants used to treat attention-deficit/
hyperactivity disorder

Drug (trade name)	Half-life, hours	Dosage range, mg/kg/day (mg/day)	Comments
Dextroamphetamine (Dexedrine)	6–7	0.3–1.25 (5–40)	Possibly associated with growth retardation
Methylphenidate (Ritalin)	2–4	0.6–1.7 (10–60)	Most commonly used and best studied; high doses (1 mg/kg) may impair cognitive performance
Pemoline (Cylert)	Acute: 2–12	0.5–3.0 (37.5–112.5)	May take weeks for effects to become apparent; less abuse potential than other agents
	Chronic: 14–34		

should be monitored during the initial titration, and weight and height should be measured several times each year.

Common side effects that usually disappear within 2–3 weeks of initiating therapy, or in response to a dose reduction, include appetite suppression, weight loss, irritability, abdominal pain, and insomnia. Mild dysphoria and social withdrawal may occur at higher doses in some patients. In rare cases, children can develop a mild to moderate depression requiring drug discontinuation. A major concern has been the potential for these drugs to cause growth retardation. Recent research shows that the decrease in expected weight gain is small and probably not significant. This effect appears greater with dextroamphetamine than with methylphenidate or pemoline. The effect on growth can be minimized by using drug holidays; this side effect does not appear to be mediated by effects on growth hormone. Some researchers have even suggested that growth delay is caused by processes inherent to ADHD itself.

Other miscellaneous side effects of the stimulants include dizziness, nausea, nightmares, dry mouth, constipation, lethargy, anxiety, hyperacusis, and fearfulness. Further information about the use of stimulants in children with ADHD is found in Chapter 23.

Electroconvulsive Therapy

ECT is a procedure in which an electric current is applied across scalp electrodes to induce a grand mal seizure. The procedure was introduced in 1938 in Italy by Cerletti and Bini to replace less reliable convulsive therapies that used liquid chemicals. ECT is one of the oldest medical treatments still in regular use, a fact that attests to its safety and efficacy. Its mechanism of action remains a mystery, yet it is known to produce multiple effects on the CNS, including the downregulation of β-receptors, a property that ECT has in common with most antidepressants. No alternative therapy has been shown to be more effective than ECT in the treatment of depression.

Indications for Electroconvulsive Therapy

ECT is used almost exclusively for the treatment of mood disorders and is generally reserved for patients who fail one or more trials of antidepressant medication, patients who are at high risk for suicide, patients who are debilitated by their failure to take in adequate food and fluids, and patients who are at risk for cardiovascular collapse. Patients at high risk for suicide and in need of rapid treatment should receive ECT because it tends to work more quickly than antidepressant medication. Most patients receive a course of 6–12 treatments (mean=9) at a rate of 3 per week, although the number is individualized based on the patient's response.

Research shows that approximately 70%–80% of depressed patients receiving ECT improve. Certain depressive symptoms are associated with a good response to ECT, including psychomotor agitation or retardation; nihilistic, somatic, or paranoid delusions; and acute onset of illness. ECT is relatively ineffective in patients with chronic depression or in patients with severe personality disorders.

Mania refractory to medication also responds well to ECT. Predictors of response to ECT include mixed manic and depressive symptoms and severe manic behavior. Schizophrenic patients are sometimes treated with ECT, particularly when a superimposed major depression or a catatonic syndrome is present. Catatonia often responds to fewer than five treatments, and we have seen catatonic patients respond to a single treatment. Patients with schizophrenia of relatively brief duration (i.e., less than 18 months) who have not adequately responded to antipsychotic medication may respond to ECT. Once the schizophrenic illness has become chronic, ECT is of little benefit. Indications for ECT are summarized in Table 27–9.

TABLE 27–9. Indications for electroconvulsive therapy (ECT)

Medication-refractory depression

Suicidal depression

Depression accompanied by refusal to eat or take fluids

Depression during pregnancy

History of positive response to ECT

Catatonic syndromes

Acute forms of schizophrenia

Mania unresponsive to medication

Psychotic or melancholic depression unresponsive to medication

Pre–Electroconvulsive Therapy Workup

ECT is classified as a surgical procedure, yet it is relatively uncomplicated. Routine laboratory tests, including a complete blood count, serum electrolytes, urinalysis, and an electrocardiogram, and a physical examination are performed to rule out physical disorders that may contraindicate ECT. Spine films are no longer routinely obtained but may be of value in documenting the condition of the vertebrae before ECT, especially in the elderly and patients with arthritis. Relative contraindications include recent myocardial infarction (i.e., within 6 months), unstable coronary artery disease, uncompensated congestive heart failure, uncontrolled hypertensive cardiovascular disease, and venous thrombosis. Other conditions that increase the risk of ECT treatment include space-occupying brain lesions and other causes of increased intracranial pressure, recent intracerebral hemorrhage, bleeding or otherwise unstable aneurisms or vascular malformations, and other conditions associated with increased anesthetic risk.

Electroconvulsive Therapy Procedure

To minimize the risk of aspiration, patients cannot have food or fluids after midnight. At the ECT site the next morning, patients are anesthetized with a short-acting anesthetic (e.g., methohexital), receive oxygen to prevent hypoxia, receive succinylcholine as a muscle relaxant to attenuate convulsions, and receive atropine or glycopyrrolate to reduce secretions and to prevent bradyarrhythmias. After the patient is anesthetized, electrodes are placed on the scalp. Bitemporal electrode placement is still widely used, but unilateral leads placed on the nondominant hemisphere are becoming more commonplace because they are less likely to cause cognitive impairment after treatment.

A brief electrical stimulus is applied after placement of the electrodes. The amount of electricity used is approximately equivalent to that required to light a 20-watt bulb for 2 seconds (40 joules). A brief pulse of electrical stimulus is given, rather than a continuous sinusoidal waveform because brief pulse stimulation is associated with less cognitive impairment. Stimulation usually produces a 30- to 60-second tonicoclonic seizure. The seizure is accompanied by a period of bradycardia and transient drop in blood pressure, followed by tachycardia and a rise in blood pressure. A rise in cerebrospinal fluid pressure parallels the rise in blood pressure. These physiological responses are attenuated by the pre-ECT medications. Minor arrhythmias are frequent but are seldom a problem.

Adverse Effects of Electroconvulsive Therapy

During ECT, adverse effects can include brief episodes of hypotension or hypertension, bradyarrhythmias, and tachyarrhythmias; these effects are rarely serious. Fractures were widely reported to occur during ECT-induced seizures in the past but are uncommon now because of the use of muscle relaxants. Other possible adverse effects include prolonged seizures, laryngospasm, and prolonged apnea due to pseudocholinesterase deficiency, a rare genetic disorder. When a seizure is prolonged (i.e., more than 90 seconds), it can be easily terminated with intravenous lorazepam (e.g., 1–2 mg). Immediately after treatment, patients experience postictal confusion. Headache, nausea, and muscle pain also may be experienced after ECT.

The most troublesome long-term effect of ECT is memory impairment. Because ECT disrupts new memories that have not been incorporated into long-term memory stores, ECT can cause a retrograde amnesia involving a short period before and during the hospitalization. This process can sensitize patients to the normal process of forgetting, so that patients who have undergone ECT may be more aware of minor memory disturbances than are patients who have not had these treatments. There is no evidence that ECT affects anterograde memory and subsequent learning. Not all patients experience amnesia, and modifications in ECT, including unilateral electrode placement and brief-pulse stimulation, help to minimize any memory loss that occurs.

Surveys of patients receiving ECT generally have found high acceptance levels. In one study, nearly 80% of the patients believed that they were helped by ECT, and 80% said that they would not be reluctant to have it again. A substantial minority reported approaching the treatment with anxiety. In retrospect, more than 80% of the respondents found that it produced no more anxiety than a dental appointment.

Amobarbital Sodium (Amytal) Interview

For more than 50 years, sedative-hypnotic drugs have been used to produce a sedated state during which an interview is conducted. Despite its long history, indications for the amobarbital sodium (Amytal) interview have not been well established, and its value has not been adequately proven. Yet, many psychiatrists still consider it a valuable procedure.

The usual method consists of administering 200–500 mg of amobarbital sodium intravenously at a rate of 25–50 mg/minute, although other drugs (including thiopental, pentobarbital, or one of the benzodiazepines) can be used. The interviewer talks with the patient as the drug is being administered and halts drug administration when the desired level of sedation is obtained (i.e., when lateral nystagmus appears at light sedation and slurred speech develops during a deeper state of sedation). The interview continues for 30–60 minutes or until sufficient material has been produced for diagnostic purposes or therapeutic goals have been reached. Vital signs are monitored throughout the interview, and the patient is carefully observed by nursing staff until he or she is fully alert.

One indication for the Amytal interview is the evaluation of mute patients. Patients whose muteness is due to a catatonic syndrome often recover spontaneously and begin to speak. The patient's speech may show a formal thought disorder, hallucinations, or delusions that are useful in diagnosing the underlying disorder. Muteness returns when the sedation wears off. Sometimes patients who are immobilized by acute anxiety or panic may begin to talk about their concerns when sedated. Dissociative amnesia and fugue and conversion disorders are often temporarily relieved by amobarbital sodium; useful information then may be obtained (e.g., amnesic patients may reveal their name and address). The interview also has been thought to be helpful in separating cognitive impairment associated with a delirium or dementing illness from that caused by a mood or psychotic disorder. Patients who are confused or disoriented from a delirium or dementia tend to worsen with amobarbital sodium. Patients whose impairment is due to a major depression or a psychotic disorder will often temporarily improve.

There are several medical and psychiatric contraindications to the use of the Amytal interview. Medical contraindications include a history of barbiturate allergy or addiction; severe liver, renal, or cardiac disorders; and severe bronchopulmonary disease. A thorough psychiatric history, physical examination, and screening laboratory examination should identify these conditions. The interview should be avoided both in paranoid patients, who may misinterpret its use, and in unwilling patients because cooperation is important to the success of the procedure. Patients who are overenthusiastic about the interview are poor candidates because they may use the test for their own (possibly manipulative) purposes or may have unrealistic expectations.

Bibliography

American Psychiatric Association: Practice guidelines for the treatment of patients with bipolar disorder. Am J Psychiatry 151 (suppl):12, 1994

American Psychiatric Association: Practice guidelines for the treatment of patients with schizophrenia. Am J Psychiatry 154 (suppl):4, 1997

American Psychiatric Association: Practice guidelines for the treatment of patients with major depressive disorder (revision). Am J Psychiatry 157 (suppl):4, 2000

Arana GW: An overview of side effects caused by typical antipsychotics. J Clin Psychiatry 61 (suppl 8):5–11, 2000

Ashton AK, Rosen RC: Bupropion as an antidote for serotonin reuptake inhibitor-induced sexual dysfunction. J Clin Psychiatry 59:112–115, 1998

Barak Y, Swartz M, Shamir E: Vitamin E (α-tocopherol) in the treatment of tardive dyskinesia: a statistical meta-analysis. Ann Clin Psychiatry 10:101–106, 1998

Busto U, Sellers EM, Naranjo CA, et al: Withdrawal reaction after long-term therapeutic use of benzodiazepines. N Engl J Med 315:854–859, 1986

Cabras PL, Hardoy J, Hardoy MC, et al: Clinical experience with gabapentin in patients with bipolar or schizoaffective disorder: results of an open label study. J Clin Psychiatry 6:245–248, 1999

Chiarello RJ, Cole JO: The use of psychostimulants in general psychiatry: a reconsideration. Arch Gen Psychiatry 44:286–295, 1987

Clary C, Schweizer E: Treatment of MAOI hypertensive crisis with sublingual nifedipine. J Clin Psychiatry 48:249–250, 1987

Fawcett J, Baskin RL: A meta-analysis of eight randomized, double-blind controlled clinical trials of mirtazapine for the treatment of patients with major depression and symptoms of anxiety. J Clin Psychiatry 59:123–127, 1998

Feigher JP: Mechanism of action of antidepressant medications. J Clin Psychiatry 60 (suppl 4):4–11, 1999

Gorman JM: Mirtazapine: clinical overview. J Clin Psychiatry 60 (suppl 17):9–13, 1999

Hirschfeld RMA: Efficacy of SSRIs and newer antidepressants in severe depression: comparison with TCAs. J Clin Psychiatry 60:326–335, 1999

Hyman SE, Arana GW: Handbook of Psychiatric Drug Therapy. Boston, MA, Little, Brown, 1987

Ichim L, Berk M, Brook S: Lamotrigine compared with lithium in mania: a double-blind randomized controlled trial. Ann Clin Psychiatry 12:5–10, 2000

Igbal MM: Effect of antidepressants during pregnancy and lactation. Ann Clin Psychiatry 11:237–256, 1999

Jones KL, Lacro RV, Johnson KA, et al: Pattern of malformations in the children of women treated with carbamazepine during pregnancy. N Engl J Med 320:1661–1666, 1989

Lipinsky JF, Zubenko G, Cohen BM, et al: Propranolol in the treatment of neuroleptic induced akathisia. Am J Psychiatry 141:412–415, 1984

Nemeroff CB, DeVane CL, Pollock BG: Newer antidepressants and the cytochrome P450 system. Am J Psychiatry 153:311–320, 1996

Noyes R, Garvey MJ, Cook BL, et al: Benzodiazepine withdrawal: a review of the evidence. J Clin Psychiatry 49:382–389, 1988

Olajide D, Lader M: A comparison of buspirone, diazepam, and placebo in patients with chronic anxiety states. J Clin Psychopharmacol 75:148–152, 1987

Perry JC, Jacobs D: Overview: clinical applications of the Amytal interview in psychiatric emergency settings. Am J Psychiatry 139:552–559, 1982

Perry PJ, Alexander B, Liskow BI: Psychotropic Drug Handbook, 7th Edition. Washington, DC, American Psychiatric Press, 1997

Small JG, Klapper MH, Kellams JJ, et al: Electroconvulsive treatment compared with lithium in the management of manic states. Arch Gen Psychiatry 45:727–732, 1988

Tyrer P, Murphy S: The place of benzodiazepines in psychiatric practice. Br J Psychiatry 151:719–723, 1987

Zajecka J, Tracy KA, Mitchell S: Discontinuation syndromes after treatment with serotonin reuptake inhibitors: a literature review. J Clin Psychiatry 58:291–297, 1997

Self-Assessment Questions

1. What is the mechanism of action of the antipsychotics?
2. What are the common indications for antipsychotics?
3. How are the antipsychotics used in the treatment of acute psychosis? How are they used in maintenance treatment?
4. What are the common extrapyramidal side effects that occur with antipsychotics? Describe the syndromes and discuss their clinical management.
5. What disorders can be treated with antidepressants? Why is the term *antidepressant* a misnomer?

6. What is the putative mechanism of action of the TCAs? Of the MAOIs? Of the SRIs? Of the newer agents?
7. Are blood levels of TCAs meaningful? When should they be obtained?
8. What are the common side effects of the TCAs? Of the MAOIs? Of the SRIs? Of the newer agents?
9. What agent is associated with the occurrence of priapism? Why is this worrisome?
10. What are the typical plasma level ranges for lithium carbonate for acute treatment of mania? For prophylaxis?
11. What are the common side effects of lithium carbonate? Of valproate?
12. What is carbamazepine used to treat? What are its side effects?

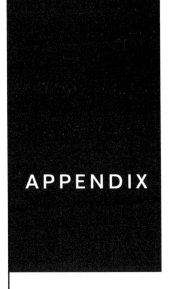

APPENDIX

Brief Psychiatric Rating Scale (BPRS)

DIRECTIONS: Place an X in the appropriate box to represent level of severity of each symptom.

	Not present	Very mild	Mild	Moderate	Moderately severe	Severe	Extremely severe
SOMATIC CONCERN—preoccupation with physical health, fear of physical illness, hypochondriasis.	❑	❑	❑	❑	❑	❑	❑
ANXIETY—worry, fear, overconcern for present or future, uneasiness.	❑	❑	❑	❑	❑	❑	❑
EMOTIONAL WITHDRAWAL—lack of spontaneous interaction, isolation deficiency in relating to others.	❑	❑	❑	❑	❑	❑	❑
CONCEPTUAL DISORGANIZATION—thought processes confused, disconnected, disorganized, disrupted.	❑	❑	❑	❑	❑	❑	❑
GUILT FEELINGS—self-blame, shame, remorse for past behavior.	❑	❑	❑	❑	❑	❑	❑
TENSION—physical and motor manifestations of nervousness, overactivation.	❑	❑	❑	❑	❑	❑	❑
MANNERISMS AND POSTURING—peculiar, bizarre unnatural motor behavior (not including tic).	❑	❑	❑	❑	❑	❑	❑
GRANDIOSITY—exaggerated self-opinion, arrogance, conviction of unusual power or abilities.	❑	❑	❑	❑	❑	❑	❑
DEPRESSIVE MOOD—sorrow, sadness, despondency, pessimism.	❑	❑	❑	❑	❑	❑	❑
HOSTILITY—animosity, contempt, belligerence, disdain for others.	❑	❑	❑	❑	❑	❑	❑
SUSPICIOUSNESS—mistrust, belief others harbor malicious or discriminatory intent.	❑	❑	❑	❑	❑	❑	❑
HALLUCINATORY BEHAVIOR—perceptions without normal external stimulus correspondence.	❑	❑	❑	❑	❑	❑	❑
MOTOR RETARDATION—slowed, weakened movements or speech, reduced body tone.	❑	❑	❑	❑	❑	❑	❑
UNCOOPERATIVENESS—resistance, guardedness, rejection of authority.	❑	❑	❑	❑	❑	❑	❑
UNUSUAL THOUGHT CONTENT—unusual, odd, strange, bizarre thought content.	❑	❑	❑	❑	❑	❑	❑
BLUNTED AFFECT—reduced emotional tone, reduction in formal intensity of feelings, flatness.	❑	❑	❑	❑	❑	❑	❑
EXCITEMENT—heightened emotional tone, agitation, increased reactivity.	❑	❑	❑	❑	❑	❑	❑
DISORIENTATION—confusion or lack of proper association for person, place, or time.	❑	❑	❑	❑	❑	❑	❑

Global Assessment Scale (Range 1–100)_____

Source. Reprinted from Overall JE: "The Brief Psychiatric Rating Scale (BPRS): Recent Developments in Ascertainment and Scaling." *Psychopharmacology Bulletin* 24:97–99, 1988. Used with permission.

Scale for the Assessment of Negative Symptoms (SANS)

0=None	1=Questionable	2=Mild	3=Moderate	4=Marked	5=Severe

AFFECTIVE FLATTENING OR BLUNTING

1   *Unchanging Facial Expression*   0 1 2 3 4 5
The patient's face appears wooden, changes less than
expected as emotional content of discourse changes.

2   *Decreased Spontaneous Movements*   0 1 2 3 4 5
The patient shows few or no spontaneous movements,
does not shift position, move extremities, etc.

3   *Paucity of Expressive Gestures*   0 1 2 3 4 5
The patient does not use hand gestures, body position,
etc., as an aid to expressing his ideas.

4   *Poor Eye Contact*   0 1 2 3 4 5
The patient avoids eye contact or "stares through" interviewer even when speaking.

5   *Affective Nonresponsivity*   0 1 2 3 4 5
The patient fails to smile or laugh when prompted.

6   *Lack of Vocal Inflections*   0 1 2 3 4 5
The patient fails to show normal vocal emphasis patterns,
is often monotonic.

7   *Global Rating of Affective Flattening*   0 1 2 3 4 5
This rating should focus on overall severity of symptoms,
especially unresponsiveness, eye contact, facial expression, and vocal inflections.

ALOGIA

8   *Poverty of Speech*   0 1 2 3 4 5
The patient's replies to questions are restricted in *amount*,
tend to be brief, concrete, and unelaborated.

9   *Poverty of Content of Speech*   0 1 2 3 4 5
The patient's replies are adequate in amount but tend to
be vague, overconcrete, or overgeneralized, and convey
little information.

10   *Blocking*   0 1 2 3 4 5
The patient indicates, either spontaneously or with
prompting, that his train of thought was interrupted.

Scale for the Assessment of
Negative Symptoms (SANS) *(continued)*

0=None	1=Questionable	2=Mild	3=Moderate	4=Marked	5=Severe

11	*Increased Latency of Response*	0 1 2 3 4 5

The patient takes a long time to reply to questions; prompting indicates the patient is aware of the question.

12	*Global Rating of Alogia*	0 1 2 3 4 5

The core features of alogia are poverty of speech and poverty of content.

AVOLITION-APATHY

13	*Grooming and Hygiene*	0 1 2 3 4 5

The patient's clothes may be sloppy or soiled, and he may have greasy hair, body odor, etc.

14	*Impersistence at Work or School*	0 1 2 3 4 5

The patient has difficulty seeking or maintaining employment, completing school work, keeping house, etc. If an inpatient, cannot persist at ward activities, such as occupational therapy, playing cards, etc.

15	*Physical Anergia*	0 1 2 3 4 5

The patient tends to be physically inert. He may sit for hours and does not initiate spontaneous activity.

16	*Global Rating of Avolition-Apathy*	0 1 2 3 4 5

Strong weight may be given to one or two prominent symptoms if particularly striking.

ANHEDONIA-ASOCIALITY

17	*Recreational Interests and Activities*	0 1 2 3 4 5

The patient may have few or no interests. Both the quality and quantity of interests should be taken into account.

18	*Sexual Activity*	0 1 2 3 4 5

The patient may show a decrease in sexual interest and activity, or enjoyment when active.

19	*Ability to Feel Intimacy and Closeness*	0 1 2 3 4 5

The patient may display an inability to form close or intimate relationships, especially with the opposite sex and family.

Scale for the Assessment of Negative Symptoms (SANS) *(continued)*

0=None 1=Questionable 2=Mild 3=Moderate 4=Marked 5=Severe

20	*Relationships With Friends and Peers* The patient may have few or no friends and may prefer to spend all of his time isolated.	0 1 2 3 4 5
21	*Global Rating of Anhedonia-Asociality* This rating should reflect overall severity, taking into account the patient's age, family status, etc.	0 1 2 3 4 5

ATTENTION

22	*Social Inattentiveness* The patient appears uninvolved or unengaged. He may seem spacey.	0 1 2 3 4 5
23	*Inattentiveness During Mental Status Testing* Tests of "serial 7s" (at least five subtractions) and spelling *world* backwards: Score: 2=1 error; 3=2 errors; 4=3 errors.	0 1 2 3 4 5
24	*Global Rating of Attention* This rating should assess the patient's overall concentration, clinically and on tests.	0 1 2 3 4 5

Source. Available from Nancy C. Andreasen, M.D., Ph.D., Department of Psychiatry, College of Medicine, The University of Iowa, Iowa City, IA 52242. Copyright 1984 by Nancy C. Andreasen. Reprinted with permission.

Scale for the Assessment of Positive Symptoms (SAPS)

| 0=None | 1=Questionable | 2=Mild | 3=Moderate | 4=Marked | 5=Severe |

HALLUCINATIONS

1 *Auditory Hallucinations*　　　　　　　　　0 1 2 3 4 5
The patient reports voices, noises, or other sounds that
no one else hears.

2 *Voices Commenting*　　　　　　　　　　　0 1 2 3 4 5
The patient reports a voice which makes a running
commentary on his behavior or thoughts.

3 *Voices Conversing*　　　　　　　　　　　0 1 2 3 4 5
The patient reports hearing two or more voices
conversing.

4 *Somatic or Tactile Hallucinations*　　　　　0 1 2 3 4 5
The patient reports experiencing peculiar physical
sensations in the body.

5 *Olfactory Hallucinations*　　　　　　　　　0 1 2 3 4 5
The patient reports experiencing unusual smells which
no one else notices.

6 *Visual Hallucinations*　　　　　　　　　　0 1 2 3 4 5
The patient sees shapes or people that are not actually
present.

7 *Global Rating of Hallucinations*　　　　　　0 1 2 3 4 5
This rating should be based on the duration and severity
of the hallucinations and their effects on the patient's
life.

DELUSIONS

8 *Persecutory Delusions*　　　　　　　　　0 1 2 3 4 5
The patient believes he is being conspired against or
persecuted in some way.

9 *Delusions of Jealousy*　　　　　　　　　　0 1 2 3 4 5
The patient believes his spouse is having an affair with
someone.

10 *Delusions of Guilt or Sin*　　　　　　　　0 1 2 3 4 5
The patient believes that he has committed some terrible
sin or done something unforgivable.

Scale for the Assessment of
Positive Symptoms (SAPS) *(continued)*

0=None	1=Questionable	2=Mild	3=Moderate	4=Marked	5=Severe

11 *Grandiose Delusions*   0 1 2 3 4 5
The patient believes he has special powers or abilities.

12 *Religious Delusions*   0 1 2 3 4 5
The patient is preoccupied with false beliefs of a
religious nature.

13 *Somatic Delusions*   0 1 2 3 4 5
The patient believes that somehow his body is diseased,
abnormal, or changed.

14 *Delusions of Reference*   0 1 2 3 4 5
The patient believes that insignificant remarks or events
refer to him or have some special meaning.

15 *Delusions of Being Controlled*   0 1 2 3 4 5
The patient feels that his feelings or actions are controlled by some outside force.

16 *Delusions of Mind Reading*   0 1 2 3 4 5
The patient feels that people can read his mind or know
his thoughts.

17 *Thought Broadcasting*   0 1 2 3 4 5
The patient believes that his thoughts are broadcast so
that he himself or others can hear them.

18 *Thought Insertion*   0 1 2 3 4 5
The patient believes that thoughts that are not his own
have been inserted into his mind.

19 *Thought Withdrawal*   0 1 2 3 4 5
The patient believes that thoughts have been taken away
from his mind.

20 *Global Rating of Delusions*   0 1 2 3 4 5
This rating should be based on the duration and
persistence of the delusions and their effect on the
patient's life.

BIZARRE BEHAVIOR

21 *Clothing and Appearance*   0 1 2 3 4 5
The patient dresses in an unusual manner or does other
strange things to alter his appearance.

Scale for the Assessment of Positive Symptoms (SAPS) *(continued)*

0=None	1=Questionable	2=Mild	3=Moderate	4=Marked	5=Severe

22	*Social and Sexual Behavior* The patient may do things considered inappropriate according to usual social norms (e.g., masturbating in public).	0	1	2 3	4	5
23	*Aggressive and Agitated Behavior* The patient may behave in an aggressive, agitated manner, often unpredictably.	0	1	2 3	4	5
24	*Repetitive or Stereotyped Behavior* The patient develops a set of repetitive actions or rituals that he must perform over and over.	0	1	2 3	4	5
25	*Global Rating of Bizarre Behavior* This rating should reflect the type of behavior and the extent to which it deviates from social norms.	0	1	2 3	4	5

POSITIVE FORMAL THOUGHT DISORDER

26	*Derailment* A pattern of speech in which ideas slip off track onto ideas obliquely related or unrelated.	0	1	2 3	4	5
27	*Tangentiality* Replying to a question in an oblique or irrelevant manner.	0	1	2 3	4	5
28	*Incoherence* A pattern of speech which is essentially incomprehensible at times.	0	1	2 3	4	5
29	*Illogicality* A pattern of speech in which conclusions are reached which do not follow logically.	0	1	2 3	4	5
30	*Circumstantiality* A pattern of speech which is very indirect and delayed in reaching its goal idea.	0	1	2 3	4	5
31	*Pressure of Speech* The patient's speech is rapid and difficult to interrupt; the amount of speech produced is greater than that considered normal.	0	1	2 3	4	5

Scale for the Assessment of
Positive Symptoms (SAPS) *(continued)*

0=None	1=Questionable	2=Mild	3=Moderate	4=Marked	5=Severe

32	*Distractible Speech* The patient is distracted by nearby stimuli which interrupt his flow of speech.	0 1 2 3 4 5
33	*Clanging* A pattern of speech in which sounds rather than meaningful relationships govern word choice.	0 1 2 3 4 5
34	*Global Rating of Positive Formal Thought Disorder* This rating should reflect the frequency of abnormality and degree to which it affects the patient's ability to communicate.	0 1 2 3 4 5

INAPPROPRIATE AFFECT

35	*Inappropriate Affect* The patient's affect is inappropriate or incongruous, not simply flat or blunted.	0 1 2 3 4 5

Source. Available from Nancy C. Andreasen, M.D., Ph.D., Department of Psychiatry, College of Medicine, The University of Iowa, Iowa City, IA 52242. Copyright 1984 Nancy C. Andreasen. Reprinted with permission.

Beck Depression Inventory (BDI)

Name_____   Date _____

On this questionnaire are groups of statements. Please read each group of statements carefully. Then pick out the one statement in each group that best describes the way you have been feeling the PAST WEEK, INCLUDING TODAY! Circle the number beside the statements you picked. If several statements in the group seem to apply equally well, circle each one. **Be sure to read all statements in each group before making your choice.**

1
0   I do not feel sad.
1   I feel sad.
2   I am sad all the time and I can't snap out of it.
3   I am so sad or unhappy that I can't stand it.

2
0   I am not particularly discouraged about the future.
1   I feel discouraged about the future.
2   I feel I have nothing to look forward to.
3   I feel that the future is hopeless and that things cannot improve.

3
0   I do not feel like a failure.
1   I feel I have failed more than the average person.
2   As I look back on my life, all I can see is a lot of failures.
3   I feel I am a complete failure as a person.

4
0   I get as much satisfaction out of things as I used to.
1   I don't enjoy things the way I used to.
2   I don't get real satisfaction out of anything anymore.
3   I am dissatisfied or bored with everything.

5
0   I don't feel particularly guilty.
1   I feel guilty a good part of the time.
2   I feel quite guilty most of the time.
3   I feel guilty all of the time.

6
0   I don't feel I am being punished.
1   I feel I may be punished.
2   I expect to be punished.
3   I feel I am being punished.

7
0   I don't feel disappointed in myself.
1   I am disappointed in myself.
2   I am disgusted with myself.
3   I hate myself.

8
0   I don't feel I am any worse than anybody else.
1   I am critical of myself for my weaknesses or mistakes.
2   I blame myself all the time for my faults.
3   I blame myself for everything bad that happens.

9
0   I don't have any thoughts of killing myself.
1   I have thoughts of killing myself, but I would not carry them out.
2   I would like to kill myself.
3   I would kill myself if I had the chance.

10
0   I don't cry any more than usual.
1   I cry more now than I used to.
2   I cry all the time now.
3   I used to be able to cry, but now I can't cry even though I want to.

11
0   I am no more irritated now than I ever am.
1   I get annoyed or irritated more easily than I used to.
2   I feel irritated all the time now.
3   I don't get irritated at all by the things that used to irritate me.

12
0   I have not lost interest in other people.
1   I am less interested in other people than I used to be.
2   I have lost most of my interest in other people.
3   I have lost all of my interest in other people.

Beck Depression Inventory (BDI) *(continued)*

13 0 I make decisions about as well as
       I ever could.
    1 I put off making decisions more than
       I used to.
    2 I have greater difficulty in making
       decisions than before.
    3 I can't make decisions at all anymore.

14 0 I don't feel I look any worse than
       I used to.
    1 I am worried that I am looking old or
       unattractive.
    2 I feel that there are permanent changes
       in my appearance.
    3 I believe that I look ugly.

15 0 I can work about as well as before.
    1 It takes an extra effort to get started
       at doing something.
    2 I have to push myself very hard to do
       anything.
    3 I can't do any work at all.

16 0 I can sleep as well as usual.
    1 I don't sleep as well as I used to.
    2 I wake up 1–2 hours earlier than usual
       and find it hard to get back to sleep.
    3 I wake up several hours earlier than I
       used to and cannot get back to sleep.

17 0 I don't get more tired than usual.
    1 I get tired more easily than I used to.
    2 I get tired from doing almost anything.
    3 I am too tired to do anything.

18 0 My appetite is no worse than usual.
    1 My appetite is not as good as it used to be.
    2 My appetite is much worse now.
    3 I have no appetite at all anymore.

19 0 I haven't lost much weight, if any, lately
    1 I have lost more than 3 pounds.
    2 I have lost more than 10 pounds.
    3 I have lost more than 15 pounds.
       I am purposely trying to lose weight by
       eating less Yes____ No ____.

20 0 I am no more worried about my health
       than usual.
    1 I am worried about physical problems
       such as aches and pains, upset stomach,
       or constipation.
    2 I am very worried about physical prob-
       lems, and it's hard to think of much else.
    3 I am so worried about my physical prob-
       lems that I cannot think about anything
       else.

21 0 I have not noticed any recent changes in
       my interest in sex.
    1 I am less interested in sex than I used to be.
    2 I am much less interested in sex now.
    3 I have lost interest in sex completely.

Source.   Reprinted from Beck AT, Ward CH, Mendelsohn M, et al.: "An Inventory for Measuring Depression." *Archives of General Psychiatry* 4:561–571, 1961. Copyrighted 1961, American
Medical Association. Used with permission.

Hamilton Rating Scale for Depression (HRSD)

For each item select the "cue" which best characterizes the patient.

1: DEPRESSED MOOD (Sadness, hopeless, helpless, worthless)

    0   Absent

    1   These feeling states indicated only on questioning

    2   These feeling states spontaneously reported verbally

    3   Communicates feeling states nonverbally—i.e., through facial expression, posture, voice, and tendency to weep

    4   Patient reports VIRTUALLY ONLY these feeling states in his spontaneous verbal and nonverbal communication

2: FEELINGS OF GUILT

    0   Absent

    1   Self-reproach, feels he has let people down

    2   Ideas of guilt or rumination over past errors or sinful deeds

    3   Present illness is a punishment. Delusions of guilt

    4   Hears accusatory or denunciatory voices and/or experiences threatening visual hallucinations

3: SUICIDE

    0   Absent

    1   Feels life is not worth living

    2   Wishes he were dead or any thoughts of possible death to self

    3   Suicide ideas or gestures

    4   Attempts at suicide (any serious attempt rates 4)

4: INSOMNIA EARLY

    0   No difficulty falling asleep

    1   Complains of occasional difficulty falling asleep—i.e., more than ¼ hour

    2   Complains of nightly difficulty falling asleep

5: INSOMNIA MIDDLE

    0   No difficulty

    1   Patient complains of being restless and disturbed during the night

    2   Waking during the night—any getting out of bed rates 2 (except for purpose of voiding)

Hamilton Rating Scale for
Depression (HRSD) *(continued)*

For each item select the "cue" which best characterizes the patient.

6: INSOMNIA LATE

   0   No difficulty

   1   Waking in early hours of the morning but goes back to sleep

   2   Unable to fall asleep again if gets out of bed

7: WORK AND ACTIVITIES

   0   No difficulty

   1   Thoughts and feelings of incapacity, fatigue or weakness related to activities, work, or hobbies

   2   Loss of interest in activity, hobbies, or work—either directly reported by patient, or indirect in listlessness, indecision and vacillation (feels he has to push self to work or activities)

   3   Decrease in actual time spent in activities or decrease in productivity. In hospital, rate 3 if patient does not spend at least three hours a day in activities (hospital job or hobbies) exclusive of ward chores

   4   Stopped working because of present illness. In hospital, rate 4 if patient engages in no activities except ward chores, or if patient fails to perform ward chores unassisted

8: RETARDATION (Slowness of thought and speech; impaired ability to concentrate; decreased motor activity)

   0   Normal speech and thought

   1   Slight retardation at interview

   2   Obvious retardation at interview

   3   Interview difficult

   4   Complete stupor

9: AGITATION

   0   None

   1   "Playing with" hands, hair, etc.

   2   Hand-wringing, nail biting, hair pulling, biting of lips

10: ANXIETY PSYCHIC

   0   No difficulty

   1   Subjective tensions and irritability

   2   Worrying about minor matters

   3   Apprehensive attitude apparent in face or speech

   4   Fears expressed without questioning

Hamilton Rating Scale for Depression (HRSD) *(continued)*

For each item select the "cue" which best characterizes the patient.

11: ANXIETY SOMATIC

0	Absent	Physiological concomitants of anxiety, such as:
1	Mild	Gastrointestinal—dry mouth, wind, indigestion, diarrhea, cramps, belching
2	Moderate	Cardiovascular—palpitations, headaches
3	Severe	Respiratory—hyperventilation, sighing
4	Incapacitating	Urinary frequency
		Sweating

12: SOMATIC SYMPTOMS GASTROINTESTINAL

0   None

1   Loss of appetite but eating without staff encouragement. Heavy feelings in abdomen

2   Difficulty eating without staff urging. Requests or requires laxatives or medication for bowels or medication for G.I. symptoms

13: SOMATIC SYMPTOMS GENERAL

0   None

1   Heaviness in limbs, back or head. Backaches, headache, muscle aches. Loss of energy and fatigability

2   Any clear cut symptoms rates 2

14: GENITAL SYMPTOMS

0	Absent	Symptoms such as:
1	Mild	Loss of libido
2	Severe	Menstrual disturbances

15: HYPOCHONDRIASIS

0   Not present

1   Self-absorption (bodily)

2   Preoccupation with health

3   Frequent complaints, requests for help, etc.

4   Hypochondriacal delusions

16: LOSS OF WEIGHT

A: WHEN RATING BY HISTORY

0   No weight loss

1   Probable weight loss associated with present illness

2   Definite (according to patient) weight loss

Hamilton Rating Scale for
Depression (HRSD) *(continued)*

For each item select the "cue" which best characterizes the patient.

    B: ON WEEKLY RATINGS BY WARD PSYCHIATRIST, WHEN ACTUAL WEIGHT CHANGES ARE MEASURED

    0 Less than 1 lb. weight loss in week

    1 Greater than 1 lb. weight loss in week

    2 Greater than 2 lb. weight loss in week

17: INSIGHT

    0 Acknowledges being depressed and ill

    1 Acknowledges illness but attributes cause to bad food, climate, overwork, virus, need for rest, etc.

    2 Denies being ill at all

18: DIURNAL VARIATION

A.M. P.M.

0 0 Absent   If symptoms are worse in the morning or evening, note which it is and rate severity of variation

1 1 Mild

2 2 Severe

19: DEPERSONALIZATION AND DEREALIZATION

    0 Absent   Such as:

    1 Mild   Feelings of unreality

    2 Moderate   Nihilistic ideas

    3 Severe

    4 Incapacitating

20: PARANOID SYMPTOMS

    0 None

    1 Suspiciousness

    2 Ideas of reference

    3 Delusions of reference and persecution

21: OBSESSIONAL AND COMPULSIVE SYMPTOMS

    0 Absent

    1 Mild

    2 Severe

Hamilton Rating Scale for
Depression (HRSD) *(continued)*

For each item select the "cue" which best characterizes the patient.

22: HELPLESSNESS

- 0   Not present
- 1   Subjective feelings which are elicited only by inquiry
- 2   Patient volunteers his helpless feelings
- 3   Requires urging, guidance, and reassurance to accomplish ward chores or personal hygiene
- 4   Requires physical assistance for dress, grooming, eating, bedside tasks, or personal hygiene

23: HOPELESSNESS

- 0   Not present
- 1   Intermittently doubts that "things will improve" but can be reassured
- 2   Consistently feels "hopeless" but accepts reassurances
- 3   Expresses feelings of discouragement, despair, pessimism about future, which cannot be dispelled
- 4   Spontaneously and inappropriately perseverates "I'll never get well" or its equivalent

24: WORTHLESSNESS (Ranges from mild loss of esteem, feelings of inferiority, self-deprecation to delusional notions of worthlessness)

- 0   Not present
- 1   Indicates feelings of worthlessness (loss of self-esteem) only on questioning
- 2   Spontaneously indicates feelings of worthlessness (loss of self-esteem)
- 3   Different from 2 by degree. Patient volunteers that he is "no good," "inferior," etc.
- 4   Delusional notions of worthlessness—i.e., "I am a heap of garbage" or its equivalent

Source.   Reprinted from Hamilton M: "A Rating Scale for Depression." *Journal of Neurology, Neurosurgery and Psychiatry* 23:56–62, 1960. Used with permission.

Hamilton Anxiety Rating Scale

Patient's Name _____   Date of First Report _____

Diagnosis _____   Date of This Report _____

Current Therapy _____

Instructions   This checklist is to assist the physician in evaluating each patient with respect to degree of anxiety and pathological condition. Please fill in the appropriate rating.

0   None
1   Mild
2   Moderate
3   Severe
4   Severe, grossly disabling

Item		Rating	Item		Rating
Anxious Mood	Worries, anticipation of the worst, fearful anticipation, irritability		Somatic (Sensory)	Tinnitus, blurring of vision, hot and cold flushes, feelings of weakness, picking sensation.	
Tension	Feelings of tension, fatigability, startle response, moved to tears easily, trembling, feelings of restlessness, inability to relax.		Cardiovascular Symptoms	Tachycardia, palpitations, pain in chest, throbbing of vessels, fainting feelings, missing beat.	
Fear	Of dark, of strangers, of being left alone, of animals, of traffic, of crowds.		Respiratory Symptoms	Pressure or constriction in chest, choking feelings, sighing, dyspnea.	
Insomnia	Difficulty in falling asleep, broken sleep, unsatisfying sleep and fatigue on waking, dreams, nightmares, night terrors.		Gastrointestinal Symptoms	Difficulty in swallowing, wind, abdominal pain, burning sensations, abdominal fullness, nausea, vomiting, borborygmi, looseness of bowels, loss of weight, constipation.	
Intellectual (Cognitive)	Difficulty in concentration, poor memory.		Genitourinary Symptoms	Frequency of micturition, urgency of micturition, amenorrhea, menorrhagia, development of frigidity, premature ejaculation, loss of libido, impotence.	
Depressed Mood	Loss of interest, lack of pleasure in hobbies, depression, early waking, diurnal swing.		Autonomic Symptoms	Dry mouth, flushing, pallor, tendency to sweat, giddiness, tension headache, raising of hair.	
Behavior at Interview	Fidgeting, restlessness or pacing, tremor of hands, furrowed brow, strained face, sighing or rapid respiration, facial pallor, swallowing, belching, brisk tendon jerks, dilated pupils, exophthalmos.		Somatic (Muscular)	Pains and aches, twitchings, stiffness, myoclonic jerks, grinding of teeth, unsteady voice, increased muscular tone.	
		Total Score			

Source. Reprinted from Hamilton M: "The Assessment of Anxiety States by Rating." *British Journal of Medical Psychology* 32:50–55, 1959. Used with permission.

Abnormal Involuntary Movement Scale (AIMS)

		None	Minimal	Mild	Moderate	Severe
FACIAL AND ORAL MOVEMENTS	1: Muscles of Facial Expression e.g., movements of forehead, eyebrows, periorbital area, cheeks; include frowning, blinking, smiling, grimacing	0	1	2	3	4
	2: Lips and Perioral Area e.g., puckering, pouting, smacking	0	1	2	3	4
	3: Jaw e.g., biting, clenching, chewing, mouth opening, lateral movement	0	1	2	3	4
	4: Tongue Rate only increase in movement both in and out of mouth, NOT in ability to sustain movement	0	1	2	3	4
EXTREMITY MOVEMENTS	5: Upper (arms, wrists, hands, fingers) Include choreic movements (i.e., rapid, objectively purposeless, irregular, spontaneous), athetoid movements (i.e., slow, irregular, complex, serpentine). Do NOT include tremor (i.e., repetitive, regular, rhythmic)	0	1	2	3	4
	6: Lower (legs, knees, ankles, toes) e.g., lateral knee movement, foot tapping, heel dropping, foot squirming, inversion and eversion of foot	0	1	2	3	4
TRUNK MOVEMENTS	7: Neck, shoulders, hips e.g., rocking, twisting, squirming, pelvic gyrations	0	1	2	3	4
	8: Severity of abnormal movements	0	1	2	3	4

Abnormal Involuntary Movement Scale (AIMS) *(continued)*

		None	Minimal	Mild	Moderate	Severe
		0	1	2	3	4
GLOBAL JUDGMENT	9: Incapacitation due to abnormal movements					
	10: Patient's awareness of abnormal movements Rate only patient's report	No awareness 0 Aware, no distress 1 Aware, mild distress 2 Aware, moderate distress 3 Aware, severe distress 4				
	11: Current problems with teeth and/or dentures	No 0 Yes 1				
	12: Does patient usually wear dentures?	No 0 Yes 1				

Examination Procedures for AIMS

Either before or after completing the Examination Procedure observe the patient unobtrusively, at rest (e.g., in waiting room). The chair to be used in this examination should be a hard, firm one without arms.

1: Ask patient whether there is anything in his/her mouth (i.e., gum, candy, etc.) and if there is, to remove it.

2: Ask patient about the *current* condition of his/her teeth. Ask patient if he/she wears dentures. Do teeth or dentures bother patient *now?*

3: Ask patient whether he/she notices any movements in mouth, face, hands, or feet. If yes, ask to describe and to what extent they *currently* bother patient or interfere with his/her activities.

4: Have patient sit in chair with hands on knees, legs slightly apart, and feet flat on floor. (Look at entire body for movements while in this position.)

5: Ask patient to sit with hands hanging unsupported. If male, between legs, if female and wearing a dress, hanging over knees. (Observe hands and other body areas.)

6: Ask patient to open mouth. (Observe tongue at rest within mouth.) Do this twice.

7: Ask patient to protrude tongue. (Observe tongue at rest within mouth.) Do this twice.

*8: Ask patient to tap thumb, with each finger, as rapidly as impossible for 10–15 seconds; separately with right hand, then with left hand. (Observe facial and leg movements.)

9: Flex and extend patient's left and right arms (one at a time). (Note any rigidity and rate on NOTES.)

10: Ask patient to stand up. (Observe in profile. Observe all body areas again, hips included.)

*11: Ask patient to extend both arms outstretched in front with palms down. (Observe trunk, legs, and mouth.)

*12: Have patient walk a few paces, turn, and walk back to chair. (Observe hands and gait.) Do this twice.

---

* Activated movements.

Source. Reprinted from Guy W: *ECDEU: Assessment Manual for Psychopharmacology* (DHEW Publ No 76-338). Washington, DC, Department of Health, Education, and Welfare, Psychopharmacology Research Branch, 1976.

Simpson-Angus Rating Scale

1. **GAIT:** The patient is examined as he walks into the examining room; his gait, the swing of his arms, his general posture, all form the basis for an overall score for this item. This is rated as follows:

   0   Normal.

   1   Diminution in swing while the patient is walking.

   2   Marked diminution in swing with obvious rigidity in the arm.

   3   Stiff gait with arms held rigidly before the abdomen.

   4   Stooped shuffling gait with propulsion and retropulsion.

2. **ARM DROPPING:** The patient and the examiner both raise their arms to shoulder height and let them fall to their sides. In a normal subject a stout slap is heard as the arms hit the sides. In the patient with extreme Parkinson's syndrome the arms fall very slowly.

   0   Normal, free fall with loud slap and rebound.

   1   Fall slowed slightly with less audible contact and little rebound.

   2   Fall slowed, no rebound.

   3   Marked slowing, no slap at all.

   4   Arms fall as though against resistance; as though through glue.

3. **SHOULDER SHAKING:** The subject's arms are bent at a right angle at the elbow and are taken one at a time by the examiner who grasps one hand and also clasps the other around the patient's elbow. The subject's upper arm is pushed to and fro and the humerus is externally rotated. The degree of resistance from normal to extreme rigidity is scored as follows:

   0   Normal.

   1   Slight stiffness and resistance.

   2   Moderate stiffness and resistance.

   3   Marked rigidity with difficulty in passive movement.

   4   Extreme stiffness and rigidity with almost a frozen shoulder.

4. **ELBOW RIGIDITY:** The elbow joints are separately bent at right angles and passively extended and flexed, with the subject's biceps observed and simultaneously palpated. The resistance to this procedure is rated. (The presence of cogwheel rigidity is noted separately.) Scoring is from 0 to 4, as in the Shoulder Shaking test.

   0   Normal

   1   Slight stiffness and resistance.

   2   Moderate stiffness and resistance.

   3   Marked rigidity with difficulty in passive movement.

   4   Extreme stiffness and rigidity with almost a frozen shoulder.

Simpson-Angus Rating Scale *(continued)*

5. **FIXATION OF POSITION OR WRIST RIGIDITY:** The wrist is held in one hand and the fingers held by the examiner's other hand, with the wrist moved to extension flexion and both ulnar and radial deviation. The resistance to this procedure is rated as in Items 3 and 4.

    0   Normal.

    1   Slight stiffness and resistance.

    2   Moderate stiffness and resistance.

    3   Marked rigidity with difficulty in passive movement.

    4   Extreme stiffness and rigidity with almost a frozen shoulder.

6. **LEG PENDULOUSNESS:** The patient sits on a table with his legs hanging down and swinging free. The ankle is grasped by the examiner and raised until the knee is partially extended. It is then allowed to fall. The resistance to falling and the lack of swinging form the basis for the score on this item:

    0   The legs swing freely.

    1   Slight diminution in the swing of the legs.

    2   Moderate resistance to swing.

    3   Marked resistance and damping of swing.

    4   Complete absence of swing.

7. **HEAD DROPPING:** The patient lies on a well-padded examining table and his head is raised by the examiner's hand. The hand is then withdrawn and the head allowed to drop. In the normal subject the head will fall upon the table. The movement is delayed in extrapyramidal system disorder, and in extreme Parkinsonism it is absent. The neck muscles are rigid and the head does not reach the examining table. Scoring is as follows:

    0   The head falls completely, with a good thump as it hits the table.

    1   Slight slowing in fall, mainly noted by lack of slap as head meets the table.

    2   Moderate slowing in the fall, quite noticeable to the eye.

    3   Head falls stiffly and slowly.

    4   Head does not reach examining table.

8. **GLABELLA TAP:** Subject is told to open his eyes wide and not to blink. The glabella region is tapped at a steady, rapid speed. The number of times patient blinks in succession is noted:

    0   0 to 5 blinks.

    1   6 to 10 blinks.

    2   11 to 15 blinks.

    3   16 to 20 blinks.

    4   21 or more blinks.

Simpson-Angus Rating Scale *(continued)*

9. **TREMOR:** Patient is observed walking into examining room and then is reexamined for this item:

   0   Normal.

   1   Mild finger tremor, obvious to sight and touch.

   2   Tremor of hand or arm occurring spasmodically.

   3   Persistent tremor of one or more limbs.

   4   Whole body tremor.

10. **SALIVATION:** Patient is observed while talking and then asked to open his mouth and elevate his tongue. The following ratings are given:

   0   Normal.

   1   Excess salivation to the extent that pooling takes place if the mouth is open and the tongue raised.

   2   When excess salivation is present and might occasionally result in difficulty in speaking.

   3   Speaking with difficulty because of excess salivation.

   4   Frank drooling.

Source.   Reprinted from Simpson GM, Angus JWS: "A Rating Scale for Extrapyramidal Side Effects." *Acta Psychiatrica Scandinavica Supplementum* 212:11–19, 1970. Used with permission.

Mini-Mental State Exam (MMSE)

Maximum Score	Score	
		ORIENTATION
5	( )	What is the (year) (season) (day) (month)?
5	( )	Where are we: (state) (country) (town) (hospital) (floor)?
		REGISTRATION
3	( )	Name 3 objects: 1 second to say each. Then ask the patient all 3 after you have said them. Give 1 point for each correct answer. Then repeat them until he learns all 3. Count trials and record. Trials _____
		ATTENTION AND CALCULATION
5	( )	Serial 7s. 1 point for each correct. Stop after 5 answers. Alternatively spell "world" backwards.
		RECALL
3	( )	Ask for the 3 objects repeated above. Give 1 point for each correct.
		LANGUAGE
9	( )	Name a pencil, and watch (2 points).

Repeat the following, "No ifs, ands, or buts." (1 point)

Follow a 3-stage command:

"Take a paper in your right hand, fold it in half, and put it on the floor." (3 points)

Read and obey the following:

CLOSE YOUR EYES (1 point)

Write a sentence (1 point)

Copy design (1 point)

Total score _____

ASSESS level of consciousness along a continuum _____
           Alert   Drowsy   Stupor   Coma

INSTRUCTIONS FOR ADMINISTRATION OF
MINI-MENTAL STATE EXAMINATION

ORIENTATION

(1) Ask for the date. Then ask specifically for parts omitted, e.g., "Can you also tell me what season it is?" One point for each correct.

(2) Ask in turn "Can you tell me the name of this hospital?" (town, county, etc.). One point for each correct.

REGISTRATION

Ask the patient if you may test his memory. Then say the names of 3 unrelated objects, clearly and slowly, about one second for each. After you have said all 3, ask him to repeat them. This first repetition determines his score (0–3) but keep saying them until he can repeat all 3, up to 6 trials. If he does not eventually learn all 3, recall cannot be meaningfully tested.

ATTENTION AND CALCULATION

Ask the patient to begin with 100 and count backwards by 7. Stop after 5 subtractions (93, 86, 79, 72, 65). Score the total number of correct answers.

If the patient cannot or will not perform this task, ask him to spell the word "world" backwards. The score is the number of letters in correct order, e.g., dlrow = 5, dlorw = 3.

RECALL

Ask the patient if he can recall the 3 words you previously asked him to remember. Score 0–3.

LANGUAGE

Naming: Show the patient a wrist watch and ask him what it is. Repeat for pencil. Score 0–2.

Repetition: Ask the patient to repeat the sentence after you. Allow only one trial. Score 0 or 1.

3-Stage command: Give the patient a piece of plain blank paper and repeat the command. Score 1 point for each part correctly executed.

Reading: On a blank piece of paper print the sentence "Close your eyes," in letters large enough for the patient to see clearly. Ask him to read it and do what it says. Score 1 point only if he actually closes his eyes.

Writing: Give the patient a blank piece of paper and ask him to write a sentence for you. Do not dictate a sentence, it is to be written spontaneously. It must contain a subject and verb and be sensible. Correct grammar and punctuation are not necessary.

Copying: On a clean piece of paper, draw intersecting pentagons, each side about 1 in., and ask him to copy it exactly as it is. All 10 angles must be present and 2 must intersect to score 1 point. Tremor and rotation are ignored.

Estimate the patient's level of sensorium along a continuum, from alert on the left to coma on the right.

Source.   Reprinted from Folstein MF, Folstein SE, McHugh PR: "'Mini-Mental State': A Practical Method for Grading the Cognitive State of Patients for the Clinician." *Journal of Psychiatric Research* 12:189–198, 1975. Copyright 1975 Pergamon Press PLC. Used with permission.

Global Assessment Scale (GAS)

Rate the subject's lowest level of functioning in the last week by selecting the lowest range which describes his functioning on a hypothetical continuum of mental health-illness. For example, a subject whose "behavior is considerably influenced by delusions" (range 21–30) should be given a rating in that range even though he has "major impairment in several areas" (range 31–40). Use intermediary levels when appropriate (e.g., 35, 58, 63). Rate actual functioning independently of whether or not subject is receiving and may be helped by medication or some other form of treatment.

100 | No symptoms, superior functioning in a wide range of activities, life's problems never
| | seem to get out of hand, is sought out by others because of his warmth and integrity.
91 |

90 | Transient symptoms may occur, but good functioning in all areas, interested and
| | involved in a wide range of activities, socially effective, generally satisfied with life,
81 | "everyday" worries that only occasionally get out of hand.

80 | Minimal symptoms may be present but no more than slight impairment in function-
| | ing, varying degrees of "everyday" worries and problems that sometimes get out of
71 | hand.

70 | Some mild symptoms (e.g., depressive mood and mild insomnia) OR some difficulty
| | in several areas of functioning, but generally functioning pretty well, has some mean-
61 | ingful interpersonal relationships and most untrained people would not consider
| | him "sick."

60 | Moderate symptoms OR generally functioning with some difficulty (e.g., few friends
| | and flat affect, depressed mood, and pathological self-doubt, euphoric mood and
51 | pressure of speech, moderately severe antisocial behavior).

50 | Any serious symptomatology or impairment in functioning that most clinicians
| | would think obviously requires treatment or attention (e.g., suicidal preoccupation
41 | or gesture, severe obsessional rituals, frequent anxiety attacks, serious antisocial be-
| | havior, compulsive drinking).

40 | Major impairment in several areas, such as work, family relations, judgment, think-
| | ing, or mood (e.g., depressed woman avoids friends, neglects family, unable to do
31 | housework), OR some impairment in reality testing or communication (e.g., speech
| | is at times obscure, illogical, or irrelevant), OR single serious suicide attempt.

30 | Unable to function in almost all areas (e.g., stays in bed all day), OR behavior is
| | considerably influenced by either delusions or hallucinations, OR serious impairment
21 | in communication (e.g., sometimes incoherent or unresponsive) or judgment (e.g.,
| | acts grossly inappropriate).

20 | Needs some supervision to prevent hurting self or others, or to maintain minimal
| | personal hygiene (e.g., repeats suicide attempts, frequently violent, manic excite-
11 | ment, smears feces), OR gross impairment in communication (e.g., largely incoherent
| | or mute).

10 | Needs constant supervision for several days to prevent hurting self or others, or
| | makes no attempt to maintain minimal personal hygiene.
1 |

Source.   Reprinted from Endicott J, Spitzer RL, Fleiss JL, et al.: "The Global Assessment Scale: A Procedure for Measuring Overall Severity of Psychiatric Disturbance." *Archives of General Psychiatry* 33:766–771, 1976. Copyright 1976/78, American Medical Association. Used with permission.

Yale-Brown
Obsessive Compulsive Scale (Y-BOCS)

For each item circle the number identifying the response which best characterizes the patient.

1. **Time Occupied by Obsessive Thoughts**

   How much of your time is occupied by obsessive thoughts? How frequently do the obsessive thoughts occur?

   0 = None

   1 = Mild (less than 1 hr day) or occasional (intrusion occurring no more than 8 times a day)

   2 = Moderate (1 to 3 hrs day) or frequent (intrusion occurring more than 8 times a day, but most of the hours of the day are free of obsessions)

   3 = Severe (greater than 3 and up to 8 hrs day) or very frequent (intrusion occurring more than 8 times a day and occurring during most of the hours of the day)

   4 = Extreme (greater than 8 hrs day) or near consistent intrusion (too numerous to count and an hour rarely passes without several obsessions occurring)

2. Interference Due to Obsessive Thoughts

   How much do your obsessive thoughts interfere with your social or work (or role) functioning? Is there anything that you don't do because of them?

   0 = None

   1 = Mild, slight interference with social or occupational activities, but overall performance not impaired.

   2 = Moderate, definite interference with social or occupational performance but still manageable

   3 = Severe, causes substantial impairment in social or occupational performance

   4 = Extreme, incapacitating

3. **Distress Associated With Obsessive Thoughts**

   How much distress do your obsessive thoughts cause you?

   0 = None

   1 = Mild, infrequent and not too disturbing

   2 = Moderate, frequent and disturbing but still manageable

   3 = Severe, very frequent and very disturbing

   4 = Extreme, near constant and disabling distress

Yale-Brown
Obsessive Compulsive Scale (Y-BOCS) *(continued)*

4. **Resistance Against Obsessions**

How much of an effort do you make to resist the obsessive thoughts? How often do you try to disregard or turn your attention away from these thoughts as they enter your mind?

0 = Makes an effort to always resist, or symptoms so minimal doesn't need to actively resist

1 = Tries to resist most of the time

2 = Makes some effort to resist

3 = Yields to all obsessions without attempting to control them, but does so with some reluctance

4 = Completely and willingly yields to all obsessions

5. **Degree of Control Over Obsessive Thoughts**

How much control do you have over your obsessive thoughts? How successful are you in stopping or diverting your obsessive thinking?

0 = Complete control

1 = Much control, usually able to stop or divert obsessions with some effort and concentration

2 = Moderate control, sometimes able to stop or divert obsessions

3 = Little control, rarely successful in stopping obsessions

4 = No control, experienced as completely involuntary, rarely able to even momentarily divert thinking

6. **Time Spent Performing Compulsive Behaviors**

How much time do you spend performing compulsive behaviors? How frequently do you perform compulsions?

0 = None

1 = Mild (less than 1 hr day performing compulsions) or occasional (performance of compulsions occurring no more than 8 times a day)

2 = Moderate (1 to 3 hrs day performing compulsions) or frequent (performance of compulsions occurring more than 8 times a day, but most of the hours of the day are free of compulsive behaviors)

3 = Severe (greater than 3 and up to 8 hrs day performing compulsions) or very frequent (performance of compulsions occurring more than 8 times a day and occurring during most of the hours of the day)

4 = Extreme (greater than 8 hrs day performing compulsions) or near consistent performance of compulsions (too numerous to count and an hour rarely passes without several compulsions being performed)

Yale-Brown
Obsessive Compulsive Scale (Y-BOCS) *(continued)*

7. **Interference Due to Compulsive Behaviors**

How much do your compulsive behaviors interfere with your social or work (or role) functioning? Is there anything that you don't do because of the compulsions?

0 = None

1 = Mild, slight interference with social or occupational activities, but overall performance not impaired

2 = Moderate, definite interference with social or occupational performance but still manageable

3 = Severe, causes substantial impairment in social or occupational performance

4 = Extreme, incapacitating

8. **Distress Associated With Compulsive Behavior**

How would you feel if prevented from performing your compulsions?
How anxious would you become? How anxious do you get while performing compulsions until you are satisfied they are completed?

0 = None

1 = Mild, only slightly anxious if compulsions prevented or only slightly anxious during performance of compulsions

2 = Moderate, reports that anxiety would mount but remain manageable if compulsions prevented or that anxiety increases but remains manageable during performance of compulsions

3 = Severe, prominent and very disturbing increase in anxiety if compulsions interrupted or prominent and very disturbing increases in anxiety during performance of compulsions

4 = Extreme, incapacitating anxiety from any intervention aimed at modifying activity or incapacitating anxiety develops during performance of compulsions

9. **Resistance Against Compulsions**

How much of an effort do you make to resist the compulsions?

0 = Makes an effort to always resist, or symptoms so minimal doesn't need to actively resist

1 = Tries to resist most of the time

2 = Makes some effort to resist

3 = Yields to all compulsions without attempting to control them, but does so with some reluctance

4 = Completely and willingly yields to all compulsions

Yale-Brown
Obsessive Compulsive Scale (Y-BOCS) *(continued)*

---

10. **Degree of Control Over Compulsive Behavior**

    0 = Complete control

    1 = Much control, experiences pressure to perform the behavior but usually able to exercise voluntary control over it

    2 = Moderate control, strong pressure to perform behavior, can control it only with difficulty

    3 = Little control, very strong drive to perform behavior, must be carried to completion, can only delay with difficulty

    4 = No control, drive to perform behavior experienced as completely involuntary

---

Source. Reprinted from Goodman WK, Price LH, Rasmussen SA, et al.: "The Yale-Brown Obsessive Compulsive Scale, I: Development, Use, and Reliability." *Archives of General Psychiatry* 46:1006–1011, 1989. Used with permission.

Index

Page numbers printed in **boldface** type refer to tables or figures.

Affective nonresponsivity, 74
Aggressive behavior, 66. *See also*
    Violent behavior
Aggressive obsessions, **350**
Agitated behavior, 66
Agitation, psychomotor, in major
    depressive disorders, 274
Agoraphobia, 83, 317–319, 321, 329
    clinical management of, 324–326
    course and outcome of, 323–324
    differential diagnosis of, 324, 325
    DSM-IV-TR criteria for, 320
    epidemiology and clinical findings
        in, 321, 322
    etiology and pathophysiology of,
        321, 323
Agranulocytosis, antipsychotics
    and, 718
AIDS, 569. *See also* HIV infection
    diagnosis of, 571, 573
AIDS dementia complex, 575
AIDS-related complex (ARC), 572
Ailurophobia, **333**
Akathisia, antipsychotics and, 717
Alcoholics Anonymous (AA), 418, 452
Alcohol-related disorders, 403–420
    clinical findings in, 407–408
    clinical management of, 413, 414,
        415–417, 417
    complications of, 408–411, 409
    course and outcome of, 412
    definition of, 404, 404, 405, 406
    dementia due to, 202
    diagnosis of, 412, 412–413
    epidemiology of, 406–407
    etiology of, 411–412
    intoxication and, DSM-IV-TR
        criteria for, 414
    magnetic resonance imaging in,
        111–112, 114, 115
    rehabilitation for, 417–420
    in schizophrenia, 222
    sleep in, 661, 662–663

Alcohol withdrawal, 413, 415–417
    delirium tremens and, 415–417
    DSM-IV-TR criteria for, 414
    hallucinosis and, 415
    management of, 416–417, 417
    seizures and, 413, 415
    uncomplicated, 413
Aliphatics, **711**
Alogia, 71, 219
Alprazolam (Xanax), **744**, 745
Altruism, as coping mechanism, 700
Alzheimer's disease, 194–195, **196**, 197
    APOE in, 177
    clinical management of, 199–200
    differentiation from dementia
        praecox, 12–13
    DSM-IV-TR criteria for, 196
    neuroimaging in, 95
Amantadine (Symmetrel)
    for akathisia, 717
    for extrapyramidal syndromes,
        749, 750
Amathophobia, **333**
The American Journal of Psychiatry, 9
American Law Institute standard, 675
American Psychiatric Association,
    founding of, 9
Amiloride, for lithium side effects, 738
Amitriptyline (Elavil), **722**
    for generalized anxiety disorder, 329
Amnestic disorder, 37, 203–204, **204**
Amnestic states, 390–393, **391**
Amobarbital sodium (Amytal)
    interviews, 756–757
Amotivational syndrome, with
    marijuana use, 447
Amoxapine (Asendin), **723**
Amphetamine
    abuse of
        intoxication and, DSM-IV-TR
            criteria for, **441**
        withdrawal and, DSM-IV-TR
            criteria for, **442**